Gerontological Nursing

Gerontological Nursing

EIGHTH EDITION

Charlotte Eliopoulos, PhD, MPH, RNC

Specialist in Holistic Gerontological Care
Executive Director, American Association
for Long Term Care Nursing

Wolters Kluwer | Lippincott Williams & Wilkins

Philadelphia · Baltimore · New York · London
Buenos Aires · Hong Kong · Sydney · Tokyo

Acquisitions Editor: Patrick Barbera
Associate Product Manager: Dawn Lagrosa
Editorial Assistant: Zack Shapiro
Production Project Manager: Priscilla Crater
Design Coordinator: Joan Wendt
Illustration Coordinator: Brett MacNaughton
Manufacturing Coordinator: Karin Duffield
Production Services/Compositor: Integra Software Services Pvt. Ltd.

8th Edition

Printed in China

Library of Congress Cataloging-in-Publication Data
Eliopoulos, Charlotte.
  Gerontological nursing/Charlotte Eliopoulos.—8th ed.
     p.; cm.
  Includes bibliographical references and index.
  ISBN 978-1-4511-7277-5
  I. Title.
  [DNLM: 1. Geriatric Nursing. WY 152]
  618.970231–dc23

                                                                                    2012041586

9 8 7 6 5 4 3 2 1

This book is dedicated to my husband, George Considine, for his unending patience, support, and encouragement and to Manuel Eliopoulos Jr., who has taught me many lessons in unconditional love, acceptance, and service to our elders.

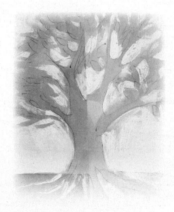

Reviewers

Nancy Henne Batchelor, MSN, RN, CNS
Assistant Professor of Clinical Nursing
University of Cincinnati
Cincinnati, Ohio

Laurie Bird, RN, BSN, MSN
Instructor in PN Program
Department Chair of PN and Health Care
    Assistant Programs
North Island College
Port Alberni, British Columbia, Canada

Beryl Cable-Williams, RN, BNSc, MN, PhD
Faculty Member
Trent/Fleming School of Nursing
    Trent University
Peterborough, Ontario, Canada

Catherine Cole, PhD, ACNS-BC
Assistant Professor
University of Arkansas for Medical Sciences/
    College of Nursing
Little Rock, Arkansas

Julia Henderson Gist, PhD, RN
Visiting Assistant Professor
Arkansas Tech University
Russellville, Arkansas

Judy A. Kopka, RN, MSN
Assistant Professor
Columbia College of Nursing
Milwaukee, Wisconsin

Susan J. Lamanna, RN, MA, MS, ANP, CNE
Professor
Onondaga Community College
Syracuse, New York

Sharon Livingstone, MSc
Coordinator of Gerontology and
    Dementia Studies
Conestoga College ATT
Kitchener, Ontario, Canada

Carol M. Patton, DrPH, APRN, BC, CRNP, CNE, Parish Nurse
Professor and Founding Director
Chatham University Nursing Programs
    Chatham University
Pittsburgh, Pennsylvania

Diane I. Ruppel, MS, RN, CNS-BC
Clinical Associate Professor
University of Memphis School of Nursing
Memphis, Tennessee

Pamela D. Thomas, MSN
Nursing Instructor
Mississippi University for Women
Columbus, Mississippi

Mary Ellen Hill Yonushonis, MS, RN, CNE
Instructor in Nursing
The Pennsylvania State University
University Park, Pennsylvania

Reviewers

Nancy Hanna Batchelor, MSN, RN, CNS
Assistant Professor of Clinical Nursing
University of Cincinnati
Cincinnati, Ohio

Laurie Bird, RN, BSN, MSN
Instructor in PN Program
Department of PN and Health Care
Transition Program
North Island College
Port Alberni, British Columbia, Canada

Beryl Cable-Williams, RN, BNSc, MN, PhD
Faculty Member
Trent/Fleming School of Nursing
Trent University
Peterborough, Ontario, Canada

Catherine Cole, PhD, ACNS-BC
Assistant Professor
University of Arkansas for Medical Sciences
College of Nursing
Little Rock, Arkansas

Julie Henderson Gist, PhD, RN
Visiting Assistant Professor
Alabama Tech University
Boaz, Alabama

Jody A. Kopec, RN, MSN
Assistant Professor
Columbus College of Nursing
Milwaukee, Wisconsin

Susan J. Lorenzana, RN, MA, MS, ANP, CNE
Professor
Onondaga Community College
Syracuse, New York

Sharon Livingstone, MSc
Coordinator of Gerontology and
Death Studies
Cenotaph College H
Ontario, Canada

Carol M. Patton, DrPH, APRN, RC, CRNP, CNE, Parish Nurse
Professor and Founding Doctoral
Chatham University Nursing Programs
Chatham University
Pittsburgh, Pennsylvania

Diane L. Ruppel, MS, RN, CMS-BC
Clinical Associate Professor
Loewenberg/UT Memphis School of Nursing
Memphis, Tennessee

Pamela D. Thomas, MSN
Nursing Instructor
Mississippi University for Women
Columbus, Mississippi

Mary Ellen Hill Yannaccone, MS, RN, CNE
Instructor in Nursing
The Pennsylvania State University
University Park, Pennsylvania

Preface

The specialty of gerontological nursing continues to grow in the body of evidence supporting practice and in the population served. Whereas there was a time that older adults were considered a homogenous group, expected to become sick, sexless, and senile, there now is recognition that they are a highly diverse group who can lead healthy, productive lives for many years after their 65th birthday. Normality from pathology increasingly is better understood through research that sheds light on the normal aging process. And, older adults have grown from a hidden minority to a significant and powerful segment of the total population who demand choice, respect, and high-quality services.

In this 8th edition, *Gerontological Nursing* continues to bridge the growing body of specialty knowledge with relevancy for practice. A wide range of topics is presented, providing comprehensive information to serve as a strong foundation for gerontological nursing practice. One of the positive features of this book is that it continues to be written by one author, thereby offering a consistent level and style—which have been appreciated as practical and user-friendly in previous editions—throughout all chapters.

TEXT ORGANIZATION

Gerontological Nursing, 8th edition, is organized into seven units. The first unit, *Understanding the Aging Experience*, provides basic knowledge about the older population and the aging experience. The growing culture and sexual diversity of this population is discussed, along with the navigation of life transitions and the changes that typically are experienced to the body and mind.

Unit 2, *Foundations of Gerontological Nursing*, provides an understanding of the development and scope of the specialty, along with descriptions of the various settings in which nurses can care for older persons. Legal and ethical issues that are relevant to gerontological nursing are reviewed, and there is guidance in applying a holistic model to gerontological care. A chapter is devoted to self-care for the gerontological nurse in recognition of the need for a healer to care for self in order to provide optimum care to others.

Unit 3, *Fostering Connection and Gratification*, provides a broad perspective on sexuality and intimacy; current thinking on menopause is included. The significance of spirituality and measures to support spiritual needs are discussed.

Some of the major care issues confronting gerontological nurses are offered in Unit 4, *General Care Considerations*. Chapters dedicated to nutrition and hydration, rest and sleep, comfort and pain management, safety, and medications guide the nurse in promoting basic health and preventing avoidable complications.

Unit 5, *Facilitating Physiological Balance*, addresses the basic functions that assure health and life. The chapters are dedicated to respiration, circulation, digestion and bowel elimination, urinary elimination, reproductive system health, movement, neurologic function, sensation, and endocrine, integumentary, and immune function. A review of the impact of aging, interventions to promote health, the unique presentation and treatment of illnesses, and integrative approaches to illness are discussed with each of these areas.

Issues and nursing care related to infections, cancer, mental health disorders, delirium, and dementia in older adults are addressed in Unit 6, *Multisystem Disorders*. Guidance is offered to assist the gerontological nurse with the unique challenges and presentations of these diseases and illnesses.

Unit 7, *Gerontological Care Issues*, discusses common challenges faced in practice, including helping people live effectively with chronic conditions, rehabilitative care, acute care, long-term care, family caregiving, and end-of-life care. With the growing concern on reducing hospital readmissions and facilitating transitions of care, an understanding of the issues impacting quality of care and quality of life is important.

FEATURES

New features offer students a greater understanding for application and include the following:

- Terms to Know defines new terms pertaining to the topic
- Bringing Research to Life not only presents current research but also describes how to apply that knowledge in practice

- Practice Realities poses real-life examples of challenges that could be faced by a nurse in practice

In addition, the features that have been welcomed by students in the past have been expanded to add appeal and include the following:

- Learning Objectives to prepare the reader for outcomes anticipated in reading the chapter
- Chapter Outlines to present an overview of content
- Highlighted Key Concepts to emphasize significant facts
- Points to Ponder boxes that pose questions to stimulate thinking related to the content
- Tables that offer facts
- Boxed information to emphasize specific points
- Assessment Guides that outline the components of general observations, interview, and physical assessment of major body systems
- Nursing Diagnoses Highlights that provide an overview of selected nursing diagnoses common in older adults
- Nursing Care Plans to demonstrate the steps in developing nursing diagnoses, goals, and actions from identified needs
- Consider This Case examples of clinical situations that offer opportunities for critical thinking
- Critical Thinking Exercises to guide application
- Resources at the end of every chapter to assist with additional exploration of the topic
- References to expand the network of available information
- Plentiful figures to complement the text

TEACHING AND LEARNING PACKAGE

Resources for Instructors

Tools to assist you with teaching your course are available upon adoption of this text at: http://thePoint.lww.com/Eliopoulos8e.

- An e-book on thePoint gives you access to the book's full text and images online.
- The Test Generator lets you put together exclusive new tests from a bank containing hundreds of questions to help you in assessing your students' understanding of the material. Test questions link to chapter learning objectives. This test generator comes with a bank of more than 900 questions.

- PowerPoint presentations provide an easy way for you to integrate the textbook with your students' classroom experience, via either slide shows or handouts. Multiple choice and true/false questions are integrated into the presentations to promote class participation and allow you to use i-clicker technology.
- An Image Bank lets you use the photographs and illustrations from this textbook in your PowerPoint slides or as you see fit in your course.
- Journal articles, updated for the new edition, offer access to current research available in Lippincott Williams & Wilkins journals.

New for this edition!

- Clinical Scenarios posing What If questions (and suggested answers) give your students an opportunity to apply their knowledge to a client case similar to the one they might encounter in practice.
- Assignments (and suggested answers) include group, written, clinical, and Web assignments.
- QSEN Competency Map shows you how content connects with the QSEN competencies of Quality and Safety Education for Nurses: Patient-Centered Care, Teamwork and Collaboration, Evidence-Based Practice, Quality Improvement, Safety, and Informatics.
- Suggested Answers to Critical Thinking Exercises allow you to gauge whether students' answers are on the right track, by giving you main points that students are expected to address in the answers.
- DocuCare offers a true-to-life EHR with a real-world format designed to prepare your students for successful practice. Its tools let you create, modify, and add patients to practice documents as well as review student documentation.

Resources for Students

Students can access all these resources at: http://thePoint.lww.com/Eliopoulos8e using the codes printed in the front of their textbooks.

- An e-book on thePoint allows access to the book's full text and images online.
- Watch & Learn Video Clips on How to Assist a Person Who Is Falling, Alternatives to Restraints, and the Five Stages of Grief. (Icons appear in the textbook to direct readers to relevant videos.)
- Recommended Readings to expand the network of available information

■ A Spanish–English Audio Glossary provides helpful terms and phrases for communicating with patients who speak Spanish.

SUMMARY

If practiced competently, gerontological nursing is among the most complex and dynamic specialties nurses could select. A wide range of knowledge and skills is demanded, along with an appreciation for the richness of unique life experiences and the wisdom to understand that true healing comes from sources beyond medications and procedures. Hopefully, this book will equip nurses to assist older adults to live with optimum health, purpose, and fullness in this season of their lives.

CHARLOTTE ELIOPOULOS RN, MPH, PHD

Acknowledgments

There are many individuals who played important roles in the birth and development of this book. I will always be grateful to Bill Burgower, a Lippincott editor, who decades ago responded to my urging that the new specialty of gerontological nursing needed resources by encouraging me to write the first edition of *Gerontological Nursing*. Many fine members of the Lippincott team have guided and assisted me since, including Patrick Barbera, Acquisitions Editor, who consistently offered encouragement and direction; Dawn Lagrosa, Associate Product Manager, who brought a new set of eyes to the book and ironed out the rough edges through her fine editorial skills; and Priscilla Crater, Production Project Manager, who shepherded the book from manuscripts through printed pages.

Lastly, I am deeply indebted to those mentors and leaders in gerontological care who generously offered encouragement and the many older adults who have touched my life and showed me the wisdom and beauty of aging. The education these individuals provided could have never been learned in a book!

CHARLOTTE ELIOPOULOS

Brief Contents

Contents

UNIT 5

Facilitating Physiological Balance   251

Index of Selected Features

UNIT 1

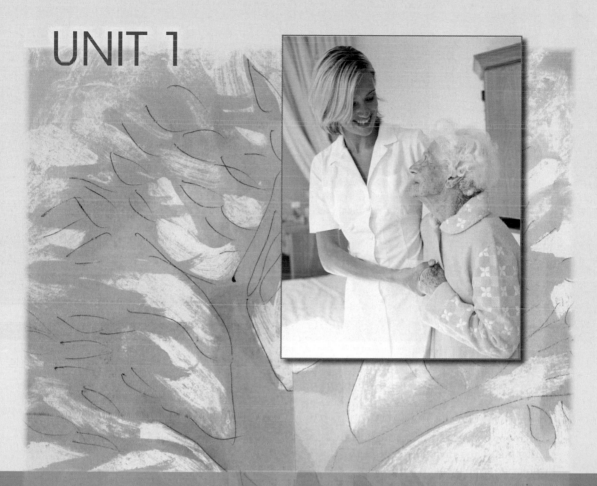

Understanding the Aging Experience

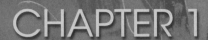

The Aging Population

CHAPTER OUTLINE

LEARNING OBJECTIVES

After reading this chapter, you should be able to:

1. Explain the different ways in which older adults have been viewed throughout history.

2. Describe characteristics of today's older population in regard to:
   - life expectancy
   - marital status
   - living arrangements
   - income and employment
   - health status

3. Discuss projected changes in future generations of older people and the implications for health care.

TERMS TO KNOW

Comorbidity: the simultaneous presence of multiple chronic conditions

Compression of morbidity: delaying or compressing the years in which serious illness and decline occur so that an extended life expectancy results in more functional, healthy years

Life expectancy: the length of time that a person can be predicted to live

Life span: the maximum years that a person has the potential to live

"Families forget their older relatives ... most people become senile in old age ... Social Security provides every older person with a decent retirement income ... a majority of older people reside in nursing homes ... Medicare covers all health care–related costs for older people." These and other myths continue to be perpetuated about older people. Misinformation about the older population is an injustice not only to this age group but also to persons of all ages who need accurate information to prepare realistically for their own senior years. Gerontological nurses must know the facts about the older population to effectively deliver services and educate the general public.

VIEWS OF OLDER ADULTS THROUGH HISTORY

The members of the current older population in the United States have offered the sacrifice, strength, and spirit that made this country great. They were the proud GIs in world wars, the brave immigrants who ventured into a new country, the bold entrepreneurs who took risks that created wealth and opportunities for employment, and the unselfish parents who struggled to give their children a better life. They have earned respect, admiration, and dignity. Today older adults are viewed with positivism rather than prejudice, knowledge rather than myth, and concern rather than neglect. This positive view was not always the norm, however.

Historically, societies have viewed their elder members in a variety of ways. In the time of Confucius, there was a direct correlation between a person's age and the degree of respect to which he or she was entitled. The early Egyptians dreaded growing old and experimented with a variety of potions and schemes to maintain their youth. Opinions were divided among the early Greeks. Plato promoted older adults as society's best leaders, whereas Aristotle denied older people any role in governmental matters. In the nations conquered by the Roman Empire, the sick and aged were customarily the first to be killed. And, woven throughout the Bible is God's concern for the well-being of the family and desire for people to respect elders (*Honor your father and your mother* ... Exodus 20:12). Yet, the honor bestowed on older adults was not sustained.

Medieval times gave rise to strong feelings regarding the superiority of youth; these feelings were expressed in uprisings of sons against fathers. Although England developed Poor Laws in the early 17th century that provided care for the destitute and enabled older persons without family resources to have some modest safety net, many of the gains were lost during the Industrial Revolution. No labor laws protected persons of advanced age; those unable to meet the demands of industrial work settings were placed at the mercy of their offspring or forced to beg on the streets for sustenance.

The first significant step in improving the lives of older Americans was the passage of the Federal Old Age Insurance Law under the Social Security Act in 1935, which provided some financial security for older persons. The profound

BOX 1-1   Publicly Supported Programs of Benefit to Older Americans

1900	Pension laws passed in some states
1935	Social Security Act
1961	First White House Conference on Aging
1965	Older Americans Act: nutrition, senior employment, and transportation programs Administration on Aging Medicare (Title 18 of Social Security Act) Medicaid (Title 19 of Social Security Act) for poor and disabled of any age
1972	Supplemental Security Income (SSI) enacted
1991	Omnibus Budget Reconciliation Act (nursing home reform law) implemented

"graying" of the population started to be realized in the 1960s, and the United States responded with the formation of the Administration on Aging, enactment of the Older Americans Act, and the introduction of Medicaid and Medicare, all in 1965 (Box 1-1).

Since that time, American society has demonstrated a profound awakening of interest in older persons as their numbers have grown. A more humanistic attitude toward all members of society has benefited older adults, and improvements in health care and general living conditions ensure that more people have the opportunity to attain old age and live longer, more fruitful years in later adulthood than previous generations (Fig. 1-1).

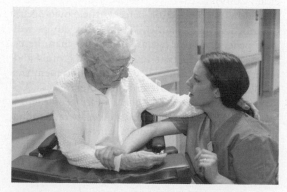

FIGURE 1-1 ■ It is important for gerontological nurses to be as concerned with adding quality to the lives of older adult, as they are with increasing the quantity of years.

CHARACTERISTICS OF THE OLDER ADULT POPULATION

Older adults are generally defined as individuals aged 65 years and older. At one time, all persons over 65 years of age were grouped together under the category of "old." Now it is recognized that much diversity exists among different age groups in late life, and older individuals can be further categorized as follows:

- young-old: 60 to 74 years
- old-old: 75 to 100 years
- centenarians: over 100 years

Some also include a fourth category of middle-old, comprising ages 75 to 84 years, shortening the old-old group to 85 to 100 years. The profile, interests, and health care challenges of each of these subsets can be vastly different. For example, a 66-year-old may desire cosmetic surgery to stay competitive in the executive job market; a 74-year-old may have recently remarried and want to do something about her dry vaginal canal; an 82-year-old may be concerned that his arthritic knees are limiting his ability to play a round of golf; and a 101-year-old may be desperate to find a way to correct her impaired vision so that she can enjoy television.

In addition to chronological age, or the years a person has lived since birth, functional age is a term used by gerontologists to describe physical, psychological, and social function; this is relevant in that how older adults feel and function may be more indicative of their needs than their chronological age. Perceived age is another term that is used to describe how people estimate a person's age based on appearance. Studies have shown a correlation between perceived age and health (Christensen et al., 2009).

How people feel or perceive their own age is described as age identity. Some older adults will view peers of similar age as being older than themselves and be reluctant to join senior groups and other activities because they see the group members as "old people" and different from themselves.

Any stereotypes held about older people must be discarded; if anything, greater diversity rather than homogeneity will be evident. Further, generalizations based on age need to be eliminated as behavior, function, and self-image can reveal more about priorities and needs than chronological age alone.

Population Growth and Increasing Life Expectancy

There was a significant growth in the number of older people for most of the 20th century. Except for the 1990s, the older population grew at a rate faster than that of the total population under age 65. The U.S. Census Bureau projects that a substantial increase in the number of individuals over age 65 will occur between 2010 and 2030 due to the impact of the baby boomers, who began to enter this group in 2011. In 2030, it is projected that this group will represent nearly 20% of the total U.S. population.

Currently, persons older than 65 years represent more than 12% of the population in the United States. This growth of the older adult population is due in part to increasing life expectancy. Advancements in disease control and health technology, lower infant and child mortality rates, improved sanitation, and better living conditions have increased life expectancy for most Americans. More people are surviving to their senior years than ever before. In 1930, slightly more than 6 million persons were aged 65 years or older, and the average life expectancy was 59.7 years. The life expectancy in 1965 was 70.2 years, and the number of older adults exceeded 20 million. Life expectancy has now reached 77.9 years, with over 34 million persons exceeding age 65 years (Table 1-1). Not only are more people reaching old age but they are living longer once they do; the number of people in their seventies and eighties has been steadily increasing and is expected to continue to increase (Fig. 1-2). The life span currently is 116 years for humans. The population over age 85 years represents approximately 40% of the older population, and the number of centenarians is steadily growing.

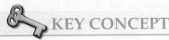 KEY CONCEPT

More people are achieving and spending longer periods of time in old age than ever before in history.

Although life expectancy has increased, it still differs by race and gender, as Table 1-1 shows. From the late 1980s to the present, the gap in life expectancy between white people and black people has widened because the life expectancy of the black population has declined. The U.S. Department of Health and Human Services attributes the declining life expectancy of black people to an increase in deaths from homicide and acquired immunodeficiency syndrome. This reality underscores the need for nurses to be concerned with health and social issues of persons of all ages because these impact a population's aging process.

Whereas the gap in life expectancy has widened among the races, the gap is narrowing between the sexes. Throughout the 20th century, the ratio of

		White Population			Black Population		
Year	Total U.S. Population	Total	Men	Women	Total	Men	Women
1920	54.1	54.9	54.4	55.6	45.3	45.5	45.2
1950	68.2	69.1	66.5	72.2	60.8	59.1	62.9
1975	72.6	73.4	69.5	77.3	68.0	63.7	72.4
2000	77.1	77.7	74.8	80.4	72.4	68.9	75.6
2007	77.0	78.4	79.5	80.8	75.6	70.0	76.8
2010 (projected)	78.5	79.0	76.1	81.8	74.5	70.9	77.8

TABLE 1-   Life Expectancy at Birth From 1920 to 2000 with Projections to 2010

From Center for Disease Control and Prevention, National Center for Health Statistics. (2011). *Health, United States, 2010: With special feature on death and dying. Table 22, Life expectancy at birth by race and sex.* Hyattsville, MD: National Center for Health Statistics.

men to women had steadily declined to the point where there were fewer than 7 older men for every 10 older women (Table 1-2). The ratio declined with each advanced decade. However, in the 21st century, this trend is changing, and the ratio of men to women is increasing.

Although living longer is desirable, of significant importance is the quality of those years. More years to life means little if those additional years consist of discomfort, disability, and a poor quality of life; therefore, compression of mortality becomes important. This means that the onset of serious illness and decline would be delayed, or compressed, into a few years prior to death; therefore, one could live a long life and enjoy a healthy, functional state for most of those years.

POINT TO PONDER

A higher proportion of older adults in our society means that younger age groups will be carrying a greater tax burden to support the older population. Should young families sacrifice to support services for older adults? Why or why not?

Marital Status and Living Arrangements

The higher survival rates of women, along with the practice of women marrying men older than themselves, make it no surprise that more than half of women older than 65 years are widowed, and most

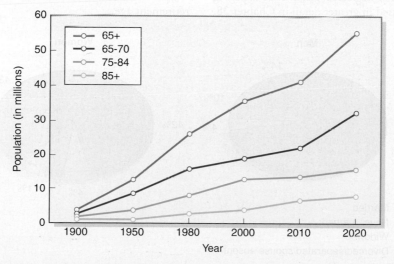

FIGURE 1-2 ■ The older population from 1900 to 2020 (in millions). (From U.S. Bureau of the Census. General Population Characteristics. Tables 42 and 45; projections for 2010 and 2020 from Census Bureau International Data Base. http://www.aoa.gov/AoARoot/Aging_Statistics/Profile/2010/4.aspx).

TABLE 1-2	Gender Ratio in the Population 65 years of Age and Older

Year	Number of Men per 100 Women
1910	101.1
1920	101.3
1930	100.5
1940	95.5
1950	89.6
1960	82.8
1970	72.1
1980	67.6
1985	67.9
1990	67.2
1995	69.1
2000	70.4
2011	75.0
2025 (projected)	82.9

From CIA World Factbooks 18, December 2003 to 28 March 2011.

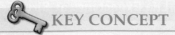

KEY CONCEPT

Women are more likely to be widowed and living alone in late life than their male counterparts.

Income and Employment

The percentage of older people living below the poverty level has been declining, with about 10% now falling into this category. However, older adults still do face financial problems. Most older people depend on Social Security for more than half of their income (Box 1-2). Women and minority groups have considerably less income than white men. Although the median net worth of older households is nearly twice the national average because of the high prevalence of home ownership by elders, many older adults are "asset rich and cash poor." The recent decline in housing prices, however, has made that asset a less valuable one for many older adults.

Although the percentage of the total population that older adults represent is growing, they constitute a steadily declining percentage of workers in the labor force. The withdrawal of men from the workforce at earlier ages has been one of the most significant labor force trends since World War II. There has been, however, a significant rise in the percentage of middle-aged women who are employed, although there has been little change in the labor force participation of women 65 years of age and older. Most baby boomers are expressing a desire and need to continue working as they enter retirement age.

of their male contemporaries are married (Fig. 1-3). Married people have a lower mortality rate than unmarried people at all ages, with men having a larger advantage.

Most older adults live in a household with a spouse or other family member, although more than twice the number of women than men live alone in later life. The likelihood of living alone increases with age for both sexes (Fig. 1-4). Most older people have contact with their families and are not forgotten or neglected. Realities of the aging family are discussed in greater detail in Chapter 38.

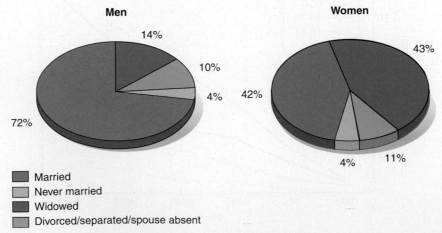

FIGURE 1-3 ■ Marital status of the population 65 years of age and older (%). (From U.S. Department of Commerce. (2005). *Current population survey, annual social and economic supplement of the U.S. Bureau of the Census.* Washington, DC: Bureau of the Census).

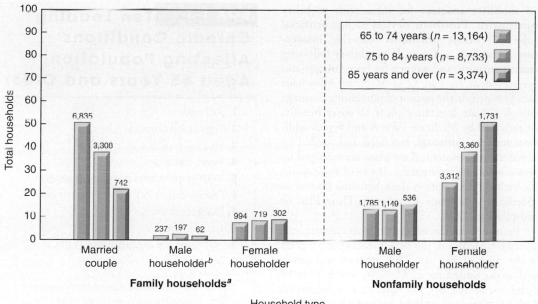

aHouseholds in which at least one member is related to the person who owns or rents the occupied housing unit (householder).

bNo spouse present.

FIGURE 1-4 ■ Living arrangements of people aged 65 years and older. (From U.S. Census Bureau, [2010]. *Current population survey, annual social and economic supplement.* Washington, DC: Bureau of the Census).

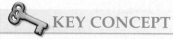KEY CONCEPT

Although Social Security was intended to be a supplement to other sources of income for older adults, it is the main source of income for more than half of all these individuals.

HEALTH INSURANCE

This decade has shaken the health care reimbursement systems in the United States and changes will be unfolding as the need to assure that every American will have access to health care is balanced against unsustainable costs to support that care. Passed in 1965 as Title 18 of the Social Security Act, Medicare is the health insurance program for older adults who are eligible for Social Security benefits. This federally funded program primarily covers hospital and physician services with very limited skilled home health and nursing home services under Part A. Preventive services and nonskilled care (e.g., personal care assistance) are not covered. To supplement the basic coverage, a person can purchase Medicare Part B, which includes physician and nursing services, **x-rays,** laboratory and diagnostic tests, influenza and pneumonia vaccinations,

blood **transfusions**, renal **dialysis**, **outpatient hospital procedures**, limited ambulance transportation, **immunosuppressive drugs** for **organ transplant** recipients, **chemotherapy**, hormonal treatments, and other outpatient medical treatments administered in a doctor's office. Part B also assists with the payment of **durable medical equipment**, including **canes**, **walkers**, **wheelchairs**,

BOX 1-2   Social Security and Supplemental Security Income

Social Security: a benefit check paid to retired workers of specific minimum age (e.g., 65 years), disabled workers of any age, and spouses and minor children of those workers. Benefits are not dependent on financial need. It is intended to serve as supplement to other sources of income in retirement.

Supplemental Security Income (SSI): a benefit check paid to persons over age 65 and/or persons with disabilities based on financial need.

and **mobility scooters** for those with **mobility impairments**. **Prosthetic devices** such as **artificial limbs** and **breast prosthesis** following **mastectomy**, as well as one pair of **eyeglasses** following **cataract surgery**, and **oxygen** for home use are also covered. Medicare Part C or Medicare Advantage Plans give people the option of purchasing coverage through private insurance plans to cover benefits not provided by Medicare Parts A and B plus additional services. Although regulated and funded by the federal government, these plans are managed by private insurance companies. Some of these plans also include prescription drug benefits, known as a Medicare Advantage Prescription Drug Plan or Medicare Part D.

Persons who meet the income criteria can qualify for Medicaid, the health insurance program for the poor of any age. This program was developed at the same time as Medicare and is Title 19 of the Social Security Act. Medicaid supplements Medicare for poor elderly individuals and most nursing home care is paid for by this program. Medicaid is supported by federal and state funding. Provisions in the Affordable Care Act expand Medicaid benefits to many older persons who did not previously qualify for the program.

People of any age can purchase long-term care insurance to cover health care costs not paid by Medicare or other health insurance. These policies can provide benefits for home care, respite, adult day care, nursing home care, assisted living, and other services. Policies vary in waiting periods, amount of funds paid per day or month, and types of services that qualify. Although beneficial, long-term care insurance has not attracted a significant number of subscribers. Part of the reason for this is that policies are expensive for older adults and although less costly for persons of younger age groups, younger and healthier individuals tend not to think about long-term care.

Health Status

The older population experiences fewer acute illnesses than younger age groups and a lower death rate from these problems. However, older people who do develop acute illnesses usually require longer periods of recovery and have more complications from these conditions.

Chronic illness is a major problem for the older population. Most older adults have at least one chronic disease, and typically they have multiple chronic conditions, termed comorbidity, that requires them to manage the care of several conditions simultaneously (Box 1-3). Chronic conditions result in some limitations in activities of daily living and instrumental activities of daily living for many individuals. The older the person is, the greater the

BOX 1-3 **Ten Leading Chronic Conditions Affecting Population Aged 65 Years and Older**
1. Arthritis
2. High blood pressure
3. Hearing impairments
4. Heart conditions
5. Visual impairments (including cataracts)
6. Deformities or orthopedic impairments
7. Diabetes mellitus
8. Chronic sinusitis
9. Hay fever and allergic rhinitis (without asthma)
10. Varicose veins
Source: Centers for Disease Control and Prevention, Chronic Disease Prevention and Health Promotion. Retrieved April 14, 2012 from http://www.cdc.gov/chronicdisease/index.html.

likelihood of difficulty with self-care activities and independent living.

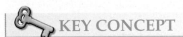

KEY CONCEPT

The chronic disorders most prevalent in the older population are ones that can have a significant impact on independence and the quality of daily life.

Chronic diseases are also the leading causes of death (Table 1-3). A shift in death rates from various causes of death has occurred over the past three decades; deaths from heart disease have declined, whereas those from cancer have increased.

Despite the advances in the health status of the older population, disparities exist. Studies have found that older minorities have lower levels of health and function and, when in need of nursing home care, are more likely to reside in facilities that offer a poor quality of care (Cai, Mukamel, & Temkin-Greener, 2010).

IMPLICATIONS OF AN AGING POPULATION

The growing number of persons older than 65 years impacts health and social service agencies and health care providers—including gerontological nurses—that serve this group. As the older adult population grows,

TABLE I-3	Leading Causes of Death for Persons 65 Years of Age and Older

Heart disease
Malignant neoplasms (cancer)
Chronic lower respiratory disease
Cerebrovascular disease
Alzheimer's disease
Diabetes mellitus
Influenza and pneumonia
Nephritis, nephrotic syndrome, nephrosis
Accidents
Septicemia

From National Center for Health Statistics. (2012). *Table 7, Death and death rates for the 10 leading causes of death in specified age groups. U.S., preliminary 2010.* National Vital Statistics Reports, Vol. 60, No.4.

these agencies and providers must anticipate future needs of services and payment for these services.

Impact of the Baby Boomers

In anticipating needs and services for future generations of older adults, gerontological nurses must consider the realities of the baby boomers—those born between 1946 and 1964—who will be the next wave of senior citizens. Their impact on the growth of the older population is such that it has been referred to as a demographic tidal wave. Baby boomers began entering their senior years in 2011 and will continue to do so until 2030 (Fig. 1-5). Although they are a highly diverse group, representing people as different

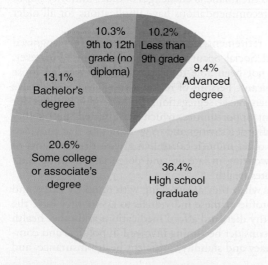

FIGURE I-5 ■ Education of population aged 65 and older. (From U.S. Census Bureau, (2010), current population survey, annual social and economic supplement, 2010. Washington, DC: Bureau of the census.

as Bill Clinton, Bill Gates, and Cher, they do have some clearly defined characteristics that set them apart from other groups:

- Most have children, but this generation's low birth rate means that they will have fewer biologic children available to assist them in old age.
- They are better educated than preceding generations.
- Their household incomes tend to be higher than other groups, partly due to two incomes (three out of four baby boomer women are in the labor force).
- They favor a more casual dress code than previous generations of older adults.
- They are enamored with "high-tech" products and are likely to own and use a home computer.
- Their leisure time is scarcer than other adults, and they are more likely to report feeling stressed at the end of the day.
- As inventors of the fitness movement, they exercise more frequently than other adults.

Some assumptions can be made concerning the baby boomer population as senior adults. They are informed consumers of health care and desire a highly active role in their care; their ability to access information often enables them to have as much knowledge as their health care providers on some health issues. They are most likely not going to be satisfied with the conditions of today's nursing homes and will demand that their long-term care facilities be equipped with bedside Internet access, gymnasiums, juice bars, pools, and alternative therapies. Their blended families may need special assistance because of the potential caregiving demands of several sets of stepparents and stepgrandparents. Plans for services and architectural designs must take these factors into consideration.

Provision of and Payment for Services

The growing number of persons older than 65 years also impacts the government that is the source of payment for many of the services older adults need. The older population has higher rates of hospitalization, surgery, and physician visits than other age group (Table 1-4), and this care is more likely to be paid by federal dollars than private insurers or older adults themselves.

Less than 5% of the older population is in a nursing home, assisted living community, or other institutional setting at any given time. Approximately one in four older adults will spend some time in a nursing home during the last years of their lives. Most people who enter nursing homes as private-pay

TABLE 1-4	Average Length of Hospital Stay					
Age (years)	<18	18–44	45–64	65–74	75–84	85+
Days of Stay	4.8	3.7	5.1	5.4	5.7	5.6

National Center for Health Statistics (2010). Health, United States, 2010. Table 102. Average length of stay in nonfederal short-stay hospitals, by sex, age, and selected first-listed diagnosis: United States, selected years 1990–2007.

residents spend their assets by the end of 1 year and require government support for their care; most of the Medicaid budget is spent on long-term care.

As the percentage of the advanced-age population grows, society will face an increasing demand for the provision of and payment for services to this group. In this era of budget deficits, shrinking revenue, and increased competition for funding of other special interests, questions may arise about the ongoing ability of the government to provide a wide range of services for older adults. There may be concern that the older population is using a disproportionate amount of tax dollars and that limits should be set.

Gerontological nurses must be actively involved in discussions and decisions pertaining to the rationing of services so that the rights of older adults are expressed and protected. Likewise, gerontological nurses must assume leadership in developing cost-effective methods of care delivery that do not compromise the quality of services to older adults.

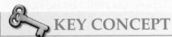

KEY CONCEPT

Gerontological nurses need to be advocates in ensuring that cost-containment efforts do not jeopardize the welfare of older adults.

BRINGING RESEARCH TO LIFE

THE ECONOMIC CRISIS FACING SENIORS OF COLOR: BACKGROUND AND POLICY RECOMMENDATIONS

Dumez, J., & Derbew, H. (2011). Berkeley, CA: Greenlining Institute.

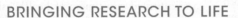

The researchers analyzed data pertaining to the financial challenges of older minority populations in California. Their findings and recommendations have implications for all older Latino and African Americans.

In considering financial security in retirement, financial planners have recognized employee pensions, personal savings, and Social Security as critical elements. However, today's older minority populations have not been able to accrue benefits from all those sources to the same extent as white Americans. Persons of retirement age today may have entered the workforce during a time when racial segregations limited opportunities for educational advancement and employment opportunities, which has affected their ability to have high-paying jobs that could have afforded savings and to work in jobs that provided pensions. Despite improvements, today's older minorities are living with the remnants of these realities, leading them to continue working in late life and potentially limiting their ability to have a quality of life that promotes health.

Nurses need to consider these realities when they are working with minority elders and take special effort to assess the financial profile of these individuals to assure they have the means to live in safe conditions, eat a healthy diet, and afford medications and other health care measures. In addition, nurses should consider becoming involved in political and community efforts that promote financial literacy and stability, sufficient health insurance, and adequate resources for all older adults.

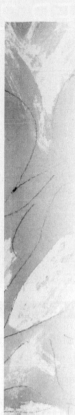

PRACTICE REALITIES

You are in the break room of a hospital unit where several of the nurses are eating the birthday cake of Nurse Clark who is celebrating her 66th birthday. "I'm so glad to have coworkers like you and work that gives me a sense of purpose," Nurse Clark commented as she thanked everyone and left the room.

Nurse Blake, in a low voice commented to the person sitting next to her, "I just don't get it. I'm half her age and this job drains me, so you know it's got to be taking its toll on her. Plus, we often get stuck doing the heavy work that she can't do."

"I know she doesn't have the physical capabilities that some others may," says Nurse Edwards, "but she sure is a storehouse of information and the patients love her."

"Yes, but that isn't helping my back when I have to pick up the slack for her," responds Nurse Blake.

What are the challenges of having different generations in the workplace. Should allowances be made for older workers, and if so, what can be done to support these?

CRITICAL THINKING EXERCISES

1. What factors influence a society's willingness to provide assistance to and display a positive attitude toward older individuals (e.g., general economic conditions for all age groups)?

2. List the anticipated changes in the characteristics of the older population of the future and describe the implications for nursing.

3. What problems may older women experience as a result of gender differences in life expectancy and income?

4. What are some of the differences between older white and black Americans?

RESOURCE

National Center for Health Statistics
http://www.cdc.gov/nchs

REFERENCES

Cai, S., Mukamel, D., & Temkin-Greener, H. (2010). Pressure ulcer prevalence among black and white nursing home residents in New York state. Evidence of racial disparity. *Medical Care, 48*(3), 233–239.

Christensen, K., Thinggaard, M., McGue, M., Rexby, H., Hjelmborg, J. V. B., Aviv, A., Vaupel, J. W., et al. (2009). Young and old. Perceived age as clinically useful biomarker of ageing. Cohort study. *British Medical Journal, 339,* b5262, doi:10.1136/bmj.b5262.

RECOMMENDED READINGS

Recommended Readings associated with this chapter can be found on the web site that accompanies the book. Visit **http://thepoint.lww.com/Eliopoulos8e** to access the recommended readings and other additional resources associated with this chapter.

Theories of Aging

CHAPTER OUTLINE

LEARNING OBJECTIVES

After reading this chapter, you should be able to:

1. Discuss the change in focus regarding learning about factors influencing aging.

2. List the major biological theories of aging.

3. Describe the major psychosocial theories of aging.

4. Identify factors that promote a healthy aging process.

TERMS TO KNOW

Aging: the process of growing older that begins at birth

Nonstochastic theories: explain biological aging as resulting from a complex, predetermined process

Stochastic theories: view the effects of biological aging as resulting from random assaults from both the internal and external environment

For centuries, people have been intrigued by the mystery of aging and have sought to understand it, some in hopes of achieving everlasting youth, others seeking the key to immortality. Throughout history there have been numerous searches for a fountain of youth, the most famous being that of Ponce de León. Ancient Egyptian and Chinese relics show evidence of concoctions designed to prolong life or achieve immortality, and various other cultures have proposed specific dietary regimens, herbal mixtures, and rituals for similar ends. Ancient life extenders, such as extracts prepared from tiger testicles, may seem ludicrous until they are compared with more modern measures such as injections of embryonic tissue and Botox. Even persons who would not condone such peculiar practices may indulge in nutritional supplements, cosmetic creams, and exotic spas that promise to maintain youth and delay the onset or appearance of old age.

No single known factor causes or prevents aging; therefore, it is unrealistic to think that one theory can explain the complexities of this process. Explorations into biological, psychological, and social aging continue, and although some of this interest focuses on achieving eternal youth, most sound research efforts aim toward a better understanding of the aging process so that people can age in a healthier fashion and postpone some of the negative consequences associated with growing old. In fact, recent research has concentrated on learning about keeping people healthy and active for a longer period of time, rather than on extending their lives in a state of long-term disability (Hubert, Bloch, Oehlert, & Fries, 2002). Recognizing that theories of aging offer varying degrees of universality,

validity, and reliability, nurses can use this information to better understand the factors that may positively and negatively influence the health and well-being of persons of all ages.

BIOLOGICAL THEORIES OF AGING

The process of biological aging differs not only from species to species but also from one human being to another. Some general statements can be made concerning anticipated organ changes, as described in Chapter 5; however, no two individuals age identically (Fig. 2-1). Varying degrees of physiologic changes, capacities, and limitations will be found among peers of a given age group. Further, the rate of aging among different body systems within one individual may vary, with one system showing marked decline while another demonstrates no significant change.

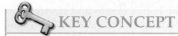 **KEY CONCEPT**

The aging process varies not only among individuals but also within different body systems of the same person.

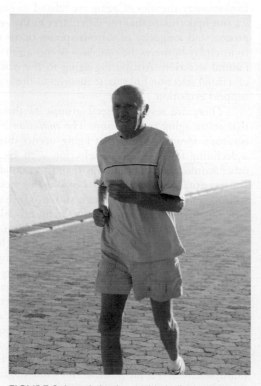 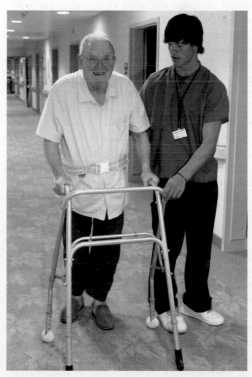

FIGURE 2-1 ■ Aging is a highly individualized process, demonstrated by the differences between persons of similar ages.

To explain biological aging, theorists have explored many factors, both internal and external to the human body, and have divided them into two categories: stochastic and nonstochastic. Stochastic theories view the effects of aging as resulting from random assaults from both the internal and external environment. Nonstochastic theories see aging changes resulting from a complex, predetermined process.

Stochastic Theories

Cross-Linking Theory

The cross-linking theory proposes that cellular division is threatened as a result of radiation or a chemical reaction in which a cross-linking agent attaches itself to a DNA strand and prevents normal parting of the strands during mitosis. Over time, as these cross-linking agents accumulate, they form dense aggregates that impede intracellular transport; ultimately, the body's organs and systems fail. An effect of cross-linking on collagen (an important connective tissue in the lungs, heart, blood vessels, and muscle) is the reduction in tissue elasticity associated with many age-related changes.

Free Radicals and Lipofuscin Theories

Free radicals are highly unstable, reactive molecules containing an extra electrical charge that are generated from oxygen metabolism. They can result from normal metabolism, reactions with other free radicals, or oxidation of ozone, pesticides, and other pollutants. These molecules can damage proteins, enzymes, and DNA by replacing molecules that contain useful biological information with faulty molecules that create genetic disorder. It is believed that these free radicals are self-perpetuating; that is, they generate other free radicals. Physical decline of the body occurs as the damage from these molecules accumulates over time. However, the body has natural antioxidants that can counteract the effects of free radicals to an extent. Also, beta-carotene and vitamins C and E are antioxidants that can offer protection against free radicals.

There has been considerable interest in the role of lipofuscin "age pigments," a lipoprotein by-product of oxidation that can be seen only under a fluorescent microscope, in the aging process. Because lipofuscin is associated with the oxidation of unsaturated lipids, it is believed to have a role similar to that of free radicals in the aging process. As lipofuscin accumulates, it interferes with the diffusion and transport of essential metabolites and information-bearing molecules in the cells. A positive relationship exists between an individual's age and the amount of lipofuscin in the body. Investigators have discovered the presence of lipofuscin in other species in amounts proportionate to the life span of the species (e.g., an animal with one tenth the life span of a human being accumulates lipofuscin at a rate approximately 10 times greater than human beings).

Wear and Tear Theories

The comparison of the body's wearing down to machines that lost their ability to function over time arose during the Industrial Revolution. Wear and tear theories attribute aging to the repeated use and injury of the body over time as it performs its highly specialized functions. Like any complicated machine, the body will function less efficiently with prolonged use and numerous insults (e.g., smoking, poor diet, and substance abuse).

In recent years, the effects of stress on physical and psychological health have been widely discussed. Stresses to the body can have adverse effects and lead to conditions such as gastric ulcers, heart attacks, thyroiditis, and inflammatory dermatoses. However, because individuals react differently to life's stresses—one person may be overwhelmed by a moderately busy schedule, whereas another may become frustrated when faced with a slow, dull pace—the role of stress in aging is inconclusive.

Evolutionary Theories

Evolutionary theories of aging are related to genetics and hypothesize that the differences in the aging process and longevity of various species occur due to interplay between the processes of mutation and natural selection. Attributing aging to the process of natural selection links these theories to those that support evolution.

There are several general groups of theories that relate aging to evolution. The *mutation accumulation theory* suggests that aging occurs due to a declining force of natural selection with age. In other words, genetic mutations that affect children will eventually be eliminated because the victims will not have lived long enough to reproduce and pass this to future generations. Genetic mutations that appear late in life, however, will accumulate because the older individuals they affect will have already passed these mutations to their offspring.

The *antagonistic pleiotropy theory* suggests that accumulated mutant genes that have negative effects in late life may have had beneficial effects in early life. This is assumed to occur either because the effects of the mutant genes occur in opposite ways in late life as compared with their effects in early life or because a particular gene can have multiple effects—some positive and some negative.

The *disposable soma theory* differs from other evolutionary theories by proposing that aging is related to the use of the body's energy rather than to genetics. It claims that the body must use energy for metabolism, reproduction, maintenance of functions, and repair, and with a finite supply of energy from food to perform these functions, some compromise occurs. Through evolution, organisms have learned to give priority of energy expenditure to reproductive functions over those functions that could maintain the body indefinitely; thus, decline and death ultimately occur.

KEY CONCEPT

Evolutionary theories suggest that aging "is fundamentally a product of evolutionary forces, not biochemical or cellular quirks ... a Darwinian phenomenon, not a biochemical one" (Rose, 1998).

Biogerontology

The study of the connection between aging and disease processes has been termed *biogerontology* (Miller, 1997). Bacteria, fungi, viruses, and other organisms are thought to be responsible for certain physiologic changes during the aging process. In some cases, these pathogens may be present in the body for decades before they begin to affect body systems. Although no conclusive evidence exists to link these pathogens with the body's decline, interest in this theory has been stimulated by the fact that human beings and animals have enjoyed longer life expectancies with the control or elimination of certain pathogens through immunization and the use of antimicrobial drugs.

Nonstochastic Theories

Apoptosis

Apoptosis is the process of programmed cell death that continuously occurs throughout life due to biochemical events (Green, 2011). In this process, the cell shrinks and there is nuclear and DNA fragmentation, although the membrane maintains its integrity. It differs from cell death that occurs from injury in which there is swelling of the cell and loss of membrane integrity. According to this theory, this programmed cell death is part of the normal developmental process that continues throughout life.

Genetic Theories

Among the earliest genetic theories was the *programmed theory of aging* that proposed that animals and humans are born with a genetic program or biological clock that predetermines the life span (Hayflick, 1965). Various studies support this idea

of a predetermined genetic program for life span. For example, studies have shown a positive relationship between parental age and filial life span. Additionally, studies of in vitro cell proliferation have demonstrated that various species have a finite number of cell divisions. Fibroblasts from embryonic tissue experience a greater number of cell divisions than those derived from adult tissue, and among various species, the longer the life span, the greater the number of cell divisions. These studies support the theory that senescence—the process of becoming old—is under genetic control and occurs at the cellular level (Harvard Gazette Archives, 2001; Martin, 2009; University of Illinois at Urbana-Champaign, 2002).

The *error theory* also proposes a genetic determination for aging. This theory holds that genetic mutations are responsible for aging by causing organ decline as a result of self-perpetuating cellular mutations:

Mutation of DNA
⇩
Perpetuation of mutation during cell division
⇩
Increasing number of mutant cells in body
⇩
Malfunction of tissues, organs, and systems
⇩
Decline in body functions

Other theorists think that aging results when a growth substance fails to be produced, leading to the cessation of cell growth and reproduction. Others hypothesize that an aging factor responsible for development and cellular maturity throughout life is excessively produced, thereby hastening aging. Some hypothesize that the cell's ability to function and divide is impaired. Although minimal research has been done to support the theory, aging may be the result of a decreased ability of RNA to synthesize and translate messages.

POINT TO PONDER

What patterns of aging are apparent in your biological family? What can you do to influence these?

Autoimmune Reactions

The primary organs of the immune system, the thymus and bone marrow, are believed to be affected by the aging process. The immune response declines after young adulthood. The weight of the thymus decreases throughout adulthood, as does the ability to produce T-cell differentiation. The level of thymic hormone declines after age 30 and is undetectable in the blood of persons older than 60 years (Goya, Console, Herenu, Brown, & Rimoldi, 2002; Williams, 1995). Related to this is a decline in the humoral immune response, a delay in the skin allograft rejection time, a reduction in the intensity of delayed hypersensitivity, and a decrease in the resistance to tumor cell challenge. The bone marrow stem cells perform less efficiently. The reduction in immunologic functions is evidenced by an increase in the incidence of infections and many cancers with age.

Some theorists believe that the reduction in immunologic activities also leads to an increase in autoimmune response with age. One hypothesis regarding the role of autoimmune reactions in the aging process is that the cells undergo changes with age, and the body misidentifies these aged, irregular cells as foreign agents and develops antibodies to attack them. An alternate explanation for this reaction could be that cells are normal in old age, but a breakdown of the body's immunochemical memory system causes it to misinterpret normal cells as foreign substances. Antibodies are formed to attack and rid the body of these "foreign" substances, and cells die.

Neuroendocrine and Neurochemical Theories

Neuroendocrine and neurochemical theories suggest that aging is the result of changes in the brain and endocrine glands. Some theorists claim that specific anterior pituitary hormones promote aging. Others believe that an imbalance of chemicals in the brain impairs healthy cell division throughout the body.

Radiation Theories

The relationship between radiation and age continues to be explored. Research using rats, mice, and dogs has shown that a decreased life span results from nonlethal doses of radiation. In human beings, repeated exposure to ultraviolet light is known to cause solar elastosis, the "old age" type of skin wrinkling that results from the replacement of collagen by elastin. Ultraviolet light is also a factor in the development of skin cancer. Radiation may induce cellular mutations that promote aging.

Nutrition Theories

The importance of good nutrition throughout life is a theme hard to escape in our nutrition-conscious society. It is no mystery that diet impacts health and aging. Obesity is shown to increase the risk of many diseases and shorten life (NIDDK, 2001; Preston, 2005; Taylor & Ostbye, 2001).

The quality of diet is as important as the quantity. Deficiencies of vitamins and other nutrients and excesses of nutrients such as cholesterol may cause various disease processes. Recently, increased attention has been given to the influence of nutritional supplements on the aging process; vitamin E, bee pollen, ginseng, gotu kola, peppermint, and kelp are among the nutrients believed to promote a healthy, long life (Margolis, 2000; Smeeding, 2001). Although the complete relationship between diet and aging is not well understood, enough is known to suggest that a good diet may minimize or eliminate some of the ill effects of the aging process.

KEY CONCEPT

It is beneficial for nurses to advise aging persons to scrutinize products that claim to cause, stop, or reverse the aging process.

Environmental Theories

Several environmental factors are known to threaten health and are thought to be associated with the aging process. The ingestion of mercury, lead, arsenic, radioactive isotopes, certain pesticides, and other substances can produce pathologic changes in human beings. Smoking and breathing tobacco smoke and other air pollutants also have adverse effects. Finally, crowded living conditions, high noise levels, and other factors are thought to influence how we age.

POINT TO PONDER

Do you believe nurses have a responsibility to protect and improve the environment? Why or why not?

SOCIOLOGIC THEORIES OF AGING

Disengagement Theory

Sociologic theories address the impact of society on older adults and vice versa. These theories often reflect the view held about older adults at the time they were developed. The norms of society affected how the older adult's roles and relationships were viewed.

Developed by Elaine Cumming and William Henry, the disengagement theory (Cumming, 1964; Cumming & Henry, 1961) has been one of the earliest, most controversial, and most widely discussed theories of aging. It views aging as a process in which society and the individual gradually withdraw, or disengage, from each other, to the mutual satisfaction and benefit of both. The benefit to individuals is that they can reflect and be centered on themselves, having been freed from societal roles. The value of disengagement to society is that some orderly means is established for the transfer of power from the old to the young, making it possible for society to continue functioning after its individual members die. The theory does not indicate whether society or the individual initiates the disengagement process.

Several difficulties with this concept are obvious and this theory has now been discredited (Johnson, 2009). Many older persons desire to remain engaged and do not want their primary satisfaction to be derived from reflection on younger years. Senators, Supreme Court justices, college professors, and many senior volunteers are among those who commonly derive satisfaction and provide a valuable service to society by not disengaging. Because the health of the individual, cultural practices, societal norms, and other factors influence the degree to which a person will participate in society during his or her later years, some critics of this theory claim that disengagement would not be necessary if society improved the health care and financial means of older adults and increased the acceptance, opportunities, and respect afforded them.

A careful examination of the population studied in the development of the disengagement theory hints at its limitations. The disengagement pattern that Cumming and Henry described was based on a study of 172 middle class persons between 48 and 68 years of age. This group was wealthier, better educated, and of higher occupational and residential prestige than the general aged population. No black people or chronically ill people were involved in the study. Caution is advisable in generalizing findings for the entire aged population based on fewer than 200 persons who are generally not representative of the average aged person. (This study exemplifies some of the limitations of gerontological research before the 1970s.) Although nurses should appreciate that some older individuals may wish to disengage from the mainstream of society, this is not necessarily a process to be expected from all aged persons.

Activity Theory

At the opposite pole from the disengagement theory, the activity theory asserts that an older person should continue a middle-aged lifestyle, denying the existence of old age as long as possible, and that society should apply the same norms to old age as it does to middle age and not advocate diminishing activity, interest, and involvement as its members grow old (Havighurst, 1963). This theory suggests ways of maintaining activity in the presence of multiple losses associated with the aging process, including substituting intellectual activities for physical activities when physical capacity is reduced, replacing the work role with other roles when retirement occurs, and establishing new friendships when old ones are lost. Declining health, loss of roles, reduced income, a shrinking circle of friends, and other obstacles to maintaining an active life are to be resisted and overcome instead of being accepted.

This theory has some merit. Activity is generally assumed to be more desirable than inactivity because it facilitates physical, mental, and social well-being. Like a self-fulfilling prophecy, the expectation of a continued active state during old age may be realized to the benefit of older adults and society. Because of society's negative view of inactivity, encouraging an active lifestyle among the aged is consistent with societal values. Also supportive of the activity theory is the reluctance of many older persons to accept themselves as old.

A problem with the activity theory is its assumption that most older people desire and are able to maintain a middle-aged lifestyle. Some aging persons want their world to shrink to accommodate their decreasing capacities or their preference for less active roles. Many older adults lack the physical, emotional, social, or economic resources to maintain active roles in society. Aged people who are expected to maintain an active middle-aged lifestyle on an income of less than half that of middle-aged people may wonder if society is giving them conflicting messages. More research and insights are needed regarding the effects on the older adults of not being able to fulfill expectations to remain active.

Continuity Theory

The continuity theory of aging, also referred to as the developmental theory, relates personality and predisposition toward certain actions in old age to similar factors during other phases of the life cycle (Neugarten, 1964). Personality and basic patterns of behavior are said to remain unchanged as the individual ages. For instance, activists at 20 years of age will most likely be activists at 70 years of age, whereas young recluses will probably not be active in the mainstream of society when they age. Patterns developed over a lifetime will determine whether individuals remain engaged and active or become disengaged and inactive.

The recognition that the unique features of each individual allow for multiple adaptations to aging and that the potential exists for a variety of reactions gives this theory validity and support. Aging is a complex process, and the continuity theory considers these complexities to a greater extent than most other theories. Although the full implications and impact of this promising theory are at the stage of research, it offers a reasonable perspective. Also, it encourages the young to consider that their current activities will lay a foundation for their own future old age.

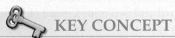
KEY CONCEPT

Basic psychological patterns are consistent throughout the life span.

Subculture Theory

This theory views older adults as a group with distinct norms, beliefs, expectations, habits, and issues that separate them from the rest of society (Rose, 1965). Their formation of a subculture is a response to the negative attitudes and treatment by society. Older persons are accepted by and more comfortable among their own age group. A component of this theory is the argument for social reform and greater empowerment of the older populations so that their rights and needs can be respected.

As the population of older adults becomes more diverse, their needs better addressed, and their power recognized, the question can be raised that this theory is less relevant today than it was in the 1960s when it was first offered.

Age Stratification Theory

This theory, appearing in the 1970s, suggests that society is stratified by age groups (Riley, Johnson, & Foner, 1972). Persons within a similar age group generally have similar experiences, beliefs, attitudes, and life transitions that offer them a unique shared history. New age groups are continually being formed with the birth of new individuals; thus, the interaction between society and the aging population is dynamic. As each group ages, they have their own unique experience with and influence on society, and there is an interdependence between society and the group.

PSYCHOLOGICAL THEORIES OF AGING

Developmental Tasks

Psychological theories of aging explore the mental processes, behavior, and feelings of persons throughout the life span, along with some of the mechanisms people use to meet the challenges they face in old age. Among these theories are those that describe the process of healthy psychological aging as the result of the successful fulfillment of developmental tasks. Developmental tasks are the challenges that must be met and adjustments that must be made in response to life experiences that are part of an adult's continued growth through the life span.

Erik Erikson (1963) described eight stages through which human beings progress from infancy to old age and the challenges, or tasks, that confront individuals during each of these stages (Table 2-1). The challenge of old age is to accept and find meaning in the life the person has lived; this gives the individual ego integrity that aids in adjusting and coping with the reality of aging and mortality. Feelings of anger, bitterness, depression, and inadequacy can result in inadequate ego integrity (e.g., despair).

Refining Erikson's description of old age tasks in the eighth stage of development, Robert Peck (1968) detailed three specific challenges facing the older adults that influence the outcome of ego integrity or despair:

- *ego differentiation versus role preoccupation:* to develop satisfactions from oneself as a person rather than through parental or occupational roles
- *body transcendence versus body preoccupation:* to find psychological pleasures rather than become absorbed with health problems or physical limitations imposed by aging
- *ego transcendence versus ego preoccupation:* to achieve satisfaction through reflection on one's past life and accomplishments rather than be preoccupied with the finite number of years left to live

TABLE 2-1	Erikson's Developmental Tasks	
Stage	**Satisfactorily Fulfilled**	**Unsatisfactorily Fulfilled**
Infancy	Trust	Mistrust
Toddler	Autonomy	Shame
Early childhood	Initiative	Guilt
Middle childhood	Industry	Inferiority
Adolescence	Identity	Identity diffusion
Adulthood	Intimacy	Isolation
Middle age	Generativity	Self-absorption
Old age	Integrity	Despair

Robert Butler and Myrna Lewis (1982) outlined additional developmental tasks of later life:

- adjusting to one's infirmities
- developing a sense of satisfaction with the life that has been lived
- preparing for death

Gerotranscendence

Gerotranscendence is a recent theory that suggests aging entails a transition from a rational, materialistic metaperspective to a cosmic and transcendent vision (Tornstam, 2005). As people age, they are less concerned with their physical bodies, material possessions, meaningless relationships, and self-interests and instead desire a life of more significance and a greater connection with others. There is a desire to shed roles and invest time in discovering hidden facets of oneself.

POINT TO PONDER

How do you see examples of gerotranscendence in the lives of others and yourself?

KEY CONCEPT

Nurses can promote joy and a sense of purpose in the older adults by viewing old age as an opportunity for continued development and satisfaction rather than a depressing, useless period of life.

APPLYING THEORIES OF AGING TO NURSING PRACTICE

The number, diversity, and complexity of factors that potentially influence the aging process show that no one theory can adequately explain the cause of this phenomenon. Even when studies have been done with populations known to have a long life expectancy, such as the people of the Caucasus region in southern Russia, longevity has not been attributable to any single factor.

The biological, psychological, and social processes of aging are interrelated and interdependent. Frequently, loss of a social role affects an individual's sense of purpose and speeds physical decline. Poor health may force retirement from work, promoting social isolation and the development of a weakened self-concept. Although certain changes occur independently as separate events, most are closely associated with other age-related factors. Wise nurses will be open-minded in choosing the aging theories they use in the care of older adults; they will also be cognizant of the limitations of these theories.

Nurses can adapt these theories by identifying elements known to influence aging and using them as a foundation to promote positive practices. Box 2-1 highlights some factors to consider in promoting a healthy aging process.

In addition, gerontological nurses play a significant role in helping aging persons experience health, fulfillment, and a sense of well-being. In addition to specific measures that can assist the older adults in meeting their psychosocial challenges (Box 2-2), nurses must be sensitive to the tremendous impact their own attitudes toward aging can have on patients. Nurses who consider aging as a progressive decline ending in death may view old age as a depressing, useless period and foster hopelessness and helplessness in older patients. However, nurses who view aging as a process of continued development may appreciate late life as an opportunity to gain new satisfaction and understanding, thereby promoting joy and a sense of purpose in patients.

POINT TO PONDER

How would you evaluate the quality of the factors that promote longevity in your own life?

BOX 2-1   Factors Contributing to a Long and Healthy Life

Diet. A positive health state that can contribute to longevity is supported by reducing saturated fats in the diet, limiting daily fat consumption to less than 30% of caloric intake, avoiding obesity, decreasing the amount of animal foods eaten, substituting natural complex carbohydrates for refined sugars, and increasing the consumption of whole grains, vegetables, and fruits.

Activity. Exercise is an important ingredient to good health. It increases strength and endurance, promotes cardiopulmonary function, and has other beneficial effects that can affect a healthy aging process.

Play and laughter. Laughter causes a release of endorphins, stimulates the immune system, and reduces stress. Finding humor in daily routines and experiencing joy despite problems contributes to good health. It has been suggested since the time of Solomon that "a cheerful heart is good medicine, but a crushed spirit dries up the bones" (Proverbs 17:22).

Faith. A strong faith, church attendance, and prayer are directly related to lower rates of physical and mental illness. Religion and spirituality can have a positive effect on the length and quality of life.

Empowerment. Losing control over one's life can threaten self-confidence and diminish self-care independence. Maximum control and decision making can have a positive effect on morbidity and mortality.

Stress management. It is the rare individual who is unaware of the negative consequences of stress. The unique stresses that may accompany aging, such as the onset of chronic conditions, retirement, deaths of significant others, and change in body appearance, can have significantly detrimental effects. Minimizing stress when possible and using effective stress management techniques are useful interventions.

BOX 2-2   Assisting Individuals in Meeting the Psychosocial Challenges of Aging

OVERVIEW

As individuals progress through their life span, they face challenges and adjustments in response to life experiences called developmental tasks. These developmental tasks can be described as:

- coping with losses and changes
- establishing meaningful roles
- exercising independence and control
- finding purpose and meaning in life

Satisfaction with oneself and the life one has lived is gained by successfully meeting these tasks; unhappiness, bitterness, and fear of one's future can result from not adjusting to and rejecting the realities of aging.

GOAL

Aging persons will express a sense of ego integrity and psychosocial well-being.

ACTIONS

- Learn about patients' life stories; ask about family backgrounds, faith, work histories, hobbies, achievements, and life experiences. Encourage patients to discuss these topics, and listen with sincere interest.
- Build on lifelong interests and offer opportunities for patients to experience new pleasures and interests.
- Accept patients' discussions of their regrets and dissatisfactions. Help them to put these in perspective of their total lives and accomplishments.
- Encourage reminiscence activities between patients and their families. Help families and staff to understand the therapeutic value of reminiscence.
- Respect patients' faith and assist them in the fulfillment of spiritual needs (e.g., help them locate a church of their religious affiliation, request visits from clergy, pray with or for them, and obtain a Bible or other religious book).
- Use humor therapeutically.
- If patients reside in an institutional setting, personalize the environment to the maximum degree possible.
- Recognize the unique assets and characteristics of each patient.

EMOTIONAL EXPERIENCE IMPROVES WITH AGE: EVIDENCE BASED ON OVER 10 YEARS OF EXPERIENCE SAMPLING

Carstensen, L. L., Turan, B., Scheibe, S., Ram, N., Ersner-Hershfield, H., Samanez-Larkin, G. R., Nesselroade, J. R., et al. (2011). Psychology and Aging, 26(1), 21–33.

This study followed a representative sample of adults spanning from early to very late adulthood to examine the developmental course of the individuals' emotional experience. The participants reported their emotional states at five randomly selected times daily for a 1-week period; this was repeated 5 and then 10 years later.

Data analyses indicated that aging is associated with more positive overall emotional well-being, with greater emotional stability, and with more complexity than typically assumed. The findings also revealed that emotional experience predicted mortality in that (controlling for age, sex, and ethnicity) individuals who experienced relatively more positive than negative emotions in everyday life were more likely to have survived over a 13-year period.

Four main findings emerged from these analyses: there is improvement in overall emotional well-being with age; emotional experiences become more stable with advancing age; emotional experience appears to become more mixed as people age; and individuals who experienced relatively more positive than negative emotions in everyday life were more likely to have survived to older ages.

The observation that emotional well-being is maintained and in some ways improves across adulthood is among the most surprising findings about human aging to emerge in recent years and challenges assumptions about emotional states and aging. This cautions nurses to avoid promoting stereotypes about aging, appreciate individual patterns of aging, and clarify beliefs that emotional well-being declines with age. In addition, nurses need to assist aging persons in achieving emotional well-being as this positively impacts health and longevity.

PRACTICE REALITIES

You are presenting a class on positive health practices to a group at a local senior center. At the end of the class there is a lively discussion and one of the older participants comments, "No matter what you do, how you age is decided by your ancestors. My grandparents ate tons of fatty foods and never exercised and they lived to their 90s."

"Oh, you're wrong," offers another member of the group. "I've been taking a supplement that my neighbor sells that will override the problems you inherited and I'm much healthier than my parents were at my age."

How would you react to these comments and guide the discussion?

CRITICAL THINKING EXERCISES

1. What disease processes are caused by or related to factors believed to influence aging?
2. You are asked to speak to a community group regarding environmental issues. What recommendations could you make for promoting a healthy environment?
3. Think about everyday life in your community. What examples do you see of opportunities to engage and disengage older adults?
4. What specific methods could you use to assist an older adult in achieving ego integrity?

REFERENCES

Butler, R. N., & Lewis, M. I. (1982). *Aging and mental health* (3rd ed., pp. 142, 376). St. Louis, MO: Mosby.

Cumming, E. (1964). New thoughts on the theory of disengagement. In R. Kastenbaum (Ed.), *New thoughts on old age*. New York, NY: Springer-Verlag.

Cumming, E., & Henry, E. (1961). *Growing old: The process of disengagement*. New York, NY: Basic Books.

Erikson, E. (1963). *Childhood and society* (2nd ed.). New York, NY: Norton.

Goya, R. G., Console, G. M., Herenu, C. B., Brown, O. A., & Rimoldi, O. J. (2002). Thymus and aging: Potential of gene therapy for restoration of endocrine thymic function in thymus-deficient animal models. *Gerontology, 48*(5), 325–328.

Green, D. (2011). Means to an end. New York, NY: Cold Spring Harbor Laboratory Press.

Harvard Gazette Archives. (2001). *Scientists identify chromosome location of genes associated with long life*. Harvard University Gazette. Retrieved August 28, 2001 from http://www.news.harvard.edu/gazette/2001/08.16/chromosomes.html

Havighurst, J. (1963). Successful aging. In R. H. Williams, C. Tibbitts, & W. Donahue (Eds.), *Processes of aging* (Vol. 1, p. 299). New York, NY: Atherton Press.

Hayflick, L. (1965). The limited in vitro lifetime of human diploid cell strains. *Experimental Cell Research, 37*, 614–636.

Hubert, H. B., Bloch, D. A., Oehlert, J. W., & Fries, J. F. (2002). Lifestyle habits and compression of morbidity. *Journals of Gerontology. Series A, Biological Sciences and Medical Sciences, 57*(6), M347–M351.

Johnson, M. (2009). Spirituality, finitude, and theories of the life span. In V. I. Bengston, M. Silverstein, N. M. Putney, & D. Gans (Eds.), *Handbook of theories of aging* (2nd ed., pp. 659–674). New York, NY: Springer Publishing Co.

Margolis, S. (Ed.). (2000). Vitamin E recommendations. *The Johns Hopkins Medical Letter: Health After 50, 12*(1), 8.

Martin, G. M. (2009). Modalities of gene action predicted by the classical evolutional theories of aging. In V. I. Bengston, M. Silverstein, N. M. Putney, & D. Gans (Eds.), *Handbook of theories of aging* (2nd ed., pp. 179–191). New York, NY: Springer Publishing Co.

Miller, R. A. (1997). When will the biology of aging become useful? Future landmarks in biomedical gerontology. *Journal of the American Geriatrics Society, 45*, 1258–1267.

National Institute of Diabetes and Digestive and Kidney Diseases of the National Institutes of Health. (2001). *Understanding adult obesity*. Bethesda, MD: Author, NIH Publication No. 01-3680.

Neugarten, L. (1964). *Personality in middle and late life*. New York, NY: Atherton Press.

Peck, R. (1968). Psychological developments in the second half of life. In B. Neugarten (Ed.), *Middle age and aging* (p. 88). Chicago, IL: University of Chicago.

Preston, S. H. (2005). Deadweight? The influence of obesity on longevity. *New England Journal of Medicine, 352*(11), 1135–1137.

Riley, M. M., Johnson, M., & Foner, A. (1972). *Aging and society, vol. 3: A sociology of age stratification*. New York, NY: Russell Sage Foundation.

Rose, A. M. (1965). The subculture of the aging: A framework for research in social gerontology. In A. M. Rose & W. Peterson (Eds.), *Older people and their social worlds*. Philadelphia, PA: F.A. Davis.

Rose, M. R. (1998). Darwinian anti-aging medicine. *Journal of Anti-Aging Medicine, 1*, 106.

Smeeding, S. J. W. (2001). Nutrition, supplements, and aging. *Geriatric Nursing, 22*(4), 219–224.

Taylor, D. H., & Ostbye, T. (2001). The effect of middle- and old-age body mass index on short-term mortality in older people. *Journal of the American Geriatrics Society, 49*(10), 1319–1326.

Tornstam, L. (2005). *Gerotranscendence: A developmental theory of positive aging*. New York, NY: Springer.

University of Illinois at Urbana-Champaign. (2002). *Study backs theory that accumulating mutations of "quiet" genes foster aging*. Science News Daily. Retrieved October 15, 2002 from http://www.sciencedaily.com/releases/2002/10/021015073143.htm

Williams, M. E. (1995). *The American Geriatrics Society's complete guide to aging and health* (p. 13). New York, NY: Harmony Books.

RECOMMENDED READINGS

Recommended Readings associated with this chapter can be found on the web site that accompanies the book. Visit **http://thepoint.lww.com/Eliopoulos8e** to access the recommended readings and other additional resources associated with this chapter.

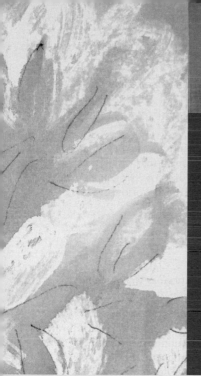

CHAPTER 3

Diversity

CHAPTER OUTLINE

LEARNING OBJECTIVES

After reading this chapter, you should be able to:

1. Describe projected changes in the diversity of the older population in the United States.

2. Describe unique views of health and healing among major ethnic groups.

3. Identify ways in which nursing care may need to be modified to accommodate persons of diverse ethnic backgrounds.

TERMS TO KNOW

Bisexual: someone sexually attracted to persons of both sexes

Culture: shared beliefs and values of a group: the beliefs, customs, practices, and social behavior of a particular group of people

Ethnic: a group of people sharing a common racial, national, religious, linguistic, or cultural heritage

Ethnocentrism: the belief that one's own race, ethnic group, or nation of origin is superior to that of other persons

Gay: someone sexually attracted to a person of the same sex; homosexual

(Continued)

Health disparity: a specific group's difference in access to health care, health status, mortality, health services utilization, or health care outcomes

Lesbian: a woman who is sexually attracted to other women

Nationality: identity based on geographic country of birth

Race: a group of people that share some biological characteristics

Racism: negative views toward another person or group based on race

Transgender: a person whose identity, appearance, and/or behavior varies from that which the culture views as conventional for his or her gender; sometimes referred to as transsexual or transvestite

INCREASING DIVERSITY OF THE OLDER ADULT POPULATION

Population projections support the view that the older population in the United States is becoming more ethnically and racially diverse. In 2000, approximately 84% of older Americans were non-Hispanic white, while it is projected that this population will decrease to 64% by 2050. During this same period, there will be a dramatic growth among Hispanic older adults, who will represent nearly 20% of the older population. Black individuals will grow from 8% to 11% of the older population during this time. By 2020, one quarter of America's older population will belong to a minority racial or ethnic group (Administration on Aging, 2012; U.S. Census Bureau, 2012). And, in addition to racial and ethnic diversity, there will be growing numbers of lesbian, gay, bisexual, and transgender persons entering their senior years who will present a unique set of challenges.

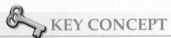

KEY CONCEPT

In the future, the percentage of white older adults will decrease as society experiences a growth in minority seniors.

The growing diversity of the older population presents challenges for gerontological nursing in providing culturally competent care. Essential to the provision of culturally competent care is an understanding of:

- the experiences of individuals of similar ethnic or racial backgrounds
- beliefs, values, traditions, and practices of various ethnic and racial groups
- unique health-related needs, experiences, and risks of various ethnic and racial groups and persons of similar sexual orientation
- one's own attitudes and beliefs toward people of various ethnic and racial groups, and persons of

similar sexual orientation, as well as those attitudes of copractitioners

- language barriers that can affect the ability of patients to communicate health-related information, understand instructions, provide informed consent, and fully participate in their care

An understanding of cultural, ethnic, and sexual orientation differences can help to erase the stereotypes and biases that can interfere with effective care and demonstrate an appreciation for the unique characteristics of each individual.

OVERVIEW OF DIVERSE GROUPS OF OLDER ADULTS IN THE UNITED STATES

People from a variety of countries have ventured to America to seek a better life in a new land. To an extent, they assimilated and adopted the American way of life; however, the values and customs instilled in them by their native cultures are often deeply ingrained, along with their language and biological differences. The unique backgrounds of these newcomers to America influence the way they react to the world around them and the manner in which that world reacts to them. To understand the uniqueness of each older adult encountered, consideration must be given to the influences of ethnic origin.

Members of an ethnic or cultural group share similar history, language, customs, and characteristics; they also hold distinct beliefs about aging and older adults. Ethnic norms can influence diet, response to pain, compliance with self-care activities and medical treatments, trust in health care providers, and other factors. The traditional responsibilities assigned to the aged of some ethnic groups can afford them opportunities for meaningful roles and high status.

Studies of cultural influences on aging and effects on older adults have been sparse but are growing. Experiences and observations can provide insight into the unique characteristics of specific ethnic groups.

Although individual differences within a given ethnic group exist and stereotypes should not be made, an understanding of the general characteristics of various ethnic groups can assist nurses in providing more individualized and culturally sensitive care.

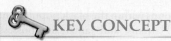

KEY CONCEPT

Although ethnic origin is important, the nurse needs to remember that not all individuals conform to the beliefs, values, roles, and traditions of the group of which they are a part. Stereotyping individuals who belong to the same cultural or ethnic group runs contrary to individualized care.

Hispanic Americans

The term *Hispanic* encompasses a variety of Spanish-speaking persons in America, including those from Spain, Mexico, Cuba, and Puerto Rico. Hispanic people now represent approximately 6% of the older population in the United States, but this percentage is expected to increase. Today, there are approximately 250,000 Hispanic Americans living in the United States, and the fastest growing segment of the U.S. population is Hispanic Americans older than 65 years.

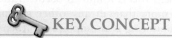

KEY CONCEPT

The terms *Hispanic* and *Latino* are often used interchangeably, and in the United States, Latino has become equated with Hispanics. However, technically, there are differences in that Latino refers to persons from countries once under Roman rule (e.g., Spain, Italy, and Portugal), whereas Hispanic describes persons from countries once under Spanish rule (e.g., Mexico, Central America, and most of South America).

Although Mexican people inhabited the Southwest United States for decades before the arrival of the Pilgrims, most Mexican immigration occurred during the 20th century as a result of the Mexican Revolution and the poor economic conditions in Mexico. Poor economic conditions continue to cause Mexicans to immigrate to the United States. The Mexican population in this country totals more than 8 million, plus an estimated 3 to 5 million illegal immigrants; most reside in California and Texas.

Most Puerto Rican immigration occurred after the United States granted citizenship to all Puerto Ricans. After World War II, nearly one third of all Puerto Rico's inhabitants immigrated to America; in the 1970s, "reverse immigration" began as growing numbers of Puerto Rican people left the United States to return to their home island. An estimated 1 million Puerto Ricans live in New York City, where most of them have settled.

Most Cuban immigrants are recent newcomers to America; the majority of the greater than 1 million Cuban Americans fled Cuba after Castro seized power. More than 25% of the Cuban American population resides in Florida, with other large groups in New York and New Jersey. Among all Hispanics, Cuban people are the most highly educated and have the highest earnings.

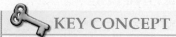

KEY CONCEPT

Although cancer deaths have declined for all persons, they remain disproportionately high among Hispanic Americans and African Americans (National Cancer Institute, 2012).

Many Hispanic people view states of health and illness as the actions of God; by treating one's body with respect, living a good life, and praying, one will be rewarded by God with good health. Illness results when one has violated good practices of living or is being punished by God. Medals and crosses may be worn at all times to facilitate well-being, and prayer plays an important part in the healing process. Illness may be viewed as a family affair, with multiple family members involved with the care of the sick individual. Rather than using practitioners of Western medicine to treat their health problems, some Hispanic persons may prefer traditional practitioners, such as:

- *Curanderos*: women who have special knowledge and charismatic qualities
- *Sobadoras*: persons who give massages and manipulate bones and muscles
- *Espiritualistas*: persons who analyze dreams, cards, and premonitions
- *Brujos*: women who practice witchcraft
- *Senoras*: older women who have learned special healing measures

The Hispanic population holds older relatives in high esteem. Old age is viewed as a positive time in which the older person can reap the harvest of his or her life. Hispanic people may expect that children will take care of their aging parents, and families may try to avoid institutionalization at all costs. Indeed, this group has a lower rate of nursing home use than the general population; less than 7% of nursing home residents are Hispanic.

Nurses may find that English is a second language for some Hispanic people, which becomes particularly apparent during periods of illness when stress causes a retreat to the native tongue.

Although older Hispanic and non-Hispanic persons have similar types of chronic conditions, older Hispanic individuals are less likely to visit physicians or obtain preventive services (e.g., mammograms and vaccines) and more likely to have difficulty obtaining care (Georgetown University Center on an Aging Society, 2012).

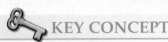

> **KEY CONCEPT**
>
> Nearly one in eight people in the United States speak a language other than English at home, with one third of these people speaking Spanish (Wan, Sengupta, Velkoff, & DeBarros, 2005).

Black Americans

Although nearly 14% of the entire U.S. population is black, they represent only 8.4% of the older population. Most of this group is of African descent. Historically, black Americans have experienced a lower standard of living and less access to health care than their white counterparts. This is reflected in the lower life expectancy of black Americans (see demographics in Chapter 1). However, once a black individual reaches the seventh decade of life, survival begins to equal that of similarly aged white people.

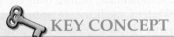

> **KEY CONCEPT**
>
> After reaching their seventh decade of life, black older adults can hope to enjoy a life expectancy equal to their white counterparts.

To survive to old age is considered by this ethnic group as a major accomplishment that reflects strength, resourcefulness, and faith; thus, old age may be considered a personal triumph by black people, not a dreaded curse. Considering their history, it should not be surprising to find that many black older adults:

- possess many health problems that have accumulated over a lifetime due to a poor standard of living and limited access to health care services
- hold health beliefs and practices that may be unconventional to stay healthy and treat illness
- are twice as likely to live in poverty compared with other older adults, which can influence their utilization of health care services

- look to family members for decision making and care rather than using formal service agencies
- may have a degree of caution in interacting with and using health services, as a defense against prejudice (Egede, 2006)

Diverse subgroups within the black population, such as Africans, Haitians, and Jamaicans, possess their own unique customs and beliefs. Differences can be apparent even among black Americans from various regions of the United States. Nurses should be sensitive to the fact that the lack of awareness and respect for these differences can be interpreted as a demeaning or prejudicial sign.

Black skin color is the result of high melanin content and can complicate the use of skin color for the assessment of health problems. To diagnose cyanosis effectively, for instance, examine the nail beds, palms, soles, and gums and under the tongue. The absence of a red tone or glow to the skin can indicate pallor. Petechiae are best detected on the conjunctiva, abdomen, and buccal mucosa.

Hypertension is a prevalent health problem among black Americans and occurs at a higher rate than in the white population. One of the factors responsible for this problem is blunted nocturnal response. Only a minor decline in blood pressure occurs during sleep, which increases the strain on the heart and vessels; this is found to occur in the black population more than in any other group. Blood pressure monitoring is an important preventive measure for black clients (Fig. 3-1).

In addition to hypertension, other health conditions are more prevalent in the black population than in the white population. For instance, as compared with the white population (National Center for Health Statistics, 2008), African Americans have a higher prevalence of heart disease, cancer,

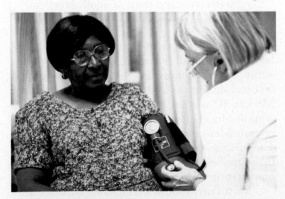

FIGURE 3-1 ■ Blood pressure monitoring is an important intervention for populations at higher risk for hypertension.

and diabetes and a higher death rate from these diseases (Office of Minority Health, 2007a).

In recent years, HIV and AIDS have become the third leading cause of death among African American males; the African American population has a rate of AIDS that is nine times that of the white population (HealthReform.gov, 2012; Office of Minority Health, 2007a). The high prevalence of these diseases among African American males suggests the need for education and counseling of younger adults in order to promote a healthy lifestyle and longevity.

According to the U.S. Centers for Disease Control and Prevention (2012), African American individuals when compared with the white population are more likely to smoke, be obese, and have a poor health status. Many causes of morbidity and mortality among black Americans can be prevented and effectively controlled by lifestyle changes (e.g., good nutrition, regular exercise, and effective stress management) and regular health screening. These are important considerations in planning health services to communities.

Despite the health problems of aged black Americans, their rate of institutionalization is lower than that of the white population: about 13% of older black people experience institutional health care in their lifetimes compared with 23% of older white people (Centers for Disease Control and Prevention, 2011).

Asian Americans

More than 10 million Asian Americans reside in the United States, representing approximately 4% of the population. Asian Americans are a diverse group comprised of individuals from countries such as China, Japan, the Philippines, Korea, Vietnam, and Cambodia.

Chinese Americans

Although Chinese laborers probably lived in America for centuries before the mid-1800s, it was not until then that large-scale Chinese immigration occurred. The largest American Chinese populations are in California, New York, Texas, New Jersey, Massachusetts, and Illinois.

Care of the body and health are of utmost importance in traditional Chinese culture, but their approach may be vastly different from that of conventional Western medicine (Box 3-1). Chinese medicine is based on the belief of the balance of yin and yang; yin is the female negative energy that protects the inner body and yang is the male positive energy that protects the body from external forces. Traditionally, Chinese people have used the senses for assessing medical problems (touching, listening to sounds, and detecting odors) rather than machinery or invasive procedures. Herbs, acupuncture, acupressure, and other treatment modalities, which are just being recognized by the Western world, continue to be treatments of choice for many Chinese individuals. These traditional treatments may be selected as alternatives or adjuncts to the use of modern treatment modalities. Ivory figurines of reclining women, now collectors' items, were used by female patients to point to the area of their problems because it was inappropriate for the male physician to touch a woman; although modern Chinese women may have forfeited this practice, they still may be embarrassed to receive a physical examination or care from

BOX 3-1 Chinese Medicine

For thousands of years, the Chinese have practiced a form of medicine that appears very different from medicine in the Western world. It is based on a system of balance; illness is seen as an imbalance and disharmony of the body. One of the theories that explains this balance is that of yin and yang. Yin is the negative female energy that is represented by that which is soft, dark, cold, and wet. Organs associated with yin qualities include the lungs, kidneys, liver, heart, and spleen. Yang is the positive, male energy that is represented by that which is hard, bright, hot, and dry. The gallbladder, small intestine, stomach, colon, and bladder are yang organs. Daytime activity is considered more of a yang state, whereas sleep is more of an yin state.

Chinese medicine also considers the body's balance in relation to the five elements or phases: wood (spring), fire (summer), earth (long summer), metal (autumn), and water (winter).

Qi is the life force that circulates throughout the body in invisible pathways called meridians. A deficiency or blockage of qi can cause symptoms of illnesses. Acupuncture and acupressure can be applied to various points along the meridians to stimulate the flow of qi.

In addition to acupuncture and acupressure, traditional Chinese medicine uses herbs, massage, and therapeutic exercises (such as t'ai chi) to promote a free flow of chi and achieve balance and harmony. These modalities are gaining increasing acceptance in the United States, and research supporting their effectiveness is increasing rapidly.

CONSIDER THIS CASE

Mrs. C is a very traditional Chinese woman who began living with her son and daughter-in-law 3 years ago, after her husband's death. Mrs. C and her husband had lived in a "Chinatown" part of the city where they could freely communicate in Chinese and interact with other Chinese individuals. She never developed fluency in English and has experienced considerable difficulty communicating with neighbors since moving into her son's suburban community. Mrs. C's son has assimilated American values and practices and has been critical of his mother for her traditional ways; he would not acknowledge her when she spoke in Chinese and refused to allow her to cook Chinese foods. His wife is not Chinese but has been sympathetic to the elder Mrs. C.

Last week Mrs. C suffered a stroke that left her with weakness and some aphasia. She will require care and supervision. Mrs. C's son states that he does not want his mother in a nursing home, but that he is not sure he can manage her; his wife says she is willing to take a leave of absence from work and help care for her mother-in-law, if that is what her husband wants.

THINK CRITICALLY

- What problems do you anticipate for each of the C family members?
- What can be arranged to assist the family?
- How could you assist Mrs. C in preserving her ethnic practices?

---

a man. Typically, disagreement or discomfort is not aggressively or openly displayed by Chinese persons. Nurses may need to observe more closely and ask specific questions (e.g., Can you describe your pain? How do you feel about the procedure you are planning to have done? Do you have any questions?) to ensure that the quiet nature of the patient is not misinterpreted to imply that no problems exist.

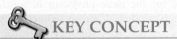

KEY CONCEPT

Traditional Chinese medicine is based on the belief that the female negative energy (yin) and the male positive energy (yang) must be in balance.

In Chinese culture, achieving old age is a blessing, and older adults are held in high esteem. They are respected and sought for advice. The family unit is expected to take care of its elder members; thus, there may be a reluctance to use service agencies for older adults.

Japanese Americans

In the past when they first immigrated to the United States, many Japanese Americans had held jobs as gardeners and farmers. Today they, like Chinese Americans, have a lower unemployment rate and a higher percentage of professionals than the national average. Today, there are approximately 796,700 Japanese Americans, most of whom live in California and Hawaii.

Although Japanese Americans have not tended to live in separate subcommunities to the same extent as Chinese Americans, they have preserved many of their traditions. They are bonded by their common heritage, and their culture places a high value on the family. The following terms describe each generation of Japanese American: *Issei*, first generation (immigrant to America); *Nisei*, second generation (first American born); *Sansei*, third generation; and *Yonsei*, fourth generation. It is expected that families will take care of their elder members. As in the Chinese culture, the aged are viewed with respect.

Similar to the Chinese, Japanese Americans may subscribe to traditional health practices either to supplement or replace modern Western technology. They may not express their feelings openly or challenge the health professional; therefore, nursing sensitivity to covert needs is crucial.

Other Asian Groups

In the early 1700s, Filipino people began immigrating to America, but most Filipino immigrants arrived in the early 1900s to work as farm laborers. In 1934, an annual immigration quota of 50 was enacted; this quota stayed in place until 1965.

In the early 1900s, Korean people immigrated to America to work on plantations. Many of these individuals settled in Hawaii. Another large influx of Koreans, many of whom were wives of American servicemen, immigrated after the Korean War.

The most recent Asian American immigrants have been from Vietnam and Cambodia. Most of these individuals came to the United States to seek political refuge after the Vietnam War.

Although differences among various Asian American groups exist, some similarities are strong family networks and the expectation that family members will care for their older relatives at home. Asian Americans represent about 2% of the total nursing home population.

 POINT TO PONDER

What attitudes toward people of different cultures were you exposed to as a child, and how has this molded your current attitudes?

Jewish Americans

In the sense that they come from a variety of nations, with different customs and cultures, Jewish people are not an ethnic group per se. However, the strength of the Jewish faith forms a bond that crosses national origin and gives this group a strong sense of identity and shared beliefs.

Jewish Americans have demonstrated profound leadership in business, arts, and sciences and have made positive contributions to American life. Scholarship is important in the Jewish culture; more than 80% of all Jewish Americans have attended college. Approximately 6.5 million Jewish people reside in the United States, representing 2.2% of the total population, with most living in urban areas of the Middle Atlantic states. It is estimated that half of the world's Jewish population resides in America.

Religious traditions are important in the Jewish faith (Fig. 3-2). Sundown Friday to sundown Saturday is the Sabbath, and medical procedures may be opposed during that time (exceptions may be made for seriously ill individuals). Because of a belief that the head and feet should always be covered, some Jewish people may desire to wear a skullcap and socks at all times. Orthodox Jews may oppose shaving. The Kosher diet (e.g., exclusion of pork and shellfish, prohibition of serving milk and meat products at the same meal or from the same dishes) is a significant aspect of Jewish religion and may be strictly adhered to by some. Fasting on holy days, such as Yom Kippur and Tisha B'Av, and the replacement of matzo for leavened bread during Passover may occur.

Modern medical care is encouraged. Rabbinical consultation may be desired for decisions involving organ transplantation or life-sustaining measures. Certain rituals may be practiced at death, such as members of the religious group washing the body

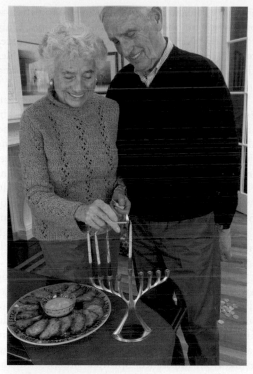

FIGURE 3-2 ■ Celebrating religious holidays may be important for certain groups, such as Jewish older adults.

and sitting with it until burial. Autopsy is usually opposed.

Family bonds are strong in Jewish American culture; they have strong and positive feelings for older adults. Illness often draws Jewish families together. Jewish communities throughout the country have shown leadership in developing a network of community and institutional services for their aged, geared toward providing service while preserving Jewish tradition.

Native Americans

Native Americans are comprised of American Indians and Alaskan Natives; together they represent 5.2 million individuals. Native Americans inhabited North America for centuries before Columbus explored the New World. An estimated 1 to 1.5 million Native Americans populated America at the time of the arrival of Columbus; however, many battles with the new settlers during the next four centuries reduced the Native American population to a quarter million. The Native American population has been steadily increasing, with the U.S. Census Bureau now showing approximately 2.9 million Native American people who belong to more than 500 recognized tribes, nations, and villages in the United States. The median age for the

American Indian and Alaska Native population is lower than for the general U.S. population. Only 8% of the Native American population is older than 65 years, representing less than 1% of all older adults; however, they are one of the fastest growing minorities of the older population.

Less than half of all American Indians live on reservations, with the highest populations found in Arizona, Oklahoma, California, New Mexico, and Alaska. The Indian Health Service, a division of the United States Public Health Service, provides free, universal access to health care to American Indians who reside on reservations. More than half live in urban areas where access to health care is inferior to that on reservations. An estimated 150 different Native American languages are spoken, although most Native American people speak English as their first language.

Native American culture emphasizes a strong reverence for the Great Creator. A person's state of health may be linked to good or evil forces or to punishment for their acts. Native American medicine promotes the belief that a person must be in balance with nature for good health and that illness results from imbalance. Spiritual rituals, medicine men, herbs, homemade drugs, and mechanical interventions such as suction cups may be used for the treatment of illness.

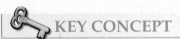

KEY CONCEPT

Spiritual rituals, medicine men, herbs, homemade drugs, and mechanical interventions can be used by Native American people to treat illness.

Close family bonds are typical among the Native American population. Family members may address each other by their family relationship rather than by name (e.g., cousin, son, uncle, and grandfather). The term *elder* is used to denote social or physical status, not just age. Elders are respected and viewed as leaders, teachers, and advisors to the young, although younger and more "Americanized" members are starting to feel that the advice of their elders is not as relevant in today's world and are breaking from this tradition. Native American people strongly believe that individuals have the right to make decisions affecting their lives. The typical nursing assessment process may be offensive to the Native American patient, who may view probing questions, validation of findings, and documentation of responses as inappropriate and disrespectful behaviors during the verbal exchange. A Native American patient may be ambivalent about accepting services from agencies and professionals.

Such assistance has provided many social, health, and economic benefits to improve the life of Native Americans, but it also conflicts with Native American beliefs of being useful, doing by oneself, and relying on spiritual powers to chart the course of life. Native American patients often remain calm and controlled, even in the most difficult circumstances; it is important that providers not mistake this behavior for the absence of feeling, caring, or discomfort.

Various tribes may have specific rituals that are performed at death, such as burying certain personal possessions with the individual. Consulting with members of the specific tribe to gain insight into special rituals during sickness and at death would be advantageous for nurses working with Native American populations.

The last part of the 20th century saw a rise in certain preventable diseases among Native Americans, attributable to their exposure to new risks, such as a poor diet, insufficient exercise, and unhealthy lifestyle choices. For example, diabetes, a disease uncommon among Native Americans at the start of the 20th century, now affects Native Americans 2.3 times as much as white Americans (Office of Minority Health, 2007b). Native Americans are more likely than the white non-Hispanic population to be obese and hypertensive and to suffer a stroke. The relatively recent high prevalence of rheumatoid diseases among Native Americans as compared with white older adults may be related to a genetic predisposition to autoimmune rheumatic disease. The cancer survival rate among Native Americans is the lowest of any U.S. population. Nurses must promote health education and early screening to aid this population in reducing risks and identifying health conditions early.

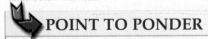

POINT TO PONDER

In what ways do you honor and celebrate your unique heritage?

Gay, Lesbian, Bisexual, and Transgender Older Adults

Despite the growing awareness and acceptance of gay, lesbian, bisexual, and transgender (LGBT) persons in society as a whole, there has been minimal consideration of the challenges and needs of these individuals when they reach late life. In fact, they are referred to as a largely invisible population (Fredriksen-Goldsen et al., 2011). This invisible population is growing, however; as much as 10% of the population identifies themselves as being lesbian, gay, bisexual, or transgender; the LGBT population is projected to double by 2030.

This generation lived through a period when considerable prejudice and discrimination existed against persons who were LGBT; therefore, these individuals may not be open about sexual orientation when seeking health services. Studies have found that LGBT older adults in community and long-term care settings reported being fearful of rejection and neglect by caregivers, not being accepted by other residents, and being forced to hide their sexual orientation (Stein, Beckerman, & Sherman, 2010). In addition, among LGBT elderly (Fredriksen-Goldsen et al., 2011):

- Nearly one half have a disability and nearly one third report depression.

- There are higher rates of mental distress and a greater likelihood of smoking and engaging in excessive drinking than heterosexual persons.

- Almost two thirds have been victimized three or more times.

- Thirteen percent have been denied health care or received inferior care.

- More than 20% do not disclose their sexual or gender identity to their physician.

Recent years have noted progress in addressing the needs of the LGBT population. The American Association of Retired Persons has created an online LGBT community, the American Society on Aging has an LGBT Aging Issues Network, and the Joint Commission has added respect for sexual orientation to the rights of residents of assisted living communities and skilled nursing homes. In addition, SAGE (Services and Advocacy for Gay, Lesbian, Bisexual, and Transgender Elders) and MAP (the Movement Advancement Project) have been aggressively addressing policy and regulatory changes that are needed to address the needs of this population.

Nurses need to appreciate that the LGBT elder population represents unique individuals with different experiences, profiles, and needs. As with any patient, individualized approaches are essential and stereotypes need to be avoided. Further, nurses need to assure that LGBT individuals can receive services without prejudice, stigmatization, or threat.

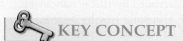

KEY CONCEPT

Culture adds to the mosaic of the older adult's life.

NURSING CONSIDERATIONS FOR CULTURALLY SENSITIVE CARE OF OLDER ADULTS

Numerous minority, ethnic, or cultural groups that have not been mentioned also possess unique histories, beliefs, and practices. Rather than viewing differences as odd and forcing patients to conform to "American" traditions, nurses should respect the beauty of this diversity and make every effort to preserve it. The beliefs, values, relationships, roles, and traditions associated with cultural and ethnic identity add a special significance to life.

The effectiveness of care can be largely influenced by the initial impression made by the nurse. Nurses need to reflect on any personal feelings or attitudes that could influence the nurse–patient relationship or convey a prejudicial attitude. For example, if a nurse comes from a religious belief that homosexuality is abnormal and sinful, the nurse may display discomfort in the nurse–patient interactions when faced with a patient who is gay. As a result, the patient may sense the nurse is prejudiced and be reluctant to share all aspects of his history and problems. Likewise, if the nurse has had limited experiences with persons of a different racial group, he or she may appear uneasy or unnatural in communicating with those individuals. Reflection on their feelings and discussing these issues with other professionals can assist in preventing personal feelings from interfering with the professional relationship.

Nurses need to be careful not to stereotype patients based on race, ethnicity, sexual orientation, or other factors. All patients should be addressed by their last name unless they request otherwise. Recognizing that based on their cultural or ethnic backgrounds some persons may be guarded with the personal information, nurses should explain the reason various questions will be asked during the interview. Ample time should be allotted for patients to share their histories and cultural or religious practices. The use of touch (e.g., patting the person's hand or touching an arm) often demonstrates caring and assists in putting a person at ease; however, be aware that in some cultural groups being touched by a stranger is viewed as inappropriate. The same holds true for the spatial distance between the nurse and the patient during the interview. This reinforces the importance of nurses becoming familiar with the beliefs and practices of various groups.

Dietary preferences should be accommodated, adaptations made for special practices, and unique ways of managing illness understood. Consideration should be given to differences in the expression of pain, fear, and other feelings. Reactions to illness and care can vary. For example, one person may view illness as punishment for wrongdoing; however, another sees it as part of the normal human experience. Some individuals may desire the active participation of family members or traditional healers in their care, whereas others, even those whose ethnic or cultural group traditionally do desire these things, do not.

If nurses are unfamiliar with a particular group, they should invite the patient and the family members to educate them or contact churches or ethnic associations (e.g., Polish National Alliance, Celtic League, Jewish Family and Children's Services, and Slovak League of America) for interpreters or persons who can serve as cultural resources. One powerful means to learn about cultural influences for individual patients is to ask them to describe their life stories (see Chapter 4). Nurses convey sensitivity and caring when they try to recognize and support patients' ethnic and cultural backgrounds. Nurses also will become enriched by gaining an appreciation and understanding of the various interesting ethnic groups.

The U.S. Department of Health and Human Services has developed standards for culturally and linguistically appropriate services that can guide clinical settings in working with diverse populations; their web site can be accessed at http://minorityhealth. hhs.gov.

The increasing diversity of future aged populations will affect services in a variety of ways. Among the needs that could present are:

- institutional meal planning that incorporates ethnic foods
- multilingual health education literature
- readily available translators
- provisions for celebration of holidays (e.g., Chinese New Year, St. Patrick's Day, Black History Month, Greek Orthodox Easter)
- special interest groups for residents of long-term care facilities and assisted living communities

An uncomfortable reality that a nurse may face is the prejudicial comment by a patient. As patients will reflect the society in which they live and with prejudices, unfortunately, being alive and well in society, it stands to reason that the nurse will encounter prejudiced patients. For example, a patient may refuse to receive care from a nurse of a different race. At times, persons who are highly stressed or who have dementias may use offensive racial language. Understandably, this can be hurtful to the nurse. The individual patient and situation, as well as the nurse's experience in handling these situations, will determine the action the nurse should take; options include requesting the patient not to make the comment, asking the patient if he or she would prefer to have someone else assigned as his or her nurse, asking to be reassigned, and discussing the situation with one's manager.

Nurses need to ensure that cultural, religious, and sexual orientation differences of older adults are understood, appreciated, and respected. Demonstrating this sensitivity honors the older adult's unique history and preserves the familiar and important. The challenges faced by older adults need not be compounded by insensitive or prejudicial behaviors by nurses.

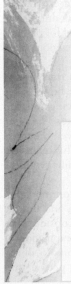

BRINGING RESEARCH TO LIFE

GROWTH OF RACIAL AND ETHNIC MINORITIES IN U.S. NURSING HOMES DRIVEN BY DEMOGRAPHICS AND POSSIBLE DISPARITIES IN OPTIONS

Feng, Z., Fennell, M. L., Tyler, D. A., Clark, M., & Mor, V. (2011). Growth of racial and ethnic minorities in US nursing homes driven by demographics and possible disparities in options. Health Affairs, 30(7), 1358.

This Brown University study suggests that there is racial disparity in the care options for older minority patients in the United States. An analysis of data showed that between 1999 and 2008, the nation's nursing home population shrank by 6.1% to just over 1.2 million people. In that time period, the number of whites in nursing homes decreased by 10.2% nationwide, while the number of blacks rose by 10.8%, the number of Hispanics rose by 54.9%, and the number of Asians rose by 54.1%. Although this could be viewed as a positive step in reducing the limited access to nursing home care that minority populations have experienced in the past, the researchers suggested that part of the reason for this was due to these minorities lacking the same access to more desirable forms of care that wealthier whites may have.

Nurses can contribute to the health and well-being of older minority populations by educating policymakers on these disparities and offering recommendations to reduce them. They should assure that every community has a continuum of resources available for persons of all income, racial, and cultural backgrounds. If quality resources are unavailable in the immediate community, patients should be assisted in locating such resources elsewhere.

This research also demonstrates the importance of evaluating data carefully. In isolation, the finding that minority patients are having an increased presence in nursing homes could be viewed as a positive sign. Seen in totality, that rise in nursing home use was related to the lack of other forms of care.

PRACTICE REALITIES

You are a nurse manager in an assisted living community that serves an affluent population. The current resident population is all white, whereas most of the caregiving staff is African American.

Some of the staff shared with the nurse manager their frustration at the way several residents treat them. Although most of the residents are courteous and polite in their manner of speaking to staff, many have a tendency to use terms like "girls," "you people," and "help." A few of the nursing assistants reported that they have heard residents make comments to each other and their visitors that "You need to watch what you keep here because these people have sticky fingers," and "Those people basically are lazy, so you need to stay on their back." In addition, staff complain that visitors often ask them to do things that really are not part of their jobs, such as having them go to visitor's cars to retrieve something or serve food that the visitor brought in for herself, the resident, and other family members.

The African American staff believe they are being treated in a prejudicial manner. One nursing assistant comments, "You would think this was their plantation and we were their slaves." Another reacts, "Yes, but if we daresay something to them they'll be running to administration. I can't afford to lose this job." Yet another adds, "Maybe we should live with it. White people have always been this way to our people."

As the nurse manager, how would you handle this situation?

CRITICAL THINKING EXERCISES

1. What are some reasons for older adults of minority groups to be suspicious or distrustful of health care services in this country?

2. What would you do if faced with a situation in which an older client refused to allow you to provide nursing care for him because you are of a different ethnic or racial group?

3. You are working in a hospital that serves a large population of immigrants who have not entered the country legally. These individuals frequently have had poor health care and present with multiple chronic conditions. The hospital is concerned that the care offered to these immigrants is placing a significant strain on its budget and may threaten its survival. The local community does not want to lose its hospital and has voiced opposition to providing free care for this group of immigrants. What do you see as concerns for all parties involved? What are the implications of either continuing or discontinuing free care to this group of immigrants? What solutions could you recommend?

4. A nursing home has a variety of ethnic groups represented in the resident population. What can the facility do to show sensitivity to their backgrounds?

RESOURCES

Bureau of Indian Affairs
http://www.bia.gov

National Asian Pacific Center on Aging
http://www.napca.org

National Association for Hispanic Elderly
http://www.anppm.org

National Caucus & Center on Black Aged
http://www.ncba-aged.org

National Hispanic Council on Aging
http://www.nhcoa.org

National Indian Council on Aging
http://www.nicoa.org

National Resource Center on Native American Aging
http://www.med.und.nodak.edu/depts/rural/nrcnaa/

Office of Minority Health Resource Center
http://www.mintorityhealth.hhs.gov

Organization of Chinese Americans
http://www.ocanational.org

SAGE (Services and Advocacy for Gay, Lesbian, Bisexual, and Transgender Elders)
http://sageusa.org/index.cfm

REFERENCES

Administration on Aging. (2012). *Minority aging.* Retrieved April 10, 2012 from http://www.aoa.gov/AoARoot/Aging_Statistics/Minority_Aging/index.aspx

Centers for Disease Control and Prevention. (2011). *U.S. census populations with bridged race categories.* Retrieved April 6, 2012 from http://www.cdc.gov/nchs/nvss/bridged_race.htm

Centers for Disease Control and Prevention. (2012). *Health of black or African American non-Hispanic population.* *FastStats.* Retrieved April 3, 2012 from http://www.cdc.gov/nchs/fastats/black_health.htm

Egede, L. (2006). Race, ethnicity, culture, and disparities in health care. *Journal of General Internal Medicine, 21*(6), 667–669.

Fredriksen-Goldsen, K. I., Kim, H.-J., Emlet, C. A., Muraco, A., Erosheva, E. A., Hoy-Ellis, C. P., Petry, H., et al. (2011). *The aging and health report: Disparities and resilience among Lesbian, Gay, Bisexual, and Transgender older adults.* Seattle, WA: Institute for Multigenerational Health.

Georgetown University Center on an Aging Society. (2012). *Older Hispanic Americans.* Data Profile, No. 9. Retrieved March 15, 2012 from http://ihcrp.georgetown.edu/agingsociety/pubhtml/hispanics/hispanics.html

HealthReform.gov. (2012). *Health disparities: A case for closing the gap.* U.S. Department of Health and Human Services. Retrieved April 5, 2012 from http://www.healthreform.gov/reports/healthdisparities

National Cancer Institute. (2012). *Cancer health disparities.* National Cancer Institute fact sheet. Retrieved April 12, 2012 from http://www.cancer.gov/cancertopics/factsheet/disparities/cancer-health-disparities#2

National Center for Health Statistics. (2011). *Rates of illness by age, sex, and race. Data warehouse on trends in aging.* Retrieved August 31, 2012 from http://www.cdc.gov/nchs/data/hus/hus11.pdf. Office of Minority Health. (2007a). *African-American profiles.* Washington, DC: U.S. Government Printing Office.

Office of Minority Health. (2007b). *American Indians/Alaska Natives profiles.* Washington, DC: U.S. Government Printing Office.

Stein, G. L., Beckerman, N. L., & Sherman, P. A. (2010). Lesbian and gay elders and long-term care: Identifying the unique psychosocial perspectives and challenges. *Journal of Gerontological Social Work, 53*(5), 421–435.

U.S. Census Bureau. (2012). Figure 11, percent distribution of population age 65 and over by race and Hispanic oridi: 1990 to 2050. *Population projections of the United States by age, sex, race, and Hispanic origin: 1995 to 2050.* Retrieved April 19, 2012 from http://www.census.gov/prod/1/pop/p25-1130.pdf

Wan, H., Sengupta, M., Velkoff, V. A., & DeBarros, K. A. (2005). *U.S. Census Bureau, current population reports, 60+ in the United States: 2005* (p. 16). Washington, DC: U.S. Government Printing Office.

RECOMMENDED READINGS

Recommended Readings associated with this chapter can be found on the web site that accompanies the book. Visit **http://thepoint.lww.com/Eliopoulos8e** to access the recommended readings and other additional resources associated with this chapter.

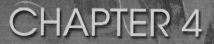
Life Transitions and Story

LEARNING OBJECTIVES

After reading this chapter, you should be able to:

1. Discuss ageism and its consequences.

2. Discuss changes that occur in aging families.

3. Describe challenges faced by widows.

4. Outline the phases and challenges of retirement.

5. Discuss the impact of age-related changes in health and functioning on roles.

6. Describe cumulative effects of life transitions.

7. List nursing measures to assist individuals in adjusting to the challenges and changes of aging.

TERMS TO KNOW

Ageism: applying prejudices to older adults due to their age

Inner resource: a strength within the person that can be drawn upon when needed

Life review: a process of reminiscing or reflecting on one's life

Retirement: the period in which one no longer works

Growing old is not easy. Various changes during the aging process demand multiple adjustments that require stamina, ability, and flexibility. Frequently, more simultaneous changes are experienced in old age than during any other period of life. Many young adults find it exhausting to keep pace with technological advances, societal changes, cost-of-living fluctuations, and labor market trends. Imagine how complex and complicated life can be for older individuals, who must also face retirement, reduced income, possible housing changes, frequent losses through deaths of significant persons, and a declining ability to function. Further, each of these life events can be accompanied by role changes that can influence behavior, attitudes, status, and psychological integrity. To promote awareness and appreciation of the complex and arduous adjustments involved in aging, this chapter considers some of the factors that affect older adults' ability to cope with multiple changes associated with aging and their achievement of satisfaction and well-being during the later years.

AGEISM

Ageism is a concept introduced decades ago and defined as "the prejudices and stereotypes that are applied to older people sheerly on the basis of their age ..." (Butler, Lewis, & Sutherland, 1991). It is not difficult to detect overt ageism in our society. Rather than showing appreciation for the vast contributions of older adults and their wealth of resources, society is beset with prejudices and lacks adequate provisions for them, thus derogating their dignity. The same members of society who object to providing sufficient income and health care benefits for the older population enjoy an affluence and standard of living that was the result of the efforts of these older persons.

Although older adults constitute the most diverse and individualized age group in the population, they continue to be stereotyped by the following misconceptions:

- Old people are sick and disabled.
- Most old people are in nursing homes.
- Dementia comes with old age.
- People are either very tranquil or very cranky as they age.
- Old people have lower intelligence and are resistant to change.
- Old people are not able to have sexual intercourse and are not interested in sex.
- There are few satisfactions in old age.

For most older persons, the above statements are not true. Increased efforts are necessary to heighten societal awareness of the realities of aging. Groups such as the Gray Panthers have done an outstanding job of informing the public about the facts regarding aging and the problems and rights of older adults. More advocates for older persons are needed.

Ageism carries several consequences. By separating people of advanced age from themselves, younger people are less likely to see the similarities between themselves and older adults. This not only leads to a lack of understanding of older people but also reduces the opportunities for the young to gain realistic insights into aging. Furthermore, separating older individuals from the rest of society makes it easier for younger individuals to minimize the socioeconomic challenges of the older population. However, systematically stereotyping and discriminating against older persons will not prevent individuals from growing old themselves and experiencing the challenges of old age.

Chapter 2 outlines Erikson's (1963) stages of life in which he describes the last stage of the life cycle as concerned with achieving integrity versus despair. Integrity results when the older individual derives satisfaction from an evaluation of his or her life. Disappointment with life and the lack of opportunities to alter the past bring despair. Ageism, unfortunately, can predispose aging persons to disappointment because they may believe stereotypical views that old age is a time of purposelessness and decline. The experiences of our entire lifetime determine whether our old age will be an opportunity for freedom, growth, and contentment or a miserable imprisonment of our human potential.

CHANGES IN FAMILY ROLES AND RELATIONSHIPS

The emergence of today's nuclear family units changed the roles and functions of the individuals in a family. Older parents are expected to have limited input into the lives of their adult children. Children are not required to meet the needs of their aging parents for financial support, health services, or housing. Parents increasingly do not depend on their children for their needs, and the belief that children are the best insurance for old age is fading. In addition, grandparenting, although satisfying, is not usually as active a role as in the past, especially because grandchildren may be scattered throughout the country. These changes in family structure and function are not necessarily negative. Older adults may enjoy the independence and freedom from responsibilities that nuclear family life offers. Adjusting to changes in responsibilities and roles over time, though, is an important challenge of aging.

Parenting

The dynamic parental role frequently changes to meet the growth and development needs of both parent and child. During middle and later life, parents must adjust to the independence of their children as they become responsible adult citizens and leave home. The first child usually leaves home and establishes an independent unit 22 to 25 years after the parents married. For persons who have invested most of their adult lives nurturing and providing for their offspring, a child's independence may have significant impact. Although parents who are freed from the responsibilities and worries of rearing children have more time to pursue their own interests, they are also freed from the meaningful, purposeful, and satisfying activities associated with child rearing, and this frequently results in a profound sense of loss.

Today's older woman has been influenced by a historical period that emphasized the role of wife and mother. For instance, to provide job opportunities for men returning from World War II, women were encouraged to focus their interests on raising a family and to forfeit the scarce jobs to men. Unlike many of today's younger women, who pursue and may equally value both a career and motherhood, these older women centered their lives on their families, from which they derived their sense of fulfillment. Having developed few roles from which to achieve satisfaction other than those of wife and mother, many of these older women feel a void when their children are grown and gone. Compounding this problem, the highly mobile lifestyle of many young persons limits the degree of direct contact an older woman has with her adult children and grandchildren.

The older man shares many of the same feelings as his wife. Throughout the years, he may have felt that he has performed useful functions that made him a valuable member of the family. Most likely, he worked hard to support his wife and children, and his masculinity was reinforced with proof of his ability to beget and provide for offspring. Now, with his children grown, he is no longer required to provide—a mixed blessing in which he may find both relief and purposelessness. In addition, he learns that the rules have changed—his ability to support a family without the need for his wife to work is now viewed by some as oppressive, his efforts to replenish the earth are scorned by zero population proponents, and his attempt to fill the masculine role for which he was socialized is considered oppressive or inane by today's standards.

However, this lessening of the parenting role and the changes in family function are not necessarily negative. Most children do not abandon or neglect their aging parents; they maintain regular contact. Separate family units may help the parent–child relationship develop on a more adult-to-adult basis, to the mutual satisfaction of both the young and the old. If older adults adjust to their new role as parents of independent, adult children, they may enjoy the freedom from previous responsibilities and the new developments in their family relationships.

POINT TO PONDER

List at least three ways that your life is different from the lives of your parents and grandparents.

Grandparenting

In addition to experiencing changes in the parenting role that come with age, many older adults enter a new role as grandparents. Americans' extended life expectancy enables more people to experience the role of grandparent and spend more years in that role than previous generations. More than 65 million Americans are grandparents, and:

- Most are baby boomers, more likely to be college educated and employed than previous generations of grandparents.
- One in five grandparents is African American, Hispanic, or Asian.
- They are spending more on grandchildren than previous generations (MetLife, 2011).

Grandchildren can bring considerable joy and meaning to the lives of older adults (Fig. 4-1). In turn, grandparents who are not burdened with the same daily childrearing responsibilities of parents can offer love, guidance, and enjoyment to the family's young. They can share lessons learned from their life experiences and family history and traditions that help the young understand their roots. There can be as many grandparenting styles as there are personalities; there is no single model of grandparenthood.

Changes in the family structure and activities present new challenges to today's grandparents. Most mothers are employed outside of the home. This is compounded by the fact that approximately one third of children are being raised by one parent. As a result, grandparents may assume childcare responsibilities to a greater extent than previous generations did. Grandparents may even provide for or share a home with their children and grandchildren. Family structures may differ from older adults' experience, with an increase in remarriage and blended families as well as homosexual households. More than one third of children under 18 years live in blended households, and an estimated 8 to 10 million children have gay or lesbian parents

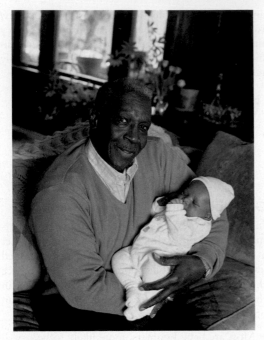

FIGURE 4-1 ■ Grandparenting offers new roles and joys for many older adults.

(Gates, Badgett, Macomber, & Chambers, 2007). As a result of an adult child's marriage or relationship, older adults may find themselves becoming step-grandparents, a role for which few are prepared. Conscious choices will be needed to love and accept these new family members.

In addition to older adults having to adapt to new family lifestyles and structures, children and grandchildren may need to adapt to grandparents who have different lifestyles from previous generations. Rather than the stay-at-home grandma who cooked elaborate family dinners and welcomed grandchildren whenever they needed a sitter, today's grandmother may have an active career and social calendar and not want to be burdened with frequent babysitting responsibilities or hosting family functions. Grandparents may be divorced, causing their children and grandchildren to face issues such as grandmother's weekend trips with her new male friend or grandpop's new, much younger wife. The family may need to be referred for counseling to help them address these issues.

Grandparenthood is a learned role and some older individuals may need guidance to become effective grandparents. Older adults may need to be guided in thinking through issues such as:

- respecting their children as parents and not interfering in the parent–child relationship
- calling before visiting

- establishing rules for babysitting
- allowing their children to establish their own traditions within their family and not expecting them to adhere to the grandparent's traditions

Nurses can help families locate resources that can assist in meeting the challenges of grandparenting. Also, nurses can suggest activities that can help grandparents be connected with their grandchildren, particularly if they are not geographically close; these can include audio- and videotapes, e-mails, videoconferencing, texting, faxes, and handwritten letters. (In addition to offering a means of communication, these can provide lasting memories that can be passed from one generation to the next.) Older adults can be encouraged to keep diaries, scrapbooks, and notebooks of family recipes and customs that can help their grandchildren and future generations have special insights into their ancestors.

In addition to fulfilling the grandparenting role, many older adults may assume primary childrearing responsibilities for their grandchildren. An increasing number of grandparents are raising grandchildren. Over six million grandparents have grandchildren under the age of 18 living with them and many more live with their grandparents off and on; a grandparent is providing care for nearly one fourth of children younger than 5 years (U.S. Census Bureau, 2012). Full-time caregiving often arises out of crises with the child's parents, such as substance abuse, teen pregnancy, or incarceration. Older persons may need help thinking through the implications of deciding to raise a grandchild; some questions that nurses can raise with grandparents contemplating this decision include:

- How will raising this child affect your own health, marriage, and lifestyle?
- Have you any health conditions that could interfere with this responsibility?
- What is your backup plan in the event that you become ill or disabled?
- Do you have the energy and physical health required to care for an active child?
- Can you afford to care for the child, pay medical and educational expenses, and the like?
- What rights and responsibilities will the child's parent(s) have?
- Do you have the legal right to serve as a surrogate parent (e.g., to give consent for medical procedures)? Have you consulted with an attorney?

Organizations exist to assist grandparents who are raising grandchildren; some are listed at the end of this chapter.

LOSS OF SPOUSE

The death of a spouse is a common event that alters family life for many older persons. The loss of that individual with whom one has shared more love and life experiences and more joys and sorrows than anyone else may be intolerable. How, after many decades of living with another person, does one adjust to his or her sudden absence? How does one adjust to setting the table for one, to coming home to an empty house, or to not touching that warm, familiar body in bed? Adjustment to this significant loss is coupled with the demand to learn the new task of living alone (Fig. 4-2).

The death of a spouse affects more women than men because women tend to have a longer life expectancy than men. In fact, most women will be widowed by the time they reach their eighth decade of life. Unlike many of today's younger women, who have greater independence through careers and changed norms, most of today's older women have led family-oriented lives and have been dependent on their husbands. Their age, limited education, lack of skills, and long period of unemployment while raising their families are limitations in a competitive job market. If these women can find employment, adjusting to the new demands of work may be difficult and stressful. The unemployed widow, however, may learn that pensions or other sources

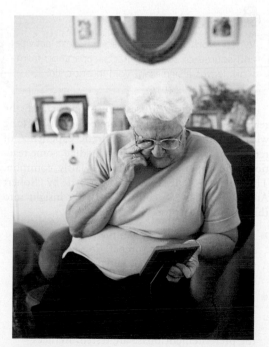

FIGURE 4-2 ■ For an older adult, the loss of a spouse means the loss of one's closest companion of many years.

of income may be reduced or discontinued when the husband dies, necessitating an adjustment to an extremely limited budget. In addition to financial dependence, the woman may have depended on her husband's achievements to provide her with gratification and identity. Frequently, the achievements of children serve this same purpose. Sexual desires may be unfulfilled because of lack of opportunity, religious beliefs regarding sex outside marriage, fear of repercussion from children and society, or residual attitudes from early teachings about sexual mores. If a woman's marriage promoted friendships with other married couples and only inactive relationships with single friends, the new widow may find that her number of single female friends is small.

For the most part, when the initial grief of the husband's death passes, most widows adjust quite well. The high proportion of older women who are widowed provides an availability of friends who share similar problems and lifestyles, especially in urban areas. Old friendships may be revived to provide sources of activity and enjoyment. Some widows may discover that the loss of certain responsibilities, such as cooking and laundering for their husbands, brings them a new, pleasant freedom. With alternative roles to develop, sufficient income, and choice over lifestyle, many women are able to make a successful adjustment to widowhood.

The likelihood of an older adult remarrying after the loss of a spouse diminishes with age. This is especially true for women who often live longer than men and find a shortage of eligible men, because men of the same age tend to marry women younger than themselves.

Nurses may facilitate the adjustment to widowhood by identifying sources of friendships and activities such as clubs, volunteer organizations, or groups of widows in the community and by helping the widow understand and obtain all the benefits to which she is entitled. This may require reassuring the widow that enjoying her new freedom and desiring relationships with other men is no reason to feel guilty and may help her to adjust to the loss of her husband and the new role of widow. (See Chapter 39 for more information on death and dying.)

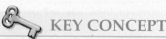

KEY CONCEPT

The high prevalence of widows provides opportunities for friendships between women who share similar challenges and lifestyles.

RETIREMENT

Retirement is another of the major adjustments of an aging individual. This transition brings the loss of a work role and is often an individual's first experience of the impact of aging. In addition, retirement can require adjusting to a reduced income.

Loss of the Work Role

Retirement is especially difficult in Western society, in which worth is commonly measured by an individual's productivity. Work is also often viewed as the dues required for active membership in a productive society. Many of today's older persons, raised to value a strong work ethic, hold the attitude that unemployment, for whatever reason, is an undesirable state.

KEY CONCEPT

Older adults often view work as the dues required for active membership in a productive society.

Occupational identity largely determines an individual's social position and social role. Although individuals function differently in similar roles, some behaviors continue to be associated with certain roles, which promote stereotypes. Certain stereotypes continue to be heard frequently—the tough construction worker, the wild exotic dancer, the fair judge, the righteous clergyman, the learned lawyer, and the eccentric artist. The realization that these associations are not consistently valid does not prevent their propagation. Too frequently, individuals are described in terms of their work role rather than their personal characteristics, for example, "the nurse who lives down the road" or "my son the doctor." Considering the extent to which social identity and behavioral expectations are derived from the work role, it is not surprising that retirement threatens an individual's sense of identity (Fig. 4-3). During childhood and adolescence, we are guided toward an independent, responsible adult role, and in academic settings we are prepared for our professional roles, but where and when are we prepared for the role of retiree?

POINT TO PONDER

What do you derive, or think you will derive, from being a nurse in terms of purpose, identity, values, relationships, activities, and so on? What similar gains are you achieving from other roles in your life?

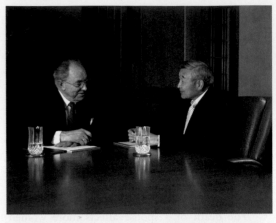

FIGURE 4-3 ■ People who defined self by their work role may have difficulty adjusting to retirement.

When one's work is one's primary interest, activity, and source of social contacts, separation from work leaves a significant void in one's life. Aging individuals should be urged to develop interests unrelated to work. Retirement is facilitated by learning how to use, appreciate, and gain satisfaction from leisure time throughout an employed lifetime. In addition, enjoying leisure time is a therapeutic outlet for life stresses throughout the aging process.

KEY CONCEPT

When work is one's primary interest, activity, and source of social contacts, separation from work leaves a significant void in one's life.

Gerontological nurses must understand the realities and reactions encountered when working with retired persons. Although the experience of retirement is unique for each individual, some reactions and experiences tend to be fairly common. The phases of retirement described by Robert Atchley decades ago continue to offer insight into this complicated process:

- *Preretirement phase.* When the reality of retirement is evident, preparation for leaving one's job begins, as does fantasy regarding the retirement role.
- *Retirement phase.* Following the retirement event, a somewhat euphoric period begins, a "honeymoon period," in which fantasies from the preretirement phase are tested. Retirees attempt to do everything they never had time for simultaneously. A variety of factors

(e.g., finances and health) limit this, leading to the development of a stable lifestyle. As contrasted with those retirees who want to engage in every fantasy, some individuals choose to rest and do very little; their activity level tends to increase after a few years.

- *Disenchantment phase.* As life begins to stabilize, a letdown, sometimes a depression, is experienced. The more unrealistic the preretirement fantasy, the greater the degree of disenchantment.

- *Reorientation phase.* As realistic choices and alternative sources of satisfaction are considered, the disenchantment with the new retirement routine can be replaced by developing a lifestyle that provides some satisfaction.

- *Retirement routine phase.* An understanding of the retirement role is achieved, and this provides a framework for concern, involvement, and action in the older person's life. Some enter this phase directly after the honeymoon phase, and some never reach it at all.

- *Termination of retirement.* The retirement role is lost as a result of either the resumption of a work role or dependency due to illness or disability (Atchley, 1975, 2000).

Different nursing interventions may be required during each phase of retirement. Assisting aging individuals with their retirement preparations during the preretirement phase is a preventive intervention that enhances the potential for health and well-being in late life. As a part of such intervention, nurses can encourage aging individuals to establish and practice good health habits such as following a proper diet; avoiding alcohol, drug, and tobacco use; and having regular physical examinations. Counseling regarding the realities of retirement may be part of retirement preparation, whereas helping retirees place their newfound freedom into proper perspective may be warranted during the honeymoon period of the retirement phase. Being supportive of retirees during the disenchantment phase without fostering self-pity and helping them identify new sources of satisfaction may facilitate the reorientation process. Appreciating and promoting the strengths of the stability phase may reinforce an adjustment to retirement. When the retirement phase is terminated due to disease or disability, the tactful management of dependency and the respectful appreciation of losses are extremely important.

As they have done with other life events, baby boomers are changing the thinking about work and retirement. Increasingly, they are replacing the model of a person being defined by his or her work with one that defines a person's work based on the totality of his or her life. Life coaches and retirement planners are helping individuals to see that the retirement stage is more meaningful when individuals create a balance of work, learning, leisure, family time, service to others, and interests and desires postponed during the active career years (Corbett, 2007). Rather than forfeit working altogether, it is suggested that people stay in the workforce, but in a different style—that is, one that leaves time for the enjoyment of other interests and a high quality of life. The baby boomers also are remaining in the workforce longer, with many finding new paths of employment that enable them to explore their passions and achieve a different sense of purpose, even if it is at lower levels of compensation.

Nurses' evaluations of their own attitudes toward retirement are beneficial. Does the nurse see retirement as a period of freedom, opportunity, and growth or as one of loneliness, dependency, and meaninglessness? Is the nurse intelligently planning for her own retirement or denying it by avoiding encounters with retirement realities? Nurses' views of retirement affect the retiree–nurse relationship. Gerontological nurses can provide especially good models of constructive retirement practices and attitudes.

Reduced Income

In addition to the adjustment in work role, retirement often requires older adults to live on a reduced income. Financial resources are important at any age because they affect our diet, health, housing, safety, and independence and influence many of our choices in life. Retirement income is less than half the income earned while fully employed. For most older Americans, Social Security income, originally intended as a supplement, is actually the primary source of retirement income—and it has not kept pace with inflation. As a result, the economic profile of many older persons is poor.

Only a minority of the older population has income from a private pension plan, and those who do often discover that the fixed benefits established when the plan was subscribed are meager by today's standards because of inflation. Of the workers who are currently active in the labor force, more than half will not have pension plans when they retire. More than one in six of all older adults live in poverty, with older African Americans and Hispanics having nearly twice the rate of poverty as older white persons. Only a minority are fully employed or financially comfortable. Few older persons have accumulated enough assets during their lifetime to provide financial security in old age.

A reduction in income is a significant adjustment for many older persons because it triggers other adjustments. For instance, an active social life and leisure pursuits may have to be markedly reduced or eliminated. Relocation to less expensive housing may be necessary, possibly forcing the aged to break many family and community ties. Dietary practices may be severely altered, and health care may be viewed as a luxury over which other basic expenses, such as food and rent, take priority. If the older parent has to depend on children for supplemental income, an additional adjustment may be necessary.

Making financial preparations for old age many years before retirement is important. Nurses should encourage aging working people to determine whether their retirement income plans are keeping pace with inflation. Also, older individuals need assistance in obtaining all the benefits they are entitled to and in learning how to manage their income wisely. Nurses should be aware of the impact of economic welfare on health status and should actively involve themselves in political issues that promote adequate income for all individuals.

POINT TO PONDER

What are you doing to prepare for your own retirement?

CHANGES IN HEALTH AND FUNCTIONING

The changes in appearance and bodily function that occur during the aging process make it necessary for the aging individual to adjust to a new body image. Colorful soft hair turns gray and dry, flexible straight fingers become bent and painful, body contours are altered, and height decreases. Stairs once climbed several times daily demand more time and energy to negotiate as the years accumulate. As subtle, gradual, and natural as these changes may be, they are noticeable and, consequently, affect body image and self-concept.

The manner in which individuals perceive themselves and their functional abilities can determine the roles they play. A construction worker who has reduced strength and energy may forfeit his work role; a club member who cannot hear conversations may cease attending meetings; fashion models may stop seeking jobs when they perceive themselves as old. Interestingly, some persons well into their seventh and eighth decades refuse to join a senior citizen club because they do not perceive themselves

as being "like those old people." The nurse will gain insight into the self-concept of older persons by evaluating what roles they are willing to accept and what roles they reject. Refer to the Nursing Diagnosis Highlight for a discussion of the possible nursing diagnosis of Ineffective Role Performance.

KEY CONCEPT

Insights into an older adult's self-concept can be gained by examining the roles that are accepted and rejected.

It is sometimes difficult for the aging person to accept the body's declining efficiency. Poor memory, slow response, easy fatigue, and altered appearance are among the many frustrating results of declining function, and they are dealt with in various ways. Some older people deny them and often demonstrate poor judgment in an attempt to make the same demands on their bodies as they did when younger. Others try to resist these changes by investing in cosmetic surgery, beauty treatments, miracle drugs, and other expensive endeavors that diminish the budget but not the normal aging process. Still others exaggerate these effects and impose an unnecessarily restricted lifestyle on themselves. Societal expectations frequently determine the adjustment individuals make to declining function.

Common results of declining function are illness and disability. As described in Chapter 1, most older people have one or more chronic diseases, and more than one third have a serious disability that limits major activities such as work and housekeeping. Older adults often fear that illness or disability may cause them to lose their independence. Becoming a burden to their family, being unable to meet the demands of daily living, and having to enter a nursing facility are some of the fears associated with dependency. Children and parents may have difficulty exchanging dependent–independent roles. The physical pain arising from an illness may not be as intolerable as the dependency it causes.

Nurses should help aging persons understand and face the common changes associated with advanced age. Factors that promote optimum function should be encouraged, including proper diet; paced activity; regular physical examination; early correction of health problems; effective stress management; and avoidance of alcohol, tobacco, and drug abuse. Nurses should offer assistance, with attention to preserving as much of the individual's independence and dignity as possible.

NURSING DIAGNOSIS HIGHLIGHT

INEFFECTIVE ROLE PERFORMANCE

Overview

Ineffectiveness in role performance exists when there is a change in the perception or performance of a role. This can be associated with a physical, emotional, intellectual, motivational, educational, or socioeconomic limitation in the ability to fill the role or restrictions in role performance imposed by others. There can be considerable distress, depression, or anger at not fulfilling the accustomed role and its associated responsibilities.

Causative or contributing factors

Illness, fatigue, pain, declining function, altered cognition, depression, anxiety, knowledge deficit, limited finances, retirement, lack of transportation, loss of significant other, ageism, and restrictions imposed by others.

Goal

The client realistically appraises role performance, adjusts to changes in role performance, and learns to perform responsibilities associated with roles.

Interventions

- Assess client's roles and responsibilities; identify deficits in role performance and reasons for deficits; review client's

perception of role and feelings associated with altered role performance.

- Assist client in realistically evaluating cause of altered role performance and potential for improvement in role performance.
- Identify specific strategies to improve role performance (e.g., instructing, negotiating with family members to allow client to perform role, counseling client to accept real limitations, referring to community resources, improving health problem, encouraging client to seek help with responsibilities, and advising for stress management).
- Encourage client to discuss concerns with family members; assist client in arranging family conference.
- Refer client to assistive resources, as appropriate, such as support groups, occupational therapist, financial counselor, Over 60 Counseling & Employment Service, visiting nurse, or social services.

CUMULATIVE EFFECTS OF LIFE TRANSITIONS

Shrinking Social World

Many of the changes associated with aging result in loss of social connections and increasing risk of loneliness. Children are grown and gone, friends and spouse may be deceased, and others who could allay the loneliness may avoid the older individual because they find it difficult to accept the changes they see or to face the fact that they too will be old someday. Living in a sparsely populated rural area can geographically isolate older persons, and fears of crime when living in an urban area may prevent older adults from venturing outside their homes.

Hearing and speech deficits and language differences can also foster loneliness. Even if in the company of others, these functional limitations can socially isolate an older person. In addition, insecurity resulting from multiple losses in communication abilities can lead to suspiciousness of others and a self-imposed isolation.

At a time of many losses and adjustments, personal contact, love, extra support, and attention—not isolation—are needed. These are essential

human needs. It is likely that a failure to thrive will occur in adults who feel unwanted and unloved just as it does in infants, who display anxiety, depression, anorexia, and behavioral and other difficulties when they perceive love and attention to be inadequate.

Nurses should attempt to intervene when they detect isolation and loneliness in an older person. Various programs provide telephone reassurance or home visits as a source of daily human contact. The person's faith community may also provide assistance. Nurses can help the older adult locate and join social groups and perhaps even accompany the individual to the first meeting. A change in housing may be necessary to provide a safe environment conducive to social interaction. If the older person speaks a language other than English, relocation to an area in which community members speak that language can often remedy loneliness. Frequently, pets serve as significant and effective companions for older adults.

Using common sense in nursing care will facilitate social activity. The nurse can review and perhaps readjust the person's schedule to conserve energy and maximize opportunities for socialization. Medication administration should be planned so that during periods of social activity analgesics will provide relief, tranquilizers will not sedate, diuretics will not reach their peak, and laxatives will not begin working. Likewise, fluid intake and bathroom visits before activities begin should be planned to reduce the fear or actual occurrence of incontinence; activities for older adults should include frequent break periods for bathroom visits. The control of these minor obstacles can often facilitate social interaction.

Nurses should also understand that being alone is not synonymous with being lonely. Periods of solitude are essential at all ages and provide the opportunity to reflect, analyze, and better understand the dynamics of one's life. Older individuals may want periods of solitude to reminisce and review their lives. Some individuals, young and old, prefer and choose to be alone and do not feel isolated or lonely in any way. Of course, nurses should always be alert to hearing, vision, and other health problems that may be the cause of social isolation.

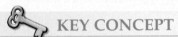

KEY CONCEPT

Periods of solitude are essential to reflect, analyze, and better understand the dynamics of life.

Awareness of Mortality

Widowhood, the death of friends, and the recognition of declining functions heighten older persons' awareness of the reality of their own deaths. During their early years, individuals intellectually understand they will not live forever, but their behaviors often deny this reality. The lack of a will and burial plans may be indications of this denial. As the reality of mortality becomes acute with advancing age, interest in fulfilling dreams, deepening religious convictions, strengthening family ties, providing for the ongoing welfare of family, and leaving a legacy are often apparent signs.

The thought of impending death may be more tolerable if people understand that their life has had depth and meaning. Unresolved guilt, unachieved aspirations, perceived failures, and other multitudinous aspects of "unfinished business" may be better understood and perhaps resolved. Although the state of old age may provide limited opportunities for excitement and achievement, satisfaction may be gained in knowing that there were achievements and excitements in other periods of life. The old woman may be frail and wrinkled, but she can still delight in remembering how she once drove young men wild. The retired old man may feel that he is useless to society now, but he realizes his worth

through the memory of wars he fought to protect his country and the pride he feels in knowing he enabled his children to obtain an education and start in life that his parents were unable to provide him. Nurses can help older adults gain this perspective on their lives through some of the interventions discussed in the following sections.

RESPONDING TO LIFE TRANSITIONS

When faced with ageism and numerous changes affecting relationships, roles, and health, older adults may respond in a variety of ways. The older adult's ability to cope and adjust to life changes determines whether they reach a stage of integrity or fall to despair. Nurses can help older adults respond to life transitions by facilitating life review and eliciting a life story, promoting self-reflection, and strengthening older adults' inner resources.

Life Review and Life Story

Life review is the process of intentionally reflecting on past experiences in an effort to resolve troublesome or traumatic life events and assess one's life in totality. The significance of a life review in interpreting and refining our past experiences as they relate to our self-concept and help us understand and accept our life history has been well discussed (Butler & Lewis, 1982; Webster & Haight, 2002). In gerontological care, life review has long been recognized as an important process to facilitate integrity in old age (i.e., to help older people appreciate that their lives have had meaning).

Rather than being a pathologic behavior, discussing the past is therapeutic and important for older individuals (Fig. 4-4). Life review can be a positive experience because older adults can reflect on the obstacles they have overcome and accomplishments they have made. It can provide the incentive to heal fractured relationships and complete unfinished business. Life review, however, can be a painful experience for older adults who realize the mistakes they've made and the lives they've hurt. Rather than conceal and avoid these negative feelings, older adults can benefit by discussing them openly and working through them; referrals to therapists and counselors may be indicated to assist with unresolved grief, depression, or anxiety.

The young can also benefit from the reminiscences of older adults by gaining a new perspective on life as they learn about their ancestry. Imagine the impact of hearing about slavery, immigration, epidemics, industrialization, or wars from an older relative who has been part of that history. What history book's description of the Great Depression can compare with hearing a grandparent describe

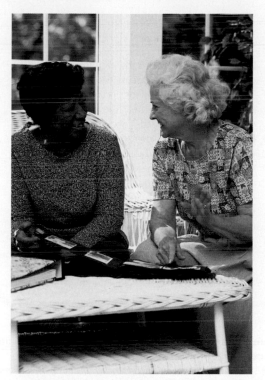

FIGURE 4-4 ■ Reminiscing is a culturally universal phenomenon of aging. It is a way for the older adult to reassess life experiences and further develop a sense of accomplishment, fulfillment, and reward in life.

events one's own family experienced, such as going to bed hungry at night? In addition to their place in the future, the young can fully realize their link with the past when the desire of older people to reminisce is appreciated and fostered.

 KEY CONCEPT

Reminiscence is not only therapeutic for older adults but bridges the past and present for the young listener.

The nurse can facilitate life review by eliciting the older adult's life story. Rich threads of life experience that create the unique fabric of one's life are accumulated with aging. When seen in isolation, some of these threads may seem to have little value or make little sense, much like a network of threads on the undersurface of a tapestry. However, when the threads are woven together and the tapestry can be viewed as a whole, a person can see the special purpose of individual life experiences—good and bad. Weaving the threads of life experiences into the tapestry of a life story can be highly beneficial to the older person and others. Successes can be appreciated and the value of trials and failures can be realized. Others are able to gain insight into the person's life in totality rather than have their understanding limited by what may be an unrepresentative segment of life that now presents. Customs, knowledge, and wisdom can be recognized, preserved, and passed to younger generations.

 POINT TO PONDER

What are the major threads that have woven your life tapestry thus far?

Eliciting life stories from older persons is not a difficult process; in fact, many older adults welcome opportunities to share their life histories and life lessons to interested listeners. Nurses can encourage older adults to discuss and analyze the dynamics of their lives, and they can be receptive and accepting listeners. Box 4-1 outlines some of the variety of approaches nurses can use to elicit life stories.

For older adults who may require some facilitation, creative activities, such as compiling a scrapbook or dictating a family history, can stimulate the process. These creative efforts, as unsophisticated as they may be, should be recognized as significant legacies from the old to the young. For example, one 75-year-old man started a family scrapbook for each of his children. Any photograph, newspaper article, or announcement pertaining to any family member was reproduced and included in every album. The family patiently tolerated this activity and sent him copies of graduation programs and photographs for every scrapbook. The family viewed the main value of this activity as providing something benign to keep him occupied. It was not until years after his death that the significance of this great task was appreciated as a priceless gift. Such tangible items may serve as an assurance to both young and old that the impact of an aged relative's life will not cease at death. Guiding older adults through this experience of compiling a life story not only provides a therapeutic exercise for them and an invaluable legacy for loved ones but also offers the gerontological nurse the gift of sharing and honoring the unique life journeys of older adults.

Self-Reflection

One of the hallmarks of successful aging is knowledge of self—that is, an awareness of the realities of who one is and one's place in the world. From infancy

---

BOX 4-1 **Eliciting Life Stories**

Older adults possess rich life histories that have accrued during the many years they have lived. These unique histories contribute to each person's identity and individuality. Learning about life histories aids nurses in understanding older adults' preferences and activities, facilitating self-actualization, and preserving identity and continuity of life experiences. Knowledge of life histories also enables caregivers to see their patients in a larger context, connected to a past full of varied roles and experiences.

A basic requisite to eliciting life stories is a willingness to listen. Often, a direct request will be sufficient to open the door to a life history. Activities to facilitate this process include the following:

- **Tree of Life.** Ask the older adult to write significant events (graduation, first job, relocations, marriages, deaths, childbirths, etc.) from the past on each branch and then discuss each.
- **Time Line.** Ask the older person to write significant events on or near the year when they occurred and then discuss each.
- **Life Map.** Ask the older adult to write significant events on the map and discuss each.
- **Oral History.** Ask the older adult to start with his or her earliest memory and record the story of his or her life into a tape recorder. (Suggest that the older person make this recording as a gift for younger family members.) If the person needs guidance in telling their history, offer a written outline or questions, or have a volunteer function as an interviewer.

---

on, we engage in dynamic experiences that mold the unique individuals we are. By adulthood, we have formed the skeleton of our identities. Continued interactions and life experiences as we journey through life further add to the development of our identities.

The self, the personal identity an individual possesses, has several dimensions that basically can be described as body, mind, and spirit. The body includes physical characteristics and functioning; the mind encompasses cognition, perception, and emotions; and the spirit consists of meaning and purpose derived from a relationship with God or other higher power. A variety of factors affect the development of body, mind, and spirit, such as genetic makeup, family composition and dynamics, roles, ethnicity, environment, education, religious experiences, relationships, culture, lifestyle, and health practices (Fig. 4-5).

POINT TO PONDER

What are the significant factors of your background that influenced your unique body, mind, and spirit?

Although a realistic appraisal of one's identity and place in the world fosters healthy aging, not all persons complete this task successfully. Some people may live with unrealistic expectations or views of themselves, going through life playing parts that are ill-suited for them and wasting time

in fruitless or unfulfilling activities. Harry is an example of this:

Harry, the eldest of five children, was raised in an inner-city community in which poverty was the norm. His father was an auto mechanic who had difficulty holding jobs. His mother didn't miss an opportunity to voice her dissatisfaction with her husband's meager income nor to emphasize to Harry that he needed to be sure to "make it big and not be like his father."

The message instilled by his mother and his desire for a better life than he enjoyed as a child fueled Harry to be a high achiever. By age 30, Harry owned

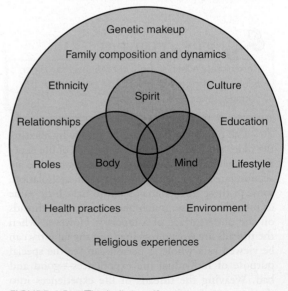

FIGURE 4-5 ■ The holistic self.

a small chain of convenience stores, a large home in the suburbs, several luxury cars, and most of the possessions that reflected an upper-middle-class lifestyle. Harry was proud that he could provide a comfortable life for his wife and expensive education for his children—quite the opposite of what his father achieved. Yet, something was missing. His business demanded most of his time and energy; therefore, he had little left of himself to offer his family. He also rarely had the time for his passion, restoring classic cars. His life seemed to consist of managing his businesses and sleeping, with an occasional social event with his family. Time for relaxation and reflection had no place in Harry's busy life.

In his late 50s, with children grown and his business worth enough to provide a comfortable retirement income, Harry was in a position where he didn't have to work the long days—or at all for that matter. His wife encouraged him to consider selling his business and spend his time "tinkering with cars and taking it easy." Although he was tempted, Harry felt that he just couldn't do this. Unfortunately, the script to "make it big," programmed into Harry's mind as a child, held him prisoner to a role that brought him little joy and fulfillment. Furthermore, he had no idea of what his purpose and identity was other than being an entrepreneur.

Like Harry, many individuals may reach their senior years without having evaluated who they really are, what drives them to behave as they do, or what their true purposes and pleasures are.

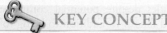

KEY CONCEPT

Some adults may not have invested the time and effort in self-evaluation and, consequently, reach old age with a lack of clarity of their identity.

Exploring and learning about one's true self are significant to holistic health in late life. Examining and coming to terms with thoughts, feelings, beliefs, and behaviors foster older adults' reaching a state of integrity rather than feeling despair over the lives they've lived. However, as important a process as it is, self-reflection does not come easily or naturally for some individuals. They may require interventions to facilitate this process; therefore, guiding aging people through self-reflective activities is an important therapeutic measure that gerontological nurses may need to offer. Life review and telling one's life story can function as self-reflective activities. In addition, other activities that facilitate self-reflection include journaling, writing letters and e-mails, and reflecting through art. These certainly do not exhaust the strategies that can be used

to foster self-reflection. Nurses are bound only by their creativity in the approaches used for promoting self-reflection.

Journaling

Whether it is done with pencil and paper or a word processing program, the process of writing often facilitates self-reflection. There is no one right way to keep a journal or diary; individuals should develop styles that are comfortable for them. Some people may make daily entries that include details about their communications, sleep patterns, mood, and activities, whereas others make periodic entries that address major emotional and spiritual issues. Nurses can assist individuals who have not kept journals and diaries by guiding them in the selection of a blank book and writing instrument. This is an important step, not only because these tools will be used often but also because the book will be a tangible compilation of significant thoughts and feelings that could have meaning to others in years to come. Novices to journaling can be encouraged to start by reflecting on their lives and beginning their journals/diaries with a summary of the past. Suggesting that feelings and thoughts be written, in addition to the events of the day, can contribute to the process being one that fosters self-reflection.

Writing Letters and E-Mails

Letters or e-mails are another means to reflect and express feelings. Often thoughts and feelings that individuals may not feel comfortable verbalizing can be expressed in writing. For some older adults, letters of explanation and apology to friends and family with whom there have been strained relationships can be a healing exercise. Older people can be encouraged to locate friends and family in other parts of the country (or world) with whom they have not had contact for a while and to initiate communication concerning what has transpired in their lives and current events. Letters to grandchildren and other younger members of the family can provide a means to share relevant family history and offer special attention (many children love to receive their own mail!). Older adults may enjoy communicating by e-mail because of the ease and relatively low cost. If older adults do not own their own computers, nurses can refer them to local senior centers or libraries that offer free or nominal cost access to the Internet.

Reflecting Through Art

Many people find that painting, sculpting, weaving, and other forms of creative expression facilitate self-reflection and expression. It is important that the process, not the finished product, be emphasized.

Arts and crafts classes and groups often are offered by local organizations dedicated to specific activities (e.g., weavers' guild and arts' council), schools, and senior centers. Nurses can assist older adults in locating such groups in their communities.

KEY CONCEPT

Producing a work of art, discussing literature, and sharing one's life story are among the many interventions that can be used to foster self-reflection.

Strengthening Inner Resources

The declines and dependencies that increasingly are present in late life can cause us to view older adults as being fragile and incapable. However, most older individuals possess significant inner resources— physical, emotional, and spiritual—that have enabled them to survive to old age. Behaviors that exemplify their survivor capabilities are described in Box 4-2.

KEY CONCEPT

By considering the strengths displayed by older adults as they navigated the aging process, nurses and others can develop an enlightened perspective of the older population.

Against the backdrop of threats to independence and self-esteem, nurses best serve older adults by maintaining and bolstering their inner strengths. Basic to this effort is ensuring physical health and well-being. It is quite challenging for persons of any age to optimally meet intellectual, emotional, socioeconomic, and spiritual challenges when their basic physical needs are not fully satisfied or they are experiencing the symptoms associated with deviations from health. Comprehensive and regular assessment of health status and interventions to promote health provide a solid base from which inner strengths can be nurtured.

POINT TO PONDER

How would you judge your "survivor competencies?" What experiences have contributed to this?

By being empowerment facilitators, nurses can support older adults' inner strengths. Nurses must begin this process by examining and strengthening their own level of empowerment. When nurses

---

| **BOX 4-2** | **Characteristics Reflective of Survivor Competencies of Aging Individuals** |

- Assumption of responsibility for self-care
- Mobilization of internal and external resources to solve problems and manage crises
- Development of support system via a network of family, friends, and professional individuals and groups (e.g., social clubs, churches, physicians, and volunteers)
- Sense of control over life events
- Adaptation to change
- Perseverance in the face of obstacles and difficulties
- Recovery from trauma
- Realization and acceptance of reality that life includes positive and negative events
- Discovery of meaning in life events
- Determination to fulfill personal, family, community, and work expectations despite difficulties and distractions
- Recognition of limitations and competencies
- Ability to trust, love, and forgive and to accept trust, love, and forgiveness

develop a mindset of seeing possibilities despite fiscal and other constraints, they are better able to help older adults see possibilities despite potential constraints imposed by age and illness. In addition to being role models, nurses can facilitate empowerment by:

- including and encouraging the active participation of older adults in care planning and caregiving activities to the maximum extent possible

- avoiding ageist attitudes that can be communicated through the manner of speaking to older adults (e.g., raising voice due to assumption all older people are hearing impaired and using terms like "Sweetie" or "Pops") and practices (e.g., having signs like "Fall Risk" or "Toilet q2h" in view of others and labeling clothing in a manner that is visible to others)

- providing a variety of options to older people and freedom to choose among them

- equipping older adults for maximum self-care and self-direction by educating, relating, coaching, sharing, and supporting them

- advocating for older adults as they seek information, make decisions, and execute their own selected self-care strategies

■ offering feedback, positive reinforcement, encouragement, and support

A sense of hope fosters empowerment and is a thread that reinforces the fabric of inner strengths. Hope is an expectation—that a problem will be resolved, relief will be obtained, and something desired will be obtained. Hope enables people to see beyond the present and make sense of the senseless. It empowers them to take action. Nurses foster hope in older people by honoring the value of their lives despite infirmities and limitations, assisting in establishing goals, supporting the use of coping strategies, building on capabilities, and displaying an optimistic, caring attitude. Spiritual beliefs and practices also provide inner strength that enables older adults to cope with current challenges and maintain hope and optimism for the future (see Chapter 13); nurses need to support older individuals in their prayers, devotional readings, church attendance, and other expressions of spirituality.

BRINGING RESEARCH TO LIFE

RISK OF ACUTE MYOCARDIAL INFARCTION AFTER THE DEATH OF A SIGNIFICANT PERSON IN ONE'S LIFE: THE DETERMINANTS OF MYOCARDIAL INFARCTION ONSET STUDY

Mostofsky, E., Maclure, M., Sherwood, J. B., Tofler, G. H., Muller, J. E., & Mittleman, M. A. (2012). Circulation, 125(3), 491–496.

Recognizing that acute psychological stress is associated with an increase in cardiovascular events, the researchers studied the role of intense grief in triggering an acute myocardial infarction (MI). They investigated persons hospitalized with an acute MI for their experience in losing a loved one within 6 months of their MI. They found that the incidence rate of acute MI onset was elevated within 24 hours of the death of a significant person, and grief over the death of a significant person was associated with an acutely increased risk of MI in the subsequent days. The impact may be greatest among individuals at high cardiovascular risk.

Nurses need to be aware of the risk of cardiovascular events in the older adult who has experienced a significant loss and assure the person is observed and has contact with others so that symptoms can be promptly addressed. If the person has no family member or friend who can provide this contact, arrangements should be made with a bereavement or other group to have someone regularly check in on the grieving person. The person also should be counseled in measures to reduce his or her stress.

PRACTICE REALITIES

Widowed 78-year-old Mrs. Knight lives in the house she was raised in and in which she raised her own family. Her 56-year-old unemployed son lives with her, and a daughter lives in a neighboring state.

Despite her independence, Mrs. Knight is a cause of concern for her daughter who believes her brother is taking advantage of their mother. The daughter has suggested to Mrs. Knight that she move in with her. Mrs. Knight has refused, stating that her son "just couldn't make it on his own."

The daughter shares her concerns with the nurse practitioner who works in the practice that manages Mrs. Knight's care.

What would be reasonable actions for the nurse practitioner to take?

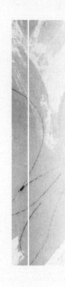

CRITICAL THINKING EXERCISES

1. What examples of ageism can be found in television programs, advertisements, and other vehicles of communication?

2. How will the life experiences of today's 30-year-old woman affect her ability to adapt to old age? What factors will enable her to cope more or less as well than her grandmother's generation of women?

3. Describe actions nurses can take to help aging individuals prepare for retirement.

4. How can you determine if an older individual's time alone is reflective of needed solitude or social isolation?

5. How can the gerontological nurse elicit life stories from older adults in the midst of caregiving demands during a busy shift?

6. In what ways will today's young generation be in a better or worse position than today's older population in developing survivor competencies?

RESOURCES

AARP Grandparent Information Center
http://www.aarp.org
AARP Retirement Calculator
http://www.aarp.org
Grandparents Raising Grandchildren
http://www.uwex.edu
International Institute for Reminiscence and Life Review
http://www.uwsuper.edu

REFERENCES

Atchley, R. C. (1975). *The sociology of retirement*. Cambridge, MA: Schenkman.

Atchley, R. C. (2000). *Social forces and aging* (9th ed.). Belmont, CA: Wadsworth.

Butler, R. H., & Lewis, M. I. (1982). *Aging and mental health* (3rd ed., p. 58). St. Louis, MO: Mosby.

Butler, R. H., Lewis, M. I., & Sutherland, T. (1991). *Aging and mental health* (4th ed.). New York: Merrill/MacMillan.

Corbett, D. (2007). *Portfolio life. The new path to work, purpose, and passion after 50*. San Francisco, CA: John Wiley and Sons.

Erikson, E. (1963). *Childhood and society* (2nd ed.). New York: Norton.

Gates, G., Badgett, L. M., Macomber, J. E., & Chambers, K. (2007). *Adoption and foster care by lesbian and gay parents in the United States*. Urban Institute. Retrieved October 17, 2007 from http://www.urban.org/url.cfm?ID=411437.

MetLife. (2011). *The MetLife report on American grandparents: new insights for a new generation of grandparents*. Westport, CT: MetLife Mature Market Institute.

U.S. Census Bureau. (2012). *2007 American community survey*. Retrieved April 9, 2012 from http://www.census.gov/acs/www/

Webster, J. D., & Haight, B. K. (2002). *Critical advances in reminiscence work: From theory to application*. New York: Springer.

RECOMMENDED READINGS

Recommended Readings associated with this chapter can be found on the web site that accompanies the book. Visit **http://thepoint.lww.com/Eliopoulos8e** to access the recommended readings and other additional resources associated with this chapter.

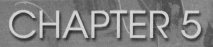

Common Aging Changes

LEARNING OBJECTIVES

After reading this chapter, you should be able to:

1. List common age-related changes at the cellular level; in physical appearance; and to the respiratory, cardiovascular, gastrointestinal, urinary, reproductive, musculoskeletal, nervous, endocrine, integumentary, and immune systems, the sensory organs, and thermoregulation.

2. Describe psychological changes experienced with age.

3. Discuss risks and nursing considerations associated with age-related changes.

TERMS TO KNOW

Crystallized intelligence: knowledge accumulated over a lifetime; arises from the dominant hemisphere of the brain

Fluid intelligence: involves new information emanating from the nondominant hemisphere; controls emotions, retention of nonintellectual information, creative capacities, spatial perceptions, and aesthetic appreciation

Immunosenescence: the aging of the immune system

Presbycusis: progressive hearing loss that occurs as a result of age-related changes to the inner ear

(Continued)

51

Presbyesophagus: a condition characterized by a decreased intensity of propulsive waves and an increased frequency of non-propulsive waves in the esophagus

Presbyopia: the inability to focus or accommodate properly due to reduced elasticity of the lens

Living is a process of continual change. Infants become toddlers, prepubescent children blossom into young men and women, and dependent adolescents develop into responsible adults. The continuation of change into later life is natural and expected.

The type, rate, and degree of physical, emotional, psychological, and social changes experienced during life are highly individualized; such changes are influenced by genetic factors, environment, diet, health, stress, lifestyle choices, and numerous other elements. The result is not only individual variations among older persons but also differences in the pattern of aging of various body systems within the same individual. Although some similarities exist in the patterns of aging among individuals, the pattern of aging is unique in each person.

CHANGES TO THE BODY

Cells

Organ and system changes can be traced to changes at the basic cellular level. The number of cells is gradually reduced, leaving fewer functional cells in the body. Lean body mass is reduced, whereas fat tissue increases until the sixth decade of life. Total body fat as a proportion of the body's composition increases (St-Onge & Gallagher, 2010; Woo, Leung, & Kwok, 2007). Cellular solids and bone mass are decreased. Extracellular fluid remains fairly constant, whereas intracellular fluid is decreased, resulting in less total body fluid. This decrease makes dehydration a significant risk to older adults.

Physical Appearance

Many physical changes of aging affect a person's appearance (Fig. 5-1). Some of the more noticeable effects of the aging process begin to appear after the fourth decade of life. It is then that men experience hair loss, and both sexes develop gray hair and wrinkles. As body fat atrophies, the body's contours gain a bony appearance along with a deepening of the hollows of the intercostal and supraclavicular spaces, orbits, and axillae. Elongated ears, a double chin, and baggy eyelids are among the more obvious manifestations of the loss of tissue elasticity throughout the body. Skin-fold thickness is significantly reduced in the forearm and on the back of the hands. The loss of subcutaneous fat content, responsible for the decrease in skin-fold thickness, is also responsible for a decline in the body's natural insulation, making older adults more sensitive to cold temperatures.

Stature decreases, resulting in a loss of approximately 2 inches in height by 80 years of age. Body shrinkage is due to reduced hydration, loss of cartilage, and thinning of the vertebrae. The decrease in stature causes the long bones of the body, which do not shrink, to appear disproportionately long. Any curvature of the spine, hips, and knees that may be present can further reduce height.

These changes in physical appearance are gradual and subtle. Further differences in physiologic structure and function can arise from changes to specific body systems.

Respiratory System

The changes to the respiratory system are apparent at the entrance to the system with changes to the nose. Connective tissue changes cause a relaxation of the tissue at the lower edge of the septum; the reduced support causes the tip of the nose to slightly rotate downward. Septal deviations can occur, as well. Mouth breathing during sleep becomes more common as a result, contributing to snoring and obstructive apnea. The submucosal glands have decreased secretions, reducing the ability to dilute mucus secretion; the thicker secretions are more difficult to remove and give the older person a sensation of nasal stuffiness.

Various structural changes occur in the chest with age that reduce respiratory activity (Fig. 5-2). The calcification of costal cartilage makes the trachea and rib cage more rigid; the anterior–posterior chest diameter increases, often demonstrated by kyphosis; and thoracic inspiratory and expiratory muscles are weaker. There is a blunting of the cough and laryngeal reflexes. In the lungs, cilia reduce in number and there is hypertrophy of the bronchial mucous gland, further complicating the ability to expel mucus and debris. Alveoli reduce in number and stretch due to a progressive loss of elasticity—a process that begins

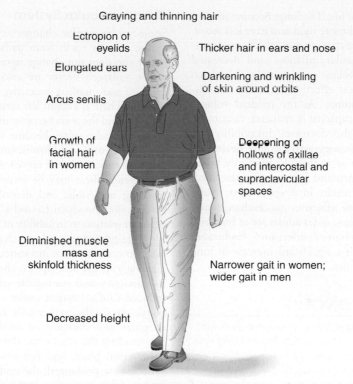

Graying and thinning hair

Ectropion of eyelids

Elongated ears

Arcus senilis

Growth of facial hair in women

Diminished muscle mass and skinfold thickness

Decreased height

Thicker hair in ears and nose

Darkening and wrinkling of skin around orbits

Deepening of hollows of axillae and intercostal and supraclavicular spaces

Narrower gait in women; wider gait in men

FIGURE 5-1 ■ Age-related changes noticeable on inspection.

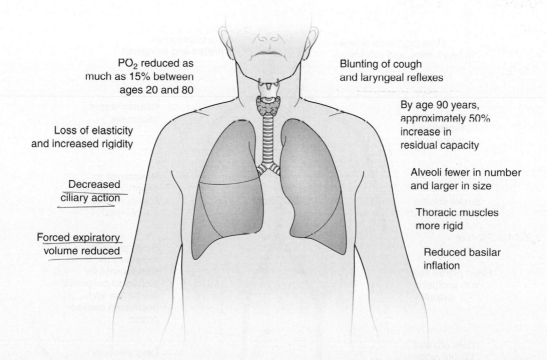

PO$_2$ reduced as much as 15% between ages 20 and 80

Loss of elasticity and increased rigidity

Decreased ciliary action

Forced expiratory volume reduced

Blunting of cough and laryngeal reflexes

By age 90 years, approximately 50% increase in residual capacity

Alveoli fewer in number and larger in size

Thoracic muscles more rigid

Reduced basilar inflation

FIGURE 5-2 ■ Respiratory changes that occur with aging.

by the sixth decade of life. The lungs become smaller, less firm, lighter, and more rigid and have less recoil.

The sum of these changes causes less lung expansion, insufficient basilar inflation, and decreased ability to expel foreign or accumulated matter. The lungs exhale less effectively, thereby increasing the residual volume. As the residual volume increases, the vital capacity is reduced; maximum breathing capacity also decreases. Immobility can further reduce respiratory activity. The decline in ventilatory capacity is noticeable primarily when an extra breathing demand is present, as the lower pulmonary reserve results in dyspnea more easily occurring. With less effective gas exchange and lack of basilar inflation, older adults are at high risk for developing respiratory infections. Endurance training can produce a significant increase in lung capacity of older adults.

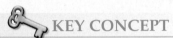
KEY CONCEPT

The reduced respiratory activity associated with advanced age puts older adults at increased risk for developing pneumonia easily, especially when they are immobile.

Cardiovascular System

Some cardiovascular changes commonly attributed to age actually result from pathological conditions. Heart size does not change significantly due to age; rather, enlarged hearts are associated with cardiac disease, and marked inactivity can cause cardiac atrophy. There is a slight left ventricular hypertrophy with age, and the aorta becomes dilated and elongated. Atrioventricular valves become thick and rigid as a result of sclerosis and fibrosis, compounding the dysfunction associated with any cardiac disease that may be present. There may be incomplete valve closure resulting in systolic and diastolic murmurs. Extra systolic sinus bradycardia and sinus arrhythmia can occur in relation to irritability of the myocardium.

Age-related physiologic changes in the cardiovascular system appear in a variety of ways (Fig. 5-3). Throughout the adult years, the heart muscle loses its efficiency and contractile strength, resulting in reduced cardiac output under conditions of physiologic stress. Pacemaker cells become increasingly irregular and decrease in number, and the shell surrounding the sinus node thickens. The isometric contraction phase and relaxation time of the left ventricle are prolonged; the cycle of diastolic filling and systolic emptying requires more time to be completed.

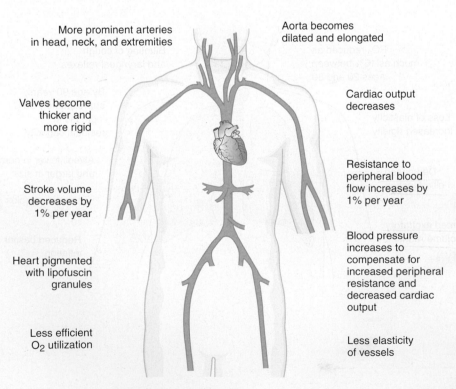

More prominent arteries in head, neck, and extremities

Aorta becomes dilated and elongated

Valves become thicker and more rigid

Cardiac output decreases

Stroke volume decreases by 1% per year

Resistance to peripheral blood flow increases by 1% per year

Heart pigmented with lipofuscin granules

Blood pressure increases to compensate for increased peripheral resistance and decreased cardiac output

Less efficient O₂ utilization

Less elasticity of vessels

FIGURE 5-3 ■ Cardiovascular changes that occur with aging.

Usually, adults adjust to changes in the cardiovascular system quite well; they learn that it is easier and more comfortable for them to take an elevator rather than the stairs, to drive instead of walking a long distance, and to pace their activities. When unusual demands are placed on the heart (e.g., shoveling snow for the first time of the season, receiving bad news, and running to catch a bus), the person feels the effects. The same holds true for older individuals who are not severely affected by less cardiac efficiency under non-stressful conditions. When older persons are faced with an added demand on their hearts, however, they note the difference. Although the peak rate of the stressed heart may not reach the levels experienced by younger persons, tachycardia in older people will last for a longer time. Stroke volume may increase to compensate for this situation, which results in elevated blood pressure, although the blood pressure can remain stable as tachycardia progresses to heart failure in older adults. The resting heart rate is unchanged.

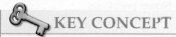

KEY CONCEPT

Age-related cardiovascular changes are most apparent when unusual demands are placed on the heart.

Maximum exercise capacity and maximum oxygen consumption vary among older people. Older adults in good physical condition have comparable cardiac function to younger persons who are in poor condition.

Blood vessels consist of three layers, each of which is affected differently by the aging process. The tunica intima, the innermost layer, experiences the most direct changes, including fibrosis, calcium and lipid accumulation, and cellular proliferation. These changes contribute to the development of atherosclerosis. The middle layer, the tunica media, undergoes a thinning and calcification of elastin fibers and an increase in collagen, which cause a stiffening of the vessels. Impaired baroreceptor function and increased peripheral resistance occur, which can lead to a rise in systolic blood pressure. Interestingly, although a gradual increase in blood pressure is common in the United States and other industrialized nations, it does not tend to occur in less industrialized societies; cross-cultural studies that currently are being conducted will help to clarify if the rise in blood pressure is a result of normal aging or other factors. The outermost layer, the tunica adventitia, is not affected by the aging process. Decreased elasticity of the arteries is responsible for vascular changes to the heart,

kidney, and pituitary gland. Reduced sensitivity of the blood pressure–regulating baroreceptors increases problems with postural hypotension and postprandial hypotension (blood pressure reduction of at least 20 mm Hg within 1 hour of eating). The reduced elasticity of the vessels, coupled with thinner skin and less subcutaneous fat, causes the vessels in the head, neck, and extremities to become more prominent.

Gastrointestinal System

Although not as life-threatening as respiratory or cardiovascular problems, gastrointestinal symptoms may be of more bother and concern to older persons. This system is altered by the aging process at all points. Changes in the teeth and mouth and accessory structures such as the liver also affect gastrointestinal function. Figure 5-4 summarizes gastrointestinal system changes.

Tooth enamel becomes harder and more brittle with age. Dentin, the layer beneath the enamel, becomes more fibrous and its production is decreased. The nerve chambers become narrower and shorter and teeth are less sensitive to stimuli. The root pulp experiences shrinkage and fibrosis, the gingiva retracts, and bone density in the alveolar ridge is lost. Increasing numbers of root cavities and cavities around existing dental work occur. Flattening of the chewing cusps is common. The bones that support the teeth decrease in density and height, contributing to tooth loss. Tooth loss is not a normal consequence of growing old, but poor dental care, diet, and environmental influences have contributed to many of today's older population being edentulous. After 30 years of age, periodontal disease is the major reason for tooth loss. More than half of all older adults must rely on partial or full dentures, which may not be worn regularly because of discomfort or poor fit. If natural teeth are present, they often are in poor condition; fracture easier; and have flatter surfaces, stains, and varying degrees of erosion and abrasion of the crown and root structure. The tooth brittleness of some older people creates the possibility of aspiration of tooth fragments.

Taste sensations become less acute with age because the tongue atrophies, affecting the taste buds; chronic irritation (as from pipe smoking) can reduce taste efficiency to a greater degree than that experienced through aging alone. The sweet sensations on the tip of the tongue tend to suffer a greater loss than the sensations for sour, salt, and bitter flavors. Excessive seasoning of foods may be used to compensate for taste alterations and could lead to health problems for older individuals. Loss of papillae and sublingual varicosities on the tongue are common findings.

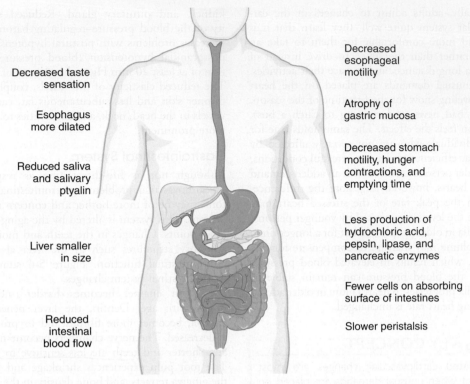

Decreased taste sensation

Esophagus more dilated

Reduced saliva and salivary ptyalin

Liver smaller in size

Reduced intestinal blood flow

Decreased esophageal motility

Atrophy of gastric mucosa

Decreased stomach motility, hunger contractions, and emptying time

Less production of hydrochloric acid, pepsin, lipase, and pancreatic enzymes

Fewer cells on absorbing surface of intestines

Slower peristalsis

FIGURE 5-4 ■ Gastrointestinal changes that occur with aging.

Older adults produce approximately one third of the amount of saliva they produced in younger years (Gupta, Epstein, & Sroussi, 2006). Saliva often is diminished in quantity and is of increased viscosity as a result of some of the medications commonly used to treat geriatric conditions. Salivary ptyalin is decreased, interfering with the breakdown of starches. Because of subtle changes in the swallowing mechanism, swallowing can take twice as long (Shaker et al., 2003). Diminished muscle strength and tongue pressure can interfere with mastication and swallowing (Ney, Weiss, Kind, & Robinson, 2009).

Esophageal motility is affected by age. Presbyesophagus occurs, a condition characterized by a decreased intensity of propulsive waves and an increased frequency of non-propulsive waves in the esophagus. The esophagus tends to become slightly dilated, and esophageal emptying is slower, which can cause discomfort because food remains in the esophagus for a longer time. Relaxation of the lower esophageal sphincter may occur; when combined with the older person's weaker gag reflex and delayed esophageal emptying, aspiration becomes a risk.

The stomach is believed to have reduced motility in old age, along with decreases in hunger contractions. Studies regarding changes in gastric emptying time have been inconclusive, with some claiming delayed gastric emptying to occur with normal aging and others attributing it to other factors. The gastric mucosa atrophies. Hydrochloric acid and pepsin decline with age; the higher pH of the stomach contributes to an increased incidence of gastric irritation in the older population.

Some atrophy occurs throughout the small and large intestines, and fewer cells are present on the absorbing surface of intestinal walls. There is a gradual reduction in the weight of the small intestine and shortening and widening of the villi, leading to them developing the shape of parallel ridges rather than the finger-like projections of earlier years. Functionally, there is no significant change in mean small bowel transit time with age. Fat absorption is slower, and dextrose and xylose are more difficult to absorb. Absorption of vitamin B, vitamin B$_{12}$, vitamin D, calcium, and iron is faulty. The large intestine has reductions in mucous secretions and elasticity of the rectal wall. Normal aging does not interfere with the motility of feces through the bowel, although other factors that are highly prevalent in late life do contribute to constipation. An age-related loss of tone of the internal sphincter can affect bowel elimination. Slower transmission of neural impulses to the lower bowel reduces awareness of the need to evacuate the bowels.

With advancing age, the liver has reduced weight and volume but this seems to produce no ill effects. The older liver is less able to regenerate damaged cells. Liver function tests remain within a normal range. Less efficient cholesterol stabilization and absorption cause an increased incidence of gallstones. The pancreatic ducts become dilated and distended, and often the entire gland prolapses.

Urinary System

The urinary system is affected by changes in the kidneys, ureters, and bladder (Fig. 5-5). The renal mass becomes smaller with age, which is attributable to a cortical loss rather than a loss of the renal medulla. Renal tissue growth declines and atherosclerosis may promote atrophy of the kidney. These changes can have a profound effect on renal function, reducing renal blood flow and the glomerular filtration rate by approximately one half between the ages of 20 and 90 years (Kielstein et al., 2003; Lerma, 2009).

Tubular function decreases. There is less efficient tubular exchange of substances, conservation of water and sodium, and suppression of antidiuretic hormone secretion in the presence of hypo-osmolality. Older kidneys have less ability to conserve sodium in response to sodium restriction. Although these changes can contribute to hyponatremia and nocturia, they do not affect specific gravity to any significant extent. The decrease in tubular function also causes decreased reabsorption of glucose from the filtrate, which can cause 1+ proteinurias and glycosurias not to be of major diagnostic significance.

Urinary frequency, urgency, and nocturia accompany bladder changes with age. Bladder muscles weaken and bladder capacity decreases. Emptying of the bladder is more difficult; retention of large volumes of urine may result. The micturition reflex is delayed. Although urinary incontinence is not a normal outcome of aging, some stress incontinence may occur because of a weakening of the pelvic diaphragm, particularly in multiparous women.

Reproductive System

As men age, the seminal vesicles are affected by a smoothing of the mucosa, thinning of the epithelium, replacement of muscle tissue with connective tissue, and reduction of fluid-retaining capacity. The seminiferous tubules experience increased fibrosis, thinning of the epithelium, thickening of the basement membrane, and narrowing of the lumen. The structural changes can cause a reduction in sperm count in some men. Increases in follicle-stimulating and luteinizing hormone levels occur, along with decreases in both serum and bioavailable testosterone levels. Venous and arterial sclerosis and

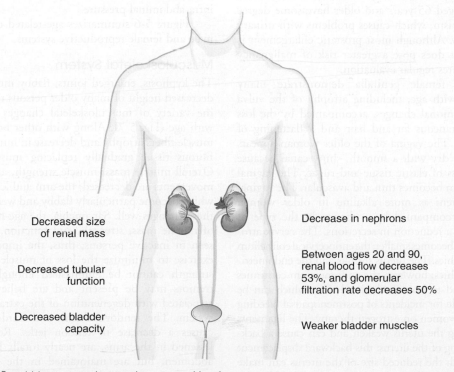

Decreased size of renal mass

Decreased tubular function

Decreased bladder capacity

Decrease in nephrons

Between ages 20 and 90, renal blood flow decreases 53%, and glomerular filtration rate decreases 50%

Weaker bladder muscles

FIGURE 5-5 ■ Urinary tract changes that occur with aging.

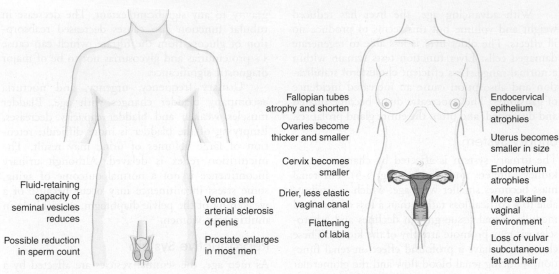

Fallopian tubes
atrophy and shorten

Ovaries become
thicker and smaller

Cervix becomes
smaller

Drier, less elastic
vaginal canal

Flattening
of labia

Endocervical
epithelium
atrophies

Uterus becomes
smaller in size

Endometrium
atrophies

More alkaline
vaginal
environment

Loss of vulvar
subcutaneous
fat and hair

Fluid-retaining
capacity of
seminal vesicles
reduces

Possible reduction
in sperm count

Venous and
arterial sclerosis
of penis

Prostate enlarges
in most men

FIGURE 5-6 ■ Changes in the male and female reproductive structures that occur with aging.

fibroelastosis of the corpus spongiosum can affect the penis with age. The older man does not lose the physical capacity to achieve erections or ejaculations, although orgasm and ejaculation tend to be less intense (Sampson, Untergasser, Plas, & Berger, 2007). There is some atrophy of the testes.

Prostatic enlargement occurs in most older men (Marks, Roehrborn, & Andiole, 2006). The rate and type vary among individuals. Three fourths of men aged 65 years and older have some degree of prostatism, which causes problems with urinary frequency. Although most prostatic enlargement is benign, it does pose a greater risk of malignancy and requires regular evaluation.

The female genitalia demonstrate many changes with age, including atrophy of the vulva from hormonal changes, accompanied by the loss of subcutaneous fat and hair and a flattening of the labia. The vagina of the older woman appears pink and dry with a smooth, shiny canal because of the loss of elastic tissue and rugae. The vaginal epithelium becomes thin and avascular. The vaginal environment is more alkaline in older women and is accompanied by a change in the type of flora and a reduction in secretions. The cervix atrophies and becomes smaller; the endocervical epithelium also atrophies. The uterus shrinks and the endometrium atrophies; however, the endometrium continues to respond to hormonal stimulation, which can be responsible for incidents of postmenopausal bleeding in older women on estrogen therapy. The ligaments supporting the uterus weaken and can cause a backward tilting of the uterus; this backward displacement along with the reduced size of the uterus can make it difficult to palpate during an exam. The fallopian

tubes atrophy and shorten with age, and the ovaries atrophy and become thicker and smaller. The ovaries can shrink to such a small size that they are not palpable during an exam. Despite these changes, the older woman does not lose the ability to engage in and enjoy intercourse or other forms of sexual pleasure. Estrogen depletion also causes a weakening of pelvic floor muscles, which can lead to an involuntary release of urine when there is an increase in intra-abdominal pressure.

Figure 5-6 summarizes age-related changes in male and female reproductive systems.

Musculoskeletal System

The kyphosis, enlarged joints, flabby muscles, and decreased height of many older persons result from the variety of musculoskeletal changes occurring with age (Fig. 5-7). Along with other body tissue, muscle fibers atrophy and decrease in number, with fibrous tissue gradually replacing muscle tissue. Overall muscle mass, muscle strength, and muscle movements are decreased; the arm and leg muscles, which become particularly flabby and weak, display these changes well. Sarcopenia, the age-related loss of muscle mass, strength, and function, is mostly seen in inactive persons; thus, the importance of exercise to minimize the loss of muscle tone and strength cannot be emphasized enough. Muscle tremors may be present and are believed to be associated with degeneration of the extrapyramidal system. The tendons shrink and harden, which causes a decrease in tendon jerks. Reflexes are lessened in the arms, are nearly totally lost in the abdomen, but are maintained in the knee. For various reasons, muscle cramping frequently occurs.

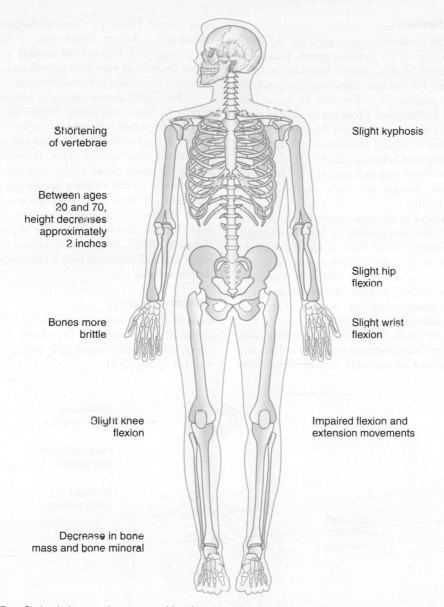

Shortening
of vertebrae

Slight kyphosis

Between ages
20 and 70,
height decreases
approximately
2 inches

Slight hip
flexion

Bones more
brittle

Slight wrist
flexion

Slight knee
flexion

Impaired flexion and
extension movements

Decrease in bone
mass and bone mineral

FIGURE 5-7 ■ Skeletal changes that occur with aging.

KEY CONCEPT

Regular exercise helps maintain muscle strength and tone and reduces some of the negative functional consequences of aging.

Bone mineral and bone mass are reduced, contributing to the brittleness of the bones of older people, especially older women who experience an accelerated rate of bone loss after menopause. Bone density decreases at a rate of 0.5% each year after the third decade of life. There is diminished calcium absorption, a gradual resorption of the interior surface of the long bones, and a slower production of new bone on the outside surface. These changes make fractures a serious risk to the older adults. Although long bones do not significantly shorten with age, thinning disks and shortening vertebrae reduce the length of the spinal column, causing a reduction in height with age. Height may be further shortened because of varying degrees of kyphosis, a backward tilting of the head, and some flexion at the hips and knees. A deterioration of the cartilage surface of joints and the formation of points and spurs may limit joint activity and motion.

Nervous System

It is difficult to identify with accuracy the exact impact of aging on the nervous system because of the dependence of this system's function on other body systems. For instance, cardiovascular problems can reduce cerebral circulation and be responsible for cerebral dysfunction. There is a decline in brain weight and a reduction in blood flow to the brain; however, these structural changes do not appear to affect thinking and behavior (Rabbitt et al., 2007). Declining nervous system function may be unnoticed because changes are often nonspecific and slowly progressing.

A reduction in neurons, nerve fibers, cerebral blood flow, and metabolism is known to occur. Reduced cerebral blood flow is accompanied by a reduction in glucose utilization and metabolic rate of oxygen in the brain. Although β-amyloid and neurofibrillary tangles are associated with Alzheimer's disease, they can be present in older adults with normal cognitive function.

The nerve conduction velocity is lower (Fig. 5-8). These changes are manifested by slower reflexes and delayed response to multiple stimuli. Kinesthetic sense lessens. There is a slower response to changes in balance, a factor contributing to falls. Slower recognition and response to stimuli is associated with a decrease in new axon growth and nerve reinnervation of injured peripheral nerves.

The hypothalamus regulates temperature less effectively. Brain cells slowly decline over the years, the cerebral cortex undergoes some loss of neurons, and there is some decrease in brain size and weight, particularly after age 55 years. Because the brain affects the sleep–wake cycle, and circadian and homeostatic factors of sleep regulation are altered with aging, changes in the sleep pattern occur, with stages III and IV of sleep becoming less prominent (Munch, Knoblauch, Blatter, Wirz-Justice, & Cajochen, 2007). Frequent awakening during sleep is not unusual, although only a minimal amount of sleep is actually lost.

Sensory Organs

Each of the five senses becomes less efficient with advanced age, interfering in varying degrees with safety, normal activities of daily living, and general well-being (Fig. 5-9).

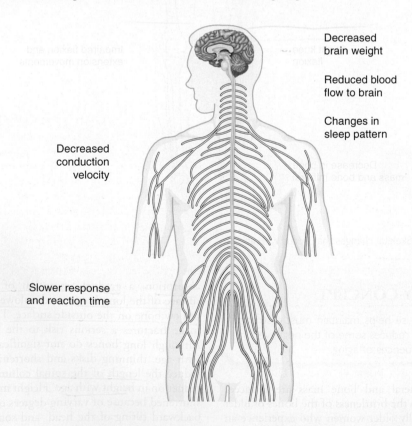

Decreased brain weight

Reduced blood flow to brain

Changes in sleep pattern

Decreased conduction velocity

Slower response and reaction time

FIGURE 5-8 ■ Neurologic changes that occur with aging.

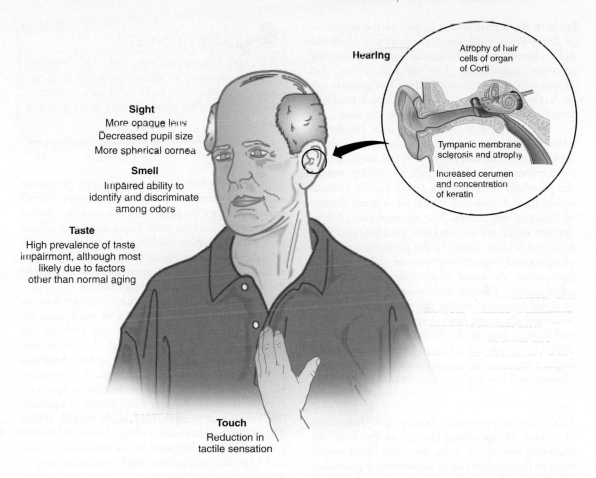

Hearing

Atrophy of hair cells of organ of Corti

Tympanic membrane sclerosis and atrophy

Increased cerumen and concentration of keratin

Sight
More opaque lens
Decreased pupil size
More spherical cornea

Smell
Impaired ability to identify and discriminate among odors

Taste
High prevalence of taste impairment, although most likely due to factors other than normal aging

Touch
Reduction in tactile sensation

FIGURE 5-9 ■ Effects of sensory changes that occur with aging.

Vision

Perhaps the sensory changes having the greatest impact are changes in vision. Presbyopia, the inability to focus or accommodate properly due to reduced elasticity of the lens, is characteristic of older eyes and begins in the fourth decade of life. The stiffening of the muscle fibers of the lens that occurs with presbyopia decreases the eye's ability to change the shape of the lens to focus on near objects and decreases the ability to adapt to light. This vision problem causes most middle-aged and older adults to need corrective lenses to accommodate close and detailed work. The visual field narrows, making peripheral vision more difficult. There is difficulty maintaining convergence and gazing upward. The pupil is less responsive to light because the pupillary sphincter hardens, the pupil size decreases, and rhodopsin content in the rods decreases. As a result, the light perception threshold increases and vision in dim areas or at night is difficult; older individuals require more light than younger persons to see adequately.

Alterations in the blood supply of the retina and retinal pigmented epithelium can cause macular degeneration, a condition in which there is a loss in central vision. Changes in the retina and retinal pathway interfere with critical flicker fusion (the point at which a flickering light is perceived as continuous rather than intermittent).

The density and size of the lens increase, causing the lens to become stiffer and more opaque. Opacification of the lens, which begins in the fifth decade, leads to the development of cataracts, which increases sensitivity to glare, blurs vision, and interferes with night vision. Exposure to the ultraviolet rays of the sun contributes to cataract development. Yellowing of the lens (possibly related to a chemical reaction involving sunlight with amino acids) and alterations in the retina that affect color perception make older people less able to differentiate the low-tone colors of the blues, greens, and violets.

Depth perception becomes distorted, causing problems in correctly judging the height of curbs and steps. This change results from a disparity between the retinal images caused by the separation of the two eyes and is known as stereopsis. Dark and light adaptation takes longer, as does the processing of visual information. Less efficient reabsorption of intraocular fluid increases the older person's risk of developing glaucoma. The ciliary muscle gradually atrophies and is replaced with connective tissue.

The appearance of the eye may be altered; reduced lacrimal secretions can cause the eyes to look dry and dull, and fat deposits can cause a partial or complete glossy white circle to develop around the periphery of the cornea (arcus senilis). Corneal sensitivity is diminished, which can increase the risk of injury to the cornea. The accumulation of lipid deposits in the cornea can cause a scattering of light rays, which blurs vision. In the posterior cavity, bits of debris and condensation become visible and may float across the visual field; these are commonly called floaters. Vitreous decreases and the proportion of liquid increases, causing the vitreous body to pull away from the retina; blurred vision, distorted images, and floaters may result. Visual acuity progressively declines with age due to decreased pupil size, scatter in the cornea and lens, opacification of the lens and vitreous, and loss of photoreceptor cells in the retina.

Hearing

Presbycusis is progressive hearing loss that occurs as a result of age-related changes to the inner ear, including loss of hair cells, decreased blood supply, reduced flexibility of basilar membrane, degeneration of spiral ganglion cells, and reduced production of endolymph. This degenerative hearing impairment is the most serious problem affecting the inner ear and retrocochlea. High-frequency sounds of 2,000 Hz and above are the first to be lost; middle and low frequencies also may be lost as the condition progresses. A variety of factors, including continued exposure to loud noise, may contribute to the occurrence of presbycusis. This problem causes speech to sound distorted as some of the high-pitched sounds (s, sh, f, ph, and ch) are filtered from normal speech and consonants are less able to be discerned. This change is so gradual and subtle that affected persons may not realize the extent of their hearing impairment. Hearing can be further jeopardized by an accumulation of cerumen in the middle ear; the higher keratin content of cerumen as one ages contributes to this problem. The acoustic reflex, which protects the inner ear and filters auditory distractions from sounds made by one's own body and voice, is diminished due to a weakening and stiffening of the middle ear muscles and ligaments. In addition to hearing problems, equilibrium can be altered because of degeneration of the vestibular structures and atrophy of the cochlea, organ of Corti, and stria vascularis.

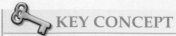

KEY CONCEPT

Although hearing declines with age, impaired hearing can occur at younger ages due to exposure to loud music, traffic, and other environmental noise. This noise-induced hearing loss is preventable.

Taste and Smell

Approximately half of all older persons experience some loss of their ability to smell. The sense of smell reduces with age because of a decrease in the number of sensory cells in the nasal lining and fewer cells in the olfactory bulb of the brain. By age 80 years, the detection of scent is almost half as sensitive as it was at its peak. Men tend to experience a greater loss in the ability to detect odors than women.

As most of the taste acuity is dependent on smell, the reduction in the sense of smell alters the sense of taste. Atrophy of the tongue with age can diminish taste sensations, although there is no conclusive evidence that the number or responsiveness of taste buds decreases (Fukunaga, A., Uematsu, H., & Sugimoto, K., 2005). A decrease in taste perception of food is thought to be related to a perceptual loss of taste (Gupta, Epstein, & Sroussi, 2006). The ability to detect salt is affected more than other taste sensations. Reduced saliva production, poor oral hygiene, medications, and conditions such as sinusitis can also affect taste.

Touch

A reduction in the number of and changes in the structural integrity of touch receptors occurs with age. Tactile sensation is reduced, as observed in the reduced ability of older persons to sense pressure and pain and differentiate temperatures. These sensory changes can cause misperceptions of the environment and, as a result, profound safety risks.

Endocrine System

The endocrine system has groups of cells and glands that produce the chemical messengers known as hormones. With age, the thyroid gland undergoes fibrosis, cellular infiltration, and increased nodularity. The resulting decreased thyroid gland activity causes a lower basal metabolic rate, reduced radioactive iodine uptake, and less thyrotropin secretion and release. Protein-bound iodine levels in the blood do not change, although total serum iodide is reduced. The release of thyroidal iodide decreases with age, and excretion of the 17-ketosteroids declines. The thyroid gland progressively atrophies, and the loss of adrenal function can further decrease thyroid activity. Secretion of thyroid-stimulating hormone (TSH) and the serum concentration of thyroxine (T4) do not change, although there is a significant reduction in triiodothyronine (T3), believed to be a result of the reduced conversion of T4 to T3. Overall, the thyroid function remains adequate.

Much of the secretory activity of the adrenal cortex is regulated by adrenocorticotropic hormone (ACTH), a pituitary hormone. As ACTH secretion decreases with age, secretory activity of the adrenal gland also decreases. Although the secretion of ACTH does not affect aldosterone secretion, it has been shown that less aldosterone is produced and excreted in the urine of older persons. The secretion of glucocorticoids, 17-ketosteroids, progesterone, androgen, and estrogen, also influenced by the adrenal gland, is reduced as well.

The pituitary gland decreases in volume by approximately 20% in older persons. Somatotropic growth hormone remains present in similar amounts, although the blood level may be reduced with age. Decreases are seen in ACTH, TSH, follicle-stimulating hormone, luteinizing hormone, and luteotropic hormone to varying degrees. Gonadal secretion declines with age, including gradual decreases in testosterone, estrogen, and progesterone. With the exception of alterations associated with changes in plasma calcium level or dysfunction of other glands, the parathyroid glands maintain their function throughout life.

There is a delayed and insufficient release of insulin by the beta cells of the pancreas in older people, and there is believed to be decreased tissue sensitivity to circulating insulin. The older person's ability to metabolize glucose is reduced, and sudden concentrations of glucose cause higher and more prolonged hyperglycemia levels; therefore, it is not unusual to detect higher blood glucose levels in nondiabetic older persons.

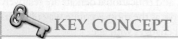

KEY CONCEPT

Higher blood glucose levels than are normal in the general adult population are not unusual in nondiabetic older people.

Integumentary System

Diet, general health, activity, exposure, and hereditary factors influence the normal course of aging of the skin. This system's changes are often the most bothersome because they are obvious and clearly reflect advancing years. Flattening of the dermal–epidermal junction, reduced thickness and vascularity of the dermis, slowing of epidermal proliferation, and an increased quantity and degeneration of elastin fibers occur. Collagen fibers become coarser and more random, reducing skin elasticity. The dermis becomes more avascular and thinner. As the skin becomes less elastic and more dry and fragile, and as subcutaneous fat is lost, lines, wrinkles, and sagging become evident. Skin becomes irritated and breaks down more easily. There is a reduction in the number of melanocytes by 10% to 20% each decade beginning by the third decade of life, and the melanocytes cluster, causing skin pigmentation, commonly referred to as age spots; these are more prevalent in areas of the body exposed to the sun. The reduction in melanocytes causes older adults to tan more slowly and less deeply. Skin immune response declines, causing older people to be more prone to skin infections. Benign and malignant skin neoplasms occur more with age.

Scalp, pubic, and axillary hair thins and grays due to a progressive loss of pigment cells and atrophy and fibrosis of hair bulbs; hair in the nose and ears becomes thicker. By age 50 years, most white men have some degree of baldness and about half of all people have evidence of gray hair. Growth rate of scalp, pubic, and axillary hair declines; the growth of facial hair may occur in older women. An increased growth of eyebrow, ear, and nostril hair occurs in older men. Fingernails grow more slowly, are fragile and brittle, develop longitudinal striations, and experience a decrease in lunula size. Perspiration is slightly reduced because the number and function of the sweat glands are lessened.

Immune System

The aging of the immune system, known as immunosenescence, includes a depressed immune response, which can cause infections to be a significant risk of older adults. After midlife, thymic mass decreases steadily, to the point that serum activity of thymic hormones is almost undetectable in the aged. T-cell activity declines and more immature T cells are present in the thymus. A significant decline in cell-mediated immunity occurs, and T lymphocytes are less able to proliferate in response to mitogens. Changes in the T cells contribute to the reactivation of varicella zoster and *Mycobacterium* tuberculosis, infections that are witnessed in many older individuals. Serum immunoglobulin (Ig) concentration is not significantly altered; the concentration of IgM is lower, whereas the concentrations of IgA and IgG are higher. Responses to influenza, parainfluenza, pneumococcus, and tetanus vaccines are less effective (although vaccination is recommended because of the serious potential consequences of infections for older adults). Inflammatory defenses decline and, often, inflammation presents atypically in older individuals (e.g., low-grade fever and minimal pain). In addition, an increase in proinflammatory cytokines occurs with age, which is believed to be linked to atherosclerosis, diabetes, osteoporosis, and other diseases that increase in prevalence with age.

Thermoregulation

Normal body temperatures are lower in later life than in younger years. Mean body temperature ranges from 96.9°F to 98.3°F orally and 98°F to 99°F rectally. Rectal and auditory canal temperatures are the most accurate and reliable indicators of body temperature in older adults.

There is a reduced ability to respond to cold temperatures due to inefficient vasoconstriction, decreased cardiac output, diminished shivering, and reduced muscle mass and subcutaneous tissue. At the other extreme, differences in response to heat are related to impaired sweating mechanisms and decreased cardiac output.

CHANGES TO THE MIND

Psychological changes can be influenced by general health status, genetic factors, educational achievement, activity, and physical and social changes. Sensory organ impairment can impede interaction with the environment and other people, thus influencing psychological status. Feeling depressed and socially isolated may obstruct optimum psychological function. Recognizing the variety of factors potentially affecting psychological status and the range of individual responses to those factors, some generalizations can be discussed.

Personality

Drastic changes in basic personality normally do not occur as one ages. The kind and gentle old person was most likely that way when young; likewise, the cantankerous old person probably was not mild and meek in earlier years. Excluding pathologic processes, the personality will be consistent with that of earlier years; possibly, it will be more openly and honestly expressed. The alleged rigidity of older persons is more a result of physical and mental limitations than a personality change. For example, an older person's insistence that her furniture not be rearranged may be interpreted as rigidity, but it may be a sound safety practice for someone coping with poor memory and visual deficits. Changes in personality traits may occur in response to events that alter self-attitude, such as retirement, death of a spouse, loss of independence, income reduction, and disability. No personality type describes all older adults. Morale, attitude, and self-esteem tend to be stable throughout the life span.

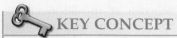

KEY CONCEPT

Personality in late life is a reflection of lifelong personality.

Memory

The three types of memory are short term, lasting from 30 seconds to 30 minutes; long term, involving that learned long ago; and sensory, which is obtained through the sensory organs and lasts only a few seconds. Retrieval of information from long-term memory can be slowed, particularly if the information is not used or needed on a daily basis. The ability to retain information in the consciousness while manipulating other information—working memory function—is reduced. Older adults can improve some age-related forgetfulness by using memory aids (mnemonic devices) such as associating a name with an image, making notes or lists, and placing objects in consistent locations. Memory deficits can result from a variety of factors other than normal aging.

Intelligence

In general, it is wise to interpret the findings related to intelligence and the older population with much caution because results may be biased from the measurement tool or method of evaluation used. Early gerontological research on intelligence and aging was guilty of such biases. Sick old people cannot be compared with healthy persons; people with different educational or cultural backgrounds cannot be compared; and one group of individuals who are skilled and capable of taking an IQ test cannot be compared with those who have sensory deficits and may not have ever taken this type of test. Longitudinal studies that measure changes in a specific generation as it ages and that compensate for sensory, health, and educational deficits are relatively recent, and they serve as the most accurate way of determining intellectual changes with age.

Basic intelligence is maintained; one does not become more or less intelligent with age. The abilities for verbal comprehension and arithmetic operations are unchanged. Crystallized intelligence, which is the knowledge accumulated over a lifetime and arises from the dominant hemisphere of the brain, is maintained through the adult years; this form of intelligence enables the individual to use past learning and experiences for problem solving. Fluid intelligence, involving new information and emanating from the nondominant hemisphere, controls emotions, retention of nonintellectual information, creative capacities, spatial perceptions, and aesthetic appreciation; this type of intelligence is believed to decline in later life. Some decline in intellectual function occurs in the moments preceding death. High levels of chronic psychological stress have been found to be associated with an increased incidence of mild cognitive impairment (Wilson et al., 2007).

Learning

Although learning ability is not seriously altered with age, other factors can interfere with the older person's ability to learn, including motivation, attention span, delayed transmission of information to the brain, perceptual deficits, and illness. Older persons may display less readiness to learn and depend on previous experience for solutions to problems rather than experiment with new problem-solving techniques. Differences in the intensity and duration of the older person's physiologic arousal may make it more difficult to extinguish previous responses and acquire new material. The early phases of the learning process tend to be more difficult for older persons than younger individuals; however, after a longer early phase, they are then able to keep equal pace. Learning occurs best when the new information is related to previously learned information. Although little difference is apparent between the old and young in verbal or abstract ability, older persons do show some difficulty with perceptual motor tasks. Some evidence indicates a tendency toward simple association rather than analysis. Because it is generally a greater problem to learn new habits when old habits exist and must be unlearned, relearned, or modified, older persons with many years of history may have difficulty in this area.

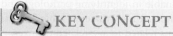

KEY CONCEPT

Older adults maintain the capacity to learn, although a variety of factors can easily interfere with the learning process.

Attention Span

Older adults demonstrate a decrease in vigilance performance (i.e., the ability to retain attention longer than 45 minutes). They are more easily distracted by irrelevant information and stimuli and are less able to perform tasks that are complicated or require simultaneous performance.

POINT TO PONDER

In the past 10 years, what changes have you experienced in regard to appearance, behaviors, and attitudes? How do you feel about these changes?

NURSING IMPLICATIONS OF AGE-RELATED CHANGES

An understanding of common aging changes is essential to ensure competent gerontological nursing practice. Such knowledge can aid in promoting practices that enhance wellness, thereby reducing risks to health and well-being. Differentiating normal from unusual findings in older adults and the atypical presentation of

CONSIDER THIS CASE

Mr. G is a 72-year-old retired truck driver admitted to the hospital for the treatment of acute glomerulonephritis. His height is 5 feet 11 inches and his weight is 180 lb. You note from the record that he weighed 220 lb last year and has experienced a reduction in weight at each of his monthly physician's visits. Although he has a moderate degree of chronic obstructive pulmonary disease, he continues to smoke one pack of cigarettes daily. He has varicosities on both lower extremities and hemorrhoids. Mr. G is coherent and responds appropriately. His wife comments that he has always had a sharp mind, although in the past few years he has become considerably quieter and less gregarious. As you observe Mr. G throughout the day, you note that he:

- becomes short of breath with minimal exertion
- develops edema
- has urinary hesitancy and scanty urine output
- adds considerable salt to his food before tasting it
- has difficulty hearing normal conversation
- moves very little when in bed

THINK CRITICALLY

- Which signs and observations are related to normal aging and which can you attribute to pathology?
- What factors contributed to the health conditions possessed by Mr. G?
- Describe the risks that are high for Mr. G and list nursing measures that could minimize them.

illness can be invaluable in identifying pathology and obtaining treatment in a timely manner. Table 5-1 lists some nursing actions related to age-related changes.

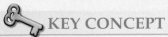

KEY CONCEPT

By promoting positive practices in persons of all ages, nurses can help greater numbers of individuals enter late life with high levels of health and function.

Nurses caring for older adults must realize that, despite the numerous changes commonly experienced with age, most older adults function admirably well and live normal, satisfying lives. Although nurses need to acknowledge factors that can alter function with aging, they should also emphasize the capabilities and assets possessed by older adults and assist persons of all ages in achieving a healthy aging process.

TABLE 5-1	Nursing Actions Related to Age-Related Changes
Age-Related Change	**Nursing Action**
Reduction in intracellular fluid	Prevent dehydration by ensuring fluid intake of at least 1,500 mL daily
Decrease in subcutaneous fat content, decline in natural insulation	Ensure adequate clothing is worn to maintain body warmth; maintain room temperatures between 70°F (21°C) and 75°F (24°C)
Lower oral temperatures	Use thermometers that register low temperatures; assess baseline norm for body temperature when patient is well to be able to identify unique manifestations of fever
Decreased cardiac output and stroke volume; increased peripheral resistance	Allow rest between activities, procedures; recognize the longer time period required for heart rate to return to normal following a stress on the heart, and evaluate presence of tachycardia accordingly; ensure blood pressure level is adequate to meet circulatory demands by assessing physical and mental function at various blood pressure levels
Decreased lung expansion, activity, and recoil; lack of basilar inflation; increased rigidity of lungs and thoracic cage; less effective gas exchange and cough response	Encourage respiratory activity; recognize that atypical symptoms and signs can accompany respiratory infection; monitor oxygen administration closely, keep oxygen infusion rate under 4 mL, unless otherwise prescribed
Brittleness of teeth; retraction of gingiva	Encourage daily flossing and brushing; ensure patient visits dentist annually; inspect oral cavity for periodontal disease, jagged-edged teeth, other pathologies
Reduced acuity of taste sensations	Observe for overconsumption of sweets and salt; be sure foods are served attractively; season food healthfully
Drier oral cavity	Offer fluids during meals; have patient drink before swallowing tablets and capsules, and examine oral cavity after administration to ensure drugs have been swallowed
Decreased esophageal and gastric motility; decreased gastric acid	Assess for indigestion; encourage five to six small meals rather than three large ones; advise patient not to lie down for at least 1 hour following meals

TABLE 5-1	Nursing Actions Related to Age-Related Changes (Continued)

Age-Related Change	Nursing Action
Decreased colonic peristalsis; duller neural impulses to lower bowel	Encourage toileting schedule to provide adequate time for bowel elimination; monitor frequency, consistency, and amount of bowel movements
Decreased size of renal mass, number of nephrons, renal blood flow, glomerular filtration rate, tubular function	Ensure age-adjusted drug dosages are prescribed; observe for adverse responses to drugs; recognize that urine testing for glucose can be unreliable, urinary creatinine excretion and creatinine clearance are decreased, and blood urea nitrogen level is higher
Decreased bladder capacity	Assist patient with need for frequent toileting; ensure safety for visits to bathroom during the night
Weaker bladder muscles	Observe for signs of urinary tract infection; assist patient to void in upright position
Enlargement of prostate gland	Ensure patient has prostate examined annually
Drier, more fragile vagina	Advise patient in safe use of lubricants for comfort during intercourse
Increased alkalinity of vaginal canal	Observe for signs of vaginitis
Atrophy of muscle; reduction in muscle strength and mass	Encourage regular exercise; advise patient to avoid straining or overusing muscles
Decreased bone mass and mineral content	Instruct patient in safety measures to prevent falls and fractures; encourage good calcium intake and exercise
Less prominent stages III and IV of sleep	Avoid interruptions at night; assess quantity and quality of sleep
Decreased visual accommodation; reduced peripheral vision; less effective vision in dark and dimly lit areas	Ensure patient has ophthalmologic exam annually; use night lights; avoid drastic changes in level of lighting; ensure objects used by patient are within visual field
Yellowing of lens	Avoid using shades of greens, blues, and violets together
Decreased corneal sensitivity	Advise patient to protect eyes
Presbycusis	Ensure patient has audiometric exam if problem exists, speak to patient in loud, low-pitched voice
Reduced capacity to sense pain and pressure	Ensure patient changes positions before tissue reddens; inspect body for problems that patient may not sense; recognize unique responses to pain
Reduced immunity	Prevent persons who have infectious diseases from infection early; recommend pneumococcal, tetanus, and annual influenza vaccinations; promote good nutritional status to improve host defenses
Slower metabolic rate	Advise patient to avoid excess calorie consumption
Altered secretion of insulin and metabolism of glucose	Advise patient to avoid high carbohydrate intake, observe for unique manifestations of hyper- or hypoglycemia
Flattening of dermal–epidermal junction; reduced thickness and vascularity of dermis; degeneration of elastin fibers	Use principles of pressure ulcer prevention
Skin drier	Recognize need for less frequent bathing; avoid use of harsh soaps; use skin softeners
Slower response and reaction time	Allow adequate time for patient to respond, process information, and perform tasks

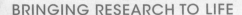

BRINGING RESEARCH TO LIFE

COMPARISON OF AGE AND TIME-TO-DEATH IN THE DEDIFFERENTIATION OF LATE-LIFE COGNITIVE ABILITIES

Batterham, P.J., Christensen, H., & Mackinnon, A.J. (2011). Psychology and Aging, 26(4), 844–851.

The *dedifferentiation hypothesis* proposes that specific cognitive abilities become more highly associated with general ability in old age and that this results from pathology that affects fluid intelligence. Because the evidence supporting this hypothesis was found by the researchers to be limited, they examined cognitive abilities of aging individuals.

The Canberra Longitudinal Study community-based cohort, consisting of 896 Australian adults aged 70 and older, provided data from 687 persons who were followed for up to 17 years prior to their death. Changes in cognitive ability were found to be related to dementia and other pathologies rather than normal aging. It was suggested that theories of cognitive function need to account for the diversity of late-life abilities and pathology.

This study demonstrates that there remains much to be learned about "normal aging." When changes in intellectual function are noted, even when assumed to be consistent with normal aging, nurses should review the history for previous intellectual function, any recent changes noted, and the presence of conditions that could affect intellectual ability. Although upon initial assessment an older adult may be found to have evidence of decreased fluid intelligence, if the history reveals good fluid intelligence until recently, this finding could be an abnormality for this individual, reflective of a pathological condition, despite the fact that it is assumed to be a common finding in many older adults.

PRACTICE REALITIES

You are working in an office with a group of medical doctors who have had some of the same patients in their practice for nearly two decades. Although many of their patients have aged, the physicians use basically the same approach, reorder the same medications, and include no review of psychosocial issues.

What could you suggest to update the practice to assure the needs of the aging patients are adequately being addressed?

CRITICAL THINKING EXERCISES

1. What efforts do you see to educate persons of all ages in practices that will foster a healthy aging experience?

2. What age-related changes can you identify in yourself and in your parents?

3. Consider recommendations that you would give young adults for promotion of a healthy aging process.

REFERENCES

Fukunaga, A., Uematsu, H., & Sugimoto, K. (2005). Influences of aging on taste perception and oral somatic sensation. *Journal of Gerontology, Series A, Biological Sciences, 60*(1), 109–113.

Gupta, A., Epstein, J. B., & Sroussi, H. (2006). Hyposalivation in elderly patients. *Journal of the Canadian Dental Association, 72*(9), 841–846.

Kielstein, J. T., Body-Boger, S. M., Frolich, J. C., Ritz, E., Haller, H., & Fliser, D. (2003). Asymmetric dimethyl-

arginine, blood pressure, and renal perfusion in elderly subjects. *Circulation, 107*(14), 1891–1895.

Lerma, E.V. (2009). Anatomic and physiologic changes of the aging kidney. *Clinics in Geriatric Medicine, 25,* 325–329.

Marks, L. S., Roehrborn, C. G., & Andiole, G. L. (2006). Prevention of benign prostatic hyperplasia disease. *Journal of Urology, 176*(4), 1299–1406.

Munch, M., Knoblauch, V., Blatter, K., Wirz-Justice, A., & Cajochen, C. (2007). Is homeostatic sleep regulation under low sleep pressure modified by age? *Sleep, 30*(6), 781–792.

Ney, D., Weiss, J, Kind, A., & Robinson, J. A. (2009). Senescent swallowing: Impact, strategies and interventions. *Nutrition in Clinical Practice, 24*(3), 395–413.

Rabbitt, P., Scott, M., Lunn, M., Thacker, N., Lowe, C., Pendleton, N., Jackson, A., et al. (2007). White matter lesions account for all age-related declines in speed but not in intelligence. *Neuropsychology, 21*(3), 363–370.

Sampson, N., Untergasser, G., Plas, E., & Berger, P. (2007). The aging male reproductive tract. *Journal of Pathology, 211*(2), 206–218.

Shaker, R., Ren, J., Bardan, E., Easterling, C., Dua, K., Xie, P., & Kern, M. (2003). Pharyngoglottal closure reflex: Characterization in healthy young, elderly and dysphagic patients with predeglutitive aspiration. *Gerontology, 49*(1), 12–20.

St-Onge, M. P., & Gallagher, D. (2010). Body composition changes with aging: The cause or the result of alternations in metabolic rate and macronutrient oxidation? *Nutrition, 26*(2), 152–155.

Wilson, R. S., Schneider, J. A., Boyle, P. A., Arnold, S. E., Tang, Y., & Bennett, D. A. (2007). Chronic distress and incidence of mild cognitive impairment. *Neurology, 68*(24), 2085–2092.

Woo, J., Leung, J., & Kwok, T. (2007). BMI, body composition, and physical functioning in older adults. *Obesity, 15*(7), 1886–1894.

RECOMMENDED READINGS

Recommended Readings associated with this chapter can be found on the web site that accompanies the book. Visit **http://thepoint.lww.com/Eliopoulos8e** to access the recommended readings and other additional resources associated with this chapter.

UNIT 2

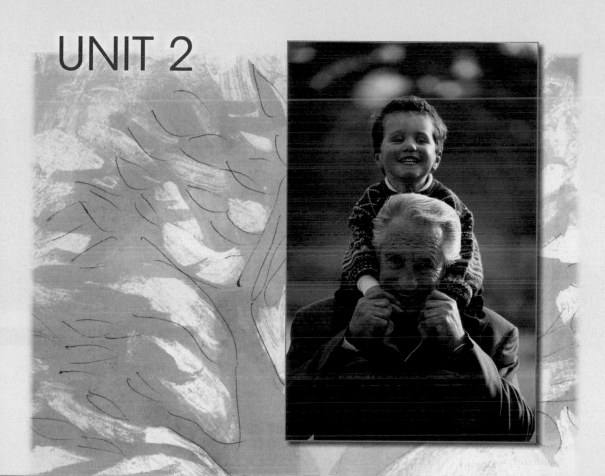

Foundations of Gerontological Nursing

The Specialty of Gerontological Nursing

LEARNING OBJECTIVES

After reading this chapter, you should be able to:

1. Describe the importance of evidence-based practice in gerontological nursing.

2. Identify standards used in gerontological nursing practice.

3. List principles guiding gerontological nursing practice.

4. Discuss major roles for gerontological nurses.

5. Discuss future challenges for gerontological nursing.

TERMS TO KNOW

Competency: having skill, knowledge, and ability to do something according to a standard

Evidence-based practice: using research and scientific information to guide actions

Geriatric nursing: nursing care of sick older adults

Gerontological nursing: nursing practice that promotes wellness and highest quality of life for aging individuals

Standard: desired, evidence-based expectations of care that serve as a model against which practice can be judged

The specialty of gerontological nursing was not always a popular or well-respected area of practice. However, over the past few decades, the specialty has experienced profound growth and has benefited from societal recognition of the importance of the older segment of the population. Nurses have many opportunities to play significant roles in the care of the aging population today and to shape the future of gerontological nursing.

DEVELOPMENT OF GERONTOLOGICAL NURSING

Nurses, long interested in the care of older adults, seem to have assumed more responsibility than other professional disciplines for this segment of the population. In 1904, the *American Journal of Nursing* printed the first nursing article on the care of the aged, presenting many principles that continue to guide gerontological nursing practice today (Bishop, 1904): "You must not treat a young child as you would a grown person, nor must you treat an old person as you would one in the prime of life." Interestingly, this same journal featured an article entitled "The Old Nurse," which emphasized the value of the aging nurse's years of experience (DeWitt, 1904).

After the Federal Old Age Insurance Law (better known as Social Security) was passed in 1935, many older persons had an alternative to alms houses and could independently purchase room and board. Because many of the homes that offered these services for older persons were operated by women who called themselves nurses, such residences later became known as nursing homes.

For many years, care of older adults was an unpopular branch of nursing practice. Geriatric nurses—those nurses who care for ill older adults—were thought to be somewhat inferior in capabilities, neither good enough for acute care settings nor ready to retire. Geriatric facilities may have further discouraged many competent nurses from working in these settings by paying low salaries. Little existed to counter the negativism in educational programs, where experiences with older persons were inadequate in both quantity and quality and attention focused on the sick rather than the well, who were more representative of the older population. Although nurses were among the few professionals involved with older adults, gerontology was missing from most nursing curriculums until recently.

Frustration over the lack of value placed on geriatric nursing led to an appeal to the American Nurses Association (ANA) for assistance in promoting the status of this area of practice. After years of study, in 1961 the ANA recommended that a specialty group for geriatric nurses be formed. In 1962, the ANA's Conference Group on Geriatric Nursing Practice held its first national meeting. This group became the Division of Geriatric Nursing in 1966, gaining full recognition as a nursing specialty. An important contribution by this group was the development in 1969 of *Standards for Geriatric Nursing Practice*, first published in 1970. Certification of nurses for excellence in geriatric nursing practice followed, with the first 74 nurses achieving this recognition in 1975. The birth of the *Journal of*

Gerontological Nursing, the first professional journal to meet the specific needs and interests of gerontological nurses, also occurred in 1975.

Through the 1970s, nurses became increasingly aware of their role in promoting a healthy aging experience for all individuals and ensuring the wellness of older adults. As a result, they expressed interest in changing the name of the specialty from geriatric to gerontological nursing to reflect a broader scope than the care of the ill aged. In 1976, the Geriatric Nursing Division became the Gerontological Nursing Division. Box 6-1 lists landmarks in the development and growth of gerontological nursing.

 KEY CONCEPT

Gerontological nursing involves the care of aging people and emphasizes the promotion of the highest possible quality of life and wellness throughout the life span. Geriatric nursing focuses on the care of sick older persons.

In the past few decades, the specialty of gerontological nursing has experienced profound growth. Whereas only 32 articles on the topic of the nursing care of older adults were listed in the *Cumulative Index to Nursing Literature* in 1956, and only twice that number appeared a decade later, the number of articles published has grown considerably since. Gerontological nursing texts grew from a few in the 1960s to dozens currently, and the quantity and quality of this literature has been rising as well. Growing numbers of nursing schools are including gerontological nursing courses in their undergraduate programs and offering advanced degrees with a major in this area. Certification offers a means by which the nurse's knowledge and competencies are validated through a professional nursing organization. Registered nurses can receive certification as a generalist in gerontological nursing with a basic nursing degree and 2 years of experience in the specialty or advanced certification as a clinical nurse specialist in gerontological nursing or gerontological nurse practitioner with graduate education and additional experience. (For information on certification, see the Resource listing for the American Nurses' Credentialing Center at the end of this chapter.) Nursing administration in long-term care, geropsychiatric nursing, geriatric rehabilitation, and other areas of subspecialization have evolved; many nursing specialty associations have developed position papers related to the integration of geriatric nursing into their unique specialty practice (these often are posted on the association web sites). The Hartford Institute for Geriatric Nursing, established in the 1990s, has

BOX 6-1   Landmarks in the Growth of Gerontological Nursing

1902   First article on care of aged in *American Journal of Nursing* written by a physician

1904   First article on care of aged in *American Journal of Nursing* written by a nurse

1950   First gerontological nursing text published (*Geriatric Nursing*, K. Newton)

First master's thesis on care of aged (Eleanor Pingrey)

Geriatrics recognized as an area of specialization in nursing

1952   First nursing study on care of aged published in *Nursing Research*

1961   American Nurses Association (ANA) recommends specialty group for geriatric nurses

1962   First national meeting of ANA Conference on Geriatric Nursing Practice

1966   Formation of Geriatric Nursing Division of ANA

First gerontological nursing clinical specialist nursing program (Duke University)

1968   First nurse makes presentation at International Congress of Gerontology (Laurie Gunter)

1969   Development of standards for geriatric nursing practice

1970   First publication of *ANA Standards of Gerontological Nursing Practice*

1973   First offering of ANA Certification in Gerontological Nursing (74 nurses certified)

1975   First specialty publication for gerontological nurses, *Journal of Gerontological Nursing*

First nursing conference at International Congress of Gerontology

1976   ANA changes name from Geriatric Nursing Division to Gerontological Nursing Division

1976   Publication of *ANA Standards of Gerontological Nursing*

ANA Certification of Geriatric Nurse Practitioners initiated

1980   *Geriatric Nursing* journal launched by *American Journal of Nursing* company

1981   First International Conference on Gerontological Nursing

ANA Division of Gerontological Nursing develops statement on scope of practice

1982   Development of Robert Wood Johnson Teaching Home Nursing Program

1983   First university chair in gerontological nursing in the United States (Case Western Reserve)

1984   National Gerontological Nursing Association (NGNA) formed

ANA Division of Gerontological Nursing Practice becomes Council on Gerontological Nursing

1986   National Association for Directors of Nursing Administration in Long-Term Care (NADONA/LTC) formed

1989   ANA Certification of Gerontological Clinical Specialists first offered

1990   Division of Long-Term Care established within ANA Council of Gerontological Nursing

1996   Hartford Gerontological Nursing Initiatives funding launched by John A. Hartford Foundation

2001   ANA publishes revised *Standards and Scope of Gerontological Nursing Practice*

2002   Nurse Competence in Aging initiative to provide gerontological education and activities within specialty nursing associations

2004   American Association of Colleges of Nursing publishes competencies for advanced practice programs in gerontological nursing

2007   American Association for Long-Term Care Nursing formed

---

significantly contributed to the advancement of the specialty by identifying and developing best practices and facilitating the implementation of these practices (for more information, visit http://www.hartfordign.org). In 2003, the Hartford Institute for Geriatric Nursing collaborated with the American Academy of Nursing and the American Association of Colleges of Nursing to develop the Hartford Geriatric Nursing Initiative that has significantly contributed to the growth of evidence-based practice in the specialty. Gerontological nursing has indeed

advanced rapidly, and all indications are that this growth will continue.

Along with the growth of the specialty there has been a heightened awareness of the complexity of gerontological nursing. Older people exhibit great diversity in terms of health status, cultural background, lifestyle, living arrangement, socioeconomic status, and other variables. Most have chronic conditions that uniquely affect acute illnesses, reactions to treatments, and quality of life. Symptoms of illness can be atypical. Multiple health conditions can coexist and muddle the ability to chart the course of a single disease or identify the underlying cause of symptoms. The conditions that older adults experience can cut across many clinical specialties, thereby challenging gerontological nurses to have a broad knowledge base. The risk of complications is high. Other factors, such as limited finances or social isolation, affect the state of health and well-being. Also, the elective status of geriatrics in many medical and nursing schools can limit the pool of colleagues who are knowledgeable about the unique aspects of caring for older adults.

CORE ELEMENTS OF GERONTOLOGICAL NURSING PRACTICE

With the formalization and growth of the gerontological nursing specialty, nurses and nursing organizations have developed informal and formal guidelines for clinical practice. Some of these core elements include evidence-based practice and standards and principles of gerontological nursing.

Evidence-Based Practice

There was a time when nursing care was guided more by trial and error than sound research and knowledge. Fortunately, that has changed, and nursing now follows a systematic approach that uses existing research for clinical decision making—a process known as evidence-based practice. Testing, evaluating, and using research findings in the nursing care of older adults is of such importance that it is among the ANA Standards of Professional Gerontological Nursing Performance.

Evidence-based practice relies on the synthesis and analysis of available information from research. Among the more popular ways to report this information are the meta-analysis and cost-analysis (Agency for Healthcare Research and Quality, 2008). *Meta-analysis* is a process of analyzing and compiling the results of published research studies on a specific topic. This process combines the results of many small studies to allow more significant conclusions to be made. With *cost-analysis* reporting, cost-related data are gathered on outcomes to make comparisons. Performance also can be compared with best practices or industry averages through a process of *benchmarking*. For instance, the rate of pressure ulcers in one facility may be compared with another facility that has similar characteristics. The data can be used to stimulate improvements.

KEY CONCEPT

Best practices are evidence based and are built on the expertise of the nurse.

Standards

Professional nursing practice is guided by standards. Standards reflect the level and expectations of care that are desired and serve as a model against which practice can be judged. Thus, standards serve to both guide and evaluate nursing practice.

Standards arise from a variety of sources. State and federal regulations outline minimum standards of practice for various health care workers (e.g., nurse practice acts) and agencies (e.g., nursing homes). The Joint Commission has developed standards for various clinical settings that strive to describe the maximum attainable performance levels. The ANA Scope and Standards of Practice for Gerontological Nursing, as listed in Box 6-2, are the only standards developed by and for gerontological nurses. Nurses must regularly evaluate their actual practices against all standards governing their practice areas to ensure their actions reflect the highest quality care possible.

Competencies

Nurses who work with older adults need to have competencies specific to gerontological nursing to promote the highest possible quality of care to older adults. Although they can vary based on educational preparation, level of practice, and practice setting, some basic competencies of the gerontological nurse include the ability to:

- differentiate normal from abnormal findings in the older adult
- assess the older adult's physical, emotional, mental, social, and spiritual status and function
- engage the older adult in all aspects of care to the maximum extent possible
- provide information and education on a level and in a language appropriate for the individual
- individualize care planning and implementation of the plan
- identify and reduce risks
- empower the older adult to exercise maximum decision making
- identify and respect preferences arising from the older adult's culture, language, race, gender, sexual preference, lifestyle, experiences, and roles
- assist the older adult in evaluating, deciding, locating, and transitioning to environments that fulfill living and care needs
- advocate for and protect the rights of the older person
- facilitate discussion of and honor advance directives

To maintain and improve competencies, nurses need to stay abreast of new research, resources, and

BOX 6-2 ANA Standards of Practice for Gerontological Nursing

STANDARD 1. ASSESSMENT

The gerontological nurse collects comprehensive data pertinent to the older adult's physical and mental health or situation.

STANDARD 2. DIAGNOSIS

The gerontological nurse analyzes the assessment data to determine the diagnoses or issues.

STANDARD 3. OUTCOME IDENTIFICATION

The gerontological nurse identifies expected outcomes for a plan individualized to the older adult or situation.

STANDARD 4. PLANNING

The gerontological nurse develops a plan to attain expected outcomes.

STANDARD 5. IMPLEMENTATION

The gerontological nurse implements the identified plan.

STANDARD 5A: COORDINATION OF CARE

The gerontological nurse coordinates care delivery.

STANDARD 5B: HEALTH TEACHING AND HEALTH PROMOTION

The gerontological registered nurse employs strategies to promote health and a safe environment.

STANDARD 5C: CONSULTATION

The gerontological advanced practice registered nurse provides consultation to influence the identified plan, enhance the abilities of others, and effect change.

STANDARD 5D: PRESCRIPTIVE AUTHORITY AND TREATMENT

The gerontological advanced practice registered nurse uses prescriptive authority, procedures, referrals, treatments, and therapies in accordance with state and federal laws and regulations.

STANDARD 6. EVALUATION

The gerontological nurse evaluates the older adult's progress toward attainment of expected outcomes.

Source: From American Nurses Association. (2010). *Gerontological nursing scope and standards of practice.* Silver Spring, MD: Nursebooks.org. (A full copy of the standards that includes the measurement criteria and Standards of Professional Performance for Gerontological Nursing can be ordered from the American Nurses Association, http://www.nursesbooks.org.)

best practices. This is a personal responsibility of the professional nurse.

Principles

Scientific data regarding theories, life adjustments, normal aging, and pathophysiology of aging are combined with selected information from psychology, sociology, biology, and other physical and social sciences (Fig. 6-1) to develop nursing principles. Nursing principles are those proven facts or widely accepted theories that guide nursing actions. Professional nurses are responsible for using these principles as the foundation for nursing practice and ensuring through educational and managerial means that other caregivers use a sound knowledge base.

In addition to the basic principles that direct the delivery of care to persons in general, specific and unique principles guide care for individuals of certain age groups or those who possess particular

health problems. Some of the principles guiding gerontological nursing practice are listed in Box 6-3 and are discussed below.

Aging: A Natural Process

Every living organism begins aging from the time of conception. The process of maturing or aging helps the individual achieve the level of cellular, organ, and system function necessary for the accomplishment of life tasks. Constantly and continuously, every cell of every organism ages. Despite the normality and naturalness of this experience, many people approach aging as though it were a pathologic experience. For example, commonly heard comments associate aging with:

- "looking gray and wrinkled"
- "losing one's intellectual function"
- "becoming sick and frail"
- "obtaining little satisfaction from life"

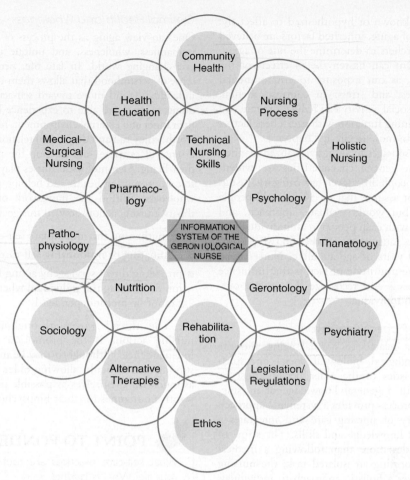

FIGURE 6-1 ■ Information system of the gerontological nurse.

- "returning to childlike behavior"
- "being useless"

These are hardly valid descriptions of the outcomes of aging for most people. Aging is not a crippling disease; even with limitations that could be imposed by pathologies of late life, opportunities for usefulness, fulfillment, and joy are readily present. A realistic understanding of the aging process can promote a positive attitude toward old age.

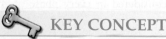

KEY CONCEPT

Aging is a natural experience, not a pathologic process.

Factors Influencing the Aging Process

Heredity, nutrition, health status, life experiences, environment, activity, and stress produce unique effects in each individual. Among the variety of

---

BOX 6-3   Principles of Gerontological Nursing Practice

- Aging is a natural process common to all living organisms.
- Various factors influence the aging process.
- Unique data and knowledge are used in applying the nursing process to the older population.

- Older adults share similar self-care and human needs with all other human beings.
- Gerontological nursing strives to help older adults achieve wholeness by reaching optimum levels of physical, psychological, social, and spiritual health.

factors either known or hypothesized to affect the usual pattern of aging, inherited factors are believed by some researchers to determine the rate of aging. Malnourishment can hasten the ill effects of the aging process, as can exposure to environmental toxins, diseases, and stress. In contrast, mental, physical, and social activity can reduce the rate and degree of declining function with age. These factors are examined in more detail in Chapter 2.

Every person ages in an individualized manner, although some general characteristics are evident among most people in a given age category. Just as one would not assume that all 30-year-old people are identical but would evaluate, approach, and communicate with each person in an individualized manner, nurses must recognize that no two persons 60, 70, or 80 years of age are alike. Nurses must understand the multitude of factors that influence the aging process and recognize the unique outcomes for each individual.

The Nursing Process Framework

Scientific data related to normal aging and the unique psychological, biological, social, and spiritual characteristics of the older person must be integrated with a general knowledge of nursing. The nursing process provides a systematic approach to the delivery of nursing care and integrates a wide range of knowledge and skills. The scope of nursing includes more than following a medical order or performing an isolated task; the nursing process involves a holistic approach to individuals and the care they require. The unique physiologic, psychological, social, and spiritual challenges of older adults are considered in every phase of the nursing process.

Common Needs

Core needs that promote health and optimum quality of life for all patients are:

- *Physiological balance*: respiration, circulation, nutrition, hydration, elimination, movement, rest, comfort, immunity, and risk reduction
- *Connection:* familial, relational, societal, cultural, environmental, spiritual, and self
- *Gratification*: purpose, pleasure, and dignity

Through self-care practices, people usually perform activities independently and voluntarily to meet these life requirements. When an unusual circumstance interferes with an individual's ability to meet these demands, nursing intervention could be warranted. The requirements for these needs and specific problems that older persons may experience in fulfilling them are discussed in Units III through V.

Optimal Health and Wholeness

One can view aging as the process of realizing one's humanness, wholeness, and unique identity in an ever-changing world. In late life, people achieve a sense of personhood that allows them to demonstrate individuality and move toward self-actualization. By doing so, they are able to experience harmony with their inner and external environment, realize their self-worth, enjoy full and deep social relationships, achieve a sense of purpose, and develop the many facets of their being. Gerontological nurses play an important role in promoting health and helping people achieve wholeness. Within the framework of the self-care theory, nursing actions toward this goal are:

- strengthening the individual's self-care capacity
- eliminating or minimizing self-care limitations
- providing direct services by acting for, doing for, or assisting the individual when demands cannot be met independently

The thread woven throughout the above nursing actions is the promotion of maximum independence. Although it may be more time-consuming and difficult, allowing older persons to do as much for themselves as possible produces many positive outcomes for their biopsychosocial health.

POINT TO PONDER

What self-care practices are routine parts of your life? What is lacking?

GERONTOLOGICAL NURSING ROLES

In their activities with older adults, nurses function in a variety of roles, most of which fall under the categories of healer, caregiver, educator, advocate, and innovator (Fig. 6-2).

Healer

Early nursing practice was based on the Christian concept of the intertwining of the flesh and spirit. In the mid-1800s, nursing's role as a healing art was recognized; this is apparent through Florence Nightingale's writings that nursing "puts the patient in the best condition for nature to act upon him" (Nightingale, 1860). As medical knowledge and technology grew more sophisticated and the nursing profession became grounded more in science than in healing arts, the early emphasis on nurturance, comfort, empathy, and intuition was replaced by detachment, objectivity, and scientific approaches. However, the revival of the holistic approach to health care has enabled nurses to again recognize

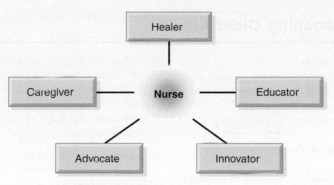

FIGURE 6-2 ■ Gerontological nursing roles.

the interdependency of body, mind, and spirit in health and healing.

Nursing plays a significant role in helping individuals stay well, overcome or cope with disease, restore function, find meaning and purpose in life, and mobilize internal and external resources. In the healer role, the gerontological nurse recognizes that most human beings value health, are responsible and active participants in their health maintenance and illness management, and desire harmony and wholeness with their environment. A holistic approach is essential, recognizing that older individuals must be viewed in the context of their biological, emotional, social, cultural, and spiritual elements. (Information on holistic nursing can be obtained from the American Holistic Nurses' Association, listed under Resources at the end of this chapter.)

POINT TO PONDER

Henri Nouwen (1990) spoke of the "wounded healer" who uses his or her own problems or wounds as a means to assist in the healing of others. What life experiences or "wounds" do you possess that enable you to assist others in their healing journeys?

For healing to be a dynamic process, nurses need to identify their own weaknesses, vulnerabilities, and need for continued self-healing. This belief is consistent with the concept of the wounded healer and suggests that by recognizing the wounds of all human beings, including themselves, nurses can provide services within a loving, compassionate framework.

Caregiver

The major role played by nurses is that of a caregiver. In this role, gerontological nurses use gerontological

theory in the conscientious application of the nursing process to the care of older adults. Inherent in this role is the active participation of older adults and their significant others and promotion of the highest degree of self-care. This is especially significant in that older adults who are ill and disabled are at risk for having decisions made and actions taken for them, in the interest of "providing care," "efficiency," and "best interest"—that rob them of their existing independence.

Although the body of knowledge of geriatrics and gerontological care has grown considerably, many practitioners lack this information. Gerontological nurses are challenged to ensure that the care of older adults is based on sound knowledge that reflects the unique characteristics, needs, and responses of older persons by disseminating gerontological principles and practices. Nurses working in this specialty area are challenged to gain the knowledge and skills that will enable them to meet the unique needs of older adults and to assure evidence-based practices are utilized.

Educator

Gerontological nurses must be prepared to take advantage of formal and informal opportunities to share knowledge and skills related to the care of older adults. This education extends beyond professionals to the general public. Areas in which gerontological nurses can educate others include normal aging, pathophysiology, geriatric pharmacology, health promotion, and available resources. With the diversity and complexities of health insurance plans, an important area for consumer education is teaching older adults how to interpret and compare various plans to enable them to make informed decisions. Essential to the educator role is effective communication involving listening, interacting, clarifying, coaching, validating, and evaluating.

BOX 6-4 Teaching Older Adults

When teaching older adults:
- Assess knowledge deficits, readiness to learn, and obstacles that could interfere with the learning process
- Organize the material prior to the teaching experience
- Plan strategies to actively engage them in the learning process
- Assure the environment is conducive to learning (e.g., comfortable room temperature, noise control, avoidance of glare, and lack of distractions and interruptions)
- Be sensitive to vision and hearing deficits that are present
- Speak on a level and in a language that is understandable
- Avoid medical jargon
- Use several different teaching methods to supplement verbal presentation (e.g., videos, demonstration, PowerPoint slides, pamphlets, and fact sheets)

- Provide written material to complement verbal instruction; as blues and greens are difficult colors for older eyes, avoid using blue print on green paper
- Summarize what has been taught and recognize knowledge gains

Be aware of potential barriers to learning:
- Stress
- Sensory deficits
- Limited educational or intellectual abilities
- Emotional state
- Pain, fatigue, and other symptoms
- Unmet physiological needs
- Attitudes or beliefs held about topic
- Prior experience with issue
- Feelings of helplessness and hopelessness

The nurse's educator role also surfaces during routine nurse–patient interactions. The nurse educates the patient to address knowledge deficits identified during the assessment process. New medications, treatments, and choices create the need for teaching to assure the patient has the knowledge and skill to competently make decisions and engage in care. Box 6-4 outlines some of the principles of adult learning and some of the barriers to learning.

Advocate

The gerontological nurse can function as an advocate in several ways. First and foremost, advocacy for individual clients is essential and can include aiding older adults in asserting their rights and obtaining required services. In addition, nurses can advocate to facilitate a community's or other group's efforts to effect change and achieve benefits for older adults and to promote gerontological nursing, including new and expanded roles of nurses in this specialty.

Innovator

Gerontological nursing continues to be an evolving specialty; therefore, nurses have opportunities to develop new technologies and different modalities of care delivery. As an innovator, the gerontological nurse assumes an inquisitive style, making conscious decisions and efforts to experiment for an end result of improved gerontological practice. This requires the nurse to be willing to think "out of the box" and take risks associated with traveling down new roads, transforming visions into reality.

These roles can be actualized in a variety of practice settings, discussed in Chapter 10, and offer opportunities for gerontological nurses to demonstrate significant creativity and leadership.

ADVANCED PRACTICE NURSING ROLES

To competently and effectively care for the clinical complexities of older adults, nurses need preparation in the unique principles and best practices of geriatric care. This requires a broad knowledge base, capacity for independent practice and leadership, and complex clinical problem-solving ability that is possible by nurses prepared for advanced practice roles. Advance practice roles include geriatric nurse practitioners, geriatric nurse clinical specialists, and geropsychiatric nurse clinicians. Most of these roles require the completion of a master's degree at a minimum.

There is strong evidence that nurses in advanced practice roles make a significant difference to the care of older adults. Gerontological nurse practitioners and clinical nurse specialists have been shown to improve the quality and reduce the cost of care for older persons in a variety of settings, including hospitals, nursing homes, and ambulatory care.

The clear positive impact on the health and well-being of older adults should encourage gerontological nurses to pursue these types of advanced practice roles and to encourage the employment of these advanced practitioners in their clinical settings.

THE FUTURE OF GERONTOLOGICAL NURSING

Historically, nurses were the major caregivers to older adults. Going forward, gerontological nurses must strive to protect both the care of older adults and the specialty of gerontological nursing. Tremendous strides have been made already. Dynamic professionals are selecting gerontological nursing as a specialty that offers a multitude of opportunities to use a wide range of knowledge and skills and one that presents many challenges that can be independently addressed within the realm of nursing practice. Excellent research for and by nurses is growing to provide a strong scientific foundation for practice. Increasing numbers of nursing schools are adding specialization in gerontological nursing. New opportunities for gerontological nurses to develop practice models are emerging in acute hospitals, assisted-living settings, health maintenance

organizations, life-care communities, adult day treatment centers, and other settings (Fig. 6-3). The future of gerontological nursing appears dynamic and exciting. Nevertheless, more challenges exist.

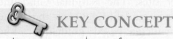

KEY CONCEPT

Increasing numbers of nurses are finding gerontological nursing to be a dynamic specialty that affords significant opportunities for independence and creativity.

Utilize Evidence-Based Practices

Considerable knowledge has been gained through research that can guide practice that is based on evidence rather than assumption; the body of knowledge continuously grows and changes. Practices that were routine in years past may have since been discovered to be ineffective or even harmful. This challenges nurses in keeping abreast of and utilizing evidence-based practices.

Gerontological nurses can access literature upon which evidence-based practice can be obtained from several sources. The Cochrane Collaboration (www.cochrane.org) publishes Cochrane Reviews,

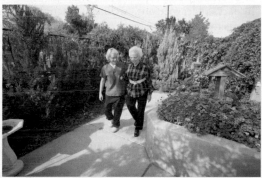

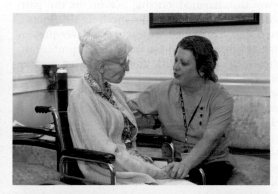

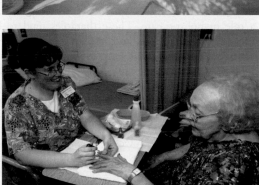

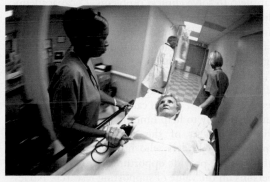

FIGURE 6-3 ■ The specialty of gerontological nursing offers multiple opportunities to use a wide range of knowledge and skills in a variety of settings. (Photo by Rick Brady.)

systematic assessments of research that meet the highest standard in evidence-based practice. Among the collaboration's valuable resources are links to databases offering online access to medical evidence from other sites. The National Guideline Clearinghouse (www.guideline.gov), as the name implies, offers evidence-based guidelines. The Hartford Institute for Geriatric Nursing (www .hartfordign.org) offers many evidence-based resources to guide geriatric nursing practice. In addition, geriatric and gerontological journals and publications of professional associations provide reports of recent research.

The gerontological nurse should assure that when new policies and procedures are being developed in the workplace, they are based on evidence. This may require the nurse to conduct a literature search and summarize and present findings to other members of the team. Bridging research to the practice setting is an important function of the gerontological nurse.

Advance Research

The growing complexity of and demand for gerontological nursing services is exciting and challenging but is accompanied by the need for a strong knowledge base on which these services can be built. There is no room for the trial and error that flavored nursing actions in the past; older adults' delicately balanced health status, increased consumer expectations, ever-present risk of litigation, and the requisites of professionalism demand scientific foundations for nursing practice. Fine nursing research is being conducted on a variety of issues, and gerontological nurses must encourage and support these efforts through various actions.

One way for nurses to advance research is to network with nurse researchers. Researchers can be important resources. Combining their research skills with the abilities of those in practice settings can help to solve clinical problems. Local academic institutions, teaching hospitals, and nursing homes may be conducting research that can be relevant to various gerontological settings or in which a service agency can participate.

Nurses can also help to support research efforts in a variety of ways. As funding is sought for research projects, nurses can write letters of support and testimony to help funding agencies understand the full benefit of the research effort. Regular contact with leaders who influence the allocation of funds can provide opportunities to educate these persons on the value of supporting research. No less significant to the support of research efforts is the assurance that protocols be followed, because the

efforts of researchers can be facilitated or thwarted by colleagues in clinical settings.

Finally, nurses must keep abreast of new findings. Gerontological nursing knowledge is continuously expanding, disproving past beliefs and offering new insights. Nurses can engage in independent study, formal courses, and continuing education programs to keep current. Equally important to acquiring knowledge is implementing evidence-based practice to improve the care of older adults.

KEY CONCEPT

Older adults' delicately balanced health status and high risk of complications, along with rising consumer expectations and a highly litigious society, reinforce the importance of evidence-based practice.

Promote Integrative Care

In the United States, conventional medicine, with an emphasis on the diagnosis and treatment of diseases, has set the tone for health care practice. Current managed care and reimbursement priorities reinforce the medical model and disease-focused care. Unfortunately, the care of medical conditions is just one aspect of the services older adults need to be healthy and experience a high quality of life. In fact, older persons' wellness practices; adjustments to life changes; sense of purpose, hopefulness, joy, connections to others; and ability to manage stress can be equally if not more significant to their health and quality of life than medical care.

Nurses must ensure that gerontological care is holistic, meaning that the physical, emotional, social, and spiritual facets of individuals are considered (see Chapter 7). This implies that nurses not only practice in a holistic manner themselves but also advocate for other disciplines to do so.

Alternative and complementary therapies play a role in holistic care. These therapies tend to be more comforting, safe, and less invasive than conventional treatments and empower older adults and their caregivers in self-care. Many people who use these therapies report positive experiences with their alternative therapists, who frequently spend more time getting to understand and address the needs of the total person than do staff in the typical medical office or hospital. However, the use of alternative therapies does not equate with holistic care. An alternative therapist with tunnel vision, believing that every malady can be corrected with the one modality he or she practices and excluding effective conventional treatments, is no different from the physician who prescribes an analgesic but does not consider imagery, massage, relaxation exercises, and other nonconventional forms of pain relief. Integrating the best of conventional and alternative/complementary therapy supports holistic care.

Part of a holistic approach to care includes care of the caregivers as well. Professional and family caregivers who are in poor health, struggling with psychosocial issues, feeling spiritually empty and disconnected, or managing stress poorly need to heal themselves before they can be effective caregivers. Nurses can assist these caregivers in identifying their needs and finding the help needed for their healing.

POINT TO PONDER

Many nurses are in poor physical condition, smoke, regularly eat junk foods, take little time for themselves, and demonstrate other unhealthy habits. What do you think are some of the reasons for this? What can be done to improve nurses' health habits?

Educate Caregivers

Be it the nursing director, a family member who cares for an older relative, a health aide who has more frequent contact with the patient than the professional nurse, or the physician who only occasionally has an older person in the caseload, caregivers at every level require competency in providing services to the older population. Gerontological nurses can influence the education of caregivers by:

■ helping nursing schools identify relevant issues for inclusion in the curricula

■ participating in the classroom and field experiences of students

■ evaluating educational deficits of personnel and planning educational experiences to eliminate deficits

■ promoting interdisciplinary team conferences

■ attending and participating in continuing education programs

■ reading current nursing literature and sharing information with colleagues

■ serving as a role model by demonstrating current practices

With increasing numbers of family members providing more complex care in the home setting than ever before, it is essential that the education of this group not be overlooked. It should not be assumed that because the family has had contact

with other providers or has been providing care they are knowledgeable in correct care techniques. The nurse must periodically evaluate and reinforce the family's knowledge and skills.

Develop New Roles

As gerontological subspecialties and settings for care grow, so will the opportunities for nurses to carve new roles for themselves. Nurses can demonstrate creativity and leadership as they break from traditional roles and settings and develop new models of practice, which may include the following:

■ geropsychiatric nurse specialist in the assisted-living setting

■ independent case manager for community-based chronically ill patients

■ columnist for local newspaper on issues pertaining to health and aging

■ owner or director of mature women's health care center, geriatric day care program, respite agency, or caregiver training center

■ preretirement counselor and educator for private industry

■ faith community nurse

■ consultant, educator, and case manager for geriatric surgical patients

KEY CONCEPT

Opportunities exist for nurses to develop new practice models in gerontological care.

This list only begins to describe opportunities awaiting gerontological nurses. It will be important for gerontological nurses to identify nontraditional roles, approach them creatively, test innovative practice models, and share their successes and failures with colleagues to aid them in their development of new roles. Nurses must recognize that their biopsychosocial sciences knowledge, clinical competencies, and human relations skills give them a strong competitive edge over other disciplines in affecting a wide range of services.

POINT TO PONDER

Based on changes in the health care system and society at large, what unique services could gerontological nurses offer in the future within your community?

Balance Quality Care and Health Care Costs

The increasing number of older adults is placing increasing demands for diverse health care services than ever before. At the same time, third-party insurers are trying to control the constantly escalating cost of services. Earlier hospital discharges, limited home health visits, increased complexity of nursing home residents, and greater out-of-pocket payment for services by patients demonstrate some of the effects of changes in reimbursement policy. There is concern that, as a result of these changes, patients are discharged from hospitals prematurely and suffer greater adverse consequences, nursing homes are confronting residents with complex problems for whom they are not adequately prepared or staffed, families are being strained by considerable caregiving burdens, and patients are being deprived of needed but unaffordable services.

Such changes are disconcerting and may cause nurses to feel overwhelmed, frustrated, or dissatisfied. Unfortunately, more cost cutting is likely to occur. Rather than experience burnout or consider a change of occupation, nurses should become involved in cost-containment efforts so that a balance between quality services and budgetary concerns can be achieved. Efforts toward this goal can include the following:

■ *Test creative staffing patterns.* Perhaps six nurses can be more productive than three nurses and three unlicensed caregivers. Or, perhaps some of the high nonproductive time costs associated with unlicensed personnel are related to poor hiring and supervision practices; improved management techniques may increase the cost-effectiveness of these workers.

■ *Use lay caregivers.* Neighbors assisting each other, a family member rooming-in during hospitalizations, and other methods to increase the resources available for service provision can be explored.

■ *Abolish unnecessary practices.* Why must nurses spend time administering medications to patients who have successfully administered them before admission and who will continue to administer them after discharge, take vital signs every 4 hours on patients who have shown no abnormalities, bathe all patients on the same schedule regardless of skin condition or state of cleanliness, or rewrite assessments and care plans at specified intervals regardless of a patient's changes or stability? Often regulations and policies are developed under the assumption that, without them, vital signs would never be taken, baths would not be given, and other facets of care would not be completed. Perhaps the time has come for nurses to aggressively convince others that they have the professional judgment to determine the need for and frequency of assessment, care planning, and care delivery.

■ *Ensure safe care.* The implementation of cost-containment efforts should be accompanied by concurrent studies of its impact on rates of complications, readmissions, incidents, consumer satisfaction, and staff turnover, absenteeism, and morale. Specific numbers and documented cases carry more weight than broad criticisms or complaints that care is suffering.

■ *Advocate for older adults.* The priorities of society and professions change. History shows us that at different times the spotlight has focused on various underserved groups, such as children, pregnant women, the mentally ill, the disabled, substance abusers, and, most recently, older adults. As interests and priorities shift to new groups, gerontological nurses must make certain that the needs of older individuals are not forgotten or shortchanged.

As gerontological nursing continues to shed its image of a less-than-challenging specialty for less-than-competent nurses and fully emerges as the dynamic, multifaceted, and opportunity-filled area of nursing that it is, it will be recognized as a specialty for the finest talent the profession has to offer. Gerontological nursing has just begun to show its true potential.

BRINGING RESEARCH TO LIFE

QUALITY GERIATRIC CARE AS PERCEIVED BY NURSES IN LONG-TERM AND ACUTE CARE SETTINGS

Barba, B. E., Hu, J., & Efird, J. (2012). Journal of Clinical Nursing, 21(5), 833–840.

This descriptive study explored the differences between acute and long-term care nurses in regard to their satisfaction with the quality of care of older adults. The self-selected sample included 298 registered nurses and licensed practical nurses who provide care to minority, underserved, and disadvantaged older populations in 89 long-term care facilities and hospitals of less than 100 beds in a southern state. All completed the Agency Geriatric Nursing Care survey, which consisted of a 13-item scale measuring nurses' satisfaction with the quality of geriatric care in their practice settings and an 11-item scale examining obstacles to providing quality geriatric care.

Significant differences were found between the two groups of nurses in regard to level of satisfaction and perceived obstacles to providing quality care. Long-term care nurses were more satisfied and perceived fewer obstacles to providing quality care than nurses in acute hospitals. The long-term care nurses believed their care was more evidence based and specialized to the geriatric population.

Although acute care nurses commonly do not identify themselves as geriatric nurses, they are engaged in geriatric nursing practice due to the large number of hospitalized older adults. These nurses need to know best practices for geriatric care. This study demonstrates that without evidence-based guidelines to assist nurses in providing care that promotes autonomy, independence, and high-quality services, they feel less satisfied with the care offered to older patients. It can be beneficial for acute care nurses to discuss this need with managerial and education staff at their hospitals and support efforts to bridge evidence-based geriatric nursing practices to their clinical setting.

PRACTICE REALITIES

Nurse Yen is a new graduate of a BSN program who has joined the staff of a subacute care unit of the local hospital. Most of the nurses on staff are diplomas and ADN graduates who have been out of school for more than a decade.

Ms. Yen notices that some of the nurses are unaware of current best practices and trends. In informal conversations she has learned that none of the nurses subscribes to professional journals or belongs to a professional association, and the rare times they have attended continuing education programs was when the hospital sent them.

What can Nurse Yen do to help these nurses understand the importance and engage in continuing education?

CRITICAL THINKING EXERCISES

1. What were some of the reasons for the poor status of gerontological nursing in the past?
2. Why is the nursing role of healer particularly meaningful to gerontological practice?
3. What theme regarding the involvement of the older adult is apparent in the ANA Standards of the Gerontological Nurse?
4. Describe several issues that could warrant gerontological nursing research activities.
5. Describe how the increased use of holistic practices could have a positive effect on cost and consumer satisfaction.
6. Outline functions that could be performed by a gerontological nurse in the roles of:

   (a) assisted-living community preadmission health screener; (b) health counselor in a retirement community; (c) caregiver trainer; (d) industrial preretirement health educator; and (e) faith community nurse.

RESOURCES

American Holistic Nurses Association
http://www.ahna.org

American Nurses Credentialing Center
http://www.nursecredentialing.org

Hartford Institute for Geriatric Nursing
http://www.hartfordign.org

REFERENCES

Agency for Healthcare Research and Quality. (2008). *Evidence-based practice centers*. Rockville, MD: Agency for Healthcare Research and Quality. Retrieved September 20, 2008 from http://www.ahrq.gov

Bishop, L. F. (1904). Relation of old age to disease with illustrative cases. *American Journal of Nursing, 4*(4), 674.

DeWitt, K. (1904). The old nurse. *American Journal of Nursing, 4*(4), 177.

Nightingale, F. (1860). *Notes on nursing: What it is, and what it is not*. New York, NY: D. Appleton and Company.

Nouwen, H. J. M. (1990). *The wounded healer*. New York, NY: Doubleday.

RECOMMENDED READINGS

Recommended Readings associated with this chapter can be found on the web site that accompanies the book. Visit **http://thepoint.lww.com/Eliopoulos8e** to access the recommended readings and other additional resources associated with this chapter.

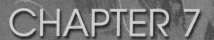

Holistic Model for Gerontological Nursing

LEARNING OBJECTIVES

After reading this chapter, you should be able to:

1. Explain holistic gerontological nursing care.

2. Describe the needs of older adults pertaining to the promotion of health and the management of health challenges.

3. List the requisites that influence older persons' abilities to meet self-care needs.

4. Describe the general types of nursing interventions that are employed when older adults present self-care deficits.

TERM TO KNOW

Holistic: pertains to whole person; body, mind, and spirit

Surviving to old age is a tremendous accomplishment. Basic life requirements such as obtaining adequate nutrition, keeping oneself relatively safe, and maintaining the body's normal functions have been met with some success to survive to this time. Older adults have confronted and overcome to varying degrees the hurdles of coping with crises, adjusting to change, and learning new skills. Throughout their lives, older individuals have faced many important decisions, such as should they:

- leave their country of birth to make a fresh start in America?

- stay in the family business or seek a job in the local factory?

- risk their lives to support a cause in which they believe?

- encourage their children to fight in an unpopular war?

- invest their entire savings in launching a business of their own?

- allow their children to continue their education when the children's employment would ease a serious financial hardship?

Too often, nurses seek external resources to meet the needs of older persons rather than recognizing that older adults have considerable inner resources for self-care and empowering them to use these strengths. Older adults then become passive recipients of care rather than active participants. This seems unreasonable because most older adults have had a lifetime of taking care of themselves and others, making their own decisions, and meeting life's most trying challenges. They may become angry or depressed at being forced to forfeit their decision-making functions to others. They may unnecessarily develop feelings of dependency, uselessness, and powerlessness. Gerontological nurses must recognize and mobilize the strengths and capabilities of older people so that they can be responsible and active participants in, rather than objects of, care. Tapping the resources of older individuals in their own care promotes normalcy, independence, and individuality; it aids in reducing risks of secondary problems related to the reactions of older adults to an unnecessarily imposed dependent role; and it honors their wisdom, experience, and capabilities.

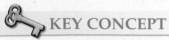 KEY CONCEPT

Older individuals have had to be strong and resourceful to navigate the stormy waters of life. Nurses should not overlook these strengths when planning care for older adults.

HOLISTIC GERONTOLOGICAL CARE

Holism refers to the integration of the biologic, psychological, social, and spiritual dimensions of an individual in which the synergy creates a sum that is greater than its parts; within this framework, healing the whole person is the goal of nursing (Dossey & Keegan, 2009). Holistic gerontological care incorporates knowledge and skills from a variety of disciplines to address the physical, mental, social, and spiritual health of individuals. Holistic gerontological care is concerned with:

- facilitating growth toward wholeness

- promoting recovery and learning from an illness

- maximizing quality of life when one possesses an incurable illness or disability

- providing peace, comfort, and dignity as death is approached

In holistic care, the goal is not to treat diseases but to serve the needs of the total person through the healing of the body, mind, and spirit.

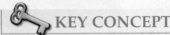 KEY CONCEPT

Gerontological nurses help older individuals achieve a sense of wholeness by guiding them in understanding and finding meaning and purpose in life; facilitating harmony of the mind, body, and spirit; mobilizing their internal and external resources; and promoting self-care behaviors.

Health promotion and healing through a balance of the body, mind, and spirit of individuals are at the core of holistic care and have particular relevance for gerontological care. The impact of age-related changes and the effects of highly prevalent chronic conditions can easily threaten the well-being of the body, mind, and spirit; therefore, nursing interventions to reduce such threats are essential. Because chronic diseases and the effects of advanced age cannot be eliminated, healing rather than curative efforts will be most beneficial in gerontological nursing practice. Equally significant is assisting older adults toward self-discovery in their final phase of life so that they find meaning, connectedness with others, and an understanding of their place in the universe.

HOLISTIC ASSESSMENT OF NEEDS

There are many evidence-based assessment tools that can be useful to gerontological nurses. One of the most comprehensive listings of these tools can be found at the Hartford Institute for Geriatric Nursing (see Resource listing), which includes resources for assessment of activities of daily living, hearing, sleep, sexuality, elder mistreatment, dementia, hospital admission risk, and other topics.

These tools can be used to supplement the holistic assessment, which has a slightly different emphasis. Holistic assessment identifies patient needs related to health promotion and health challenges and also identifies the older adult's requisites to meet these needs.

Health Promotion–Related Needs

The concept of health seems simple, yet it is quite complex. Viewing health as the *absence of disease* offers little more clarity than defining cold as the absence of hot and creates an image that begs for a more positive, broad understanding. In regard to older adults, most of whom are living with chronic conditions, this definition would relegate most of them to the ranks of the unhealthy.

When asked to describe the factors that contribute to health, most people would be likely to list the basic life-sustaining needs such as breathing, eating, eliminating, resting, being active, and protecting oneself from risks. These are essential to maintaining the physiological balance that sustains life. However, the reality that we can have all of our physiological needs satisfied, yet still not feel well, demonstrates that physiological balance is but one component of overall health. Connection with ourselves, others, a higher power, and nature are important factors influencing health. The fulfillment of physiological needs and a sense of being connected promote well-being of the body, mind, and spirit that enables us to experience gratification through achieving purpose, pleasure, and dignity. This holistic model demonstrates that optimal health includes those activities that not only enable us to exist but also help us to realize effective, enriched lives (Fig. 7-1).

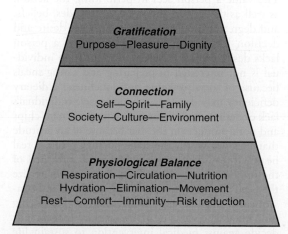

FIGURE 7-1 ■ Health promotion–related needs.

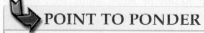

POINT TO PONDER

What does it mean to you to be healthy and whole?

An improved definition of health includes consideration of the root meaning of the word health: whole. Using this foundation, health is understood as *a state of wholeness ... an integration of body, mind, and spirit to achieve the highest possible quality of life each day* (Fig. 7-2). For some individuals, this can mean exercising at the gym, engaging in challenging work, and having a personal relationship with God; for others, it can represent propelling oneself in a wheelchair to a porch, enjoying the beauty of nature, and connecting with a universal energy.

Views of health differ not only from individual to individual but also within the same individual from one time to another. Health priorities and expectations in a 70-year-old person may not resemble what they were when that individual was half that age. Cultural and religious influences can also affect one's view of health.

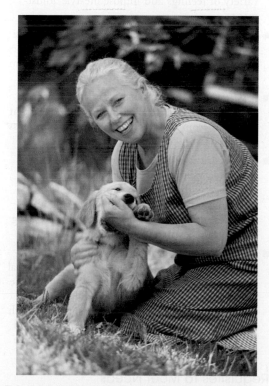

FIGURE 7-2 ■ Rather than being limited to meaning the absence of disease, health implies a wholeness and harmony of body, mind, and spirit.

Optimal health of older adults rests on the degree to which the needs for physiological balance, connection, and gratification are satisfied. There is the risk that in busy clinical settings, the less tangible needs of gratification and connection can be overlooked; as advocates for older adults, gerontological nurses must assure that comprehensive care is provided by not omitting these important needs.

Health Challenges–Related Needs

An unfortunate reality is that most older adults live with at least one chronic condition that challenges their health status. In fact, most involvement that nurses have with older adults typically involves assisting them with the demands imposed by health challenges. Older adults with acute or chronic conditions have the same basic health promotion needs as healthy individuals (i.e., physiological balance, connection, and gratification); however, their conditions may create new needs such as:

- *Education*: As individuals face a new diagnosis, they need to understand the condition and its care.
- *Counseling*: A health condition can trigger a variety of feelings and impose lifestyle adjustments.
- *Coaching*: Just as athletes and musicians require the skills of a professional who can bring out the best in them, patients, too, can benefit from efforts to improve compliance and motivation.
- *Monitoring*: The complexities of health care and the changing status of aging people warrant oversight from the nurse who can track progress and needs.
- *Coordination*: Older adults with a health condition often visit several health care providers; assistance with scheduling appointments, following multiple instructions, keeping all members of the team informed, and preventing conflicting treatments are often needed.
- *Therapies*: Often, health conditions are accompanied by the need for medications, exercises, special diets, and procedures. These therapies can include conventional ones that are commonly used in mainstream practice or complementary ones, such as biofeedback, herbal remedies, acupressure, and yoga. Patients may need partial or total assistance as they implement these treatments.

Requisites to Meet Needs

As straightforward and clear as the health promotion and health challenges–related needs may seem, these needs are met with varying degrees of success because they are dependent on several factors unique to the patient. Nurses assess older adults' requisites to meet needs to determine areas for intervention.

Physical, Mental, and Socioeconomic Abilities

An individual relies on several factors to meet even the most basic life demands. For example, to normally fulfill nutritional needs, a person must have the ability to experience hunger sensations; proper cognition to adequately select, prepare, and consume food; good dental status to chew food; a functional digestive tract to utilize ingested food; energy to shop and prepare food; and the funds to purchase food. Deficits in any of these areas can create risks to nutritional status. A variety of nursing interventions can be used to reduce or eliminate physical, mental, and socioeconomic deficits.

Knowledge, Experience, and Skills

Limitations exist when the knowledge, experience, or skills required for a given self-care action are inadequate or nonexistent. An individual with a wealth of social skills is capable of a normal, active life that includes friendship and other social interaction. People who have knowledge of the hazards of cigarette smoking will be more capable of protecting themselves from health risks associated with this habit. An older man who is widowed, however, may not be able to cook and provide an adequate diet for himself, having always depended on his wife for meal preparation. Similarly, the person who has diabetes and cannot self-inject the necessary insulin may not be able to meet the therapeutic demand for insulin administration. Specific nursing considerations for enhancing self-care capacities are offered in other chapters.

Desire and Decision to Take Action

The value a person sees in performing the action, as well as the person's knowledge, attitudes, beliefs, and degree of motivation, influences the desire and decision for action. Limitations result if a person lacks desire or decides against action. If an individual is not interested in preparing and eating meals because of social isolation and loneliness, a dietary deficiency may develop. A hypertensive individual's lack of desire and decision not to forfeit potato chips and pork products in the diet because of an attitude that it is not worth the trade-off may create a real health threat. The person who is not informed of the importance of physical activity may not realize the need to arise from bed during an illness and consequently may develop complications. The dying individual who views death as a natural process may decide against medical intervention to sustain life and may not comply with the prescribed therapies.

Values, attitudes, and beliefs are deeply established and not easily altered. Although the nurse should respect the right of individuals to make decisions affecting their lives, if limitations restrict their ability to meet self-care demands, the nurse can help by explaining the benefit of a particular action, providing information, and motivating. In some circumstances, as with an emotionally ill or mentally incompetent person, desires and decisions may have to be superseded by professional judgments.

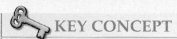

> ### KEY CONCEPT
>
> There can be vastly different reasons for older adults to have a deficit in meeting a similar need. This challenges the gerontological nurse to explore the unique and sometimes subtle dynamics of each older person's life.

GERONTOLOGICAL NURSING PROCESSES

The assessment process considers patients' effectiveness in meeting needs related to health promotion and health challenges. If the individual is successful in fulfilling needs, there is no need for nursing intervention except to reinforce the capability for self-care. When the older adult does not have the requisites to meet needs independently, however, nursing interventions are needed. Nursing interventions are directed toward empowering the older individual by strengthening self-care capacities, eliminating or minimizing self-care limitations, and providing direct services by acting for, doing for, or assisting the individual when requirements cannot be independently fulfilled (Fig. 7-3). Assessment factors pertaining to specific systems and areas of function are found in the related chapters throughout this book.

EXAMPLES OF APPLICATION

Nursing care for older persons is often associated with implementing actions when health conditions exist. When individuals face health challenges, new needs frequently arise, such as administering medications, observing for specific symptoms, and performing special treatments; these needs exceed and may affect the needs related to health promotion. In geriatric nursing, consideration must be given to assessing the impact of the health challenge on the individual's self-care capacity and identifying appropriate nursing interventions to ensure that the needs related to both health promotion and the management of health challenges are adequately met.

During the assessment, the nurse identifies the specific health challenges–related needs that are present and the requisites (e.g., physical capability, knowledge, and desire) that need to be addressed to strengthen self-care capacity.

It is significant that interventions include those actions that can empower the older individual to achieve maximum self-care in regard to health challenges–related needs. Figure 7-3 demonstrates how the holistic self-care model becomes operational in geriatric nursing practice. The cases that follow demonstrate the application of this model.

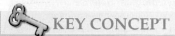

> ### KEY CONCEPT
>
> More effort may be needed to instruct and coach an older person to perform a self-care task independently, and more time may be taken for the person to perform the task independently than would be necessary if a caregiver did the task; however, the benefits of independence to the older person's body, mind, and spirit are worth the investment.

Assessing Needs: The Case of Mr. R

Mr. R, who has lived with diabetes for a long time, administers insulin daily and follows a diabetic diet. Because of a recent urologic problem, he may now need to take antibiotics daily and perform intermittent self-catheterization. During the assessment, the nurse identifies the presence of these illness-imposed needs.

After the primary assessment has revealed the presence of needs related to health challenges, the nurse will evaluate how well these needs are met.

The nurse finds that Mr. R performs self-catheterization according to procedure and is administering his antibiotics as prescribed, but is not adhering to his diabetic diet and alters his insulin dosage based on "how he feels that day."

The next level of assessment must seek the reasons for deficits in meeting the health challenges–related needs.

Mr. R has knowledge of the diabetic diet and wants to comply; however, he had depended on his wife to prepare meals, and now that she is deceased, he has difficulty cooking nutritious meals independently. He denies ever being informed of the need for regular doses of his insulin and states that he has relied on the advice of his brother-in-law, also a diabetic, who told him to "take an extra shot of insulin when he eats a lot of sweets."

Once the shortcomings in skills and knowledge behind the patient's deficits in meeting these health challenges–related needs are identified, specific nursing care plan actions can be developed.

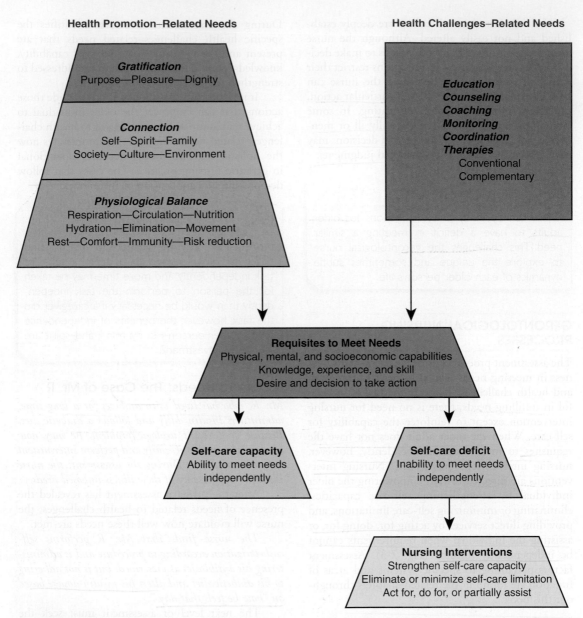

Health Promotion–Related Needs

Gratification
Purpose—Pleasure—Dignity

Connection
Self—Spirit—Family
Society—Culture—Environment

Physiological Balance
Respiration—Circulation—Nutrition
Hydration—Elimination—Movement
Rest—Comfort—Immunity—Risk reduction

Health Challenges–Related Needs

Education
Counseling
Coaching
Monitoring
Coordination
Therapies
Conventional
Complementary

Requisites to Meet Needs
Physical, mental, and socioeconomic capabilities
Knowledge, experience, and skill
Desire and decision to take action

Self-care capacity
Ability to meet needs
independently

Self-care deficit
Inability to meet needs
independently

Nursing Interventions
Strengthen self-care capacity
Eliminate or minimize self-care limitation
Act for, do for, or partially assist

FIGURE 7-3 ■ If the nurse identifies self-care deficits in the older adult for meeting health promotion– and health challenges–related needs, nursing interventions are needed.

Applying the Holistic Model: The Case of Mrs. D

The following case demonstrates how this model can work.

Mrs. D, 78 years old, was admitted to a hospital service for acute conditions with the identified problems of a fractured neck of the femur, malnutrition, and a need for a different living arrangement. Initial observation revealed a small-framed, frail-looking lady, with obvious signs of malnutrition and dehydration. She was well oriented to person, place, and time and was able to

converse and answer questions coherently. Although her memory for recent events was poor, she seldom forgot to inform anyone who was interested that she neither liked nor wanted to be in the hospital. Her previous and only other hospitalization was 55 years earlier.

Mrs. D had been living with her husband and an unmarried sister for more than 50 years when her husband died. For the 5 years following his death, she depended heavily on her sister for emotional support and guidance. Then her sister died, which promoted feelings of anxiety, insecurity, loneliness, and depression.

For the year since her sister's death she has lived alone, caring for her six-room home in the country with no assistance other than that from a neighbor who did the shopping for Mrs. D and occasionally provided her with transportation.

On the day of her admission to the hospital, Mrs. D had fallen on her kitchen floor, weak from her malnourished state. Discovering her hours later, her neighbor called an ambulance, which transported Mrs. D to the hospital. Once the diagnosis of fractured femur was established, plans were made to perform a nailing procedure, to correct her malnourished state, and to find a new living arrangement because her home demanded more energy and attention than she was capable of providing.

Nursing Care Plan 7-1 illustrates how Mrs. D's holistic needs directed nursing diagnoses and related nursing actions.

NURSING CARE PLAN 7-1

HOLISTIC CARE FOR MRS. D

NEEDS: Respiration and Circulation

Nursing Diagnoses: (1) Impaired Physical Mobility related to fracture; (2) Impaired Gas Exchange related to immobility

Goals: The patient demonstrates signs of adequate respiration; is free from respiratory distress and infection; and is free from signs of impaired circulation.

Nursing Actions	Type of Intervention
Maintain normal respirations.	
■ Prevent blockage of airway or any other interference with normal breathing.	Partially assisting
■ Observe for and detect respiratory problems early.	Partially assisting
Promote active and passive exercises.	
■ Teach and encourage turning, coughing, and deep-breathing exercises.	Strengthening self-care capacity
■ Encourage active exercises, such as using incentive spirometers and deep breathing.	Strengthening self-care capacity
■ Perform passive range-of-motion exercises.	Doing for
Avoid external interferences with respiration.	
■ Provide good room ventilation.	Doing for
■ Avoid restrictive clothing, linens, or equipment.	Doing for
■ Position in manner conducive to best respiration.	Partially assisting
■ Prevent anxiety-producing situations, such as delays in answering bell call.	Doing for

NEEDS: Nutrition and Hydration

Nursing Diagnosis: Imbalanced Nutrition: Less than Body Requirements, related to depression and loneliness

Goals: The patient consumes at least 1,500 mL of fluids and 1,800 calories of nutrients daily; increases weight to 125 lb.

Nursing Actions	Type of Intervention
Stimulate appetite.	
■ Plan diet according to the person's preferences, consistent with therapeutic requirements.	Partially assisting
■ Provide a quiet, pleasant environment that allows for socialization with others.	Doing for
■ Stimulate appetite through appearance and seasoning of foods.	Minimizing self-care limitation
Plan meals.	
■ Read menu selection to the patient.	Partially assisting
■ Guide the choice of high-protein, carbohydrate, and vitamin- and mineral-rich foods.	Minimizing self-care limitation
■ Access food preferences and include them in menu selections.	Acting for

(Continues)

NURSING CARE PLAN 7-1 (Continued)

Assist with feeding.

Nursing Actions	Type of Intervention
■ Conserve energy and promote adequate intake by preparing food tray, encouraging rest periods, and feeding when necessary.	Strengthening self-care capacity, doing for, and partially assisting

Prevent complications.

Nursing Actions	Type of Intervention
■ Do not leave solutions, medications, or harmful agents in locations where they may be mistakenly ingested (especially when assessment indicates visual limitations).	Acting for
■ Check the temperature of foods and drinks to prevent burns (especially when assessment indicates decreased cutaneous sensation).	Acting for
■ Assist in the selection of foods conducive to bone healing and correction of malnutrition.	Partially assisting
■ Observe the fluid intake and output for early detection of imbalances.	Minimizing self-care limitation
■ Assess general health status frequently to detect new problems or improvements resulting from changes in nutritional status (e.g., weight changes, skin turgor, mental status, and strength).	Acting for and minimizing self-care limitation

NEED: Elimination

Nursing Diagnoses: (1) Constipation related to immobility; (2) Risk of Infection related to malnutrition and interferences with normal bathing

Goals: The patient is free from infection; establishes a regular bowel elimination schedule; is free from constipation; and is clean and odor free.

Nursing Actions	Type of Intervention
Promote regular elimination of bladder and bowels.	
■ Guide the selection of a diet high in roughage and fluids.	Partially assisting
■ Observe and record elimination pattern.	Acting for and minimizing self-care limitation
■ Assist with exercises to promote peristalsis and urination.	Partially assisting
■ Arrange schedule to provide regular time periods for elimination.	Acting for
■ Assist with hygienic care of body surfaces.	Partially assisting
■ Provide privacy when bedpan is used.	Acting for and minimizing self-care limitation
Develop good hygienic practices.	
■ Teach the importance and method of cleansing perineal region after elimination.	Strengthening self-care capacity
Prevent social isolation.	
■ Prevent, detect, and correct body odors.	Acting for and minimizing self-care limitation

NEED: Movement

Nursing Diagnoses: (1) Activity Intolerance related to malnutrition and fracture; (2) Impaired Physical Mobility related to fracture

Goals: The patient maintains/achieves sufficient range of joint motion to engage in activities of daily living (ADL); is free from complications secondary to immobility.

Nursing Actions	Type of Intervention
Adjust hospital routines to individual's pace.	
■ Space procedures and other activities.	Acting for
■ Allow longer periods for self-care activities.	Strengthening self-care capacity

(Continues)

NURSING CARE PLAN 7-1 (Continued)

Nursing Actions	Type of Intervention
Provide for energy conservation.	
■ Promote security and relaxation through the avoidance of frequent changes of personnel.	Acting for
■ Prevent complications associated with immobility (e.g., decubiti, constipation, renal calculi, contractures, hypostatic pneumonia, thrombi, edema, and lethargy).	Minimizing self-care limitation
■ Encourage frequent change of position.	Minimizing self-care limitation
■ Motivate and reward activity.	Strengthening self-care capacity
■ Teach simple exercises to prevent complications and improve motor dexterity.	Strengthening self-care capacity
■ Plan activities to increase independence progressively.	Acting for and strengthening self care capacity

NEED: Rest

Nursing Diagnosis: Disturbed Sleep Pattern related to hospital environment and movement limitations associated with fracture
Goals: The patient obtains sufficient sleep to be free from fatigue; learns measures to facilitate sleep and rest.

Nursing Actions	Type of Intervention
Control environmental stimuli.	
■ Schedule rest periods between procedures.	Acting for
■ Instruct in progressive relaxation.	Strengthening self-care capacity

NEED: Comfort

Nursing Diagnosis: Acute Pain related to fracture
Goals: The patient is free from pain; is able to participate in ADLs without pain-related restrictions.

Nursing Actions	Type of Intervention
■ Monitor for signs of pain.	Minimizing self-care limitation
■ Assist with positioning and exercises to reduce discomfort.	Strengthening self-care capacity
■ Plan analgesic administration in collaboration with health care team.	Minimizing self care limitation

NEED: Immunity

Nursing Diagnoses: (1) Ineffective Health Maintenance; (2) Risk of Infection
Goals: The patient is free from infection.

Nursing Actions	Type of Intervention
■ Encourage good food and fluid intake.	Strengthening self-care capacity
■ Teach the client to include foods in diet that positively affect immune system, such as milk, yogurt, nonfat cottage cheese, eggs, fresh fruits and vegetables, and garlic.	Strengthening self-care capacity
■ Instruct in and assist with immune-enhancing exercises such as yoga and t'ai chi.	Strengthening self-care capacity
■ Review immunization history and arrange for immunizations as needed.	Strengthening self-care capacity
■ Instruct in stress management techniques.	Strengthening self-care capacity

(Continues)

NURSING CARE PLAN 7-1 (Continued)

NEED: Risk Reduction

Nursing Diagnoses: (1) Disturbed Sensory Perception (visual, auditory, olfactory, and tactile) related to advanced age; (2) Risk of Injury related to sensory deficits; (3) Risk of Impaired Skin Integrity related to immobility, malnutrition, and decreased sensations; (4) Impaired Home Maintenance related to altered health state, convalescence

Goals: The patient is free from injury; possesses intact skin; effectively and correctly uses assistive devices, eyeglasses, and hearing aids (as prescribed) to compensate for sensory deficits; has safe, acceptable living arrangements after discharge.

Nursing Actions	Type of Intervention
Compensate for poor vision.	
■ Read to the person.	Doing for and minimizing self-care limitation
■ Write information and label with large letters and color coding when possible.	Minimizing self-care limitation
■ Remove obstacles that could cause accidents such as foreign objects in bed, clutter on floor, and solutions that could be mistaken for water.	Minimizing self-care limitation and acting for
■ Communicate this problem to other personnel.	Acting for
■ Initiate an ophthalmology referral.	Acting for
Compensate for decreased ability to smell.	
■ Prevent and correct odors resulting from poor hygienic practices.	Partially assisting and minimizing self-care limitation
■ Detect unusual odors early (may be symptomatic of infection).	Acting for
Compensate for hearing loss.	
■ Speak clearly and loudly while facing the person.	Minimizing self-care limitation
■ Use feedback techniques to make sure the person has heard and understood.	Minimizing self-care limitation
■ Initiate referral to ear, nose, and throat clinic.	Acting for
Maintain good skin condition.	
■ Inspect for rashes, reddened areas, and sores.	Doing for
■ Assist with hygienic practices.	Partially assisting
■ Give back rubs, change the person's position frequently, and keep the person's skin soft and dry.	Doing for, partially assisting, and minimizing self-care limitation
Prevent falls.	
■ Support the person who is ambulating or being transported.	Partially assisting
■ Teach and encourage exercises to assist in maintaining muscle tone.	Strengthening self-care capacity
■ Keep bed rails up and support the person in wheelchair.	Doing for
■ Provide rest periods between activities.	Strengthening self-care capacity and minimizing self-care limitation
■ Place frequently used objects within easy reach.	Partially assisting
Maintain proper body alignment.	
■ Use sandbags, trochanter rolls, and pillows.	Minimizing self-care limitation and partially assisting
■ Support the person's affected limb when it is lifted or moved.	Partially assisting and minimizing self-care limitation

(Continues)

NURSING CARE PLAN 7-1 (Continued)

Seek safe living arrangements in preparation for the person's discharge.

Nursing Actions	Type of Intervention
■ Evaluate patient's preferences, capacities, and limitation to suggest appropriate arrangements.	Acting for and partially assisting
■ Initiate referral to social worker.	Acting for

NEED: Connection

Nursing Diagnoses: (1) Spiritual Distress, Hopelessness, and Powerlessness related to hospitalization, health state, and lifestyle changes; (2) Impaired Social Interaction related to hospitalization and health state
Goals: The patient expresses satisfaction with the amount of social interaction; identifies means for fulfilling spiritual needs; is free from signs of emotional distress.

Nursing Actions	Type of Intervention
Control environmental stimuli.	
■ Schedule the same personnel for caregiving.	Acting for
■ Maintain a regular daily schedule.	Strengthening self-care capacity
■ Arrange for a roommate with similar interests and background.	Acting for and strengthening self-care capacity
Promote meaningful social interactions.	
■ Instruct others to speak clearly and sufficiently loud while facing the person.	Strengthening self-care capacity
■ Plan meaningful activities.	Strengthening self-care capacity
■ Promote and maintain an oriented state.	Strengthening self-care capacity and minimizing self-care limitation
■ Display interest in the person's social interactions and encourage their continuation.	Strengthening self-care capacity
■ Initiate contacts with community agencies to develop relationships that can continue after discharge.	Acting for and minimizing self-care limitation
■ Assist with grooming and dressing.	Partially assisting and minimizing self-care limitation
■ Learn about the patient's spirituality and religious beliefs and incorporate this into care.	Strengthening self-care capacity
■ Arrange for pastoral/spiritual counseling.	Acting for and strengthening self-care capacity
■ Encourage verbalization of feelings concerning meaning of health state and life changes.	Strengthening self-care capacity
■ Provide opportunities for prayer.	Strengthening self-care capacity

NEED: Gratification

Nursing Diagnoses: (1) Anxiety, Fear, Hopelessness, and Powerlessness related to hospitalization and health state; (2) Impaired Social Interaction related to hospitalization; (3) Chronic Low Self-Esteem related to health problems and life situation
Goals: The patient demonstrates preinjury level of physical activity; performs self-care activities to maximum level of independence; expresses satisfaction with the amount of solitude; and is free from signs of emotional distress.

Nursing Actions	Type of Intervention
■ Control environmental stimuli.	Acting for
■ Respect privacy.	Strengthening self-care capacity

(Continues)

NURSING CARE PLAN 7-1 (Continued)

Provide opportunities for solitude.

- Provide several preplanned time periods during the day in which the person can be alone.

Acting for and strengthening self-care capacity

- Provide privacy by pulling curtains around bed and making use of facilities such as chapel.

Minimizing self-care limitation

Improve physical limitations where possible.

- Assist with re-education for ambulation.

Partially assisting and strengthening self-care capacity

- Exercise body parts to maintain function.

Partially assisting and minimizing self-care limitation

- Encourage patient to consume an adequate diet.

Strengthening self-care capacity

- Initiate referral for audiometric examination to explore utility of hearing aid.

Acting for and minimizing self-care limitation

- Initiate ophthalmology referral to explore utility of corrective lenses.

Acting for and minimizing self-care limitation

Maintain familiar components of lifestyle.

- Adjust hospital routine to the person's home routine as much as possible.

Acting for and minimizing self-care limitation

- Encourage the person to wear own clothing.

Minimizing self-care limitation

- Provide the person with personal items from home, pillow, blanket, photographs, and tea cup.

Minimizing self-care limitation

- Provide leisure activities to which the person is accustomed.

Minimizing self-care limitation and strengthening self-care capacity

Promote active participation.

- Provide the person with opportunities to make own decisions whenever possible.

Strengthening self-care capacity

- Involve the person in care.

Strengthening self-care capacity

- Stimulate and encourage communication.

Strengthening self-care capacity

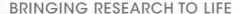

BRINGING RESEARCH TO LIFE

ADVANCED PRACTICE NURSES' PERSPECTIVES ON THE USE OF HEALTH OPTIMIZATION STRATEGIES FOR MANAGING CHRONIC DISEASE AMONG OLDER ADULTS IN DIFFERENT CARE SETTINGS: PUSHING THE BOUNDARIES OF SELF-MANAGEMENT PROGRAMS

Dickerson, J. B., Smith, M. L., Dowdy, D. M., McKinley, A., Ahn, S., & Ory, M. G. (2011). Geriatric Nursing, 32(6), 429–438.

This study examined the intention of advanced practice nurses (APNs) in various settings to use health optimization programs (HOPs). HOPs are self-management strategies that patients learn to use to improve their physical and emotional well-being despite having a disease. These self-management skills can help to prevent complications and improve the quality of life for older adults and can include clinical activities such as medication management and recreational activities.

As APNs have been shown to have an important role in facilitating the ability of older adults to manage health conditions, this study explored differences in APNs' intention to use HOPs based on work setting. APNs were given information on self-management programs and then completed a survey. APNs in nursing homes were found to be least likely to use self-management programs. Explanations for this included the APNs' views that the residents were too frail to benefit from the programs and that the structure of the nursing home placed adherence to medical practices above HOPs.

It is important for nurses in all settings to learn about HOPs and self-management techniques for use with older adults with chronic conditions. Regardless of the setting, empowering and encouraging older adults to be as active in care as possible promotes maximum independence and improved quality of life. Particularly in the nursing home setting, gerontological nurses need to carefully assess each individual and, where deficits in self-care ability exist, use individualized interventions to promote maximum engagement in self-care.

PRACTICE REALITIES

As a new staff member of a nursing home, you notice that other staff make decisions and perform activities for many residents who seem capable of doing these things for themselves. When caring for some of these residents, you give them the opportunity to make choices about their preferences, which they have been pleased and able to make. In addition, when encouraging them to feed themselves, residents have performed the task, although more time was required to complete care.

What could be the possible reasons for staff creating unnecessary dependence in the residents? How could you encourage a change in their approaches?

CRITICAL THINKING EXERCISES

1. Identify life experiences that have been unique to today's older population and that have prepared them to cope with some of the challenges of old age.

2. List age-related changes that could affect each of the health promotion–related needs.

3. What are some reasons for older adults not wanting to function independently in self-care activities?

4. Describe some situations in which older adults are at risk for losing independence as a result of nurses doing for them rather than promoting independence.

RESOURCES

American Holistic Health Association
http://www.ahha.org

American Holistic Medical Association
http://www.holisticmedicine.org

American Holistic Nurses Association
http://www.ahna.org

Hartford Institute for Geriatric Nursing Try This Assessment Tool Series
http://hartfordign.org/practice/try_this/

RECOMMENDED READINGS

Recommended Readings associated with this chapter can be found on the web site that accompanies the book. Visit **http://thepoint.lww.com/Eliopoulos8e** to access the recommended readings and other additional resources associated with this chapter.

REFERENCE

Dossey, B. M., & Keegan, L. (2009). *Holistic nursing: A handbook for practice* (5th ed.) Sudbury, MA: Jones & Bartlett Publishers.

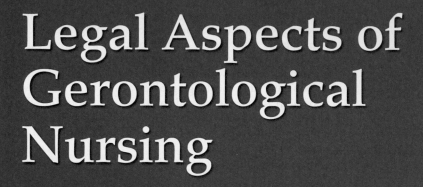

CHAPTER 8

Legal Aspects of Gerontological Nursing

CHAPTER OUTLINE

Laws Governing Gerontological Nursing Practice

Legal Risks in Gerontological Nursing
Malpractice
Confidentiality
Patient Consent
Patient Competency
Staff Supervision
Medications
Restraints
Telephone Orders
Do Not Resuscitate Orders
Advance Directives and Issues Related to Death and Dying
Elder Abuse

Legal Safeguards for Nurses

LEARNING OBJECTIVES

After reading this chapter, you should be able to:

1. Discuss laws governing gerontological nursing practice.

2. Describe legal issues in gerontological nursing practice and ways to minimize risks.

3. List legal safeguards for nurses.

TERMS TO KNOW

Consent: granting of permission to have an action taken or procedure performed

Durable power of attorney: allows competent individuals to appoint someone to make decisions on their behalf in the event that they become incompetent

Duty: a relationship between individuals in which one is responsible or has been contracted to provide service for another

Injury: physical or mental harm to another, or violation of a person's rights resulting from a negligent act

Malpractice: deviation from standard of care

(Continued)

Negligence: failure to conform to the standard of care

Private law: governs relationships between individuals and/or organizations

Public law: governs relationships between private parties and the government

Standard of care: the norm for what a reasonable individual in a similar circumstance would do

Nurses in every specialty must be cognizant of the legal aspects of their practice, and gerontological nurses are no exception. In fact, legal risks can intensify and legal questions can arise when working in geriatric care settings. Frequently, gerontological nurses are in highly independent and responsible positions in which they must make decisions without an abundance of professionals with whom to confer. They are also often responsible for supervising unlicensed staff and ultimately are accountable for the actions of those they supervise. In addition, gerontological nurses are likely to face difficult situations in which their advice or guidance may be requested by patients and families; they may be asked questions regarding how to protect the assets of the wife of a patient with Alzheimer's disease, how to write a will, what can be done to cease life-sustaining measures, and who can give consent for a patient. Also, the multiple problems faced by older adults, their high prevalence of frailty, and their lack of familiarity with laws and regulations may make them easy victims of unscrupulous practices. Advocacy is an integral part of gerontological nursing, reinforcing the need for nurses to be concerned about protecting the rights of their older patients. To fully protect themselves, their patients, and their employers, nurses must have knowledge of basic laws and ensure that their practice falls within legally sound boundaries.

LAWS GOVERNING GERONTOLOGICAL NURSING PRACTICE

Laws are generated from several sources. Because many laws are developed at the state and local levels, variation exists among the states. This variation necessitates nurses' familiarity with the unique laws within their specific states, particularly those governing professional practice, labor relations, and regulation of health care agencies.

There are both public and private laws. Public law governs relationships between private parties and the government and includes criminal law and regulation of organizations and individuals engaged in certain practices. The scope of nursing practice and the requirements for being licensed as a home health agency fall under the enforcement of public law. Private law governs relationships between individuals and organizations and involves contracts and torts (i.e., wrongful acts against another party, including assault, battery, false imprisonment, and invasion of privacy). These laws protect individual rights and also set standards of conduct, which, if violated, can result in liability of the wrongdoer.

In addition to laws, there are voluntary standards by which a nurse can be judged. The American Nurses' Association publication *Scope and Standards of Gerontological Nursing* provides guidelines for gerontological nurses that offer descriptions of what is considered safe and effective care. (See Chapter 6 for a discussion of these standards.)

LEGAL RISKS IN GERONTOLOGICAL NURSING

Most nurses do not commit wrongful acts intentionally; however, certain situations can increase the nurse's risk of liability. Such situations include working without sufficient resources, not checking agency policy or procedure, bending a rule, giving someone a break, taking shortcuts, or trying to work when physically or emotionally exhausted. Not only repeated episodes of carelessness but also the one-time deviation from standards can result in serious legal problems. Box 8-1 reviews some of the general acts that could make nurses liable for violating the law. Nurses must be alert to all the potential legal risks in their practice and make a conscious effort to minimize them. Some of the issues that could present legal risks for nurses are presented below.

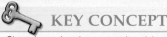

KEY CONCEPT

Situations that increase the risk of liability include working with insufficient resources, failing to follow policy and procedures, taking shortcuts, or working when feeling highly stressed.

BOX 8-1 | Acts That Could Result in Legal Liability for Nurses

ASSAULT

A deliberate threat or attempt to harm another person that the person believes could be carried through (e.g., telling a patient that he will be locked in a room without food for the entire day if he does not stop being disruptive).

BATTERY

Unconsented touching of another person in a socially impermissible manner or carrying through an assault. Even a touching act done to help a person can be interpreted as battery (e.g., performing a procedure without consent).

DEFAMATION OF CHARACTER

An oral or written communication to a third party that damages a person's reputation. Libel is the written form of defamation; slander is the spoken form. With slander, actual damage must be proven, except when:

- accusing someone of a crime
- accusing someone of having a loathsome disease
- making a statement that affects a person's professional or business activity
- calling a woman unchaste

Defamation does not exist if the statement is true and made in good faith to persons with a legitimate reason to receive the information. Stating on a reference that an employee was fired from your agency for physically abusing patients is not defamation if, in fact, the employee was found guilty of those charges. However, stating on a reference that an employee was a thief because narcotics were missing every time he or she was on duty can be considered defamation if the employee was never proved guilty of those charges.

FALSE IMPRISONMENT

Unlawful restraint or detention of a person. Preventing a patient from leaving a facility is an example of false imprisonment, unless it is shown that the patient has a contagious disease or could harm himself or herself or others. Actual physical restraint need not be used for false imprisonment to occur: telling a patient that he or she will be tied to the bed if he or she tries to leave

can be considered false imprisonment.

FRAUD

Willful and intentional misrepresentation that could cause harm or cause a loss to a person or property (e.g., selling a patient a ring with the claim that memory will be improved when it is worn).

INVASION OF PRIVACY

Invading the right of an individual to personal privacy. Can include unwanted publicity, releasing a medical record to unauthorized persons, giving patient information to an improper source, or having one's private affairs made public. (The only exceptions are reporting communicable diseases, gunshot wounds, and abuse.) Allowing a visiting student to look at a patient's pressure ulcers without permission can be an invasion of privacy.

LARCENY

Unlawful taking of another person's possession (e.g., assuming that a patient will not be using his or her personally owned wheelchair anymore and giving it away to another patient without permission).

NEGLIGENCE

Omission or commission of an act that departs from acceptable and reasonable standards, which can take several forms:
- *Malfeasance:* committing an unlawful or improper act (e.g., a nurse performing a surgical procedure)
- *Misfeasance:* performing an act improperly (e.g., including the patient in a research project without obtaining consent)
- *Nonfeasance:* failure to take proper action (e.g., not notifying the physician of a serious change in the patient's status)
- *Malpractice:* failure to abide by the standards of one's profession (e.g., not checking that a nasogastric tube is in the stomach before administering a tube feeding)
- *Criminal negligence:* disregard to protecting the safety of another person (e.g., allowing a confused patient, known to have a history of starting fires, to have matches in an unsupervised situation)

Malpractice

Nurses are expected to provide services to patients in a careful, competent manner according to a standard of care. The standard of care is considered the norm for what a reasonable individual in a similar circumstance would do. When performance deviates from the standard of care, nurses can be liable for malpractice. Examples of situations that could lead to malpractice include:

■ administering the incorrect dosage of a medication to a patient, thereby causing the patient to experience an adverse reaction

- identifying respiratory distress in a patient, but not informing the physician in a timely manner

- leaving an irrigating solution at the bedside of a confused patient, who then drinks that solution

- forgetting to turn an immobile patient during the entire shift, resulting in the patient developing a pressure ulcer

- having a patient fall because one staff member attempted to lift the patient manually when the use of a lift device was the standard

The fact that a negligent act occurred in itself does not warrant that damages be recovered; instead, it must be demonstrated that the following conditions were present:

- *Duty:* a relationship between the nurse and the patient in which the nurse has assumed responsibility for the care of the patient

- *Negligence:* failure to conform to the standard of care (i.e., malpractice)

- *Injury:* physical or mental harm to the patient, or violation of the patient's rights resulting from the negligent act

KEY CONCEPT

Duty, negligence, and injury must be present for malpractice to exist.

The complexities involved in caring for older adults, the need to delegate responsibilities to others, and the many competing demands on the nurse contribute to the risk of malpractice. As the responsibilities assumed by nurses increase, so will the risk of malpractice. Nurses should be aware of the risks in their practice and be proactive in preventing malpractice (Box 8-2). Also, it is advisable for nurses to carry their own malpractice insurance and not rely only on the insurance provided by their employers. Employers may refuse to cover nurses under their policy if it is believed they acted outside of their job descriptions; further, jury awards can exceed the limits of employers' policies.

POINT TO PONDER

In addition to the time and money involved in defending a lawsuit, what are some consequences of being accused of malpractice?

Other situations can cause nurses to be liable for negligence, if not malpractice, including the following:

- failing to take action (e.g., not reporting a change in the patient's condition or not notifying the administration of a physician's incompetent acts)

- contributing to patient injury (e.g., not providing appropriate supervision of confused patients or failing to lock the wheelchair during a transfer)

- failing to report a hazardous situation (e.g., not letting anyone know that the fire alarm system is inoperable or not informing anyone that a physician is performing procedures under the influence of alcohol)

- handling patient's possessions irresponsibly

- failing to follow established policies and procedures

POINT TO PONDER

Are you familiar with your state's nurse practice act and the regulations governing the area in which you practice or will practice?

Confidentiality

It is the rare patient who is seen by only one health care provider. More often the patient visits a variety of medical specialists, therapists, diagnostic facilities, pharmacies, and institutions. These providers often need to communicate information about the patient to ensure coordinated, quality care. However, with the potentially high number of individuals who have access to patients' personal medical information and the ease with which information is able to be transferred, there are increased opportunities for confidential information to fall into unintended hands.

In an effort to protect the security and confidentiality of patients' health information, the federal government developed the Health Insurance Portability and Accountability Act (HIPAA). HIPAA provides patients with access to their medical records and control over how their personal health information is used and disclosed. Congress authorized civil and criminal penalties for covered entities that misuse personal health information.

There can be variations in the procedures providers and facilities use to review HIPAA-related facts with patients, protect patients' information, and communicate information related to patients. It is important that nurses be familiar with and adhere to policies and procedures related to the protection of patients' privacy.

BOX 8-2 Recommendations for Reducing the Risk of Malpractice

- Be familiar with and follow the nurse practice act that governs nursing practice in the specific state.
- Keep current of and adhere to policies and procedures of the employing agency.
- Ensure that policies and procedures are revised as necessary.
- Do not discuss a patient's condition, share patient information, or allow access to a patient's medical record to anyone unless the patient has provided written consent.
- Consult with the physician when an order is unclear or inappropriate.
- Know patients' normal status and promptly report changes in status.
- Assess patients carefully and develop realistic care plans.
- Read patients' care plans and relevant nursing documentation before giving care.
- Identify patients before administering medications or treatments.
- Document observations about patients' status, care given, and significant occurrences.

- Assure that documentation by self and subordinates is accurate and that documentation reflects care that actually was provided.
- Know the credentials and assure competency of all subordinate staff.
- Discuss with supervisory staff assignments that cannot be completed due to insufficient staff or supplies.
- Do not accept responsibilities that are beyond your capabilities to perform and do not delegate assignments to others unless you are certain that they are competent to perform the delegated tasks.
- Report broken equipment and other safety hazards.
- Report or file an incident report when unusual situations occur.
- Promptly report all actual or suspected abuse to the appropriate state and local agencies.
- Attend continuing education programs and keep current of knowledge and skills pertaining to your practice.

Adapted from Eliopoulos, C. (2002). *Legal risks management guidelines and principles for long-term care facilities* (p. 28). Glen Arm, MD: Health Education Network.

Patient Consent

Patients are entitled to know the full implications of procedures and make an independent decision as to whether they choose to have them performed. This may sound simple enough, but it is easy for consent to be overlooked or improperly obtained by health care providers. For instance, certain procedures may become so routine to staff that they fail to realize patient permission must be granted, or a staff member may obtain a signature from a patient who has a fluctuating level of mental competency and who does not fully understand what he or she is signing. In the interest of helping patients and delivering care efficiently, or from a lack of knowledge concerning consent, staff members can subject themselves to considerable legal liability.

KEY CONCEPT

Patients who do not fully comprehend or who have fluctuating levels of mental function are incapable of granting legally sound consent.

Consent must be obtained before performing any medical or surgical procedure; performing procedures without consent can be considered battery. Usually when patients enter a health care facility they sign consent forms that authorize the staff to perform certain routine measures (e.g., bathing, examination, care-related treatments, and emergency interventions). These forms, however, do not qualify as *carte blanche* consent for all procedures. Even blanket consent forms that patients may sign, authorizing staff to do anything required for treatment and care, are not valid safeguards and may not be upheld in a court of law. Consent should be obtained for anything that exceeds basic, routine care measures. Particular procedures for which consent definitely should be sought include any entry into the body, either by incision or through natural body openings; any use of anesthesia, cobalt or radiation therapy, electroshock therapy, or experimental procedures; any type of research participation, invasive or not; and any procedure, diagnostic or treatment, that carries more than a slight risk. Whenever there is doubt regarding

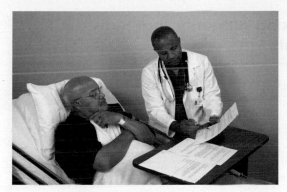

FIGURE 8-1 ■ It is important for the patient to give informed consent before any medical or surgical procedure. Written consent forms should describe the procedure, its purpose, alternatives to the procedure, expected consequences, and risks.

whether consent is necessary, it is best to err on the safe side.

Consent must be *informed*. It is unfair to the patient and legally unsound to obtain the patient's signature for a myelogram without telling the patient what that procedure entails. Ideally, a written consent that describes the procedure, its purpose, alternatives to the procedure, expected consequences, and risks should be signed by the patient, witnessed, and dated (Fig. 8-1). It is best that the person performing the procedure (e.g., the physician or researcher) be the one to explain the procedure and obtain the consent. Nurses or other staff members should not be in the position of obtaining consent for the physician because it is illegal and because they may not be able to answer some of the medical questions posed by the patient. Nurses can play an important role in the consent process by ensuring that it is properly obtained, answering questions, reinforcing information, and making the physician aware of any misunderstanding or change in the desire of the patient. Finally, nurses should not influence the patient's decision in any way.

Every conscious and mentally competent adult has the right to refuse consent for a procedure. To protect the agency and staff, it is useful to have the patient sign a release stating that consent is denied and that the patient understands the risks associated with refusing consent. If the patient refuses to sign the release, this should be witnessed, and both the professional seeking consent and the witness should sign a statement that documents the patient's refusal for the medical record.

Patient Competency

Increasingly, particularly in long-term care facilities, nurses are caring for patients who are confused, demented, or otherwise mentally impaired. Persons who are mentally incompetent are unable to give legal consent. Often in these circumstances, staff will turn to the next of kin to obtain consent for procedures; however, the appointment of a guardian to grant consent for the incompetent individual is the responsibility of the court. When the patient's competency is questionable, staff should encourage family members to seek legal guardianship of the patient or request the assistance of the state agency on aging in petitioning the court for appointment of a guardian. Unless they have been judged incompetent by a judge, people are entitled to make their own decisions.

Various forms of guardianship (also called conservatorship) can be granted when a person has been judged incompetent (Box 8-3), each with its own restrictions. The guardian is monitored by the court to ensure that he or she is acting in the best interests of the incompetent individual. In the case of a guardian of property, the guardian must file financial reports with the court.

Guardianship differs from power of attorney in that the latter is a mechanism used by competent individuals to appoint someone to make decisions for them. Usually, a power of attorney becomes invalid if the individual granting it becomes incompetent, except in the case of a durable power of attorney. A durable power of attorney allows competent individuals to appoint someone to make decisions on their behalf in the event that they become incompetent; this is a recommended procedure for individuals with dementias and other disorders in which competency can be anticipated to decline.

To ensure protection of patients' rights, nurses should recommend that patients and their families seek legal counsel for guardianship and power of attorney issues and, when such appointment has been made, clarify the type of decision-making authority that the appointed parties possess.

 KEY CONCEPT

A durable power of attorney can be useful for patients with Alzheimer's disease because they can appoint someone to make decisions on their behalf at a time when they may be incompetent to do so.

Staff Supervision

In many settings, gerontological nurses are responsible for supervising other staff, many of whom may be unlicensed personnel. In these situations, nurses are responsible not only for their own actions but also for the actions of the staff they are supervising.

BOX 8-3 **Kinds of Decision-Making Authority That Individuals Can Legally Possess Over Patients**

GUARDIANSHIP

Court appointment of an individual or organization to have the authority to make decisions for an incompetent person. Guardians can be granted decision-making authority for specific types of issues:

- Guardian of property (conservatorship): this limited guardianship allows the guardian to take care of financial matters but not make decisions concerning medical treatment.
- Guardian of person: decisions pertaining to the consent or refusal for care and treatments can be made by persons granted this type of guardianship.
- Plenary guardianship (committeeship): all types of decisions pertaining to person and property can be made by guardians under this form.

POWER OF ATTORNEY

Legal mechanism by which competent individuals appoint parties to make decisions for them; this can take the form of:

- Limited power of attorney: decisions are limited to certain matters (e.g., financial affairs) and power of attorney becomes invalid if the individual becomes incompetent.
- Durable power of attorney: provides a mechanism for continuing or initiating power of attorney in the event the individual becomes incompetent.

This falls under the doctrine of *respondeat superior* ("let the master answer"). Nurses must understand that if a patient is injured by an employee they supervise while the employee is working within the scope of the applicable job description, nurses can be liable. Various types of situations can create risks for nurses:

- permitting unqualified or incompetent persons to deliver care
- failing to follow up on delegated tasks
- assigning tasks to staff members for which they are not qualified or competent
- allowing staff to work under conditions with known risks (e.g., being short staffed and improperly functioning equipment)

These are considerations that nurses need to keep in mind when they accept responsibility for covering the house, sending an aide into a home to deliver care without knowing the aide's competency, or allowing registry or other employees to work without fully orienting them to agency policies and procedures.

KEY CONCEPT

A nurse needs to ensure that those caregivers to whom tasks are delegated are competent to perform the tasks and carry out their assignments properly.

Medications

Nurses are responsible for the safe administration of prescribed medications. Preparing, compounding, dispensing, and retailing medications fall within the practice of pharmacy, not nursing, and, when performed by nurses, can be interpreted as functioning outside their licensed scope of practice. An act as seemingly benign as going into the agency's pharmacy after hours, pouring some tablets into a container, labeling that container, and taking it to the unit so that a patient can receive the drug that is urgently needed is illegal.

Restraints

The Omnibus Budget Reconciliation Act (OBRA) heightened awareness of the serious impact of restraints by imposing strict standards on their use in long-term care facilities. This increased concern regarding and sensitivity to the use of chemical and physical restraints has had a ripple effect on other practice settings.

Anything that physically or mentally restricts a patient's movement (e.g., protective vests, trays on wheelchairs, safety belts, geriatric chairs, side rails, and medications) can be considered a restraint. Improperly used restraining devices can not only violate regulations concerning their use but also result in litigation for false imprisonment and negligence.

Older adults with deliriums and dementias can pose challenges to staff in terms of behavioral management. There are several medications (e.g., haloperidol, benzodiazepines, and lorazepam) that can be useful in reducing agitation and the need for physical restraints; however, these can result in complications such as aspiration due to depression of the gag reflex and pneumonia due to reduced respiratory activity. It must be recognized that these drugs are forms of chemical restraints and should only be employed after other measures have proven ineffective. Further, nonpharmacological strategies to manage behaviors can reduce the amount of drug needed. Consultation with geropsychiatric specialists or psychologists can prove beneficial in identifying other strategies.

Alternatives to restraints should be used when ever possible. Measures to help manage behavioral problems and protect the patient include alarmed doors, wristband alarms, bed alarm pads, beds and chairs close to the floor level, and increased staff supervision and contact. Specific patient behavior that creates risks to the patient and others should be documented. Assessment of the risk posed by the patient not being restrained and the effectiveness of alternatives should be included.

When restraints are deemed absolutely neces sary, a physician's order for the restraints must be obtained, stating the specific conditions for which the restraints are to be used, the type of restraints, and the duration of use. Agency policies should exist for the use of restraints and should be followed strictly. Detailed documentation should include the times for initiation and release of the restraints, their effectiveness, and the patient's response. The patient requires close observation while restrained.

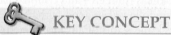

KEY CONCEPT

At no time should restraints be used for the convenience of staff.

At times, staff may assess that restraint use is required, but the patient or family objects and refuses to have a restraint used. If counseling does not help the patient and family understand the risks involved in not using the restraint, the agency may wish to have the patient and family sign a release of liability that states the risks of not using a restraint and the patient's or family's opposition. Although this may not free the nurse or agency from all responsibility, some limited protection may be afforded and, by signing the release, the patient and family may realize the severity of the situation.

Telephone Orders

In home health and long-term care settings, nurses often do not have the benefit of an on-site physician. Changes in the patient's condition and requests for new or altered treatments may be communicated over the telephone and, in response, physicians may prescribe orders accordingly. Accepting telephone orders predisposes nurses to considerable risks because the order can be heard or written incorrectly or the physician can deny that the order was given. It may not be realistic or advantageous to patient care to totally eliminate telephone orders, but nurses should minimize their risks in every way possible by taking the following precautions:

- Try to have the physician immediately fax the written order, if possible.
- Do not involve third parties in the order (e.g., do not have the order communicated by a secretary or other staff member for the nurse or the physician).
- Communicate all relevant information to the physician, such as vital signs, general status, and medications administered.
- Do not offer diagnostic interpretations or a medical diagnosis of the patient's problem.
- Write down the order as it is given and immediately read it back to the physician in its entirety.
- Place the order on the physician's order sheet, indicating it was a telephone order, the physician who gave it, time, date, and the nurse's signature.
- Obtain the physician's signature within 24 hours.

Recorded telephone orders may be a helpful way for nurses to validate what they have heard, but they may not offer much protection in the event of a lawsuit unless the physician is informed that the conversation is being recorded or unless special equipment with a 15-second tone sound is used.

Do Not Resuscitate Orders

The caseloads of many gerontological nurses contain a high prevalence of terminally ill patients. It may be understood by all parties involved that these patients are going to die and that resuscitation attempts would be inappropriate; however, unless an order specifically states that the patient should not be resuscitated, failure to attempt to save that person's life could be viewed as negligence. Nurses must ensure that DNR (do not resuscitate) orders are legally sound, remembering several points. First, DNR orders are medical orders and must be written and signed on the physician's order sheet to be valid. DNR placed on the care plan or a special symbol at the patient's bedside is not legal without the medical order. Next, unless it is detrimental to the patient's well-being or the patient is incompetent, consent for the decision not to resuscitate should be obtained; if the patient is unable to

CONSIDER THIS CASE

You are working in a nursing home that supports a restraint-free environment. In the past month, one of the residents has slipped once from her wheelchair and once off the edge of her bed; she fell onto the floor both times. Although the resident was not injured in either of these incidents, the resident's daughter is concerned that her mother has the potential to seriously hurt herself during a fall and requests that her mother be restrained while in bed and in her wheelchair. The resident has not expressed any preference but says she'll do whatever her daughter wants. You explain the rationale for not using restraints, but the daughter is insistent that her mother be restrained. "You know my mother has the tendency to slip to the floor," the daughter says, "so if you don't tie her in the chair and keep her rails up when she is in bed and she falls, I'll have my lawyers here before you can say boo!"

THINK CRITICALLY

- How do you decide if the resident's freedom to be unrestrained is worth the risk of her injuring herself during a fall?
- What dilemmas could you present for the resident if you ask her for her preference without consideration of the daughter's desires?
- How much should a facility be influenced by the threat of litigation?
- What can you do to safeguard the resident and the facility?

consent, family consent should be sought. Finally, every agency should develop a DNR policy to guide staff in these situations; this could be an excellent item for an ethics committee to review.

Advance Directives and Issues Related to Death and Dying

A variety of issues surrounding patients' deaths pose legal concern for nurses. Some of these issues arise long before death occurs, when patients choose to execute an advance directive or a living will. Advance directives express the desires of competent adults regarding terminal care, life-sustaining measures, and other issues pertaining to their dying and death.

KEY CONCEPT

There are two types of advance directives. *A durable power of attorney for health care* is a document that appoints a person selected by the patient (called a health care proxy, attorney-in-fact, surrogate, or agent) to make decisions on the patient's behalf should the patient be unable to make or communicate his or her decisions. A *living will* describes a patient's preferences and gives instructions to health care providers if at a future time he or she is unable to make or communicate decisions and has no one appointed as proxy.

In 1990, Congress passed the Patient Self-Determination Act (which went into effect from December 1, 1991), which requires all health care

institutions receiving Medicare or Medicaid funds to ask patients on admission if they possess a living will or durable power of attorney for health care. The patient's response must be recorded in the medical record. Nurses can aid by making physicians and other staff aware of the presence of a patient's advance directive, informing patients of any special measures they must take to have the document accepted into the medical record, and, unless contraindicated, following the patient's wishes (Fig. 8-2). Following an advance directive protects health care professionals from civil and criminal liability when they are followed in good faith. Nurses are advised to check the status of advance directive legislation in their individual states.

Other issues arise when patients are terminally ill and dying; one such issue involves wills. Wills are statements of individuals' desires for the

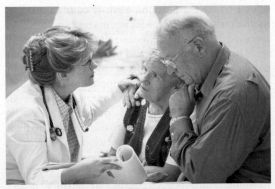

FIGURE 8-2 ■ Gerontological nurses guide older adults as they consider advance directives.

management of their affairs after their death. For a will to be valid, the person making it must be of sound mind and legal age and must not be coerced or influenced into making it. The will should be written—although under certain conditions, some states recognize oral, or nuncupative, wills—signed, dated, and witnessed by persons not named in the will. The required number of witnesses may vary among the states.

To avoid problems, such as family accusations that the patient was influenced by the nurse because of his dependency on her, nurses should avoid witnessing a will. Nurses should, however, help patients obtain legal counsel when they wish to execute or change a will. Legal aid agencies and local schools of law are also sources of assistance for older adults wishing to write their wills. If a patient is dying and wishes to dictate a will to the nurse, the nurse may write it exactly as stated, sign and date it, have the patient sign it if possible, and forward it to the agency's administrative offices for handling. It is useful for gerontological nurses to encourage persons of all ages to develop a will to avoid having the state determine how their property will be distributed in the event of their deaths.

The pronouncement of death is another area of concern. Nurses often are placed in the position and are capable of determining when a patient has died and notifying the family and funeral home. The physician is then notified of the death by telephone and signs the death certificate at a later time. This rather common and benign procedure actually may be illegal for nurses because in some states the act of pronouncing a patient dead falls within the scope of medical practice, not nursing. Nurses should safeguard their licenses by either holding physicians responsible for the pronouncement of death if they are required to do so or lobbying to have the law changed so that they are protected in these situations.

Postmortem examinations of deceased persons are useful in learning more about the cause of death. They also contribute to medical education. In some circumstances, such as when the cause of death is suspected to be associated with a criminal act, malpractice, or an occupational disease, the death may be considered a medical examiner's case and an autopsy may be mandatory. Unless it is a medical examiner's case, consent for autopsy must be obtained from the next of kin, usually in the order of spouse, children, parents, siblings, grandparents, aunts, uncles, and cousins.

Elder Abuse

Elder abuse can occur in patients' homes or in health care facilities by loved ones, caregivers, or strangers. Particularly in long-term caregiving relationships, in which family members or staff "burn out," abuse may be an unfortunate consequence. Factors contributing to abuse by family caregivers are discussed in Chapter 38.

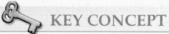

KEY CONCEPT

Caregiver stress can lead to abuse of older adults.

There are several recognized types of elder abuse (National Center for Elder Abuse, 2012), which include:

- physical abuse
- emotional abuse
- sexual abuse
- exploitation
- neglect
- abandonment

Abuse can assume many forms, including inflicting pain or injury; stealing; mismanaging funds; misusing medications; causing psychological distress; withholding food or care; or confining a person. Even threatening to commit any of these acts is considered abuse. Abuse may be undetected due to an older person's lack of contact with others (e.g., being homebound and not having communication with anyone but the relative who is the abuser) or due to the reluctance to report the problem due to fear or shame. Nurses can assess for abuse using a tool such as the Elder Assessment Instrument (Fulmer, 2003). Gerontological nurses must also be alert to indications of possible abuse or neglect during routine interactions with older adults; signs could include:

- delay in seeking necessary medical care
- malnutrition
- dehydration
- unexplained bruises
- poor hygiene and grooming
- urine odor, urine-stained clothing/linens
- excoriation or abrasions of genitalia
- inappropriate administration of medications
- repeated infections, injuries, or preventable complications from existing diseases
- evasiveness in describing condition, symptoms, problems, home life
- unsafe living environment
- social isolation
- anxiety, suspiciousness, and depression

Nurses have a legal responsibility to report all cases of known or suspected abuse. States vary regarding reporting mechanisms; nurses should thus consult specific state laws. The Resources listing includes organizations that can provide information on elder abuse and guidance on finding attorneys to assist a person who is the victim of abuse.

LEGAL SAFEGUARDS FOR NURSES

Common sense can be the best ally of sound nursing practice. Never forget that patients, visitors, and employees do not forfeit their legal rights or responsibilities when they are within the health care environment. Laws and regulations impose additional rights and responsibilities in patient–provider and employee–employer relationships. Nurses can and should protect themselves in the following ways:

- familiarize themselves with the laws and rules governing their specific care agency/facility,

their state's nurse practice act, and labor relations
- become knowledgeable about their agency's policies and procedures and adhere to them strictly
- function within the scope of nursing practice
- determine for themselves the competency of employees for whom they are responsible
- check the work of employees under their supervision
- obtain administrative or legal guidance when in doubt about the legal ramifications of a situation
- report and document any unusual occurrence
- refuse to work under circumstances that create a risk to safe patient care
- carry liability insurance

BRINGING RESEARCH TO LIFE

SCREENING FOR ABUSE AND NEGLECT OF PEOPLE WITH DEMENTIA

Wiglesworth, A., Mosqueda, L., Mulnard, R., Liao, S., Gibbs, L., & Fitzgerald, W. (2010). Journal of the American Geriatrics Society, 58(3), 493–500.

For this study, the researchers visited 129 persons who were diagnosed with dementia and their caregivers in their homes to assess for evidence of mistreatment. It was found that 47% of the participants with dementia had been mistreated by their caregivers, with psychological abuse being the most common form. When the characteristics of the individuals who were abused and their caregivers were assessed, it was found that the caregivers who abused had higher levels of anxiety, more evidence of depression, fewer social contacts, and perceived themselves to be carrying a significant burden. The persons with dementia who were abused were found to be physically and psychologically aggressive toward their caregivers.

These findings indicate a need to ask the caregivers about their perceived caregiving burden and any psychological or physical mistreatment that they experience from the person with dementia. This not only can aid in identifying the risk for the person with dementia to be abused but can also reveal the possible need for protection, support, and assistance for the caregiver. Protecting the rights of older adults sometimes means scratching below the surface to detect problems.

PRACTICE REALITIES

You are working the night shift, where there have been several call outs on the unit for postoperative patients. All staff are carrying a heavier than usual load. During tonight's shift, one of the nurses forgot to raise the side rail on a heavily sedated patient. In his confused, sedated state the patient tries to get out of bed and falls. You and the assigned nurse hurry to his aid. The other nurse tells you to help her lift the patient back to bed. You resist, stating "He should be examined and the supervisor called." The other nurse objects, stating "You know the policy. They'll either suspend or fire me and I have kids to support. I checked him out and he is fine ... and, he is too doped up to remember anything. There won't be any harm; come on."

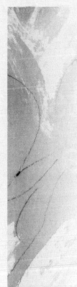

The patient doesn't appear injured and you don't want the nurse to be in jeopardy of losing her job. What should you do?

CRITICAL THINKING EXERCISES

1. Discuss the reasons why gerontological nursing is a high-risk specialty for legal liability.
2. Identify the process you would follow in your community to obtain guardianship for an incompetent older adult who has no family.
3. Describe the approach you would use to discuss the development of an advanced directive with an older adult.
4. Discuss the actions you would take if faced with the following situations:

   - A nurse whom you supervise makes repeated errors and does not seem competent to do his job
   - You begin documenting your observations but are told by your immediate supervisor to "just bite your tongue and live with it because he is the administrator's son"
   - A patient confides in you that her son is forging her name on checks and gradually emptying out her bank accounts

RESOURCES

American Association of Retired Persons (AARP) Elder Law Forum
http://www.aarp.org/research/legal-advocacy/

American Bar Association Senior Lawyers Division
http://www.abanet.org/srlawyers/home.html

Hartford Institute for Geriatric Nursing
Try This: Best Practices in Nursing Care to Older Adults
Issue Number 15 (Revised 2007), Elder Mistreatment and Abuse Assessment
http://consultgerirn.org/uploads/File/trythis/try_this_15.pdf

National Academy of Elder Law Attorneys
http://www.naela.com

National Center on Elder Abuse
http://www.elderabusecenter.org

National Senior Citizens Law Center
http://www.nsclc.org

Nursing Home Abuse/Elder Abuse Attorneys Referral Network

REFERENCES

Fulmer, T. (2003). Elder abuse and neglect assessment. *Journal of Gerontological Nursing, 29*(6), 4–5.
National Center for Elder Abuse. (2012). *Fact sheet about elder abuse.* Retrieved May 2, 2012 from http://www.ncea.aoa.gov/ncearoot/Main_Site/index.aspx

RECOMMENDED READINGS

Recommended Readings associated with this chapter can be found on the web site that accompanies the book. Visit http://thepoint.lww.com/Eliopoulos8e to access the recommended readings and other additional resources associated with this chapter.

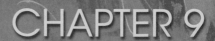

CHAPTER 9

Ethical Aspects of Gerontological Nursing

CHAPTER OUTLINE

Philosophies Guiding Ethical Thinking

Ethics in Nursing
External and Internal Ethical Standards
Ethical Principles

Ethical Dilemmas Facing Gerontological Nurses
Changes Increasing Ethical Dilemmas for Nurses
Measures to Help Nurses Make Ethical Decisions

LEARNING OBJECTIVES

After reading this chapter, you should be able to:

1. Discuss various philosophies regarding right and wrong.

2. Describe ethical standards and principles guiding nursing practice.

3. List factors that have increased ethical dilemmas for nurses.

4. Identify measures to help nurses make ethical decisions.

TERMS TO KNOW

Autonomy: to respect individual freedoms, preferences, and rights

Beneficence: to do good for patients

Confidentiality: to respect the privacy

Ethics: a system of moral principles guiding behaviors

Fidelity: to respect our words and duty to patients

Justice: to be fair, treat people equally

Nonmaleficence: to prevent harm to patients

Veracity: truthfulness

Although the concept of principles guiding right and wrong conduct is not new to nursing, professional ethics has received increasing attention in nursing circles. Gerontological nurses commonly face ethical questions regarding the provision, scope, or cost of care for older adults. Many of these questions arise in nurses' daily practice. It is important for nurses to understand both the ethics of the nursing profession and their own personal ethics and to be aware of the ethical dilemmas facing gerontological nurses today.

PHILOSOPHIES GUIDING ETHICAL THINKING

The word *ethics* originated in ancient Greece—*ethos* means those beliefs that guide life. Most current definitions of ethics revolve around the concept of accepted standards of conduct and moral judgment. Basically, ethics help determine right and wrong courses of action. As simple as this sounds, different philosophies disagree about what constitutes right and wrong; the following are some examples:

- *Utilitarianism.* This philosophy holds that good acts are those from which the greatest number of people will benefit and gain happiness.

- *Egoism.* At the opposite pole from utilitarianism, egoism proposes that an act is morally acceptable if it is of the greatest benefit to oneself and that there is no reason to perform an act that benefits others unless one will personally benefit from it as well.

- *Relativism.* This philosophy can be referred to as situational ethics, in that right and wrong are relative to the situation. Within relativism are several subgroups of thinking. Some relativists believe that there can be individual variation in what is ethically correct, whereas others feel that the individual's beliefs should conform to the overall beliefs of the society for the given time and situation.

- *Absolutism.* Under the theory of absolutism, there are specific truths to guide actions. The truths can vary depending on a person's beliefs; for example, a Christian's view may differ from an atheist's view on certain moral behaviors, and a person who supports a political view of democracy may believe in truths different from those of a communist.

To illustrate the application of these four different philosophies, consider the hypothetical situation of four poor old men who share a household. One day, one of these men finds a lottery ticket in the mailbox while checking the household's mail. The ticket holds the winning number for a million dollars. Ethically, does he owe his housemates any of the winnings? A *utilitarian* would propose that he split the winnings with his housemates because that would bring good to the greatest number of people. An *egoist* would encourage him to keep the winnings because that would do him the most good personally. A *relativist* might say that normally he should keep the winnings, but because in this situation he will have more money than he will need, he should share the winnings. An *absolutist* who happens to be Christian may say that keeping the ticket is morally wrong and an effort should be made to find the rightful owner.

Now consider the application of the philosophical approaches to the issue of federal subsidies to older adults. A *utilitarian* could say that 12% of the population should not use one third of the gross national product and that the money instead should be equally allocated on a per capita basis. An *egoist* would say that the individual old person should take whatever he feels he needs, regardless of the impact on others. A *relativist* could say that older people can use this proportion of the budget unless more is needed for dependent children or defense, at which point it would no longer be right to do so. *Absolutists* could hold various views depending on their belief systems, ranging from giving the older population whatever they need because of a moral responsibility to care for the sick and aged, to withholding funds from the older population so that finances are available to build the military and meet specific political goals.

Other philosophies guiding ethics exist, but the few that have been briefly described demonstrate the diversity of approaches to ethical thinking and reinforce the fact that determining right and wrong actions can be a complicated endeavor.

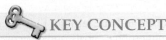

KEY CONCEPT

Individuals can be guided by a wide range of ethical philosophies that cause them to view the same situations in vastly different ways.

ETHICS IN NURSING

External and Internal Ethical Standards

Professions such as nursing require a code of ethics on which practice can be based and evaluated. A professional code of ethics is accepted by those who practice the profession as the formal guidelines for their actions. The American Nurses Association (ANA) Code of Ethics for Nurses (Box 9-1) outlines the broad values of the profession. The American Holistic Nurses' Association has developed the *Code of Ethics for Holistic Nursing* that provides guidance for nurses' actions and responsibilities for self, others, and the environment (the full document is available at http://www.ahna.org).

Nurses are also subject to ethical standards created outside of the nursing profession. Federal, state, and local standards, in the form of regulations, guide the nursing practice. In addition, various organizations such as the Joint Commission and the American Healthcare Association develop standards

BOX 9-1   Code of Ethics for Nurses

1. The nurse, in all professional relationships, practices with compassion and respect for the inherent dignity, worth, and uniqueness of every individual, unrestricted by considerations of social or economic status, personal attributes, or the nature of health problems.

2. The nurse's primary commitment is to the patient, whether an individual, family, group, or community.

3. The nurse promotes, advocates for, and strives to protect the health, safety, and rights of the patient.

4. The nurse is responsible and accountable for individual nursing practice and determines the appropriate delegation of tasks consistent with the nurse's obligation to provide optimum patient care.

5. The nurse owes the same duties to self as to others, including the responsibility to preserve integrity and safety, to maintain competence, and to continue personal and professional growth.

6. The nurse participates in establishing, maintaining, and improving health care environments and conditions of employment conducive to the provision of quality health care and consistent with the values of the profession through individual and collective action.

7. The nurse participates in the advancement of the profession through contributions to practice, education, administration, and knowledge development.

8. The nurse collaborates with other health professionals and the public in promoting community, national, and international efforts to meet health needs.

9. The profession of nursing, as represented by associations and their members, is responsible for articulating nursing values, for maintaining the integrity of the profession and its practice, and for shaping social policy.

Courtesy of American Nurses Association, Washington, DC. Developed and published by the American Nurses Association, 2001.

for specific practitioners and care settings. Individual agencies, too, have philosophies, goals, and objectives that support a specific level of nursing practice.

Most importantly, individual nurses possess values that they have developed throughout their lives that will largely influence ethical thinking. Ideally, a nurse's individual value system meshes with that of the profession, society, and employer; conflict can arise when value systems are incompatible.

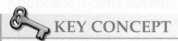 KEY CONCEPT

It is important for a nurse to understand his or her own values as conflict and distress can result when the nurse's values differ from those of the employer or population served.

Ethical Principles

Several ethical principles are used to guide health care, including the following:

- *Beneficence:* to do good for patients. This principle is based on the belief that the education and experience of nurses enable them to make sound decisions that serve patients' best interests. Nurses are challenged to take actions that are good for patients while not ignoring patients' desires. To override patients' decisions

and invoke professional authority to take actions that nurses view as in patients' best interests is viewed as paternalism and interferes with the freedom and rights of patients.

- *Nonmaleficence:* to prevent harm to patients. This principle could be viewed as a subset of beneficence because the intent is ultimately to take action that is good for patients. In addition to not directly performing an act that causes harm, actions such as informing management that staffing is inadequate to provide safe care support nonmaleficence.

- *Justice:* to be fair, treat people equally, and give patients the service they need. At the foundation of this principle is the belief that patients are entitled to services based on need, regardless of the ability to pay. Scarce resources have challenged this concept of unrestricted access and use of health care services.

- *Fidelity and veracity:* fidelity means to respect our words and duty to patients; veracity means truthfulness. This principle is central to all nurse–patient interactions because the quality of this relationship depends on trust and integrity. Older patients may have higher degrees of vulnerability than the younger adults and may be particularly dependent on the truthfulness of their caregivers.

■ *Autonomy:* to respect patients' freedoms, preferences, and rights. Ensuring and protecting older patients' right to provide informed consent are consistent with this principle.

■ *Confidentiality:* to respect the privacy of patients. Patients often share highly personal information with nurses and need to feel assured that their trust will not be violated. In addition to respecting confidentiality as being a morally sound principle, the Health Insurance Portability and Accountability Act and other laws have afforded people the legal right to privacy and consequences if this is violated.

Few nurses would argue with the value of these principles (Fig. 9-1). In fact, practices that reinforce these principles are widely promoted, such as ensuring that patients receive the care they need, respecting the rights of patients to consent to or deny consent for treatment, preventing incompetent staff from caring for patients, and following acceptable standards of practice. Actual nursing practice is seldom simple, however, and situations emerge that add new considerations to the application of moral principles to patient care. Ethical dilemmas can

emerge when other circumstances interfere with the clear, basic application of ethical principles.

POINT TO PONDER

How do you respond to and try to solve ethical dilemmas? If you are in practice, do you accept different standards in practice from what you would accept in your personal life? If so, why?

ETHICAL DILEMMAS FACING GERONTOLOGICAL NURSES

Nursing practice involves many situations that could produce conflicts—conflicts between nurses' values and external systems affecting their decisions and conflicts between the rights of patients and nurses' responsibilities to those patients. Box 9-2 presents examples of such dilemmas. These examples are typical of the decisions facing nurses everyday and for which there are no simple answers.

It is easy to say that nurses should always follow the regulations, adhere to principles, and do what is best for the patient. But can nurses realistically be expected to follow these guidelines 100% of the time? What if following the rules means they may lose the income on which their families depend, violate the rights of individuals to decide their own destinies, create problems for coworkers or their employers, or cause them to be labeled troublemakers? Is it alright to knowingly violate a regulation or law if no real harm will result? Do nurses need to limit how much of an advocacy role they can assume? Should nurses base their decisions on what is right for themselves, their patients, or their employers? To whom are nurses really most responsible and accountable?

KEY CONCEPT

Most clinical situations do not lend themselves to simple, clear-cut ethical decisions.

Changes Increasing Ethical Dilemmas for Nurses

Questions of ethics are not new to nursing. However, changes within the profession and the entire health care delivery system have introduced new areas of ethical dilemmas to nursing practice.

Expanded Role of Nurses

Nurses have gone beyond the confines of simply following doctors' orders and providing basic comfort and care. They now perform sophisticated assessments, diagnose nursing problems, monitor

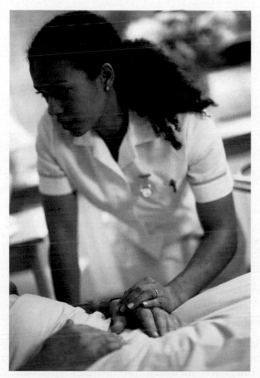

FIGURE 9-1 ■ Nurses follow the principles of doing good, treating people equally, honoring their word, and respecting older adults' rights.

BOX 9-2   Examples of Ethical Dilemmas in Gerontological Nursing Practice

While working in an outreach program to bring services to community-based older adults, you meet Mr. Brooks, a 68-year-old homeless man. Mr. Brooks asks your opinion about respiratory symptoms that he has been experiencing over the past several months. He reports a chronic cough, hemoptysis, and dyspnea. He appears thin and admits to having lost weight. He states he has smoked at least one pack of cigarettes daily for over 50 years and has no intention of changing his smoking habit. Although he is not cognitively impaired, he strongly resists efforts to find him housing and arrange for medical evaluation and treatment. You are convinced that without intervention, Mr. Brooks will not survive much longer.

Do you respect Mr. Brooks' right to make his own decisions about his life, even if those decisions run contrary to what is best for his health and well-being?

You are the new director of nursing for a nursing home and were pleased to get the job because yours has become the sole source of income for your family. Ten cases of diarrhea develop among the residents and you know that the regulations require that you report five cases or more. You bring this to the attention of the medical director and administrator, who direct you not to "cause trouble by putting the health department on their backs." The medical director assures you that the problem is not serious and will pass in a few days. You know you should notify the health department, but you also know that the administrator fired the last nursing director for opposing him on a similar issue.

Do you allow a regulation to be violated or risk losing a job that you may badly need?

Insurance coverage expires tomorrow for 76-year-old Mrs. Brady, and the physician has written an order for her discharge. Because Mrs. Brady continued to be weak and slightly confused, she was not able to be instructed in the safe use of home oxygen and medication administration during her hospitalization. Her 80-year-old husband, who is expected to be her primary caregiver, is weak and in poor health himself. The social worker tells you that arrangements have been made for a nurse to visit the home daily but that the couple does not qualify for 24-hour home care assistance. You and other nursing staff members firmly believe that Mrs. Brady's health will be in jeopardy if she is discharged tomorrow. The physician tells you that you are probably right, but "the hospital cannot be expected to eat the bills that Medicare does not want to pay."

Do you increase the hospital's financial risks by insisting that nonreimbursed care be provided?

Seventy-nine-year-old Mr. Adams lies in his bed in a fetal position, unresponsive except to deep painful stimuli. He has multiple pressure ulcers, has recurrent infections, and must be fed with a nasogastric tube. His wife and children express concern over the quality of his life and state that Mr. Adams would never have wanted to survive in this state. The children privately tell the multidisciplinary team that if their father's care expenses continue, their mother will be destitute, and they beg the staff to remove the tube. The family expresses that they do not have the emotional or financial resources to take the issue to court. The physician is sympathetic, but states he feels compelled to continue the feedings and antibiotics because he does not condone euthanasia; however, privately, the physician tells you that he will close his eyes and keep quiet if you want to pull the tube without anyone knowing.

Do you exceed your authority and discontinue a life-sustaining measure to grant the family's request?

Mrs. Smith is dying of cancer and being cared for at home by her husband. The couple has been married for 63 years and has never been apart during that time. They are highly interdependent and each one's world revolves around the other's. During your home nursing visit, the couple openly discusses their plans with you. They tell you that they have agreed that when Mrs. Smith's pain becomes too severe to tolerate, they will both ingest sufficient medication, which they have accumulated, to kill themselves, and die peacefully in each other's arms.

Do you ignore your responsibility to report suicidal intent to respect a couple's wish to end their lives together?

and give complicated treatments, use alternative modalities of care, and, particularly, in geriatric care settings, increasingly make independent judgments about patients' clinical conditions. This wider scope of functions, combined with higher salaries and greater status, has increased the accountability and responsibility of nurses for the care of patients.

Medical Technology

Artificial organs, genetic screening, new drugs, computers, lasers, ultrasound, and other innovations have increased the medical community's ability to diagnose and treat problems and to save lives that once would have been given no hope. However, new problems have accompanied these advances, such as determining on whom, when, and how this technology should be used.

New Fiscal Constraints

In the past, the major concern of health care providers and agencies was to provide quality services to help people maintain and restore health. Now, there are competing and sometimes overriding concerns, including the following: being cost effective, minimizing bad debts, and developing alternate sources of revenue. Patients' needs are weighed against economic survival, resulting in some difficult decisions. Further, in this era of rationed care and scarce resources, questions are raised regarding the right of older adults to expect a high quality and quantity of health and social services while other groups lack basic assistance.

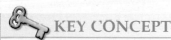

KEY CONCEPT

Increasingly, questions are raised regarding the right of older adults to expect greater benefits than other members of the society.

Conflict of Interest

Nurses can face a variety of situations that present a conflict of interest. Examples of this could include the following: a nurse, believing a resident's life could be extended with nasogastric feedings and antibiotic therapy, feeling that a resident's and family's rejection of this care is inappropriate; a patient's physical therapy discontinued due to insurance restrictions and the nurse knowing that the patient has the potential to make continued progress with the therapy; and, the nurse knowing the employer is intentionally keeping staffing levels below what is needed but not objecting or advocating for proper staffing because the nurse does not want to jeopardize his or her position.

Greater Numbers of Older Adults

Entitlement programs and services for older persons had less impact when only a small portion of the population was old, but with growing numbers of people spending more years in old age and the increasing ratio of dependent individuals to productive workers, society is beginning to feel burdened. Although older adults' problems and needs are more evident, the ability and responsibility of society to support these needs are in question.

Assisted Suicide

The ANA has been clear in its objection to assisted suicide, believing instead that nurses should provide competent, compassionate end-of-life care.

However, although participating in a patient's assisted suicide is unethical and inappropriate, nurses may care for terminally ill individuals who accept and desire assisted suicide. The situation becomes even more complicated by the fact that laws have been enacted (e.g., Oregon's Death with Dignity Act of 1997) to allow terminally ill persons to end their lives with lethal medications, and individuals have the right to refuse care under self-determination directives. Nurses may face the dilemma of knowing that a competent patient is arranging an assisted suicide and believing that they must intervene. Or, they may know that a competent patient is arranging an assisted suicide, and while understanding and respecting the patient's decision, they feel they are violating professional standards by not reporting it so that it may be halted.

POINT TO PONDER

Do you believe that gerontological nurses have an ethical responsibility to advocate for older individuals by objecting to and bringing public attention to policy and reimbursement decisions that are not in older persons' best interests?

Measures to Help Nurses Make Ethical Decisions

Although guidelines exist, no solid answers can solve all of the ethical dilemmas that nurses face. Nurses should, however, minimize their struggles in making ethical decisions by using critical thinking and employing the following measures:

- *Encourage patients to express their desires.* Advise patients to express their desires in advance directives, wills, and other legally binding documents and advocate compliance with patients' wishes. Box 9-3 offers suggestions on assisting patients in making decisions.

- *Identify significant others who impact and are impacted.* Consider family members, friends, and caregivers who are involved with the patient and the situation, and their concerns and preferences.

- *Know yourself.* The nurse should review his or her personal value system. The influences of religion, cultural beliefs, and personal experiences should be explored to understand one's unique comfort zone with specific ethical issues.

- *Read.* Review the medical literature for discussions and case experiences of other nurses to gain a wider perspective into the types of

CONSIDER THIS CASE

Seventy-nine-year-old Mr. J has been diagnosed with a rare liver cancer. The oncologist informs Mr. J that although he is willing to attempt a round of chemotherapy, no treatment has been effective in extending life for more than a few months for this aggressive type of cancer. Mr. J and his 66-year-old wife are devastated by this information and look to the Internet for help. They read testimonials of patients who have had similar liver cancers whose lives allegedly were extended for several years with an alternative treatment offered by a hospital in Germany. They make contact with the hospital and learn that Mr. J qualifies for their treatment, which consists of a 2-week-long stay at the hospital in Germany, every 2 months. Each of the hospitalizations costs $25,000 plus the couple's travel expenses. The couple has no savings but owns a very modest house; they have no children. The couple discusses this option with the oncologist, who discourages the alternative treatment, stating, "Your time and money would be better spent in enjoying the remaining time you have together and making preparations for Mr. J's declining health and ultimate death." Despite the physician's discouraging remarks, Mr. J wants to mortgage the house to pay for the alternative treatment. Mrs. J wants to help her husband extend his life but is concerned that she will face the prospect of losing the house or being required to pay off the mortgage on her limited Social Security check long after Mr. J dies. She is not comfortable with the idea, but feels that if she voices her concerns, her husband, friends, and family will consider her uncaring.

THINK CRITICALLY

- Does Mr. J have the right to deplete the couple's resources for a questionable treatment that may only extend his life for a few months?
- Does Mrs. J have the right to oppose this plan?
- Does Mr. J's physician have the right to dash Mr. J's hopes?
- How could you assist the couple?

BOX 9-3   Assisting Older Adults in Decision Making

- Assure the person is competent to make decisions. Even if the person has no diagnosis (e.g., dementia) that would interfere with decision making, the stress of a hospitalization and the effects of medications or other treatments could alter the mental ability to make competent decisions. Assess for alterations in mental status that could influence competent decision making. If competency is in question, consult with the organization's social worker or other designated professional to have a surrogate properly appointed.
- Document the assessment of factors influencing the ability to make decisions, such as mental status, ability to express preferences, mood, effects of medications, and family influence.

If the individual is competent to make decisions:

- Offer explanations and information regarding treatment options to increase the person's understanding. Offer to include family members or significant others in the discussion if the person desires.

- Ensure that the person understands the diagnosis, prognosis, treatment options, and risks and benefits of various treatments.
- Encourage the person to ask questions and express any concerns.
- If there is question or confusion about procedures for which consent is needed or has been granted, request that the provider who will perform the procedure meet with the person to discuss the issue.
- Ensure that the person is not being coerced into any decision or feels intimidated to state a refusal to give consent.
- Recognize that ability to make competent decisions can fluctuate (e.g., due to medications, pain) and ensure that explanations are provided and decisions made during times of lucidity.
- Document all assessment findings, explanations given, the person's expressed preferences and concerns, and other relevant information.

ethical problems confronted within nursing and strategies for managing them. Literature outside the field of nursing can help add new facets to one's thinking.

■ *Discuss.* In formal education programs or informal coffee breaks, talk about issues with other health team members. Members of the clergy, attorneys, ethicists, and others also can provide interesting perspectives.

■ *Form an ethics committee.* Bring together various members of the health team, clergy, attorneys, and lay persons to study ethical problems within the specific care setting, clarify legal and regulatory boundaries, develop policies, discuss ethical problems that surface, and investigate charges of ethical misconduct.

■ *Consult.* Clinical ethics consultation takes the form of an ethics committee or consultation provided by expert individuals or groups (e.g., lawyers, philosophers, and clinicians who specialize in bioethics). Clinical ethics consultants provide education, mediate moral conflict, facilitate moral reflection, and advocate for patients (American Society for Bioethics and the Humanities, 2010). (For information on the competencies and practice of Health Care Ethics Consultants, visit http://www.asbh.org/papers.)

■ *Share.* When faced with a difficult ethical decision, talk with others and seek guidance and support.

■ *Evaluate decisions.* Assess the outcomes of the actions and whether the same courses of action would be chosen in a similar situation in the future. Even the worst decision holds some lessons.

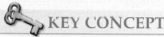

KEY CONCEPT

When facing ethical decisions, it is beneficial to be clear about one's own value system.

Gerontological nursing holds its share of ethical questions. Should resources be spent for a heart transplant for an octogenarian? Should an affluent child rather than public funds pay for a parent's care? How much sacrifice must a family endure to care for a relative at home? How much compromise in care can nurses accept to keep an agency's budget healthy? Nurses must be active participants in the process of developing ethically sound policies and practices affecting the care of older adults. The choice between being a leader or an ostrich in this arena can significantly determine the future status of gerontological nursing practice.

BRINGING RESEARCH TO LIFE

WHY DO MORE PEOPLE DIE DURING ECONOMIC EXPANSIONS?

Stevens, A.H., Miller, D.L., Page, M. & Filiski, M. (2012). Center for Retirement Research, No. 12-8.

This study examined the impact of rising employment levels on mortality. In examining the additional deaths that occurred in a year in which unemployment dropped 1.1%, the study found that working age individuals accounted for just 9% of the additional deaths, whereas 75% were among people over the age of 65. Older women alone accounted for 55% of the total additional deaths. Most of the increased deaths were among nursing home residents.

The researchers discovered that employment changes in the nursing homes contributed to the increased mortality rates of the older adults. Their analyses revealed that 1% decline in the unemployment rate caused more than a 3% drop in overall full-time employment at nursing homes; in other words, when employment opportunities became more abundant, nursing home workers left for better jobs. The fact that most nursing home residents are women accounted for the high mortality rates in females. It was concluded that low staffing can have a deadly impact on nursing home residents.

This study demonstrates the importance of adequate reimbursement to nursing homes to provide competitive salaries to staff. Without competitive wages, caregiving staff are less likely to be retained and the resultant turnover and low staffing patterns have deleterious effects. When considering nonmaleficence, the issue of advocating for and assuring adequate reimbursement and staffing patterns must be considered.

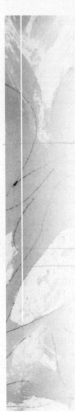

PRACTICE REALITIES

A citizen action group is concerned about taxes and is developing a list of recommendations to offer its congressional representatives. Among the recommendations is one to limit Medicaid and Medicare reimbursed expensive surgeries (e.g., hip replacements and organ transplant) to only persons under the age of 80. The rationale is that the limited funds are best used in younger persons who have more years left of life.

Although you understand that health care dollars are limited and appreciate the impact of growing tax burdens, as a gerontological nurse you feel a responsibility to advocate for the rights of older adults to have the same services available as other age groups.

How would you react to the citizens' group?

CRITICAL THINKING EXERCISES

1. What factors have influenced your personal ethics?
2. Discuss the dilemmas arising from the following situations:
   - Having a terminally ill patient confide plans to commit suicide
   - Being instructed to discharge a patient whose care is no longer being reimbursed while knowing that the patient is not ready for discharge
   - Having to terminate a nursing assistant for attendance problems, knowing that she is the sole wage earner in her family
   - Being asked by a senior citizen group to support its position of converting a local playground into a senior citizen center
   - Learning of an insurer's proposed policy of not reimbursing for dialysis and organ transplants for persons over 75 years of age

RESOURCES

American Nurses Association, Center for Ethics and Human Rights
http://www.nursingworld.org/ethics

American Society of Bioethics and Humanities
http://www.asbh.org

RECOMMENDED READINGS

Recommended Readings associated with this chapter can be found on the web site that accompanies the book. Visit **http://thepoint.lww.com/Eliopoulos8e** to access the recommended readings and other additional resources associated with this chapter.

REFERENCE

American Society for Bioethics and the Humanities. (2010). *Core competencies for health care ethics consultation* (2nd ed.). Glenview, IL: American Society for Bioethics and the Humanities. Retrieved from http://www.asbh.org

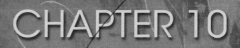

CHAPTER 10

Continuum of Care in Gerontological Nursing

CHAPTER OUTLINE

LEARNING OBJECTIVES

After reading this chapter, you should be able to:

1. Describe the continuum of services available to older adults.

2. Discuss factors that influence service selection for older adults.

3. Describe various practice settings for gerontological nurses.

4. List major functions of gerontological nurses.

TERMS TO KNOW

Adult day services: centers that provide health and social services for a portion of the day to persons with moderate physical or mental disabilities and give respite to their caregivers

Assisted living facility: residential care for persons who do not require nursing home level services but who cannot fulfill all personal care and/or health care needs independently; are referred to as assisted living communities, residential care facilities, personal care, and boarding homes.

Case management: services provided by registered nurses or social workers who assess an individual's needs, identify appropriate

(Continued)

services, and help the person obtain and coordinate these services in the community

Hospice: services that provide support and palliative care to dying individuals and their families in the home or an institutional setting

Nursing home: facility that provides 24-hour supervision and nursing care to persons with physical or mental conditions who are unable to be cared for in the community

Respite care: services to provide short-term care to individuals, thereby offering their caregivers short-term relief from their caregiving responsibilities

---

The effects of a graying population are all around us. The media report the spiraling costs of Medicare and Social Security. Banks advertise reverse annuity mortgage programs aimed at helping aging persons remain in their homes. A new retirement community is constructed. A major corporation initiates an adult day care program. A family leave law is passed. The local hospital issues a circular informing the community of new services for senior citizens. A nearby church sponsors a caregiver support group.

Even if we were not nurses and nursing students, we could not help noticing the impact of older adults on all segments of society. We are increasingly aware that older adults are major consumers of virtually all health care services. Consider the following:

- Growing numbers of Americans are interested in wellness programs that help them stay youthful, active, and healthy.

- More than one third of all surgical patients are older than 65 years of age (Centers for Disease Control and Prevention, 2006).

- The prevalence of mental health problems increases with age.

- Chronic diseases occur at a rate four times greater in old age than at other ages, with 80% of older adults having at least one chronic condition (Centers for Disease Control and Prevention, 2012).

- Approximately 40% of all older persons will spend some time in a nursing home during their lives (Centers for Medicare and Medicaid Services, 2007).

- Most beds in acute medical hospitals are filled by older patients.

- Older adults are the most significant users of home health services.

Whether working in nursing homes, health maintenance organizations (HMOs), outpatient surgical centers, hospice programs, rehabilitation units, or private practice, nurses are likely to be involved in gerontological nursing.

The diversity of the aging population and the complexity of needs it presents demands a wide range of nursing services. A continuum of care, including services for older adults who are the most independent and well at one end and the most dependent and ill at the other, is essential to meet the complex and changing needs presented by the older population.

SERVICES IN THE CONTINUUM OF CARE FOR OLDER ADULTS

The continuum of care consists of supportive and preventive services, partial and intermittent care services, and complete and continuous care services (Fig. 10-1). This continuum includes opportunities for community-based services, institution-based services, or a combination of both. Complementary and alternative services may also be included in the continuum.

To plan care for older adults effectively, nurses must be familiar with the various forms of care available. In fact, visiting various agencies to learn about their services firsthand can prove beneficial for the gerontological nurse. Although services can vary from one area to another, some general examples are described in the sections that follow.

Supportive and Preventive Services

Most older adults reside in the community and function with minimal or no formal assistance. Many of them adjust their lives to accommodate changes commonly experienced with aging; some manage complex care demands. Nurses are challenged to help older adults maintain independence, prevent risks to health and well-being, establish meaningful lifestyles, and develop self-care strategies for health and medical needs.

Supportive and preventive services support independent individuals in maintaining their self-care capacity so that they can avoid physical, emotional, social, and spiritual problems. In this

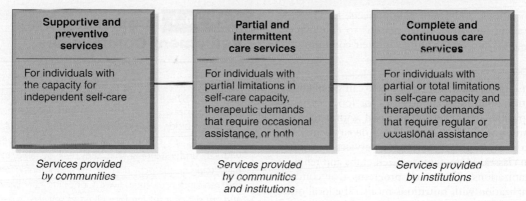

FIGURE 10-1 ■ Continuum of care services for older adults.

category of services, nurses most likely will be involved with the following:

■ identifying service needs
■ referring older adults to appropriate services
■ supporting and coordinating services

Local offices on aging, commissions on retirement education, libraries, and health departments usually provide assistance to older persons in learning about available services. Nurses should encourage older persons to use these resources for any questions and assistance needed. The Silver Pages telephone directory for older adults is also a useful resource. In addition, the Administration on Aging hosts a web site that is a gateway to a wide range of information and services for older adults and their families; this can be accessed through http://www.aoa.gov/AoARoot/Elders_Families/index.aspx. Examples of supportive and preventive services for community-based older adults are described below.

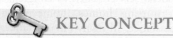

KEY CONCEPT

When working with community-based older adults, nurses focus on maintaining independence, preventing risks to health and well-being, establishing meaningful lifestyles, and developing self-care strategies for health and medical needs.

Financial Services

The Social Security Administration may be able to help older persons obtain retirement income, disability benefits, supplemental security income, and Medicare or other health insurances. The district office of the Social Security Administration can provide direct assistance and information. The Department of Veterans Affairs (VA) can provide financial aid to older veterans and their families; interested persons should be directed to the local VA office. Various communities offer discounts to senior citizens at department stores, pharmacies, theaters, concerts, restaurants, and transportation services. Lists of discounts may be obtained from the local offices on aging.

Many banks offer free checking accounts and other special services to senior citizens. By completing a direct deposit form at their bank, older adults can have the Social Security Administration deposit Social Security and Supplemental Security Income checks directly to the bank; likewise, pension checks can be deposited directly into checking accounts. This service saves older adults from having to travel to the bank and serves as a protection from crime. Reverse annuity mortgages can be arranged through banking institutions to allow older homeowners to use the equity in their homes to remain in the community. It is advisable for older persons to explore details of such services with their individual financial institution.

Financial assistance is also available for burial and funeral expenses. For instance, wartime veterans are eligible for some assistance from the VA. Also, the Social Security Administration provides a small payment for burial expenses to those who have been insured by that program. Local offices of these administrations can be contacted for information; funeral directors are also a good source of information about these benefits. Finally, social service agencies and religious organizations often provide assistance for persons with insufficient funds to pay for burial expenses.

Employment

If older adults desire to work, nurses can refer them to employment services. State employment services and the Over 60 Counseling & Employment Service conduct programs that provide employment counseling and job placement. Various states also have foster grandparent programs, older businessperson associations, and senior aide projects. Local offices on aging can direct older persons to employment programs and opportunities in their community.

Food

The departments of social services can supply information about and applications for food stamps to help older persons purchase food within the constraints of their budget. These departments may also provide grocery shopping services and nutrition classes. Many senior citizen clubs and religious organizations offer lunch programs that combine socialization with nutritious meals. The local office or department on aging or the health department can direct persons to the sites of such programs.

Housing

Local social service agencies and departments of housing and community development can assist older persons in locating adequate housing at an affordable cost. These agencies also may be able to direct the older homeowner to resources to assist in home repairs and provide information regarding property tax discounts. A variety of continuing care retirement communities (Box 10-1), villages, mobile home parks, and apartment complexes, specifically designed for older persons, are available throughout the United States. Some of these housing complexes include special security patrols, transportation services, health programs, recreational activities, and architectural adjustments (e.g., low cabinets, grab bars in bathrooms, tinted windows, slopes instead of stairs, and emergency call bells). Some of these housing options require a "buy-in fee" or purchase price, a monthly fee, or both. The older person exploring retirement housing should be advised that sound facts are more important to decision making than exciting promises. Visits to the housing complex and a full investigation of benefits and costs before making a contractual commitment are essential.

Health Care

Nurses can encourage older adults to engage in preventive health practices to avoid illness and detect health problems at an early stage. Health services for older adults are provided by health departments, HMOs, private practitioners, and hospital outpatient services. In addition to health services, these providers may help older adults obtain transportation and financial assistance for their health care. Older individuals should inquire about such services at their nearest health care office.

Social Support and Activities

Churches, synagogues, and mosques offer not only a place of worship but also a community that can

---

BOX 10-1 Continuing Care Retirement Communities

Continuing care retirement communities (CCRCs) offer a continuum of services in one location to provide various levels of housing and services to meet an older adult's changing needs. Typically, people pay an entrance fee and a monthly fee, with an understanding that they will be able to have their needs provided by the community for the remainder of their lives. Contracts can vary and consist of a set fee for unlimited services, a set fee for time-limited services, or additional charges if assisted living, home health, or skilled nursing services are required.

Healthy individuals can enter and live in independent housing units, which could consist of single-family homes, apartments, or condominiums. Housekeeping, laundry, meals, transportation, social activities, and health services can be provided for additional fees.

As individuals require more assistance they can receive assistance with personal care in their own housing unit or move to the assisted living center or nursing home section of the CCRC.

Entrance fees, conditions for refund of entrance fees, monthly costs, services available, and terms of contracts vary among CCRCs, so it is useful for older adults interested in CCRCs to visit and compare several and carefully review the contracts.

---

provide tremendous fellowship, support, and assistance to persons of all ages. Many religious groups offer health and social services such as congregate eating programs, nursing homes, home visitation, and chore assistance. In many circumstances, recipients of services need not be members of the religious group. Increasing numbers of faith communities employ nurses to assist with members' health and social needs, and Faith Community Nursing is a blossoming specialty. Individual churches and synagogues or the mother organization (e.g., Associated Jewish Charities and Catholic Charities) should be contacted for information.

Bureaus of recreation and other groups may also sponsor clubs and activities expressly for senior citizens. Local commissions or offices on aging can provide information related to the availability of such programs, their activities, schedules, and persons to contact for details. Local chapters of the American Association of Retired Persons (AARP) can provide valuable information on services that keep older persons active and independent, ranging from creative leisure endeavors at home to discount travel opportunities. Information about leisure pursuits is just one of the many services the AARP provides. Finally, art museums, libraries, theaters, concert halls, restaurants, and travel agencies should be contacted for special programs offered to senior citizens.

Volunteer Work

Nurses can also encourage older adults to participate in volunteer activities. The wealth of knowledge and experience possessed by older persons makes them especially suited for volunteer work. Not only do older volunteers provide valuable services to others, but they may also achieve a sense of self-worth from their contributions to society. Communities offer numerous opportunities for senior volunteers in hospitals, nursing homes, organizations, schools, and other sites. Older persons should be encouraged to inquire about volunteer opportunities at the agency in which they are interested in serving. Frequently, agencies without a formal volunteer program are able to use a volunteer's service if contacted. National programs also provide meaningful volunteer services in which older persons can participate. The American Red Cross, Service Corps of Retired Executives, and Retired and Senior Volunteer Program are a few such programs. Local offices of these programs should be consulted for details.

Education

Some public schools offer literacy, high school equivalency, vocational, and personal interest courses for older adults. Many colleges have free tuition for older persons. Individual schools should be contacted for more details.

Counseling

Financial problems, the need to locate new housing, strained family relationships, widowhood, adjustment to a chronic illness, and retirement are among the situations that may necessitate professional counseling. Local social service agencies, religious organizations, and private therapists are among the resources that offer assistance.

Consumer Affairs

Senior adults are frequent victims of unscrupulous people who profit by making convincing but invalid promises. It is important for older adults to investigate cure-alls, vacation programs, and get-rich-quick schemes before investing their funds. Local offices of the Better Business Bureau and consumer protection agencies provide useful information to prevent fraud and deception and offer counseling if problems do arise.

Legal and Tax Services

Local legal aid bureaus and lawyer referral services of the Bar Association may help older adults obtain competent legal assistance at a nominal cost. The Internal Revenue Service can help older people prepare federal tax returns, and the state comptroller's office can assist with state tax returns; local offices should be contacted for additional information. Various colleges and law schools should be investigated for free legal and tax services offered to senior citizens.

Transportation

Older persons often receive discounts for bus, taxicab, subway, and train services; individual agencies should be contacted for more information. Commissions or offices on aging, health and social services departments, and local chapters of the American Red Cross may be able to direct persons to services accommodating wheelchairs and other special needs. Various health and medical facilities provide transportation for persons using their services; individual facilities should be explored for specific details.

Shopping at Home

Persons who are homebound, who are geographically isolated from services, or who have busy schedules may find it useful to shop at home through mail-order catalogs, home-shopping services on television, and the Internet. Shopping by mail has a long tradition and along with its newest sibling Internet shopping reduces the inconveniences and risks associated with traveling to a shopping district, maneuvering in stores, handling large sums of money in public, and carrying packages. The shipping and handling charges may be no greater than transportation costs, not to mention the energy expended in direct shopping.

Additionally, many libraries have a service in which books and tapes can be borrowed by mail; older persons should be encouraged to inquire about such services at their local branch. The Internet offers many online books and publications, many of which are free. The U.S. Postal Service provides a service for a nominal fee in which stamps can be ordered by mail or Internet; order blanks for stamps by mail can be obtained by contacting the local postal station or postal carrier or visiting www.USPS.com.

Partial and Intermittent Care Services

Partial and intermittent care services provide assistance to individuals with a partial limitation in self-care capacity or a therapeutic demand that requires occasional assistance. Either because of the degree of the self-care limitation or the complexity of the therapeutic action required, the individual could be at risk for new or a worsening of existing physical, emotional, and social problems if some assistance were not provided at periodic intervals. These services can be provided in community or institutional settings.

Assistance with Chores

Social service agencies, health departments, private homemaker agencies, and faith communities have services for older persons that help them remain in their homes and maintain independence. These services include light housekeeping, minor repairs, errands, and shopping. Local agencies and programs should be contacted for specific information.

Home-Delivered Meals

Persons unable to shop and prepare meals independently may benefit from having meals delivered to their homes. Such a service not only facilitates good nutrition but also provides an opportunity for social contact. Meals On Wheels is the most popularly known program for home delivery of meals, although various community groups provide a similar service. If a local Meals On Wheels is unavailable, departments of social services, health departments, and commissions or offices on aging should be consulted for alternative programs.

Home Monitoring

Some hospitals, nursing homes, and commercial agencies provide home monitoring systems, whereby the older adult wears a small remote alarm that can be pressed in the event of a fall or other emergency. The alarm triggers a central monitoring station to call designated contact persons or the police to assist the individual. This type of service can be located by calling the local agency on aging or looking in the telephone directory under listings such as Medical Alarms.

A growing array of telemanagement technologies is affording the opportunity for patients to have vital signs, blood glucose levels, and other physiological measurements communicated from the home to providers. Tracking systems and sensors can enable family members or caregivers to monitor patients' activity in their homes from a distance. Two-way audio and video devices allow patients to interact with their providers from their homes. Devices can be used to signal patients when to take medications and perform other tasks. Medication administration systems exist whereby family members and caregivers in another location can be informed if a patient has not taken drugs as scheduled. An Internet search of home care and patient care technology vendors will yield many suppliers of technological aids for home care.

Telephone Reassurance

Older adults who are homebound, disabled, or lonely may benefit from a telephone reassurance program. Those who participate in the program receive a daily telephone call—usually at a mutually agreed on time—to provide them with social contact and ensure that they are safe and well. Local chapters of the American Red Cross and other health or social service agencies should be consulted for telephone reassurance programs that they may conduct.

Home Health Care

Home health care provides nursing and other therapies in individuals' homes. Visiting nurse associations have a long reputation of providing care in the home and are able to help many older persons remain in their homes rather than enter an institution. Programs vary, and services can include bedside nursing, home health aides, physical therapy, health education, family counseling, and medical services. Medicare is limited to *skilled* home care, which means that the person must:

- be homebound
- have services ordered by a primary care provider

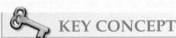 **KEY CONCEPT**

During the 1970s and the decades that followed, home health services significantly grew due to the enactment of the Older American's Act and Title XX Social Services Act in 1975 that provided federal funds for home-based services and the Federal Health Services Program that gave grants for the establishment and expansion of these services. By the 1990s home care became the fastest growing component of Medicare and the rising costs influenced Congress to place limitations on home care benefits for Medicare recipients as part of the Balanced Budget Act of 1997. At this same time, in an effort to control the rising costs of nursing home care on their Medicaid budgets, states began to develop more home care services as an alternative to nursing home care.

At present, Medicare covers skilled nursing care but not long-term nonskilled care. States have various Medicaid programs to assist in nonskilled home care; private agencies also provide these services.

The changes in home health care demonstrate the impact that government funds can have on the availability of services to older adults.

■ require skilled nursing or rehabilitative services

■ need intermittent but not full-time care

In addition to Medicare, the VA, Medicaid, and private insurers provide reimbursement for home health services, although the conditions and length of coverage vary; specific coverage should be reviewed with the insurer. These programs can be found through health departments, in telephone directories, or through social workers who assist with discharge planning.

Foster Care and Group Homes

Adult foster care and group home programs offer services to individuals who are capable of self-care but who require supervision to protect them from harm. Older persons placed in these homes may need someone to direct their self-care activities (e.g., remind them to bathe and dress and encourage and provide good nutrition); they may also need someone to oversee their judgments (e.g., financial management). Foster care and group living can serve as short- or long-term alternatives to institutionalization for older persons unable to manage independently in the community. The local department of social services can supply details about these programs.

Adult Day Services

Adult day services programs have been a growing component of community-based, long-term care, currently numbering over 4,600 centers in the United States (National Adult Day Services Association, 2012). These centers provide health and social services to persons with moderate physical or mental disabilities and give respite to their caregivers. Participants attend the program for a portion of the day and enjoy a safe, pleasant, therapeutic environment under the supervision of qualified personnel (Fig. 10-2). The programs attempt to maximize the existing self-care capacity of participants while preventing further limitations. Although the primary focus is social and recreational, there usually is some health component to these programs, such as health screening, supervision of medication administration, and monitoring of health conditions. Rest periods and meals accompany the planned therapeutic activities. Transportation to the site is provided, usually by vehicles equipped to accommodate wheelchairs and persons with other special needs.

In addition to helping older persons avoid further limitations and institutionalization, day services programs are extremely beneficial to the families of participants. Families interested in caring for their older relatives may be able to continue

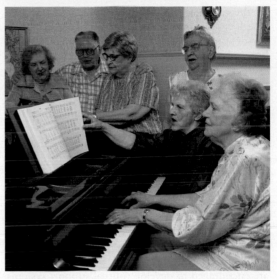

FIGURE 10-2 ■ Adult day care centers provide opportunities for a variety of recreational activities.

their routine lifestyle (e.g., maintaining a job and raising small children), knowing that they can have respite from their caregiving responsibilities for a portion of the day while the older person is cared for and safe.

Adult day services programs are sponsored by public agencies, religious organizations, and private groups, with one third being freestanding and the remaining ones affiliated with a larger parent organization; each varies in schedule, activities, costs, and program focus. The local telephone directory or information and referral service, as well as the National Adult Day Services Association, can provide information on programs in specific communities.

Day Treatment and Day Hospital Programs

Day treatment and day hospital programs offer social and health services with a primary focus on the latter. Assistance is provided with self-care activities (e.g., bathing and feeding) and therapeutic needs (e.g., medication administration, wound dressing, physical therapy, and psychotherapy). Physicians, nurses, occupational therapists, physical therapists, psychologists, and psychiatrists are among the care providers affiliated with programs for day treatment. Like adult day services programs, geriatric day treatment or day hospital programs usually provide transportation to and from the program. Sponsored by hospitals, nursing homes, or other agencies, these programs can be used as alternatives to hospitalization and nursing home admission and can facilitate earlier discharge from these care settings. Many of these programs focus on the care of persons with psychiatric conditions. The local commission or office on aging can guide persons to programs for day treatment or day hospitals in their community.

Assisted Living

Assisted living supplements independent living with special services that maximize an individual's capacity for self-care. Terminology used to describe assisted living can fall under the categories of residential care facilities, personal care, and boarding homes; different states use different regulatory designations. The housing unit is adjusted to meet the needs of older or disabled persons (e.g., wide doorways, low cabinets, grab bars in bathroom, and call-for-help light). A guard, hostess, or resident screens and greets visitors in the lobby. Various degrees of personal care assistance may be provided. Residents are encouraged to develop mutual support systems; one example is a system in which residents check on one another every morning to see if anyone needs help. Tenant councils may determine policies for the facility. Some facilities have a health professional on call or on duty during certain hours; recognizing the unique health care needs in this setting that can be appropriately addressed by nurses, nursing in assisted living communities is a developing specialty. Social programs and communal meals may also be available. State health department regulatory agencies and the local office of the Department of Housing and Urban Development may be able to direct interested persons to such facilities.

Respite Care

A variety of services can be utilized to provide short-term relief to caregivers from their caregiving responsibilities. The services depend on the need, status of the patient, and funds. For example, private home health aides/companions or nurses can be hired to live in or occasionally visit the older person while the caregiver is away; short-term admissions to assistive living communities or nursing homes can provide respite when the person's caregiving demands and/or need for supervision is 24/7.

Health Ministry and Parish Nurse Programs

Many churches and synagogues have programs to assist older adults and their caregivers such as support groups, health education classes, counseling, housekeeping and home maintenance assistance, meals, and home nursing visits. Many nurses are volunteers in these programs and some are paid to serve in these roles. These services are ideal ways to integrate health services with one's faith. As services offered vary, nurses should contact the church or synagogue of the patient, or if the patient is not a member of one a local religious organization representing the patient's faith, to learn of the availability of services.

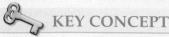
KEY CONCEPT

The American Nurses Association has recognized parish nursing as a specialty and in collaboration with the Health Ministries Association published the *Faith Community Nursing: Scope and Standards of Practice*.

Care and Case Management

The identification of needs, location and coordination of services, and maintenance of an independent lifestyle can be tremendous challenges for older persons with chronic health problems. In response to these challenges, the field of geriatric care and case management has developed.

Care and case managers most often are registered nurses or social workers who assess an individual's needs, identify appropriate services, and help the person obtain and coordinate these services. Such services include medical care, home health services, socialization programs, financial planning and management, and housing. By coordinating care and services, geriatric care and case managers assist older persons in remaining independent in the community for as long as possible. The services of care and case managers often provide peace of mind to family members who are unable to be involved with their older family members on a daily basis.

As a system of credentials within this field has surfaced, there is greater distinction between care management and case management. Both of these disciplines perform some type of assessment, develop plans, help people implement and coordinate services, and evaluate care. A distinguishing difference between the two, however, is that care management is a long-term relationship that could endure through multiple episodes of care (e.g., when a family contracts with a care manager to oversee the care of a relative on a long-term basis), whereas case management usually focuses on needs during a specific episode of care (e.g., from hospitalization through rehabilitation for a hip fracture). Case management is viewed as a means to control health care costs and may emphasize services for cost containment; care management may include case management in addition to services unrelated to health care.

Social workers, local information and referral services, and the National Association of Professional Geriatric Care Managers (http://www.caremanager.org) can provide assistance in locating care and case managers.

KEY CONCEPT

The American Nurses Association has found professional nurses to be excellent case managers because of their knowledge and skills training, their ability to deliver care that includes both physical and sociocultural components, their familiarity with the process of services referral, and the parallels between the nursing process and the process of case management.

Hospice

Although hospice care is listed here under partial and intermittent care services, it can also be included under complete and continuous care services. This is because the nature of the patient's needs determines the level at which this service is provided.

Rather than a site of care, hospice is a philosophy of caring for dying individuals. Hospice provides support and palliative care to patients and their families. Typically, an interdisciplinary team helps patients and families meet physical, emotional, social, and spiritual needs. The focus is on the quality of remaining life rather than life extension. Survivor support is also an important component of hospice care. Although hospice programs can exist within an institutional setting, most hospice care is provided in the home. Insurers vary in the conditions that must be met for reimbursement of hospice services; individual insurers should be consulted for specific information. Health care and social service agencies can be consulted for information about hospice programs in specific communities.

Complete and Continuous Care Services

At the far end of the continuum of care are services that provide regular or continuous assistance to individuals with some limitation in self-care capacity whose therapeutic needs require 24-hour supervision by a health care professional.

Hospital Care

Hospital care for older persons may be required when diagnostic procedures and therapeutic actions indicate a need for specialized technologies or frequent monitoring. Older adults can be patients of virtually all acute hospital services, except, of course, pediatrics and obstetrics (and here they may be encountered as relatives of the primary patients). Although the procedure or diagnostic problem for which they are hospitalized will dictate many of their service needs, there are some basic measures that can enhance the quality of the hospital experience, as described in Box 10-2.

Increasingly, hospitals are establishing special services for older adults, such as geriatric assessment centers, telephone hot lines, long-term care units, and home visits. Local medical societies and state hospital associations can answer inquiries about specific hospitals.

Two issues that gerontological nurses need to consider regarding the hospital care of older adults are abbreviated stays and the move toward same-day outpatient services for procedures that once would have required hospitalization. Although shortening hospital stays can be effective in lowering costs and perhaps reducing or eliminating a patient's hospital-induced complications, many older patients require a longer recovery time than younger adults and may not have adequate assistance in the home. Nurses must assess older patients' capacity to care for themselves—the ability to obtain and prepare food and manage their households—before discharge and arrange assistance as necessary. A telephone call after discharge to check on the patient's status is also useful. (Additional information on hospital care of older adults is provided in Chapter 36.)

Nursing Homes

Nursing homes provide 24-hour supervision and nursing care to persons who are unable to be cared for in the community. Chapter 37 discusses these facilities and related nursing responsibilities.

Complementary and Alternative Services

As the emphasis on holistic health and public awareness of and desire for complementary and alternative therapies grow, older adults may seek new or nonconventional types of services (Fig. 10-3). Examples of complementary and alternative services include:

- wellness and renewal centers
- education, counseling, and case management from alternative practitioners
- acupuncture and acupressure
- t'ai chi, yoga, and meditation classes
- therapeutic touch and healing touch
- medicinal herbal prescriptions
- herbal and homeopathic remedies
- guided imagery sessions
- sound, light, and aromatherapy

Nurses possess a wide range of knowledge and skills that, when combined with additional preparation in complementary and alternative therapies, makes them ideal providers of some of these

BOX 10-2 Measures That Enhance the Quality of Hospital Care for Older Adults

Perform a comprehensive assessment. It is not uncommon for the patient's diagnostic problem to be the primary and sometimes only concern during the hospitalization. However, the patient being treated for a myocardial infarction or hernia may also suffer from depression, caregiver stress, hearing deficit, or other problems that significantly affect the health status. By capitalizing on the contact with the patient during the hospitalization and conducting a comprehensive evaluation, nurses can reveal risks and problems that affect the health status and that have not been detected before. Broader problems, other than those for which the patient was admitted to the hospital, should be explored.

Recognize differences. Older patients should not be considered in the same way as younger patients: different norms may be used to interpret laboratory tests and clinical findings, the signs and symptoms of disease can appear atypically, more time is needed for care activities, and drug dosages must be age-adjusted. The priorities of older patients can differ from those of younger patients. Nurses must be able to differentiate normal pathology from pathology in older adults and understand the modifications that must be made in caring for this population.

Reduce risks. The hospital experience can be traumatic for older patients if special protection is not afforded. The elderly require more time to recover from stress; therefore, procedures and activities must be planned to provide rest. Altered function of major systems and decreased immunity make it easy for infections to develop. Reduced ability of the heart to manage major shifts in fluid load demands close monitoring of intravenous infusion rates. Lower normal body temperature, the lack of shivering, and reduced capacity to adapt to severe changes in environmental temperature require that older patients receive special protection against hypothermia. Differences in pharmacodynamics and pharmacokinetics in older adults alter their response to medications and heighten the need for close monitoring of drug therapy. The strange environment, sensory deficits, and effects of illness and medications cause falls to occur more easily and make injury prevention a priority. Confusion often emerges as a primary sign of a complication, challenging staff to detect this disorder promptly and identify its cause. Nurses should ensure that measures are taken to reduce patients' risks and recognize complications promptly when they do occur.

Maintain and promote function. Priorities addressing the primary reason for admission usually take the forefront during a patient's hospitalization. For example, the arrhythmia must be corrected, the infection controlled, and the fracture realigned. In the midst of diagnostic procedures and treatment activities, there must be consideration of factors that will ensure the older patient's optimal function and independence.

---

nonconventional services. Even if they are not direct providers of alternative therapies, nurses can advocate for older adults' rights to make informed choices about using such therapies; educate them about the benefits, risks, and limitations of therapies; and help them find reputable providers. Ideally, these therapies are used in concert with conventional ones in an integrative care model to enable patients to use the best of both worlds.

POINT TO PONDER

Increasing numbers of nurses are offering complementary therapies in independent practices. What types of factors must be considered when establishing a private practice? What do you think prevents more nurses from becoming self-employed nurse entrepreneurs?

MATCHING SERVICES TO NEEDS

The needs of the aging population are diverse and multitudinous. In addition, the needs of an individual older adult are dynamic; in other words, needs fluctuate as capacities and life demands change. These conditions require gerontological nursing services to be planned with consideration of several factors:

■ *Services must address physical, emotional, social, and spiritual factors.* Services must be available to meet the unique needs of the older population in a holistic manner. These services should be planned to address whatever problems or needs older adults are likely to develop and should be implemented in a manner relevant to the unique characteristics of this group. For instance, a local health department interested

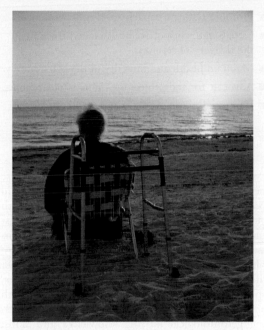

FIGURE 10-3 ■ Increasingly, older adults are turning to yoga, meditation, and other complementary health practices.

in meeting the special needs of older adults could add screening programs for hearing, vision, hypertension, and cancer to their existing services. Likewise, a social service agency with an abundance of programs for younger families may decide that a widow's support group and retirement counseling services are relevant additions. The consideration of physical, emotional, social, and spiritual factors is essential to providing holistic nursing care.

■ *Services must consider unique and changing needs.* Physical, emotional, social, and spiritual services are based on the individual's needs at a given time, recognizing that priorities are not fixed. An older adult could be seen in an outpatient medical service for hypertension control and during that visit express concern regarding a recent rent increase. Unless assistance is obtained to provide additional income or lower cost housing, the potential effects of this social problem, such as stress and dietary sacrifices, may exacerbate the individual's hypertension. Ignoring this individual's need for particular social services, then, can minimize the effectiveness of the health services provided.

■ *Care and services must be flexible.* Opportunities must exist for the older individual to move along the continuum of care, depending on his or her capacities and limitations at different times. Perhaps an older woman lives with her children and attends a senior citizen recreational program during the day. If this woman fractures her hip, she may move along the continuum to hospitalization for acute care and then to a nursing home for convalescence. As her condition improves and she becomes more independent, she moves along the continuum to home care and then possibly adult day care until she regains full independence.

■ *Services must be tailored to needs.* Individualization must be practiced to match the unique needs of the individual with specific services. Just as it is inappropriate to assume that all persons over 65 years require nursing home placement, it is equally inappropriate to assume that all older persons would benefit from counseling, sheltered housing, home-delivered meals, adult day care, or any other service. Older individuals' unique capacities and limitations and, most importantly, their preferences should be assessed to identify the most appropriate services for them.

The listing of resources at the end of the chapter can help gerontological nurses and nursing students locate and perhaps stimulate services for older adults. Nurses are encouraged to contact their local agencies on aging and information and referral services for the location of services within specific communities.

SETTINGS AND ROLES FOR GERONTOLOGICAL NURSES

Because the continuum of care includes community-based services, institution-based services, or a combination of both, gerontological nurses have an exciting opportunity to practice in a variety of settings. Some of these settings, such as long-term care facilities and home health agencies, have a long history of nursing participation. Others, such as senior housing complexes and adult day care centers, offer new opportunities for nurses to demonstrate creativity and leadership.

Although nurses' specific roles and responsibilities can differ vastly in different settings, gerontological nurses in any setting may serve similar functions (Box 10-3). These functions are varied and multifaceted and address the following goals:

■ Educate persons of all ages in practices that promote a positive aging experience.

■ Assess and provide interventions related to nursing diagnoses.

■ Identify and reduce risks.

BOX 10-3 Functions of the Gerontological Nurse

Guide persons of all ages toward a healthy aging process.
Eliminate ageism.
Respect the rights of older adults and ensure others do the same.
Oversee and promote the quality of service delivery.
Notice and reduce risks to health and well-being.
Teach and support caregivers.
Open channels for continued growth.
Listen and support.
Offer optimism, encouragement, and hope.
Generate, support, use, disseminate, and participate in research.
Implement restorative and rehabilitative measures.
Coordinate and manage care.
Assess, plan, implement, and evaluate care in an individualized, holistic manner.
Link services with needs.
Nurture future gerontological nurses for advancement of the specialty.
Understand the unique physical, emotional, social, and spiritual aspects of each older adult.
Recognize and encourage the appropriate management of ethical concerns.
Support and comfort through the dying process.
Educate to promote self-care and optimal independence.

- Promote self-care capacity and independence.
- Collaborate with other health care providers in the delivery of services.
- Maintain health and integrity of the aging family.
- Advocate for and protect the rights of older adults.
- Promote the use of ethics and standards in the care of older adults.
- Help older persons face the transition to death with peace, comfort, and dignity.

As the presence of older adults in diverse health care settings continues to increase, there will be a crucial need in such settings for nurses with gerontological nursing expertise. These nurses must understand normal aging, unique presentations and management of geriatric health problems, pharmacodynamics and pharmacokinetics in later life, psychological challenges, socioeconomic issues, spirituality, family dynamics, unique risks to health and well-being, and available resources. By possessing gerontological nursing knowledge and skills, nurses can promote efficient, effective, and appropriate health care services to older adults in a variety of settings.

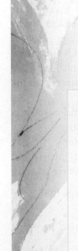

BRINGING RESEARCH TO LIFE

NURSE IDENTIFIED HOSPITAL TO HOME MEDICATION DISCREPANCIES: IMPLICATIONS FOR IMPROVING TRANSITIONS OF CARE

Corbett, C., Setter, S. M., Daratha, K. B., Neumiller, J. J., & Wood, L. D. (2010). Geriatric Nursing, 31(3), 188–196.

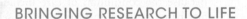

Nearly 20% of all Medicare patients are rehospitalized within 1 month after discharge and medication discrepancy is a contributing factor. This study sought to learn about medication discrepancies and nursing practices to reduce them. Medication discrepancy is defined as a difference between the medications prescribed at discharge and the medications actually taken by the patient.

A group of patients, at least 50 years of age, who were hospitalized and discharged to home care services participated in this study. They were randomly placed into intervention and control groups. Medication discrepancies were identified by the home care nurses. The discrepancies were divided by patient-level contributing factors (e.g., intentional noncompliance, intolerance, and financial barriers) and system-level factors (e.g., incomplete discharge instructions and prescription given that the patient was known to be allergic to).

Nearly 40% of the participants had at least one patient-level medication discrepancy, with the most common cause being the patient's intentional noncompliance and nonadherence. More than 69% of the participants had system-level discrepancies, with the contributing factors being incomplete or inaccurate discharge instructions, conflicting information from difference sources, and duplication of medications. The discrepancies involved all classes of medications.

Significant risks can arise in the transition from hospital to home and a common one is the lack of compliance with the medication plan. Serious complications can develop when the older adult fails to take a prescribed medication or takes one that is inappropriate. Gerontological nurses can impact the transition from one care setting to another and assure older adults receive safe, effective care by investing time in discharge planning that includes reviewing patients' medications for appropriateness, lack of interactions, and duplicative prescriptions; teaching patients about the prescribed medications; asking patients about their ability to obtain and pay for prescriptions; and encouraging patients to express any concerns or objections they have to their medication plans.

PRACTICE REALITIES

Eighty-one-year-old Ms. Jacobs has always been an independent woman. Never married, and with no surviving relatives, she lives alone in a large house located on several acres in a rural community that she has lived in for nearly 50 years. She has no interest in relocating as she enjoys her garden and the ability to have pets.

Although still independent, Ms. Jacobs can't get around as well as she once could and in the past year has had a few minor accidents when driving into town. She is competent and has the right to remain in her home, but you are concerned for her safety and welfare.

What could you do to help Ms. Jacobs? How could her changing needs be balanced with her desire for independence?

CRITICAL THINKING EXERCISES

1. How would you defend the position that nurses are ideal geriatric care managers?

2. Mrs. Johns is a 79-year-old woman who has been admitted to an acute medical hospital for a fractured femur. The orthopedic surgeon anticipates no problem in Mrs. Johns ambulating and eventually returning to the community, provided she is successful in her rehabilitation program. You learn that she lives with her son's family in a large metropolitan area. She has a dementia that requires close supervision and reminders to toilet, dress, and eat; however, with these reminders, she is physically capable of performing activities of daily living. Based on this information, what are the various types of services that can help Mrs. Johns and her family throughout the course of her recovery?

3. What could you do to stimulate the development of services for aging persons in your community? What resources could you mobilize to assist you in this effort?

RESOURCES

GENERAL

Administration on Aging Elder Page
http://www.aoa.gov/AoARoot/Elders_Families/index.
aspx
American Association of Retired Persons
http://www.aarp.org

American Geriatrics Society
http://www.americangeriatrics.org
American Health Care Association
http://www.ahca.org
American Holistic Nurses Association
http://www.ahna.org
American Nurses Association Council on Gerontological Nursing
http://www.nursingworld.org

American Society on Aging
http://www.asaging.org

Children of Aging Parents
http://www.caps4caregivers.org

Design for Aging, American Institute of Architects
http://www.aia.org/dfa

The Gerontological Society of America
http://www.geron.org

Gray Panthers
http://www.graypanthers.org

Hispanic Federation
http://www.hispanicfederation.org

National Adult Day Services Association
http://www.nadsa.org

National Association of Area Agencies on Aging
http://www.n4a.org

National Association of Professional Geriatric Care Managers
http://www.caremanager.org

National Caucus and Center on Black Aged, Inc.
http://www.ncba-aged.org

National Center for Complementary and Alternative Medicine
http://www.nccam.nih.gov

National Council on Aging
http://www.ncoa.org

National Eldercare Locator
http://www.eldercare.gov

National Gerontological Nursing Association
http://www.ngna.org

National Hospice and Palliative Care Organization
http://www.nho.org

National Institute on Aging
http://www.nia.nih.gov

NURSING HOMES

American Association of Homes and Services for the Aging
http://www.aahsa.org

American Association for Long Term Care Nursing
http://www.aaltcn.org

American Nurses Association Council on Nursing Home Nurses
http://www.nursingworld.org

American Public Health Association, Section on Aging and Public Health
http://www.apha.org/membergroups/sections/aphasections/a_ph/

National Association of Directors of Nursing Administration in Long-Term Care
http://www.nadona.org

National Association for Home Care & Hospice
http://www.nahc.org

National Consumer Voice for Quality Long Term Care
http://www.theconsumervoice.org

Visiting Nurse Associations of America
http://www.vnaa.org

ADULT DAY CARE

National Adult Day Services Association
http://www.nadsa.org

SUPPORT GROUPS

Please refer to resource listings throughout the book under the specific condition.

REFERENCES

Centers for Disease Control and Prevention. (2006). *Healthy aging*. Retrieved May 10, 2012 from http://www.cdc.gov/chronicdisease/resources/publications/aag/aging.htm

Centers for Disease Control and Prevention. (2012). *Chronic disease overview*. Retrieved May 15, 2012, from http://www.cdc.gov/nccdphp/overview.htm

Centers for Medicare and Medicaid Services. (2007). *Guide to choosing a nursing home*. Rockville, MD: U.S. Department of Health and Human Services; also available online at http://www.medicare.gov/Publications/Pubs/pdf/02174.pdf

National Adult Day Services Association. 2012. Overview and Facts. Retrieved May 8, 2012 from http://www.nadsa.org/consumers/overview-and-facts/

RECOMMENDED READINGS

Recommended Readings associated with this chapter can be found on the web site that accompanies the book. Visit **http://thepoint.lww.com/Eliopoulos8e** to access the recommended readings and other additional resources associated with this chapter.

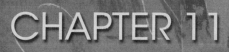

CHAPTER 11

Self-Care for the Gerontological Nurse

CHAPTER OUTLINE

Characteristics of Nurse Healers
  Presence
  Availability
  Connections
  Models of Holism
Self-Care and Nurturing
  Following Positive Health Care Practices
  Strengthening and Building Connections
  Committing to a Dynamic Process

Gerontological nursing is a unique specialty within the wide range of knowledge and skills required for providing services to aging adults. However, providing expert gerontological nursing care demands more than possessing knowledge and clinical skills. Nurses bring life experiences, unique personalities, and their very *being* to their relationships with older persons as they:

■ guide older individuals with common yet challenging life transitions

■ assist individuals in exploring the deeper meaning of the experiences they face

LEARNING OBJECTIVES

After reading this chapter, you should be able to:

1. Describe the attributes of a nurse healer.
2. Identify strategies that can be used for self-care and nurturing.

TERMS TO KNOW

Healing: facilitating optimal physical, mental, social, and spiritual function and well-being
Holistic: concern for the whole person— body, mind, and spirit
Presence: being totally "with" or engaged with another individual

- soothe the physical, emotional, and spiritual pain that frequently invade fragile territory
- provide care that facilitates individuals in becoming integrated, restored, and balanced

Offering this level of nursing care demands that nurses establish heart-to-heart connections—the kind that differentiates doing a job from authentically caring for another human being. Because of the level of personal investment and engagement required, gerontological nurses must practice self-care to optimally engage in healing relationships with patients.

CHARACTERISTICS OF NURSE HEALERS

Nurses are not merely task-doers but important instruments of their patients' healing process. If completion of tasks was all that constituted nursing care, robots could easily replace nurses. After all, technology exists that could enable a machine to administer a medication, reposition a patient, monitor vital signs, record significant events, and perform other common tasks. Yet, the nursing profession emerged as a *healing art* characterized by its practitioners offering comfort, compassion, support, and caring that were equally (and perhaps sometimes more) important to patients' healing as the procedural tasks of caregiving. The nurse serves as a healer whose interactions assist the patient in returning to wholeness (i.e., optimal function and harmony among body, mind, and spirit).

Nurses who support holism and healing do not sit on the sidelines as observers; they actively engage in patients' healing processes. This level of engagement is similar to that of the dance instructor who takes the student by the hand and demonstrates the correct steps instead of merely offering directions from the sidelines.

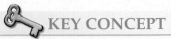

KEY CONCEPT

Nurses actively engage in the patient's dance of healing—teaching, guiding, modeling, coaching, encouraging, and helping the patient through the various steps.

Characteristics that enable nurses to engage as healers for older adults include presence, availability, willingness to form connections, and being models of holism.

Presence

The ability to be present in the moment also characterizes nurse healers. Despite the many real activities that nurses typically must complete, the "busyness" of the average clinical setting, and the unending "to do"

list lingering over them, nurse healers are able to protect their interactions with patients from distractions. When with patients, they are *with* them, giving their full, undivided attention. They actively listen; hear what patients are saying—and not saying—and use their senses to detect subtle clues about needs. Even if the time spent with individual patients is brief, the time fully belongs to their patients.

POINT TO PONDER

Reflect on an interaction in which the person with whom you were speaking seemed distracted and hurried. How did that influence your communication?

Availability

Nurse healers display availability of body, mind, and spirit. They provide the time and space for patients to express, explore, and experience. "That's not my job" are words seldom heard from nurse healers. For example, a nurse may be monitoring a patient who is recovering from cataract surgery in an outpatient surgical unit when the patient confides to the nurse that he is distressed at learning that his grandchild was arrested for possession of illegal drugs. A response from the nurse along the lines of, "You shouldn't worry about that now," gives the message that the nurse is not available to discuss the patient's concern and most likely will close the door to further discussion. By contrast, responding, "This must be very difficult for you," could be more helpful in conveying openness and interest. Although the nurse in the latter example may not be able to provide all the possible assistance that the patient may require, he or she can allow the patient the safe space to unload this burden on his mind and offer suggestions for follow-up help.

Connections

Nurse healers make connections with their patients. They engage with patients in meaningful ways that require openness, respect, acceptance, and a non-judgmental attitude. They commit to learning about what makes each patient a unique individual—the life journey that has been traveled, the story that has formed. At times, this may require that nurses offer insights from their own journeys and share some of the chapters from their lives.

KEY CONCEPT

Exploring the unique threads that have been woven into the tapestry of a patient's life facilitates connection.

Models of Holism

Effective nurse healers are models of holism, which begins with good self-care practices. They not only eat a proper diet, exercise, obtain adequate rest, and follow other positive health practices but also are attentive to their emotional and spiritual well-being. Integrity demands that nurses know what they want others to know and behave as they want others to behave. Self-care is also essential to performing any other role as a nurse healer.

SELF-CARE AND NURTURING

The depth and intensity of the nurse–patient relationship that results when nurses function as healers creates a highly therapeutic and meaningful experience that reflects the essence of professional nursing. Although the formal educational preparation of nurses offers the foundation for this level of healing relationship, the nurse's self-care influences the potential height and depth that can be realized (Fig. 11-1). Some strategies for self-care include following positive health care practices and strengthening and building connections.

Following Positive Health Care Practices

Like all human beings, nurses have basic physiological needs that include:

- respiration
- circulation
- nutrition
- hydration
- elimination
- movement
- rest
- comfort
- immunity
- safety

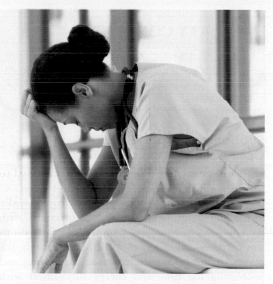

FIGURE 11-1 ■ Nurses compromise their ability to care for others when they do not care for themselves.

Most nurses are familiar with the requirements necessary to meet each of these needs (e.g., proper diet and exercise plans) but may not be applying this knowledge to their personal lives. Self-care can suffer as a result.

A periodic "checkup" of physical status can prove useful in disclosing problems that could not only minimize the ability to provide optimal services to patients but also threaten personal health and well-being. Table 11-1 provides a form that can be used to guide this self-evaluation. It could prove useful for nurses to allocate a few hours, find a quiet place, and critically review their health status.

After identifying problems, nurses can plan realistic actions to improve health. Writing the actions on an index card and placing that card in an area that is regularly seen (e.g., dresser, desk, or dashboard) can provide regular reminders of intended corrective actions.

TABLE 11-1	Taking Stock of Unhealthy Practices		
Need	**Sign/Symptom/Unhealthy Habit**	**Cause(s)/Contributing Factor(s)**	**Corrective Action**
Respiration/circulation			
Nutrition/hydration			
Elimination			
Movement			
Rest			
Solitude			
Comfort			
Immunity			
Safety			

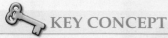

Strengthening and Building Connections

Humans are relational beings who are intended to live in a community with others. The richness of nurses' connections in their personal lives provides fertile soil to grow meaningful connections with patients. Yet, as basic and common as relationships can be, they can be quite challenging. Among the major challenges nurses may face are finding and protecting the time and energy to connect with others in meaningful ways. Like many other professionals in helping professions, nurses may find that the physical, emotional, and mental energies exerted in a typical workday leave little in reserve to invest in nurturing relationships with friends and family. The reactions to work-related stress can be displaced to significant others, thereby interfering with positive personal relationships. To compound the problems, concern for patients' welfare or employer pressure can lead to excessive overtime work, leaving precious little time and energy for nurses to do anything more in their off hours than attend to basics. Strained personal connections are the weeds of untended relationship gardens.

POINT TO PONDER

List five significant individuals in your life. Reflect on the amount of quality time you have with each of them and determine if this time is conducive to a strong relationship.

Relationships

The allocation of time and energy requires the same planning as the allocation of any finite resource. Ignoring this reality risks suffering the consequences of poor relationships. Recognizing that there always will be activities to vie for time and energy, nurses need to take control and develop practices that reflect the value of personal relationships. This can involve limiting the amount of overtime worked to no more than "x" hours each week, dedicating every Thursday evening to dining out with the family, or blocking out Sunday afternoons to visit or telephone friends. Expressing intentions through understood "personal policies" (e.g., informing a supervisor that you will work no more than one double shift per month) and committing time on your calendar (e.g., blocking off every Sunday afternoon for "friends' time") increase the likelihood that significant relationships will receive the attention they require.

Spirituality

Time and energy also must be protected to afford ample time for connecting with God or another higher power. The spiritual grounding resulting from this connection enables nurses to better understand and serve the spiritual needs of patients. Nurses can enhance spiritual connection through prayer, fasting, attending church or temple, engaging in Bible or other holy book studies, taking periodic retreats, and practicing days of solitude and silence.

Connection With Self

Connection with self is essential to nurses' self-care, and this begins with a realistic self-appraisal. Examples of strategies to facilitate this process include sharing life stories, journaling, meditating, and taking retreats.

POINT TO PONDER

What does it mean to you to be connected to self?

Sharing Life Stories

Every adult has a unique and rich storehouse of experiences that have been cemented into the life in which he or she dwells. Oral sharing of life stories with others helps people gain self-insight and puts experiences into a perspective that affords meaning. As people share stories, they begin to see that their lives are not the only ones that have been less than ideal and sprinkled with pain or have unfolded in unintended ways. Writing one's life story is a powerful means of reflection that affords a permanent record that can be revisited and reconsidered as one gains deeper wisdom about self and others. Box 11-1 provides some ideas for topics to be included in a life story. The process of sharing life stories can be particularly meaningful for gerontological nurses in their work with older adults who often have interesting life histories that they are eager to share—and that frequently can offer rich life lessons.

Journaling

Writing personal notes in a journal or diary can facilitate reflection on one's life. These writings differ from written life stories in that they record

BOX 11-1 Possible Topics for Nurses to Include in Their Life Stories

FAMILY PROFILE

- Description of parents, siblings, and extended family
- Relationship with family members
- Religious, cultural, and ethnic beliefs and practices

CHILDHOOD

- Birth: where, when, unusual events
- Reason you were given your name
- Schools attended and significant memories related to them
- Friends: roles you played in relationships
- Family dynamics
- Family health beliefs, attitudes, and practices
- Experiences with illness, hospitals, and health care professionals
- Special experiences
- Unpleasant experiences
- Religious activities; spirituality

ADOLESCENCE

- Favorite activities
- Schools attended and significant memories related to them
- Friends: role/position in peer group

- Special experiences
- Unpleasant experiences
- Religious activities; spirituality
- Experiences with illness, hospitals, and health care professionals
- Factors stimulating interest in nursing

ADULTHOOD

- Reasons for selecting nursing over other careers
- Various jobs held
- Education
- Spouse: when, how, and where you met
- Feelings about marriage
- Places you've lived
- Family dynamics
- Friends: your role in friendships
- Favorite activities, interests
- Special experiences
- Unpleasant experiences
- Spiritual growth; religious activities
- Impressions, disillusionment with nursing profession
- Goals
- Legacy you'd like to leave

---

current activities and thoughts rather than past ones. An honest written account of feelings, thoughts, conflicts, and behaviors can help people learn about themselves and work through issues.

Meditating

The ancient practice of meditation has helped people sort out thoughts and gain clarity of direction for ages. Many nurses find meditation challenging because the nature of their work consists of *doing*—and multitask doing, at that! However, periods of *being still* enable nurses to offer an optimum healing presence to their patients.

There are several techniques that can be used for meditating (see Box 13-2); individuals vary in their preference for the different forms of meditation. Some people may focus on a word or prayer, whereas others may choose to have no intentional thought and to be open to whatever thoughts drift into their minds. Essential elements to any form of meditation are a quiet environment, comfortable position, and calm and passive attitude. The physiological responses associated with the deep relaxation achieved during meditation have many health benefits (e.g., improved immunity, reduced

blood pressure, and increased peripheral blood flow). Often, issues a person has been struggling with can be clarified through meditation.

Taking Retreats

To many nurses, particularly women, taking a few days off "to do nothing" seems like a luxury that cannot be afforded. After all, there is the house to get in order, shopping that must be done, and overtime that can be worked to gather a few extra dollars for vacation. In addition to the tasks that compete for attention and time, there may be the mental script that insidiously gives the message that it is selfish to forfeit tangibly productive activities to spend time thinking, reflecting, and experiencing. Yet, unless nurses want their interactions with patients to be solely mechanical (i.e., task oriented), they must treat themselves as more than machines. Their bodies, minds, and spirits must be restored and refreshed periodically to offer holistic care—and retreats offer an ideal means to achieve that.

A retreat is a withdrawal from normal activities. It can be structured or unstructured, guided by a leader or self-directed, and taken with a group or alone. Although retreats are offered in exotic locations that offer lavish provisions, they need not be luxurious or expensive. Whatever the location or structure, key elements of the retreat experience include a respite from routine responsibilities; freedom from distractions (telephones, e-mails, children, and doorbells); no one to care for and worry about other than self; and a quiet place. During the retreat, one can spend time on activities that can aid in achieving peace and clarity, such as meditating, journaling, expressing oneself creatively through art, or praying. If life circumstances prevent a multiday or even a full-day retreat, a partial-day retreat can be planned within one's home by establishing peace and privacy (e.g., sending children off; asking roommates to stay away for the morning; unplugging telephones; turning off the computer; or placing an out-of-order sign on the doorbell) and allocating time in retreat-type activities. The charge that a retreat provides to one's physical, emotional, and spiritual batteries will more than compensate for the tasks that were postponed.

KEY CONCEPT

When nurses have strong, grounded connections to themselves, they are in a better position to have meaningful connections with patients.

Committing to a Dynamic Process

Self-care is an ongoing process that demands active attention. However, knowing the actions that support self-care is only the beginning. Committing to engaging in one's self-care completes the picture. This may mean that limits are set on the amount of overtime worked to adhere to an exercise schedule or that one is willing to face the uncomfortable feelings experienced during the process of reflecting on less than pleasant life experiences. Sacrifices, unpopular decisions, and discomfort can result when one chooses to "work on oneself." Yet, it is this inner work that contributes to nurses being effective healers and models of healthy aging practices.

KEY CONCEPT

Life changes, as does the attention it requires; therefore, self-care is dynamic. Areas that seemed to be under control may spring leaks and demand new attention. Strategies that proved successful in the past may become less effective and need replacement.

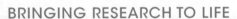

BRINGING RESEARCH TO LIFE

MINDFULNESS PRACTICE LEADS TO INCREASES IN REGIONAL BRAIN GRAY MATTER DENSITY

Hölzel, B. K., Carmody, J., Vangel, M., Congleton, C., Yerramsetti, S. M., Gard, T., & Lazar, S. W. (2011). Psychiatry Research: Neuroimaging, 191(1), 36–43.

In this study, the researchers took magnetic resonance images of the brains of 16 participants before and after their participation in a meditation group. The participants attended weekly sessions that included mindfulness meditation training exercises and received audio recordings to practice guided meditation at home. They completed a questionnaire before and after participation in the group, which measured five aspects of mindfulness: observing, describing, acting with awareness, nonjudging of inner experience, and nonreactivity to inner experience. Brain imaging and completion of the questionnaire was done similarly on a control group who did not have the intervention of meditation.

Brain images of the group who meditated revealed increases in the gray matter composition of the hippocampus, which is an area of the brain involved in memory, learning, and emotional control. The researchers concluded that meditation could influence improvements in learning and memory processes, the regulation of emotions, perspective taking, and other aspects of mental health.

Although additional studies are needed to fully understand the impact of meditation on mindfulness and mental health, this practice is worth considering. Meditation is an easy-to-perform, no-cost practice that can be done any time and place. This study suggests that meditation could improve mental health and function; therefore, nurses should consider building meditation into their daily routine as a self-care practice.

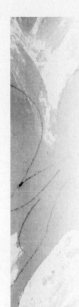

PRACTICE REALITIES

You are working with several nurses who are single parents, working part-time jobs and over-time to provide for their families. To meet the needs of work and family they often cheat on their own sleep, overload on caffeine, and consume junk food on the run rather than healthy meals. When asked what they do to relax and attend to their self-care, they just shake their heads and laugh.

Facing these realities, what could you do to help these coworkers engage in better self-care practices?

CRITICAL THINKING EXERCISES

1. Mindful care of one's body, mind, and spirit is essential to providing holistic gerontological nursing care. What does *mindful* care mean to you?

2. What would hinder you from engaging in self-care practices? What could you do to reduce obstacles to your self-care?

3. What signs, symptoms, or unhealthy habits exist in your life? What types of corrective actions could you commit to improve them?

4. How could you incorporate elements of self-care described in this chapter in an employee health program to aid people in aging well?

RESOURCE

American Holistic Nurses Association
http://www.ahna.org

RECOMMENDED READINGS

Recommended Readings associated with this chapter can be found on the web site that accompanies the book. Visit **http://thepoint.lww.com/Eliopoulos8e** to access the recommended readings and other additional resources associated with this chapter.

UNIT 3

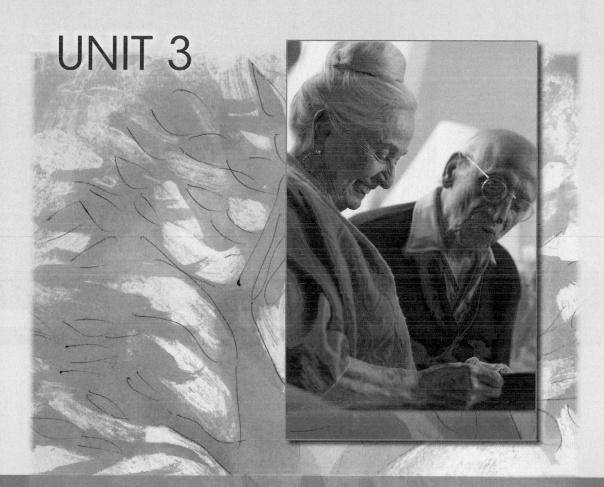

Fostering Connection and Gratification

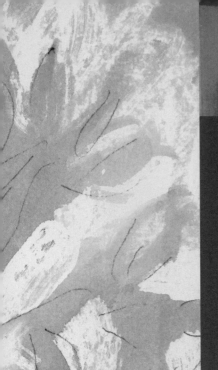

Sexuality and Intimacy

CHAPTER OUTLINE

LEARNING OBJECTIVES

After reading this chapter, you should be able to:

1. Discuss the effects of societal attitudes toward sex and older adults.

2. Identify measures to manage menopausal symptoms.

3. Explain the effects of aging on sexuality and sexual function.

4. Describe factors that can contribute to sexual dysfunction.

5. Describe ways nurses can promote healthy sexual function in older adults.

TERMS TO KNOW

Andropause: a decline in testosterone levels with aging

Dyspareunia: painful intercourse

Erectile dysfunction: the inability to attain and maintain an erection of the penis sufficient to engage in sexual intercourse

Hormone replacement therapy (HRT): replacement of estrogen and/or progestin hormone that is no longer being made by the body

Menopause: the permanent cessation of menses for at least 1 year

Perimenopause: the several years prior to the onset of menopause

Postmenopause: time beginning 12 months after the last menstrual cycle

---

ATTITUDES TOWARD SEX AND OLDER ADULTS

For many years, sex was a major conversational taboo in the United States. Discussion and education concerning this natural, normal process were discouraged and avoided in most circles. Literature on the subject was minimal and usually secured under lock and key. An interest in sex was considered sinful and highly improper. Although people were aware that sexual intercourse had more than a procreative function, the other benefits of this activity were seldom openly shared; society viewed sexual expression outside of wedlock as disgraceful and indecent. The reluctance to accept and intelligently confront human sexuality led to the propagation of numerous myths, the persistence of ignorance and prejudice, and the relegation of sex to a vulgar status.

Fortunately, attitudes have changed over the years, and sexuality has come to be increasingly understood and appreciated. Education has helped erase the mysteries of sex for both adults and children, and magazines, books, television shows, and web sites on the topic flourish. Sex courses, workshops, and counselors throughout the country are helping people gain greater insight about and enjoyment of sex. Not only has the stigma attached to premarital sex been greatly reduced but also increasing numbers of unmarried couples are living together with society's acceptance. Sex is now viewed as a natural, good, and beautiful shared experience.

However, "natural," "good," and "beautiful" are terms seldom used to describe the sexual experiences of older individuals. When the topic of sex and older adults is confronted, much ignorance and prejudice concerning sex reappear. Education about the sexuality of old age is minimal; literature abounds on the sexuality of all individuals in society with minimal attention to older individuals. Any signs of interest in sex or open discussions of sex by older persons are often mocked, discouraged, or viewed suspiciously. The same criteria that make a man a "playboy" at 30 years of age make him a "dirty old man" at 70 years of age. Unmarried young and middle-aged adults who engage in pleasurable sexual experiences are accepted, but widowed grandparents seeking the same enjoyment frequently elicit disbelief and ridicule.

 POINT TO PONDER

How comfortable are you acknowledging that your older relatives could be sexually active?

Myths about older adults and sex run rampant. How many times do we hear that women lose all desire for sex after menopause, that older men cannot achieve an erection, and that older people are not interested in sex? Respect for older adults as vital, sexual beings is minimized by the lack of privacy afforded to them; by the lack of credence given to their sexuality; and by the lack of acceptance, respect, and dignity granted to their continued sexual expression. The myths, ignorance, and vulgar status previously associated with sex in general have been conferred on the sexuality of the older population. Such misconceptions and prejudices are an injustice to persons of all ages. They reinforce any fears and aversion the young have to growing old. They impose conformity on older adults, requiring that they either forfeit warm and meaningful sexual experiences or suffer feelings of guilt and abnormality.

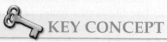 KEY CONCEPT

Often, society conveys the same attitudes regarding sex among older adults as it has in the past concerning sex in general.

One consequence of myths about sex in older adulthood is that older adults may not receive respect as sexual beings. Nurses may witness subtle or blatant violations of respect to older adults' sexual identity such as the following:

- belittling older adults' interest in clothing, cosmetics, and hairstyles
- dressing men and women residents of a nursing home in similar asexual clothing
- denying a woman's request for a female aide to bathe her
- forgetting to button, zip, or fasten clothing when dressing older persons
- unnecessarily exposing older individuals during examination or care activities
- discussing incontinent episodes when the involved individual's peers are present
- ignoring a man's desire to be cleaned and shaved before his female friend visits
- ignoring attempts by older adults to look attractive
- joking about two senior citizens' interest in and flirtation with each other

These examples demonstrate a lack of understanding of the fact that it is important to recognize and respect the sexual identity of any individual, regardless of age. It is not unusual for a 30 year old to be interested in the latest fashions; for two 35 year olds to be dating; or for a 20-year-old woman to prefer a female gynecologist. Almost any young woman would not want a new date to see her before she had time to adjust her cosmetics, hair, and clothing. No care provider would walk into the room of a 25 year old in traction and undress and bathe him in full view of other people in the room. Older adults are entitled to the same dignity and respect as sexual human beings that are afforded to persons of other ages.

POINT TO PONDER

What attitudes toward sex and older adults do you hold? What contributed to the formation of these attitudes?

An additional consequence of stereotypical views toward sex in late life is that issues pertaining to safe sex among senior adults are often ignored. The incidence of acquired immunodeficiency syndrome (AIDS) has increased more than twice as quickly in people over age 50 than in younger adults, and this older population accounts for as many as 30% of the human immunodeficiency virus (HIV)/AIDS cases in the United States (Centers for Disease Control and Prevention, 2011). Sexually active older persons who have sex with new or multiple partners may not consider using a condom because pregnancy is no longer a risk; they may also have misconceptions about sexually transmitted diseases, believing that these diseases only affect younger persons. If they do become symptomatic or learn that a sexual partner is HIV-positive, older adults may be embarrassed to seek medical attention; if they do present with symptoms to a provider, the provider may not associate the symptoms with HIV simply because the person is old (e.g., HIV-related dementia can be misdiagnosed as Alzheimer's disease). These factors contribute to HIV usually being diagnosed in a later stage in older persons. It is important for nurses to reinforce safe sex practices to older persons and to ask about safe sex practices and risk factors for HIV during the assessment.

Nurses can play a significant role in educating and counseling about sexuality in late life; they can encourage attitude changes by their own examples.

MENOPAUSE AS A JOURNEY TO INNER CONNECTION

Menopause, the permanent cessation of menses for at least 1 year, occurs for most women around the fifth decade of life. Some individuals view menopause as a time of experiencing and managing hormonal changes. In fact, to some extent, menopause has been "medicalized" because it is considered a problem or condition that must be treated. Although there are real physiological concerns to consider, menopause is broader in scope than merely a physiological experience. It is a time of important transition in a woman's life that can result in an awakening of a new wholeness of body, mind, and spirit. By the time the average woman reaches menopause, she has considerable life experience that has afforded her a special wisdom. Many cultures honor the wisdom gleaned from years of living and seek the guidance of older adults. Unfortunately, Western society tends to prize the physical beauty of youth over the inner beauty of age. Women in their fifties, sixties, and beyond can feel unattractive, unappreciated, and underused as a result.

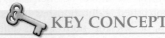

KEY CONCEPT

Menopause marks the entry into a new season of life, characterized by wisdom and groundedness.

With a generation of baby boomers—who are redefining the norms for aging—experiencing or about to experience menopause, an enlightened view of menopause is emerging. This generation of assertive, proactive women does not wish to be confined to limited roles based on physical characteristics. They desire and demand that their talents be used and that they have opportunities for continued growth. The wonder and wisdom of age may receive a long-deserved place of importance.

Symptom Management and Patient Education

Effective management of the physical aspects of menopause can enable women to experience this season of life as a positive passage rather than as a distressing detour. Gerontological nurses can serve aging women well by being knowledgeable about menopause and helping women separate myths from realities about this life transition.

Menopause occurs when estrogen levels fall and the reduced number of ovarian follicles lose their ability to respond to gonadotropic hormone stimulation. Before menopause, the main source of estrogen is estradiol, which is produced by the ovaries. When the ovaries decline in function, most estrogen is obtained through the conversion of androstenedione to estrone in the skin and adipose tissue. A variety of factors can cause estrogen levels to vary among postmenopausal women. Box 12-1 lists symptoms that may be associated with estrogen loss.

It has long been known that hormone therapy can reduce symptoms associated with menopause; however, less certain have been the issues of risks and benefits for various women. In 1991, the National Institutes of Health (NIH) launched the Women's Health Initiative, which studied the effects of hormones in more than 27,000 women. In 2002, NIH stopped the part of the study in which women received estrogen and progestin due to

HRT = Hormone replacement therapy + look up

BOX 12-1　Symptoms Associated with Menopause

PHYSICAL SYMPTOMS

- Hot flashes
- Fatigue
- New onset of migraines
- Symptoms of arthritis, fibromyalgia
- Heart palpitations, atypical angina
- Restless leg syndrome
- Vaginal dryness, itchiness
- Loss of subcutaneous fat in labia
- Insomnia
- Decreased metabolic rate, weight gain
- Increased fat on stomach and hips
- Lower urinary tract symptoms (urinary frequency, stress incontinence, urgency, and nighttime voiding)

- Bladder and vaginal infections
- Increased risks of osteoporosis, heart disease, and colon cancer *Estrogen is protective to the heart*

EMOTIONAL/COGNITIVE SYMPTOMS

- Moodiness
- Depression
- Memory problems
- Fuzzy thinking
- Lack of concentration
- Lower tolerance for annoyance
- Quick to anger
- Greater impatience
- Anxiety, restlessness, new onset of panic disorder
- Paranoia, psychotic symptoms

findings that these women experienced higher heart risks; the portion of the study in which women received only estrogen continued. Concerned about their risks, many women discontinued hormone replacement therapy (HRT) when the study results were announced. Shortly thereafter, however, additional research findings suggested that women who started HRT within 10 years of menopause appeared to have a lower risk of heart attack and breast cancer, whereas women who began taking hormones 10 or more years past menopause had a significantly higher risk of heart problems; these findings suggest that the age at which therapy is initiated is relevant to risks (Rossouw et al., 2007). Although this study showed that estrogen may protect younger women's hearts and may reduce the risks of hip fracture, diabetes, and colon cancer, it also revealed that the hormones increase the risk of other problems, such as blood clots and stroke. Although women can feel reassured that they are not increasing their risk of cardiovascular disease by using hormones to treat symptoms as they go through menopause, it is not wise to extrapolate from the data that women should take hormones for the prevention of heart disease.

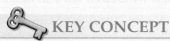

KEY CONCEPT

The benefits and risks associated with hormone replacement therapy depend on the age at which a woman starts therapy and her unique health profile.

Currently, it is recommended that if estrogen is used to treat menopausal symptoms, it is prescribed at the lowest effective dose for the shortest period of time, and only for the treatment of moderate to severe symptoms and for the prevention of osteoporosis (the benefits in preventing osteoporosis are lost when the hormone is no longer used). It is contraindicated in women with breast cancer, a history of breast cancer, suspected or known estrogen-sensitive cancers, coronary artery disease, untreated hypertension, active liver disease, pulmonary embolism, undiagnosed vaginal bleeding, or high sensitivity to hormone therapy. It is not recommended that hormone therapy be used for the prevention of cardiovascular conditions, dementia, depression, or other chronic diseases (Rouse, 2012).

The use of bioidentical, custom-compounded hormones is not recommended. There is no scientific evidence that they, and many of the herbal and other "natural" products to address menopause symptoms, are safer or more effective than the conventional hormone therapy (Endocrine Society, 2012). Although many of the herbs recommended for the management of menopausal symptoms lack scientific evidence, a standardized extract of rhapontic rhubarb (*Rheum rhaponticum*) has been shown through a placebo-controlled study to significantly reduce hot flashes and other symptoms of menopause (Geller, 2009).

In addition to HRT, natural and alternative therapies for managing symptoms are available (Box 12-2). The effectiveness of these therapies varies among women.

BOX 12-2 Complementary and Alternative Approaches to Aid in Controlling Menopausal Symptoms

- Acupuncture
- Diet:
  - Foods rich in plant estrogens: apples, beans, carrots, celery, nuts, seeds, soy products (approximately 100 to 160 mg/day of soy is needed to obtain significant relief), wheat, and whole grains
  - Foods rich in boron to increase estrogen retention: asparagus, beans, broccoli, cabbage, peaches, prunes, strawberries, and tomatoes
  - Avoidance of adrenal-stimulating foods: alcohol, caffeine, refined carbohydrates, salt, and sugar
- Exercise
- Imagery
- Herbs such as a standardized extract of rhapontic rhubarb (R. rhaponticum) and American ginseng as a general tonic
- Meditation

- Homeopathic remedies:
  - Vaginal lubrication: bryonia
  - General symptoms: amyl nitrosum, natrum muriaticum, sepia, and sulfur
- Regular, adequate sleep
- Stress management practices
- T'ai chi
- Vaginal moisturizing agents:
  - Commercial vaginal moisturizing creams (e.g., Replens), water-based gels
  - Herbal salves made with marshmallow root, calendula blossom, comfrey, licorice root, and wild yam
  - St. John's wort oil
- Vitamins and minerals such as calcium, chromium, magnesium, selenium, and vitamins C, D, and E
- Yoga

Aging women can benefit from basic education about menopause and methods for managing symptoms. Box 12-3 outlines some of the major topics that could be included in a menopausal educational program.

Self-Acceptance

Nurses can help women appreciate menopause as a time to take stock and rechart their life course. Emotions and symptoms can be used as teachers that show areas of one's self that beg for expression. Women can unleash creative energies and discover new interests. They can realize the significance of caring for and nurturing self. Whether it is their maturation or a desire to not waste the precious limited time one has remaining in life, older adults tend to understand themselves and their lives. Impossible expectations and pretense can be let go, unleashing more meaningful and creative aspects of later life. Older individuals can live in truth and love as who they truly are. This self-acceptance can provide the security to broaden their perspectives and purposes and deepen their connections with others and a higher power.

POINT TO PONDER

Do you view menopause as a time marking the loss of youthfulness and beauty or the beginning of a journey into new creativity and wisdom? What has influenced your opinion?

Andropause

Women are not the only ones to experience hormonal changes with age. Some men experience a decline in testosterone levels, known as andropause. It differs from menopause in that it does not occur in all men and, when it does occur, it is a slower process. When testosterone levels fall to low levels, the body increases the production of follicle-stimulating hormone (FSH) and luteinizing hormone (LH) in an effort to increase testosterone.

Low testosterone levels in older men can result in reduced muscle mass, energy, strength, and stamina. Erectile dysfunction can occur, along with breast enlargement, osteopenia, osteoporosis, and shrinkage of the testes. Emotional and cognitive changes can also occur. The low testosterone levels are not only associated with reduced sexual function but also a higher risk for type 2 diabetes and cardiovascular disease (Feeley, Saad, Guay, & Traish, 2009). Again, it is important to recognize that this is not a normal occurrence in all aging men.

REALITIES OF SEX IN OLDER ADULTHOOD

Until the work by Kinsey (1948) and Masters and Johnson (1966), there had been minimal exploration into the realities of sex in old age. Several possible factors have contributed to this lack of research and information. One is the acceptance and expansion of sexology that has occurred within the past few decades. Another is that impropriety

BOX 12-3 Topics for Inclusion in a Menopause Education Program

- Menopause is a naturally occurring process, not a disease. It is characterized by the absence of menstrual periods for at least 12 consecutive months.
- Menopause is a gradual process. Most women experience *perimenopause* about 3 to 6 years before menopause when menstrual periods permanently cease. By age 40, most women begin having irregular periods.
- Menopause is a multihormone process. In addition to estrogen, progesterone declines although not in a direct proportion. In fact, some of the symptoms associated with menopause can be the result of declining progesterone with estrogen dominance. One outcome of estrogen dominance over progesterone is the blocking of the action of thyroid hormone. Although it does not occur in all menopausal women, some can have declines in testosterone, which affects libido and sexual pleasure. Factors such as stress and obesity affect the hormonal secretion.
- Estrogen affects functions beyond those of reproduction. Estrogen:
  - increases the chemical enzyme choline acetyltransferase needed to synthesize the neurotransmitter acetylcholine (which is critical for memory);
  - promotes the growth of dendritic spines on neurons;
  - enhances the availability of the neurotransmitters serotonin, norepinephrine, and dopamine; and
  - acts like an antioxidant to protect nerve cells from free radical damage.
- Many physical, cognitive, and emotional symptoms can be associated with low estrogen levels (see Box 12-1).
- Diagnostic blood tests should be done to properly assess the menopausal state; these include follicle-stimulating hormone (FSH), leutienizing hormone (LH), estradiol (estrogen), testosterone, and free testosterone levels. If sexual dysfunction or low libido is present, evaluate thyroid function (T_3, T_4, free T_4, and TSH), platelet monoamine oxidase, and prolactin.
- Hormonal replacement therapy (HRT) carries the risks and benefits that must be weighed for each individual.
- Complementary therapies and practices can assist in controlling symptoms in some women (see Box 12-2).

was formerly associated with open discussions of sex. Furthermore, there was a misconception on the part of many professionals, older people, and the general public that older individuals are neither interested in nor capable of sex. In addition, practitioners lacked experience in and did not have an inclination toward discussing sex with any age group. Even today, medical and nursing assessments frequently do not reflect inquiry into sexual history and activity.

Nurses should be aware of recent interest and research in the area of sex in late life and communicate these research findings to colleagues and clients to promote a more realistic understanding of the older population's sexuality.

Sexual Behavior and Roles

Research, reinforced by creative advertisements for erectile dysfunction drugs, has disproved the belief that older persons are not interested in or capable of engaging in sex; older adults can and do enjoy the pleasures of sexual foreplay and intercourse. Because the general pattern of sexual behavior is basically consistent throughout the life, individuals who were disinterested in sex and had infrequent intercourse throughout their lifetime will not usually develop a sudden insatiable desire for sex in old age. Similarly, a couple who has maintained an interest in sex and continued regular coitus throughout their adult life will most likely not forfeit this activity at any particular age. Homosexuality, masturbation, a desire for a variety of sexual partners, and other sexual patterns also continue into old age. Sexual styles, interests, and expression must be viewed in the context of the individual's total life experience.

The same is true for identification with sexual roles. Perceptions of male and female roles have changed over time. Many of today's older population were socialized to accept certain masculine and feminine roles—older individuals have had a lifetime of experience with the expectation that men are to be aggressive, independent, and strong and that women are to be pretty, gentle, and dependent on their male counterparts. The baby boomers changed those views as the women's liberation movement encouraged women to be independent, strong, and on equal terms with men in the home and workplace. In addition, there was an acceptance and expectation that men should share household and family nurturing responsibilities that once were thought to be within the realm of women. The result is diversity in sex role identity and expectations among the older population. Such differences, based on socialization and decades of living, need to be recognized and respected.

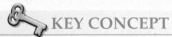

KEY CONCEPT

Sexuality and sexual interest in late life reflect lifelong patterns.

Intimacy

Sexuality also encompasses much more than physical acts. It includes love, warmth, caring, and sharing between individuals; seeing beyond gray hair, wrinkles, and other manifestations of aging; and the intimate exchange of words and touches by sexual human beings. Feeling important to and wanted by another person promotes security, comfort, and emotional well-being (Fig. 12-1).

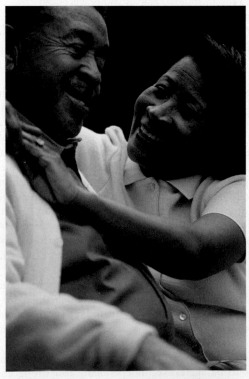

FIGURE 12-1 ■ In addition to physical means of expression, older adults express their sexuality emotionally in intimate relationships.

With the multiple losses that older adults experience, the comfort and satisfaction derived from a meaningful relationship are especially significant.

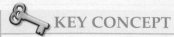

KEY CONCEPT

Sexuality includes love, warmth, caring, and sharing between people and identification with a sexual role.

Age-Related Changes and Sexual Response

Despite the physical ability to remain sexually active in old age, various factors and age-related changes do impact the older person's sexual function. Although clinical data are minimal and additional research is necessary, some general statements can be made about sex and the older person:

- There is a decrease in sexual responsiveness and a reduction in the frequency of orgasm (Greenberg, 2001; Masters & Johnson, 1981; Sand & Fisher, 2007).
- Older men are slower to erect, mount, and ejaculate.
- Older women may experience dyspareunia (painful intercourse) as a result of less lubrication, decreased distensibility, and thinning of the vaginal walls.
- Many older women gain a new interest in sex, possibly because they no longer have to fear an unwanted pregnancy or because they have more time and privacy with their children grown and gone.

Although individual differences occur in the intensity and duration of sexual response in older people, regular sexual expression for both sexes is important in promoting sexual capacity and maintaining sexual function. With good health and the availability of a partner, sexual activity can continue well into the seventh decade and beyond. The frequency of sexual activity may decrease, but that is not necessarily accompanied by a reduction in sexual interest or ability.

The work of Masters and Johnson (1966) provided the first major insight into the sexual responses of older persons. Table 12-1 summarizes their findings.

IDENTIFYING BARRIERS TO SEXUAL ACTIVITY

In addition to the impact of age-related changes, various physical, emotional, and social variables can

TABLE 12-1	Human Sexual Response Cycle in Late Life	
Phase	**Older Women**	**Older Men**
Excitement: results from stimulation from any source	Same clitoral response and nipple erection as younger women; breast less engorged; sex flush (vasocongestive skin response) occurs less frequently; less muscle tension elevation in response to sexual stimuli; unlike in younger women, labia majora does not separate, flatten, and elevate; reduced reactions of labia minora; less secretory activity of Bartholin's gland; less vaginal lubrication and wall expansion	Takes longer for erection to be achieved; less firm erection; increased difficulty regaining erection if lost or maintaining erection before ejaculation; less sex flush; reduced scrotal and testicular vasocongestion
Plateau: sexual tensions intensified; if they reach an extreme, orgasm will be achieved; if tension level drops, resolution phase will be entered	Reduced intensity; less degree of engorgement of areolae; decreased vasocongestion of labia; reduced secretions of Bartholin's gland; less uterine elevation; less intense sexual flush	Slower; full erection may not occur until just prior to ejaculation; less intense muscle tension and sexual flush; delayed and diminished testicular elevation
Orgasm: lasts a few seconds; sexual stimuli released; although entire body is involved to varying degrees, primarily concentrated in genitalia	Same vaginal contractions as younger woman but of decreased intensity and duration; similar slight degree of involuntary distention of external urinary meatus	Similar response as younger man but only slower; during ejaculation, more of a seepage of semen rather than a forceful emission; fewer and less intense ejaculatory contractions; orgasm may not occur with every intercourse, especially if it is frequent
Resolution: sexual tensions subside	Nipple erection can continue for hours; urinary symptoms may be present	Longer duration; slower loss of nipple erection; rapid penile detumescence

threaten the older person's ability to remain sexually active (Nursing Diagnosis Table 12-2 and Nursing Diagnosis Highlight: Sexual Dysfunction). A comprehensive nursing assessment includes a sexual history, which can reveal these problems. Assessment Guide 12-1 offers sample questions that can be incorporated into the assessment to identify issues pertaining to sexual function. Sensitive attention to the maintenance of sexual function and identity is significant in promoting wellness.

NURSING DIAGNOSIS

TABLE 12-2	Aging and Risks to Sexuality
Causes or Contributing Factors	**Nursing Diagnosis**
Wrinkling and sagging of tissues; age spots; graying and loss of hair; arthritic joints; loss of muscle tone; high prevalence of tooth loss; increased incidence of disabling disease	Disturbed Body Image and Sexual Dysfunction related to altered appearance
Increased physical stimulation required to achieve erection and lubricate vagina	Sexual Dysfunction related to inadequate preparation for intercourse
Increased prevalence of chronic disabling conditions	Sexual Dysfunction related to discomfort, diseases, preoccupation with health, or positional restrictions
Higher ratio of women to men in advanced years	Sexual Dysfunction related to the unavailability of a sexual partner
Ageism	Sexual Dysfunction related to the belief that sex in old age is inappropriate

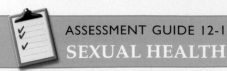

ASSESSMENT GUIDE 12-1
SEXUAL HEALTH

INTERVIEW

Begin this component of the overall assessment by explaining to the older adult that you are going to ask questions pertaining to his or her sex life to identify problems that could be improved and to learn about possible underlying conditions that could be revealed through sexual problems. Ask the older adult if he or she has your permission to ask these questions:

Are you sexually active?

If the answer is *no*, ask for reasons (e.g., no partner, not enough energy, and erectile dysfunction). Based on the reason, inquire about the older adult's interest in changing the situation to become sexually active and recommend plans accordingly (e.g., offer location of senior centers, evaluate possible causes of low energy, and refer to sexual dysfunction clinic).

If the answer is *yes*, proceed with the following questions:

- How frequently do you have sex? Is this a satisfying frequency to you? If not, how would you change the frequency of sex?
- Do you have sex with a single or multiple partners? Male or female partner?
- If you have sex with new partners, do you use a condom?
- Do you obtain pleasure from sex? If not, why not?
- Have you or your partner(s) ever been treated for a sexually transmitted infection? If yes, for what disease and when?
- Do you or your partner(s) have risk factors for HIV/AIDS, such as a history of blood transfusions, IV drug use, or sex with prostitutes?
- *Male:* Are you able to get an erection when you want to engage in sex? Do you have orgasms and ejaculate when you have sex? If not, describe what happens. Do you have any sores on your penis or any discharge?
- *Female:* Is sex comfortable for you? If not, describe. Do you have orgasms? Do you have any vaginal discharge or bleeding?
- Is your partner satisfied with your sex life? If not, why not?

- Have you ever been or are you currently being sexually abused? Raped? If yes, describe.
- *If health conditions or disabilities are present:* How has your condition affected your ability to enjoy sex?
- What concerns do you have regarding your sex life?
- Do you have any questions about your sexual function that you would like me to answer?

LABORATORY TESTS

A variety of laboratory tests can aid in identifying changes in hormone levels that can affect sexual function; these include:

- Complete blood count
- Complete metabolic panel
- Dihydrotestosterone
- Estradiol
- Mean gonadotropin-releasing hormone
- Prostate-specific antigen
- Serum prolactin
- Thyroid-stimulating hormone (TSH)
- Total serum testosterone

MEDICATIONS

A review of the prescription and over-the-counter drugs used is beneficial in identifying the relationship of medications to any sexual problems. Pay particular attention to the use of angiotensin-converting enzyme (ACE) inhibitors, alcohol, α-adrenergic blockers, antianxieties/benzodiazepines, anticholinergics, antidepressants, antihistamines, antihypertensives, antiparkinsonian agents, diuretics, dopamine agonists, monoamine oxidase inhibitors (MAOIs), nicotine, nonsteroid anti-inflammatory drugs, sedatives/hypnotics, and recreational drugs.

DIAGNOSES

Review the medical history for health conditions that could interfere with sexual function (see Table 12-3).

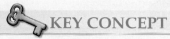

KEY CONCEPT

The unavailability of a partner, ageism, changes in body image, boredom, misconceptions, physical conditions, medications, and cognitive impairments are among the factors that can interfere with sexual function in later life.

Unavailability of a Partner

A practical interference with sexual function in later life is the lack of a partner, particularly for older women. By 65 years of age, there are only 7 men to every 10 women; by 85 years of age, the ratio becomes 1:5. Furthermore, there is a tendency for men to marry women who are younger than themselves; one third of men older than 65 years of age have wives younger than 65 years of age. Therefore, most older men are married, and most older women are widowed.

Even when an older person has a spouse or partner, that person may be too infirm to remain sexually active and, in some cases, may be institutionalized.

Psychological Barriers

Sometimes, sexual dysfunction can have psychological causes. Negative attitudes from society, fear of losing sexual abilities, concerns about body image, relationship issues, and misconceptions held by older adults themselves can impair sexual function.

Older adults are not immune to the attitudes around them. As they hear comments about the inappropriateness of older people engaging in sex and watch television shows that portray sex among older individuals in a condescending or ridiculing manner, they may feel foolish or unnatural in having sexual desires and activity. If they happen to have sexual partners who are disinterested in sex and negatively label their advances, the problem is intensified. As older adults internalize others' reactions, they may become reluctant or unable to engage in sexual activity and unnecessarily forfeit sexual function. Nurses can advocate for older adults by educating persons of all ages in the realities and importance of sexual function in later life and ensuring that nursing care does not reinforce negative attitudes about sex.

Problems may also occur when the older man believes he is losing his sexual capability, even when he is not. It is not unusual for older men to occasionally have difficulty achieving an erection; erections also may be easily lost if there is an interruption (e.g., a ringing telephone or a partner who leaves the bed to use the bathroom). These occurrences can trigger a cycle of problems, whereby an episode of impotence causes anxiety over the potential loss of sexual function permanently, and this anxiety interferes with the ability to become erect, which further heightens anxiety. Aging persons need realistic explanations—preferably before the situation arises—that occasional impotence is neither unusual nor an indication that one is "too old for sex." Open discussions and reassurance are beneficial. The partner needs to be included in this process and made aware of the importance of patience and sensitivity in helping the man deal with this problem. The couple should be encouraged to continue their efforts and, if erection is occasionally a problem, compensate with other forms of sexual gratification. Of course, chronic impotence can indicate a variety of disorders and deserves a thorough evaluation.

Body image and self-concept affect sexual activity. In a society in which beauty is youthful, older persons may believe that their wrinkles, gray hair, and sagging torsos make them physically unappealing. This can be particularly difficult for single older people who must deal with baring their bodies to new partners. The fear of being unattractive and rejected may cause older adults to avoid encountering such situations and assume a sexually inactive role.

Additional factors make developing a sexual relationship difficult for single older people. Older women were socialized during a period when sex was considered appropriate only in wedlock and, for some persons, only for the purpose of procreation. The thought of seeking sexual gratification with a partner to whom one is not married creates anxiety and guilt in many older women. The older man, who was socialized in the aggressor role, may not have had to practice his courtship skills for years if he has been monogamous for a long period, and he may feel insecure in his ability to seduce a partner or find one who understands his individual preferences. He, too, may be emotionally uncomfortable in establishing a sexual relationship. Financial considerations can affect sexual activity also when the single older adult has concern that commitment to a relationship and marriage could reduce Social Security income or create problems in sharing assets. The hurdle of building new sexual relationships can be so great that many older people may find it easier to repress their sexual needs.

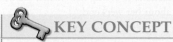

KEY CONCEPT

Some older adults may repress sexual needs rather than confront the stresses associated with establishing new sexual relationships.

NURSING DIAGNOSIS HIGHLIGHT

SEXUAL DYSFUNCTION

Overview

Sexual dysfunction implies a problem in the ability to derive sexual satisfaction. This condition can be identified through the patient's history (e.g., complaints of impotence, dyspareunia, lack of interest in sex, and changes in relationship with partner), physical findings (e.g., genital infection, prolapsed uterus, and diabetes mellitus), or behavior (e.g., depression, anxiety, and self-deprecation). Sometimes changes in the older person's life can give clues to the presence of sexual dysfunction problems, such as recent widowhood, onset of a new health problem, or moving to a child's home.

Causative or contributing factors

Age-related dryness and fragility of vaginal canal, vaginal infection, venereal disease, neurological disease, cardiovascular disease, diabetes mellitus, decreased hormone production, pulmonary disease, arthritis, pain, prostatitis, prolapsed uterus, cystocele, rectocele, medications, overeating, obesity, fatigue, alcohol consumption, fear of worsening health problem, lack of partner, unwilling or unable partner, boredom with partner, fear of failure, guilt, anxiety, depression, stress, negative self-concept, lack of privacy, religious conflict, and altered appearance.

Goal

The patient expresses satisfaction with sexual function.

Interventions

■ Obtain a sexual history from the older adult. Note the availability and quality of relationship with partner, lifelong pattern of sexual function, recent changes to sexual function, signs and symptoms of sexual dysfunction, knowledge and attitudes about sex, medical problems, drugs used, mental status, myths and misinformation, and feelings about sexual dysfunction.

■ If the cause of sexual dysfunction is not readily available through the history, refer the older person for a comprehensive physical examination.

■ Identify causative or contributing factors to sexual dysfunction and plan interventions to correct them.

■ Refer to sexual counselor or therapist as needed.

■ Clarify misconceptions (e.g., a person cannot have sex after a heart attack).

■ Provide education as to normal sexual function, measures to promote sexual function, and how to minimize impact of health problems on sexual function. (The American Heart Association, the Arthritis Foundation, and other disease-specific organizations provide literature on promoting sexual function in the presence of disease.)

■ Assist the older adult in having a good appearance and improving self-concept as needed.

■ Advise in health practices that will promote sexual function, such as regular gynecologic examinations, alcohol use in moderation, good diet, and exercise.

■ Ensure staff are nonjudgmental about the older adult's unique means of sexual expression.

■ If the older adult is hospitalized or institutionalized, provide privacy for sexual expression.

CONSIDER THIS CASE

Seventy-two-year-old Mrs. W has been widowed for 8 months. She is an attractive, active woman and desired to break up her lonely days by joining a local senior center, where she met Mr. R, a handsome 75-year-old widower. In short time, they began dating, and recently Mr. R has asked Mrs. W to join him for a long weekend at a romantic vacation spot. Mr. R has openly shared that he has had frequent sexual partners and that he envisions initiating a sexual relationship with Mrs. W during their weekend. Mrs. W is interested in taking the relationship to this new level but is nervous about the fact that she and her husband had not had intercourse during the last 8 years of his life due to his poor health, and she now wonders how much discomfort she will experience. She discusses this with a nurse friend and expresses concerns about having a new sexual partner for the first time in over 50 years, Mr. R's possible reactions to seeing her "naked old body," and what her children and grandchildren would think if they found out about her weekend.

THINK CRITICALLY

■ What advice would be helpful for the nurse friend to offer?
■ What are some of the challenges and risks that Mrs. W could face?

Married older people also may experience problems with sex. Not all marriages enjoy fulfilling sex. Some women conceded to sex because it was a "wife's duty," yet they never achieved satisfaction from this intimate experience. Some spouses may have become bored with the same partner or form of sex. Perhaps physical changes or an inattention to appearance causes dissatisfaction with the partner. Love and caring may have been lost from the marriage. Sexual interest may be diminished if one is the caregiver for a partner or if a disability causes the partner to be perceived as sexually undesirable. Older couples experience sexual problems for many of the same reasons that younger couples do.

Misconceptions are often responsible for creating obstacles to a fulfilling sex life in old age and can include the following:

- erections are not possible after prostatectomy
- penile penetration can be harmful to a woman after a hysterectomy
- menopause eliminates sexual desire
- sex is bad for a heart condition
- after a hip fracture, intercourse can refracture the bone
- sexual ability and interest are lost with age

Straightforward explanations and public education can help correct these misconceptions, as can realistic descriptions of how illness, surgery, and drugs do and do not affect sexual function.

Medical Conditions

A variety of physical conditions, many of which respond to treatment (Table 12-3), can affect sexual function in later life. A thorough evaluation is crucial in determining a realistic approach to aiding older adults with these problems. Interventions that are of value to younger people also can benefit older people, including medications, penile prostheses, lubricants, surgery, and sex counseling. Nurses should communicate their understanding of the importance of sexual functioning to older adults and a willingness to assist them in preserving sexual capabilities.

Erectile Dysfunction

Erectile dysfunction, commonly referred to as impotence, is a condition in which a man is unable to attain and maintain an erection of the penis sufficient to allow him to engage in sexual intercourse. This condition affects as many as 35% of men between the ages of 40 and 70 years, with an increased prevalence with age (Bianco et al., 2009; Hyde et al., 2012; Rosing et al., 2009). Erectile dysfunction can have multiple causes, including

atherosclerosis, diabetes, hypertension, multiple sclerosis, thyroid dysfunction, alcoholism, renal failure, structure abnormalities (e.g., Peyronie's disease), medications, and psychological factors. With the range and complexity of potential causes, a thorough physical examination is essential. (Even if the older man is not interested in being sexually active, he should be encouraged to have this dysfunction evaluated to identify underlying conditions that warrant medical attention.)

In 1998, a major breakthrough occurred in the treatment of erectile dysfunction with the Food and Drug Administration's approval of sildenafil citrate (Viagra). Within its first year on the market, nearly 4 million prescriptions were written for Viagra, demonstrating the scope of erectile dysfunction and the desire of men to correct this problem. Since then, other drugs, such as tadalafil (Cialis) and vardenafil (Levitra), have become available to treat this condition. There are other options to treat erectile dysfunction, such as alprostadil (a drug that is injected into the penis to increase blood flow), vacuum pumps, and penile implants. Men need to discuss with their physicians the options that are best for them.

Medication Adverse Effects

Frequently, medications prescribed to older people affect potency, libido, orgasm, and ejaculation. Some of these drugs include the following:

- ACE inhibitors
- alcohol
- α-adrenergic blockers
- antianxieties/benzodiazepines
- anticholinergics
- antidepressants
- antihistamines
- antihypertensives
- antiparkinsonian agents
- diuretics
- dopamine agonists
- MAOIs
- nicotine
- nonsteroid anti-inflammatories
- sedatives/hypnotics
- some recreational drugs

It is important to prepare older people for the potential changes in sexual function that drugs can produce. Imagine what it does to a patient with

TABLE 12-3	Medical Conditions Interfering with Sexual Function	
Condition	**Problem Created**	**Intervention**
Men		
Prostatitis	Discomfort, interference with ejaculation	Treat infection; prostatic massage
"Open"-type prostatectomy	Disturbed function of internal sphincter, causing impotency	Penile prosthesis
Peyronie's disease	Painful, dorsal bending of penis from fibrous scarring associated with inflammatory process	Local injections of corticosteroids Surgery
Infections of genitalia	Pain, inhibition of erection, scarring that narrows urethral outlet	Treat infection Surgical dilation of narrow outlet
Arteriosclerosis	Testicular cellular function disturbed, leading to decline in male sex hormone	Testosterone therapy
Parkinsonism	Decrease in sexual interest secondary to the loss of potency	Levodopa therapy
Cord compression from arthritic changes	Impotency	Surgery may not restore potency if reflex arc is permanently broken Penile prosthesis
Women		
Decreased level of estrogen	Excessive vaginal dryness	Local estrogens
Virginity	Thick or large hymen	Surgery Dilation
Infection of genitalia	Discomfort, itching	Treat infection and underlying cause (poor hygiene, hyperglycemia)
Prolapsed uterus	Pain, difficulty with penile penetration	Pessary Surgery
Cystocele	Discomfort, dribbling urine	Surgery
Both Sexes		
Cardiovascular, respiratory disease	Shortness of breath, coughing, discomfort, fear of heart attack or death during sex, decreased libido	Counseling on realistic restrictions necessary Instruction in alternative positions to avoid strain Advise to avoid large meals for several hours before, relax, plan medications for peak effectiveness during sex
Arthritis	Limited movement	Instruction on alternative positions
Diabetes mellitus	Local genital infection	Treat infection
	Failure of erection due to inhibition of parasympathetic nervous system	Penile prosthesis
	Absence of or difficulty achieving orgasm Delayed and decreased vaginal lubrication	Instruction in alternative positions and forms of sexual expression
Stroke	Decreased libido	Counseling
	Fear	Instruction in alternative positions
Alcoholism	Decreased potency Delayed orgasm (women)	Counseling and treatment for alcoholism

newly diagnosed hypertension when he experiences drug-related impotency and begins to feel anxious about the sudden changes in both health and sexual function. Drugs should be reviewed when new sexual dysfunction occurs and, whenever possible, nondrug treatment modalities should be used to manage health problems.

Cognitive Impairment

The sexual behavior of individuals with dementia tends to be more difficult for those around them than for the affected persons. Inappropriate behavior, such as undressing and masturbating in public areas and grabbing and making sexual comments to strangers, can occur. The cognitively impaired person may accuse his or her spouse of being a stranger improperly trying to share the bed and may misunderstand care procedures (e.g., baths and catheterization) as sexual advances. Sometimes touching and statements such as "How's my sweetheart?" or "Are you going to give me a big hug?" can be misinterpreted as invitations to become sexually intimate. Family members and caregivers need to understand that this is a normal feature of the illness. Rather than becoming upset or embarrassed, they need to learn to respond simply, for example, by taking the individual to a private area when masturbating, or stating "I'm not a stranger, I'm Mary, your wife."

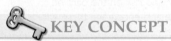

KEY CONCEPT

Unintentionally, caregivers can make comments to the cognitively impaired person that can be misinterpreted as flirtatious and trigger inappropriate sexual behaviors.

PROMOTING HEALTHY SEXUAL FUNCTION

The nurse can foster sexuality and intimacy in older persons in various ways, some of which have already been discussed. Basic education can help older adults and persons of all ages understand the effects of the aging process on sexuality by providing a realistic framework for sexual functioning. The nurse can teach about sexual functioning during routine health assessments, as part of structured health education classes, and during discharge planning when reviewing capabilities and activity restrictions.

A willingness on the nurse's part to discuss sex openly with older people demonstrates recognition, acceptance, and respect for their sexuality. A sexual history as part of the nursing assessment provides an excellent framework for launching such discussions. The nurse identifies physical, emotional, and social threats to older adults' sexuality and intimacy and

seeks solutions for problems—whether caused by the disfigurement of surgery, obesity, depression, poor self-concept, fatigue, or lack of privacy. The nurse can also promote practices that can enhance sexual function, including regular exercise, good nutrition, limited alcohol intake, ample rest, stress management, good hygiene and grooming practices, and enjoyable foreplay.

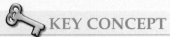

KEY CONCEPT

The nurse's willingness to discuss sex openly with older adults demonstrates recognition, acceptance, and respect for their sexuality.

Consideration must be given to the sexual needs of older persons in institutional settings. Too often, couples admitted to the same facility are not able to share a double bed, and frequently they are not even able to share the same room if they require different levels of care. It is unnatural and unfair to force a person to travel to another wing of a building to visit a spouse who has intimately shared 40, 50, or 60 years of his or her life. There are few or no places in most institutional settings where two such individuals can find a place to share intimacy where they will not be interrupted or be in full view of others. Older people in institutional settings have a right to privacy that goes beyond lip service. They should be able to close and lock a door, feeling secure that this action will be honored. They should not be made to feel guilty or foolish by their expressions of love and sexuality. Their sexuality should not be sanctioned, screened, or severed by any other person.

Masturbation is often beneficial for releasing sexual tensions and maintaining continued function of the genitalia. Nurses can convey their acceptance and understanding of the value of this activity by providing privacy and a nonjudgmental attitude. Conveying such an attitude can prevent older individuals from developing feelings of guilt or abnormality related to masturbation.

In addition, nurses must appreciate that sexual satisfaction can have different meaning to older people than to the young. To some older men and women, holding, caressing, and exchanging loving words can be as meaningful as intercourse or sexually explicit conversation.

For older adults in any setting, nurses can facilitate connections, which are essential for sexual relationships. Unfortunately, relationships can be more challenging to create and sustain in late life. The circle of friends and family gradually diminishes with each passing year; health and economic limitations decrease one's participation in social activities; and preoccupation with health conditions

BOX 12-4 Strategies to Facilitate Connections

- *Assist patients in evaluating current relationships.* Guide them in examining relationship patterns that are effective and those that could be improved. Discuss the impact of relationships on health and quality of life.
- *Guide patients in becoming aware of their behaviors and responses that impact relationships.* Help them to gain insight into roles and dynamics and impact of responses.
- *Teach strategies that promote effective expression of inner feelings.* Offer suggestions and role plays that support feeling-based communication, such as making statements that reflect how they feel rather than impersonal generalities (e.g., "I feel angry when you make my decisions for me"). Help patients to respect others' expressions of feelings.
- *Provide information on sources of social activities.* Obtain address and contact information for local senior centers, clubs, and social groups. Suggest measures that patients can use to facilitate a comfortable entry into new groups, such as asking a friend to accompany them, taking the lead in introductions, and finding a common interest that can be used as a stimulus for conversation.
- *Refer patients for hearing and/or vision examinations as needed.* Initiate audiology and ophthalmology referrals if problems are identified during the nursing assessment. Assist patients in locating financial aid if costs for examinations, glasses, or aids cannot be afforded.
- *Respect patients' interest and efforts to be sexually active.* Support efforts to enhance appearance. Listen without judgment as patients describe feelings about their sexual interests and function. Provide privacy for patients' interactions with significant others.
- *Assist patients in improving sexual function.* Refer to appropriate specialists for the treatment of conditions that affect sexual function. Support efforts to correct sexual dysfunction. Counsel patients in measures to preserve and facilitate sexual function (e.g., use of lubricating creams to compensate for vaginal dryness, alternative positions to accommodate joint pain, and timing of medication administration to maximize energy during sex).
- *Provide positive feedback for efforts patients have taken to improve the quantity and quality of connections with others.* Remember that an action that may seem minor, such as attending a community social event, could have required tremendous effort and risk on the part of patients. Recognize and encourage these efforts.

of self and significant others narrows one's sphere of interests. The risks resulting in a shrinking of older adults' social world are real and often significant; however, nurses can offer interventions that can minimize and compensate for them. Box 12-4 offers suggestions for helping older adults to maintain satisfying, healthy relationships.

Nurses must recognize, respect, and encourage sexuality in older adults. Nurses, as role models, can foster positive attitudes. Improved understanding, increased sensitivity, and humane attitudes can help the older population of today and tomorrow realize the full potential of sexuality in their later years.

BRINGING RESEARCH TO LIFE

INFLUENCE OF EXERCISE ON MOOD IN POSTMENOPAUSAL WOMEN

Villaverde Gutiérrez, C., Torres Luque, G., Ábalos Medina, G. M., Argente del Castillo, M. J., Guisado, I. M., Guisado Barrilao, R., & Ramírez Rodrigo, J. (2012). Journal of Clinical Nursing, 21(7), 923–928.

This prospective study evaluated the impact of an exercise program on symptoms of anxiety and depression in postmenopausal women. A sample of 60 postmenopausal women aged 60 to 70 years, with symptoms of depression and anxiety, was recruited. They were divided into a control group who received no intervention and a group who participated in a program of mixed physical exercise. All of the women completed questionnaires for the Hamilton Anxiety Scale and the Brink and Yesavage Geriatric Depression Scale before and after treatment.

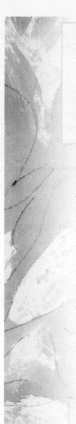

The group who participated in exercise showed statistically significant improvements in symptoms of anxiety and moderate and severe depression. No changes were noted in the control group.

Gerontological nurses should recommend and encourage aging women to engage in regular physical exercise, not only for physical health benefits but also to control the symptoms of depression and anxiety. This lifestyle practice could enhance the quality of life and reduce the need for medications.

PRACTICE REALITIES

Mrs. Jessup is a 75-year-old nursing home resident with Alzheimer's disease. Her husband visits frequently and seems caring. The nursing assistants report that on several occasions they have walked into Mrs. Jessup's room and witnessed her husband holding Mrs. Jessup's hand at his genital area. At times they have found him with his hand beneath her blanket, touching his wife in her genital region.

In addition to his behaviors with his wife, Mr. Jessup has developed a friendship with another resident who is mentally competent. The staff has noticed that when Mr. Jessup visits, this resident usually closes the door. Once, a nurse entered without knocking and found the pair together in bed.

How should the staff best handle this situation?

CRITICAL THINKING EXERCISES

1. What attitudes and actions of health care providers can have a negative effect on the sexuality of older adults? What can have a positive effect?

2. List the age-related changes that occur for men and women in the following sexual phases: excitement, plateau, orgasm, and resolution.

3. List at least six factors that can interfere with sexual function in late life.

RESOURCES

American Association of Sex Educators, Counselors, and Therapists
http://www.aasect.org

North American Menopause Society
http://www.menopause.org

Sexuality Information and Education Council of the United States
http://www.siecus.org

SAGE (Services and Advocacy for Gay, Lesbian, Bisexual, Transgender Elders)
http://www.sageusa.org/about/index.cfm

REFERENCES

Bianco, F. J., McHOne, B. R., Wagner, K., King, A., Burgess, J., Patierno, S. & Jarrett, T. W. (2009). Prevalence of erectile dysfunction in men screened for prostate cancer. *Journal of Urology*, 74(1):89–92.

Centers for Disease Control and Prevention. HIV Surveillance Report. (2011). Retrieved May 10, 2012 from http://www.cdc.gov/hiv/topics/surveillance/resources/reports/. Published February 2011

Endocrine Society, (2012). The Endocrine Society position statement on bioidentical hormones. Retrieved July 12, 2012 from http://www.menopause.org/bioidenticalHT_Endosoc.pdf

Feeley, R. J., Saad, F., Guay, A., & Traish, A. M. (2009). Testosterone in men's health: A new role for an old hormone. *Journal of Men's Health*, 6(3):169–176.

Geller, S. (2009). Improving the science for botanical and dietary supplements. *Alternative Therapies in Health and Medicine*, 15(1), 16–17.

Greenberg, S. A. (2001). Sexual health. In M. B. Mezey (Ed.), *The encyclopedia of elder care: The comprehensive resource on geriatric and social care* (pp. 589–592). New York: Springer Publishing Company.

Hyde, Z., Flicker, L., Hankey, G. J., Almeida, O. P., McCaul, K. A., Chubb, S. A., & Yeap, B. B. (2012). Prevalence and predictors of sexual problems in men aged 75–95 years: a population-based study. *Journal of Sexual Medicine*, 9(2):442–453.

Kinsey, A. (1948). *Sexual behavior in the human male*. Philadelphia, PA: Saunders.

Masters, W., & Johnson, V. (1966). *Human sexual response*. Boston, MA: Little Brown.

Masters, W., & Johnson, V. (1981). Sex and the aging process. *Journal of the American Geriatrics Society*, 9, 385.

Rosing, D., Klebingat, K. J., Berberich, H. J., Bosinski, H. A. G., Loewit, K., & Beier, K. M. (2009). Male sexual dysfunction. *Deutsches Arzteblatt International, 106*(50): 821–828.

Rossouw, J. E., Prentice, R. L., Manson, J. E., Wu, L., Barad, D., Barnabei, V. M., Stefanick, M. L., et al. (2007). Postmenopausal hormone therapy and risk of cardiovascular disease by age and years since menopause. *Journal of the American Medical Association, 297*(13), 1465–1477.

Rouse, K. (2012). Managing menopausal symptoms. *American Journal of Nursing, 112*(6), 28–35.

Sand, M., & Fisher, W. A. (2007). Women's endorsement of models of female sexual response: The nurses' sexuality study. *Journal of Sexual Medicine, 4*(3), 708–719.

RECOMMENDED READINGS

Recommended Readings associated with this chapter can be found on the web site that accompanies the book. Visit **http://thepoint.lww.com/Eliopoulos8e** to access the recommended readings and other additional resources associated with this chapter.

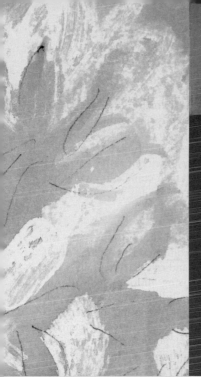

Spirituality

LEARNING OBJECTIVES

After reading this chapter, you should be able to:

1. Describe basic spiritual needs.

2. List questions that could be used for spiritual assessment.

3. Discuss measures to support spiritual needs.

TERMS TO KNOW

Religion: human-created structures, rituals, symbolism, and rules for relating to God/ higher power

Spiritual distress: a state in which one's relationship to God or other higher power is disrupted or at risk of being disrupted and/or spiritual needs cannot be fulfilled

Spirituality: relationship and feelings with that which transcends the physical world

Most people are comforted by the knowledge that they have a connection with a power that is greater than themselves. A positive, harmonious relationship with God or other higher power (the Divine) helps individuals to feel unified with other people, nature, and the environment. It offers them love and a sense of having value, despite their imperfections or errors. People derive joy, hope, peace, and purpose when they transcend beyond themselves. Suffering and hardship can have meaning and be faced with added strength.

Spirituality is the essence of our being that transcends and connects us to the Divine and other living organisms. It involves relationships and feelings. Spirituality differs from religion, which consists of human-created structures, rituals, symbolism, and rules for relating to the Divine. Religion is a significant expression of spirituality, but highly spiritual individuals may not identify with a specific religion.

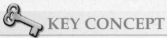

KEY CONCEPT

Spirituality and religion are not synonymous.

SPIRITUAL NEEDS

All humans have spiritual needs, regardless of whether they realize or acknowledge them. Some of these needs become particularly relevant in late life when the high prevalence of chronic illness and reality of death are evident; these needs can include love, purpose, hope, dignity, forgiveness, gratitude, transcendence, and faith.

Love

Love is probably the most important spiritual need of all. People need to feel that they are cared for and can offer caring feelings. Spiritual love is not quid pro quo in which it is offered to obtain something in return. Rather, spiritual love is unconditional—offered unselfishly, completely. In the Judeo-Christian tradition, this type of love is exemplified by the type God has for people. People need to feel loved regardless of their physical or mental condition, social position, material possessions, or productivity.

Meaning and Purpose

According to Erikson's description of the final developmental task (see Chapter 2), healthy psychological aging for the older adult involves achieving a sense of integrity. This integrity, or wholeness, is supported by the belief that life experiences—both good and bad—make sense and have served a purpose. Some individuals may believe, based on their faith, that suffering and sorrow have eternal purposes or allow God to be glorified. With this perspective, nothing is in vain and one's significance in the world is better understood.

Hope

Hope is the expectation for something in the future. For some people, hope consists of the anticipation that opportunities for new adventures, pleasures, and relationships will unfold with each tomorrow. For others, hope propels them to face the future in the presence of pain and suffering, because they believe relief and eternal reward are possible.

Dignity

In the Western society, self-worth is often judged by one's appearance, function, and productivity. Yet, every human being has intrinsic worth. When older people lack the attributes that command dignity for most of the secular society, they can derive a sense of value and worth through their connection with God or other higher power.

Forgiveness

It is human nature to err and sin. Carrying the burden of the wrongs committed by or to oneself is significantly stressful and can detrimentally affect health. Furthermore, being unforgiving can rob people of the love and fulfillment derived through relationships. Forgiving and accepting forgiveness is healing. For older adults, forgiveness can facilitate the important process of putting things in order and achieving closure to unfinished business.

Gratitude

The abundance that is so prevalent in the Western society sometimes causes much to be taken for granted. Rather than appreciating that they are not hungry or homeless, people may complain that they have not dined at certain restaurants or that their home lacks a pool. They focus on having undesirably large thighs rather than giving thanks for being able to walk. Instead of being appreciative that their children are healthy, they are distressed that they are not the parents of an honor roll student. It is easy to fall into the trap of focusing on the negatives. However, an attitude of thankfulness nourishes the spirit and strengthens the ability to cope with any situation. At a time when losses may be many, older individuals may benefit from a guided review of the positive aspects of their lives. The life review process is a good approach to use in this effort (see Chapter 4).

Transcendence

People need to feel that there is a reality beyond themselves, that they are connected to a greater power that surpasses logical thinking, and that they have a source that empowers them to achieve that which they cannot achieve independently. Transcendence affords people life beyond material existence and equips them to make sense of the difficult circumstances they face (Fig. 13-1).

Expression of Faith

Faith encompasses religious/spiritual beliefs and is expressed through religious/spiritual practices. These practices can include prayer, worship, scripture reading, rituals (e.g., fasting on certain days or

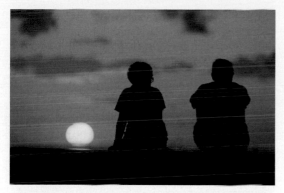

FIGURE 13-1 ■ By feeling a connection with a reality beyond their material existence, people can navigate the difficult circumstances they face.

wearing special articles of clothing), and celebration of specific holy days. Disruption in the ability to express one's faith because of illness or disability can lead to spiritual distress. Likewise, spiritual distress can arise during illness from a person feeling resentful that God has seemingly abandoned him, guilty that the illness may be a means of punishment for sin, or regretful that he lacks a strong faith to support him through the situation.

 POINT TO PONDER

Which spiritual need is most difficult for you to fulfill personally? Why?

ASSESSING SPIRITUAL NEEDS

Asking about spiritual matters as part of the initial and ongoing assessment fosters holistic care. Although various clinical settings have assessment tools preferred for use, elements that spiritual assessment should address include faith beliefs and practices; affiliation with a faith community; and the extent to which spiritual needs (e.g., love, meaning, purpose, hope, dignity, forgiveness, gratitude, transcendence, and expression of faith) are satisfied.

The nurse has several sources for gathering information about a person's spiritual needs. The person's response to spiritual/religious preference on routine admission forms can give some indication of the patient's spirituality and provide a lead for a discussion of other issues pertaining to spirituality. Visible cues, such as the wearing of a religious article or presence of religious symbols, Bible, Koran, and inspirational books, can provide insights useful in spiritual assessment. A person's comments (e.g., "All I can do now is pray" or "I can't understand why God would allow this to happen") may offer clues about spiritual needs. Depression, a flat affect, crying, and other observable signs can be a red flag for spiritual distress. In addition, the nurse can ask specific questions to explore spiritual needs. Assessment Guide 13-1 outlines questions the nurse can ask to assess a patient's spirituality.

ASSESSMENT GUIDE 13-1
SPIRITUAL NEEDS

INTERVIEW

As part of a holistic assessment, ask questions that directly address the person's spirituality and spiritual needs. Questions may include the following:

■ What is your faith or religion?

■ Are you involved with a church, temple, or faith community? What is it? Would you like to have them involved with your care?

■ Are there religious practices that are important to you? Are you able to practice them now? If not, is there a way I can assist you in practicing them?

■ Do you believe in God or a higher power? Could you please describe what that belief means to you?

■ Do you read the Bible or other religious text? Are you able to do this reading now?

■ What do you think God's role is in your illness and healing?

■ Is there anything about your faith or spiritual beliefs that is causing you distress, discomfort, or conflict?

■ What is most meaningful to you?

■ What gives your life purpose?

■ What is your source of strength or support?

■ From whom do you receive love?

■ Who are the most significant recipients of your love?

■ Do you feel like you have unfinished business? Things you need to say to someone? Forgiveness you wish to seek or offer?

■ What are your fears?

■ How can I (we) best support your spiritual beliefs and practices at this time?

ADDRESSING SPIRITUAL NEEDS

Evidence suggests that strong spiritual beliefs facilitate health and healing; therefore, it is therapeutically beneficial to support patients' spirituality and assist them in fulfilling spiritual needs. When assessment reveals specific spiritual needs or signs of spiritual distress (see Nursing Diagnosis Highlight), nurses can plan strategies to address these specific needs. In addition, nurses can use a variety of interventions to assist patients and support their spirituality; these interventions are discussed in the following sections.

Being Available

The closeness and trust that patients feel toward nurses facilitate their sharing of deep feelings with nurses more than with other members of the health care team. Nurses need to honor this trust and be available for patients to express their feelings. This means not only being physically available but also being fully present with patients without being distracted or thinking about other activities. There may

be times when nurses may not know how to respond to spiritual needs or hear expressions of beliefs that differ from their own; in these situations, attentive listening and encouraging communication remain important.

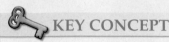

KEY CONCEPT

Being *present* with a patient implies that the nurse is not only physically with the individual but also offering undivided attention to facilitate a true connection.

Honoring Beliefs and Practices

A good spiritual assessment should reveal specific beliefs and practices that the nurse may need to facilitate. These practices can include the following special diets, refusing to participate in certain care activities on one's Sabbath, wearing of specific articles of clothing, and praying at specific times of the day. Box 13-1 outlines some common religious beliefs and practices nurses may encounter.

NURSING DIAGNOSIS HIGHLIGHT

SPIRITUAL DISTRESS

Overview

Spiritual distress is a state in which one's relationship to God or other higher power is disrupted or at risk of being disrupted and/or spiritual needs cannot be fulfilled. Illness or declining health of self or significant others, losses, awareness of mortality, and conflicts between beliefs and medical treatments are factors that could promote spiritual distress. Signs of spiritual distress could include anger, anxiety, complaints, crying, cynicism, depression, guilt, hopelessness, isolation, low self-esteem, powerlessness, refusal to make plans, sarcasm, suicidal thoughts or plans, and physical symptoms (fatigue, poor appetite, sleep disturbances, and sighing). The person may question his or her faith and beliefs.

Causative or contributing factors

Serious illness, losses, added burdens, inability to engage in religious practices, and association of current health problems with past sinful behavior or lack of faith.

Goal

The patient maintains religious practices to the maximum degree possible; discusses issues pertaining to spiritual distress; and develops support systems to promote spiritual well-being.

Interventions

- Assist the patient in identifying factors contributing to spiritual distress.
- Support the patient's religious practices: learn about the patient's religious practices and implications for care; provide Bible or other religious text, religious articles, and inspirational music; respect periods of solitude; respect and assist with practice of rituals; read scripture or arrange for a volunteer to do so.
- Pray with or for the patient if this does not violate the patient's or your own faith.
- Provide the patient with privacy and time for prayer, meditation, and solitude.
- Refer to clergy, native healer, support group, or other resources.
- Contact patient's church or temple for visitation and follow-up (e.g., via parish nurse); link the patient with community health ministry if the patient desires.
- Respect the patient's desire not to be visited by clergy or participate in religious activities.
- Do not challenge the patient's religious beliefs or attempt to change them.

BOX 13-1 | Religious Beliefs and Practices Relevant to Gerontological Nursing Practice

PROTESTANTISM

- *Assemblies of God (Pentecostal):* Encourage abstinence from tobacco, alcohol, and illegal drugs; believe in divine healing through prayer and laying on of hands; communion provided by clergy; believe in Jesus Christ as Savior; pray for God's intervention in healing
- *Baptist:* Encourage abstinence from alcohol; communion provided by clergy; Scripture reading important as Bible viewed as word of God; believe in Jesus Christ as Savior; may believe illness is God's will and respond passively to care; some believe in healing power of laying on of hands (more than two dozen different groups in United States)
- *Christian Church (Disciples of Christ):* Communion part of regular Sunday worship, provided by clergy; clergy and church elders can provide spiritual support; believe in Jesus Christ as Savior
- *Church of the Brethren:* Clergy provides anointing of sick for physical healing and spiritual well-being; communion provided by clergy
- *Church of the Nazarene:* Abstinence from tobacco and alcohol; believe in divine healing but accept medical treatment; communion provided by clergy
- *Episcopal (Anglican):* Fasting not required, although some Episcopalians may abstain from meat on Fridays; communion provided by clergy; anointing of sick may be offered although not required; believe in Jesus Christ as Savior
- *Lutheran:* Communion provided by clergy; anointing of sick by clergy; provide service of Commendation of the Dying; believe in Jesus Christ as Savior (10 different branches)
- *Mennonite:* Abstain from alcohol; prayer has important role during crisis or illness, as well as anointing with oil; may oppose medications; women may desire to wear head covering during hospitalization; simple and plain lifestyle and dress style; communion provided twice a year with foot washing part of ceremony (12 different groups)
- *Methodist:* Communion provided by clergy; anointing of sick; praying and reading Bible important during illness; organ donation encouraged; believe in Jesus Christ as Savior (more than 20 different groups)
- *Presbyterian:* Communion provided by clergy; clergy or elders can provide prayer for the dying; believe in Jesus Christ as Savior (10 different groups)
- *Quaker (Friends):* Believe God is personal and real and that any believer can achieve communion with Jesus Christ without the use of clergy or church rituals; no special death ceremony because of belief that present life is part of God's kingdom; abstain from alcohol; may oppose the use of medications
- *Salvation Army:* Follow Bible as foundation for faith; Scripture reading is important; no special ceremonies; offers social welfare programs and centers; open to medical treatment; officer of the local army can be called for visitation and assistance
- *Seventh-Day Adventist:* Healthy lifestyle practices are promoted as the body is seen as a temple of the Holy Spirit; alcohol, tobacco, coffee, tea, and recreational drugs are prohibited; pork and shellfish are avoided by most, and many are vegetarians; Sabbath is observed on Saturday; treatment may be opposed on Sabbath; communion provided by clergy; Bible reading important

ROMAN CATHOLICISM

Believe in Pope as head of the church on earth; express faith mainly in formulated creeds, such as Apostle's Creed; fasting during Lent and on Fridays optional, although older Catholics may adhere to practice; priest provides communion, Sacrament of the Sick, and hears confession; rosary beads, medals, statues, and other religious objects important.

EASTERN ORTHODOXY

Includes Greek, Serbian, Russian, and other orthodox churches; believe that Holy Spirit proceeds from Father (rather than Father and Son); therefore, reject the authority of Pope; fast from meat and dairy products on Wednesdays and Fridays during Lent and on other holy days; follow different calendar for religious celebrations; fast during Lent and before communion; holy unction administered to sick but not necessarily as last rites; last rites must be provided by ordained priest.

OTHER CHRISTIAN RELIGIONS

- *Christian Science:* Religion based on use of faith for healing; may decline drugs, psychotherapy, hypnotism, vaccination, and some treatments; use Christian Science nurses and other practitioners and may desire that they be active participants in care
- *Jehovah's Witnesses:* Discourage the use of alcohol and tobacco; blood transfusions not accepted, although alternative methods can be used

(Continues)

- *Mormons (Church of Jesus Christ of Latter Day Saints):* No professional clergy; communion and anointing of sick/laying on of hands can be provided by the member of church priesthood; abstain from alcohol; discourage the use of caffeine, alcohol, and other substances that are considered unhealthy and harmful; a sacred undergarment may be worn at all times that is only removed in absolute emergencies; prayer and reading sacred writings important; may oppose some medical treatments and use divine healing through laying on of hands
- *Unitarian:* Highly liberal branch of Christianity; belief in God as single being rather than doctrine of the Trinity; believe individuals are responsible for their own health state; advocate donation of body organs

JUDAISM

Believe in one universal God and that Jews were specially chosen to receive God's laws; observe Sabbath from sundown Friday to nightfall Saturday; three branches:

- *Orthodox (observant):* Strictly adhere to traditions of Judaism; believe in divinely inspired five Books of Moses (Torah); follow Kosher diet (not mixing of milk and meat at a meal, no pork or shellfish, no consumption of meat not slaughtered in accordance with Jewish law, use of separate cooking utensils for meat and milk products); strict restrictions during Sabbath (no riding in car, smoking, turning lights on/off, handling money, using telephone or television; medical treatments may be postponed until after Sabbath); men do not shave with razor but may use scissors or electric razor so that blade does not come in contact with skin, men wear skullcaps at all times; beard is considered sign of piety; Orthodox man will not touch any woman other than those in his family; married women cover their hair; family and friends visit and may remain with dying person; witness needs to be present when a person prays for health so that if death occurs family will be protected by God; after death body should not be left alone and only an Orthodox person should touch or wash the body; if death occurs on Sabbath, Orthodox persons cannot handle corpse but nursing staff can care for the body wearing gloves; body must be buried within 24 hours; autopsy not allowed; any removed body parts must be returned for burial with the remaining body as they believe all parts of the body need to be returned to earth; prayer and quiet time important

- *Conservative:* Follow same basic laws as Orthodox; may only cover heads during worship and prayer; some may approve of autopsy
- *Reform:* Less stringent adherence to laws; do not strictly follow Kosher diet; do not wear skullcaps; attend temples on Fridays for worship but do not follow restrictions during Sabbath; men can touch women

ISLAM (MUSLIM)

Second largest monotheistic (belief in one God) religion; founded by prophet Mohammed who was a human messenger or prophet used by God to communicate His word; Koran is a scripture; Koran cannot be touched by anyone ritually unclean and nothing should be placed on Koran; may pray five times a day facing Mecca; privacy during prayer is important; abstain from pork and alcohol; all permissible meat must be blessed and killed in a special way; cleanliness important; at prayer time, washing is required, even by the sick; accept medical practices if these do not violate religious practices; women are very modest and not allowed to sign consent or make decisions without husband; may wear a *taviz* (black string with words of Koran attached); family or any practicing Muslim can pray with dying person; prefer for family to wash and prepare body of deceased (if necessary, nurses can care for the deceased body wearing gloves); autopsy prohibited except when legally mandated; organ donation not allowed.

HINDUISM

This is considered one of the world's oldest religion; religion of most of India's residents; no scriptures, fixed doctrine, or common worship; belief in karma (every person born into position based on deeds of previous life) and reincarnation; illness may be viewed as a result of sin from past life; mostly vegetarian; abstain from alcohol and tobacco.

BUDDHISM

Offshoot of Hinduism with most followers in Japan, Thailand, and Myanmar; believe enlightenment found in individual meditation rather than communal worship; follow moral code known as Eightfold Path that leads to nirvana (form of liberation and enlightenment); vegetarian; abstain from alcohol and tobacco; may oppose medications and refuse treatments on holy days; private, uninterrupted time for meditation important.

Providing Opportunities for Solitude

Solitude can be an important aspect of the expression of spirituality. Uninterrupted time allows personal communication with one's god or other higher power. One can offer prayers, reflect, meditate, and listen for answers from the divine source (Box 13-2). Nurses must respect and protect periods of solitude for their patients.

POINT TO PONDER

Choosing solitude differs from being socially isolated. How much time do you build into your typical week for private time or solitude?

Promoting Hope

Hope is important to human beings. When people believe in the future and believe that something positive is possible, they are likely to commit to goals and actions. For older adults, especially those with serious health conditions or disabilities, maintaining hope can be challenging. The risk of feeling hopeless and depressed is real. Hopelessness can interfere with self-care and healing and drain energies that are needed to face life's challenges.

Promoting hope begins with establishing a trusting relationship with the patient so that he or she will be comfortable in expressing feelings openly. A careful assessment can assist in identifying factors that contribute to hopelessness, such as strained family relationships, unrelieved pain, and growing financial problems; interventions should be planned to address specific factors. Other beneficial actions include the following:

- assisting the patient in developing realistic short-term goals and acknowledging the achievement of goals
- guiding the patient in life review to highlight past successes in meeting life challenges that can be linked to current situations
- helping the patient to find pleasure and enjoyment in current life activities
- encouraging a relaxing, uplifting environment (e.g., flowers, fresh air, sunlight, pleasant scents, pets, and stimulating colors)
- facilitating the patient's spiritual practices; referring to clergy as needed
- assisting the patient in participating in religious services
- developing affirmations (positive statements, such as "I am a unique and special individual" or "I am loved by God") for the patient to use and recommending they be repeated daily
- suggesting that the patient maintain a personal journal to promote self-understanding and personal growth
- using music therapeutically; consulting with the music therapist for selections that promote optimism and hope
- referring to a support group
- using humor therapeutically; conveying hope and optimism

Assisting in Discovering Meaning in Challenging Situations

Patients may question the purpose of the difficulties they face or believe that God has abandoned them. Persons of faith may want to discuss their perspective on how their current situation fits into a larger plan. An open, nonjudgmental attitude when encouraging the expression of feelings can prove useful.

BOX 13-2   Meditation

Solitude provides an opportunity for meditation, an activity that calms the mind and assists in focusing thoughts to the present. It can take the form of:

- *concentrative meditation*—attention is focused on breathing, a sound, or an image; this calms and promotes mental clarity and acuity
- *mindfulness meditation*—attention is paid to sensations being experienced, such as sounds or thoughts; this promotes a calm, nonreactive mental state

- *transcendental meditation*—introduced by Maharishi Mahesh Yogi, this form involves guiding the body to a level of profound relaxation while the mind becomes more alert

Meditation has many health benefits, including stress reduction, stimulation of immune function, and pain control. Older adults may benefit from the improved self-esteem and higher levels of mental function that are allegedly achieved.

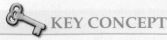

KEY CONCEPT

Some people's faith can enable them to be comforted in believing that their current challenges serve a positive purpose for God.

Facilitating Religious Practices

Patients may have a desire for communion, confession, and other religious sacraments. Nurses may contact clergy as needed. Nurses can also assist patients in wearing or displaying religious articles and ensure the safe care of these articles during nursing activities.

Praying with and for

People of faith have long understood the value of prayer, and now growing research evidence supports the positive relationship between prayer and health and healing (Butler, Koenig, Puchalski, Cohen, & Sloan, 2003; Duffin, 2007; Larson, Sawyers, & McCullough, 1998; Moberg, 2005). One need not be an ordained clergy to hold a patient's hand and offer a prayer. Prayers can be specific, for example, that the medication just administered will relieve the pain soon. The use of flowery or "religious"

vocabulary is less important than having the heart to ask a higher power to intervene on the patient's behalf. Intercessory prayers can be offered for patients. Nurses who are not comfortable in offering prayers themselves can ask the coworkers to pray with and for their patients who so desire.

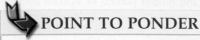

POINT TO PONDER

What would it mean to you to have someone pray for your needs or struggles?

SUMMARY: THE IMPORTANCE OF SPIRITUAL CARE

People are spiritual beings; therefore, spiritual care must be an integral component of comprehensive, holistic care. Realizing their connection to something greater than themselves—other people, nature, the universe, and a supreme being—empowers older persons to rise above their physical, intellectual, emotional, and social challenges and discover the peace and harmony that facilitates healing and well-being. Self-worth and hope can be achieved, thereby imprinting the last segment of life with integrity and joy.

BRINGING RESEARCH TO LIFE

FAITH COMMUNITY NURSES: IMPLEMENTING HEALTHY PEOPLE STANDARDS TO PROMOTE THE HEALTH OF ELDERLY CLIENTS

King, M. A., & Pappas-Roqich, M. (2011). Geriatric Nursing, 32(6), 459–464.

This study sought to determine if the faith community (parish) nurse model of practice supports the implementation of strategies that address standards contained in *Healthy People 2010*. Parish nurses were recruited to complete a questionnaire that incorporated the standards and indicators of the Healthy People 2010 Critical Health Indicators.

The study reported that faith community nurses did engage in many activities that implemented the Healthy People 2010 Critical Health Indicators. They provided services at least weekly that supported two indicators of daily physical activity and emotional health. Indicators of promoting good nutrition and healthy weight were addressed at least monthly, and at least on an annual basis the nurses provided programs related to reducing and eliminating tobacco use, reducing or eliminating substance abuse, promoting safety and reducing violence, promoting healthy environments, and encouraging immunizations—which represented 5 of the 10 indicators. The faith community nurses engaged in activities to help clients to access quality health care at least monthly. Most nurses in this survey reported that they never facilitated support groups or provided services promoting responsible sexual behavior.

The study showed that the faith community nurses serve an important role in identifying the needed services and arranging for their delivery and for helping older adults to use health services more seamlessly and efficiently. This role demonstrates how gerontological nurses can impact the lives of older adults in many nontraditional roles.

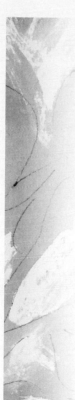

PRACTICE REALITIES

Sixty-eight-year-old Mr. Brewer has been in the shock trauma unit of the hospital for a critical condition for several weeks following a serious automobile accident. At admission, his family stated that Mr. Brewer was an atheist.

Mr. Brewer slips in and out of periods of consciousness. On several occasions during his conscious states, he has talked about God and made comments such as, "I hope God forgives me for rejecting him so many years" and "I don't want to die without getting right with God."

The nurse who regularly cares for Mr. Brewer mentions this to Mrs. Brewer, who is also an atheist, and asks if she thinks it would be useful to have a member of the hospital's clergy staff talk with her husband. Mrs. Brewer strongly objects, stating "I don't know who has been putting these crazy ideas in his head and I surely am not going to allow some religious nut to take advantage of my husband." When Mr. Brewer speaks of God in his wife's presence she says, "Tom, you've always been too intelligent for that crutch, so stop talking foolishly."

There is a strong likelihood that Mr. Brewer is not going to survive. What should the nurse do?

CRITICAL THINKING EXERCISES

1. Why may spirituality become increasingly important to people as they age?
2. Describe the ways in which spiritual needs can be difficult for older adults to meet.
3. What questions could you ask an older adult to assess his or her spiritual beliefs and needs?
4. Consider the older adult who is a patient in a hospital or a resident of a long-term care facility. What opportunities exist for that person to have periods of solitude? What could you do to facilitate periods of solitude?
5. How can the mystery inherent in life events foster spirituality?

RESOURCES

BeliefNet
http://www.beliefnet.com

Duke Center for Spirituality, Theology, and Health
http://www.dukespiritualityandhealth.org

George Washington Institute for Spirituality and Health
http://www.gwish.org

Health Ministries Association
http://www.hmassoc.org

Nurses Christian Fellowship International
http://www.ncfi.org

REFERENCES

Butler, S. M., Koenig, H. G., Puchalski, C., Cohen, C., & Sloan, R. (2003). Is Prayer Good for Your Health? A Critique of the Scientific Research. *Heritage Lecture #816,* December 22, 2003. Accessed January 2, 2008 from http://www.heritage.org/Research/Religion/HL816.cfm

Duffin, J. (2007). The doctor was surprised; or, how to diagnose a miracle. *Bulletin of the History of Medicine, 81*(4), 699–729.

Larson, D. B., Sawyers, J. P., & McCullough, M. E. (Eds.). (1998). *Scientific research on spirituality and health: A consensus report.* Rockville, MD: National Institute for Healthcare Research.

Moberg, D. O. (2005). Research in spirituality, religion and aging. *Journal of Gerontological Social Work, 45*(1–2), 11–40.

RECOMMENDED READINGS

Recommended Readings associated with this chapter can be found on the web site that accompanies the book. Visit **http://thepoint.lww.com/Eliopoulos8e** to access the recommended readings and other additional resources associated with this chapter.

UNIT 4

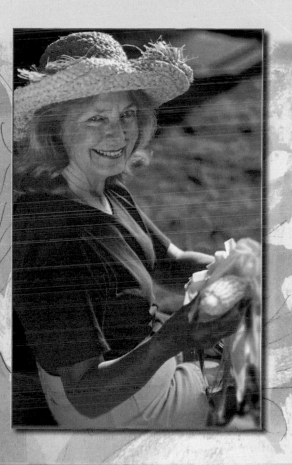

General Care
Concerns

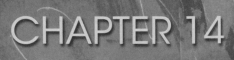

Nutrition and Hydration

CHAPTER OUTLINE

LEARNING OBJECTIVES

After reading this chapter, you should be able to:

1. List age-related factors that affect dietary requirements in late life.
2. Identify risks associated with the use of nutritional supplements.
3. List the special nutritional needs of aging women.
4. Describe age-related changes affecting hydration in older adults.
5. Identify causative factors and signs of dehydration.
6. Describe oral health problems that could influence nutritional status and recommended oral hygiene for older adults.
7. Outline threats to good nutrition in late life and ways to minimize them.

TERMS TO KNOW

Anorexia: loss of appetite

Dysphagia: difficulty swallowing due to difficulty moving food from the mouth to the esophagus (transfer dysphagia), down the esophagus (transport dysphagia), or from the esophagus into the stomach (delivery dysphagia)

Nutrition has a profound impact on health and functional capacity. Nutritional status influences one's ability to defend the body against disease, maintain anatomic and structural normality, think clearly, and possess the energy and desire to engage in social activity. Numerous age-related changes, which are often subtle and gradual, can progressively jeopardize the ability of older persons to maintain good nutritional status; these changes demand special nursing attention (Nursing Diagnosis Table 14-1).

NUTRITIONAL NEEDS OF OLDER ADULTS

Quantity and Quality of Caloric Needs

Although the body's needs for basic nutrients are consistent throughout life, the required amount of specific nutrients may vary. One of the most significant differences in nutrient requirements among people of different ages involves caloric intake. Several factors contribute to the older person's reduced need for calories:

- The older body has less lean body mass and a relative increase in adipose tissue. Adipose tissue metabolizes more slowly than lean tissue and does not burn calories as quickly.
- Basal metabolic rate declines 2% for each decade of life, which contributes to weight

increase when the same caloric intake of younger years is consumed.

- The activity level for most older adults is usually lower than that during their younger years.

Although each person has a unique caloric need based on individual body size, metabolism, health status, and activity level, some generalizations can be made. Caloric needs gradually decrease throughout adulthood as a result of age-related changes, and a reduction in calories is recommended beginning in the fourth decade of life. Quantity and quality of caloric intake must be monitored. One useful way to determine resting caloric needs that considers age and basal metabolic rate, among other factors, is the Harris-Benedict equation, also called the resting energy expenditure. With this equation, the resulting number that is obtained represents the number of calories that need to be consumed daily to maintain current body weight with no exercise expenditure.

NURSING DIAGNOSIS

TABLE 14-1	Aging and Risks to Nutritional Status

Causes or Contributing Factors	Nursing Diagnosis
Teeth have various degrees of erosion; abrasions of crown and root structure; high prevalence of tooth loss	Imbalanced Nutrition: Less Than Body Requirements related to limited ability to chew foods Acute Pain related to poor condition of teeth
Reduction in saliva to approximately one third the volume of earlier years	Imbalanced Nutrition: Less Than Body Requirements related to less efficient mixing of foods
Inefficient digestion of starch due to decreased salivary ptyalin	Imbalanced Nutrition: Less Than Body Requirements related to reduced breakdown of starches
Atrophy of epithelial covering in oral mucosa	Impaired Oral Mucous Membrane
Increased taste threshold; approximately one third the number of functioning taste buds per papilla of earlier years	Imbalanced Nutrition: More Than Body Requirements related to excessive intake of salts and sweets to compensate for taste alterations
Decreased thirst sensations; reduced hunger contractions	Imbalanced Nutrition: Less Than Body Requirements related to reduced ability to sense hunger sensations Deficient Fluid Volume related to decreased thirst
Weaker gag reflex; decreased esophageal peristalsis; relaxation of lower esophageal sphincter, reduced stomach motility	Risk of Injury from aspiration Imbalanced Nutrition: Less Than Body Requirements related to self-imposed restrictions to avoid discomfort
Less hydrochloric acid, pepsin, and pancreatic acid produced	Imbalanced Nutrition: Less Than Body Requirements related to ineffective breakdown of food
Lower fat tolerance	Acute Pain related to indigestion
Decreased colonic peristalsis: reduced sensation for signal to defecate	Imbalanced Nutrition: Less Than Body Requirements related to reduced appetite and self-imposed restrictions related to constipation
Less efficient cholesterol stabilization and absorption	Risk of Infection related to risk of gallstone formation
Increased fat content of pancreas; decreased pancreatic enzymes	Imbalanced Nutrition: Less Than Body Requirements related to problems in normal digestion

Weight in kilogram/height in centimeters:

> Males: 66 + [13.7 × weight (kg)] + [5 × height (cm)] – (6.76 × age in years)
> Females: 655 + [9.6 × weight (kg)] + [1.8 × height (cm)] – (4.7 × age in years)

Weight in pounds/height in inches:

> Males: 66 + [6.23 × weight (lbs)] + [12.7 × height (inches)] – (6.76 × age in years)
> Females: 655 + [4.35 × (lbs)] + [4.7 × height (inches)] – (4.7 × age in years)

In addition to monitoring quantity, it is important to monitor the quality of calories consumed. Because caloric requirements and intake are often reduced in later life, the ingested calories need to be of higher quality to ensure an adequate intake of other nutrients (Fig. 14-1). Limiting dietary fat intake to less than 30% of total calories consumed is a good practice for older adults. Table 14-2 lists the recommended daily allowances (RDAs) for older adults.

Fiber is particularly important in the older adult's diet. Soluble fibers, found in foods such as oats and pectin, help to lower serum cholesterol; improve glucose tolerance in diabetics; and prevent obesity, cardiovascular disease, and colorectal cancer (Dahm et al., 2010; Du et al., 2010; Hopping et al., 2010). Insoluble fibers promote good bowel activity and can be found in grains and many vegetables and fruits.

Carbohydrates provide important sources of energy and fiber. However, because of a decreased ability to maintain a regular blood glucose level, older adults need a reduced carbohydrate intake. A high-carbohydrate diet can stimulate an abnormally high release of insulin in older adults. This can cause hypoglycemia, which can first present in older adults as a confused state.

At least 1 g protein per kilogram of body weight is necessary to renew body protein and protoplasm and to maintain enzyme systems. If 10% to 20% of

	Men	Women
Protein (g)	66	66
Carbohydrates (g)	100	100
Vitamin A (mg)	625	500
Vitamin D (mg)	10	10
Vitamin E (IU)	12	12
Vitamin C (mg)	75	60
Thiamin (mg)	1.0	0.9
Riboflavin (mg)	1.1	0.9
Niacin (mg)	12	11
Vitamin B$_6$ (mg)	1.4	1.3
Folate (mg)	320	320
Vitamin B$_{12}$ (mg)	2	2
Calcium (mg)	1,000^a	1,000
Phosphorus (mg)	580	580
Magnesium (mg)	350	265
Iron (mg)	6	5
Zinc (mg)	9.4	6.8
Iodine (mg)	95	95

TABLE 14-2 Recommended Dietary Allowances for People Over 50 Years of Age

^{a}Requirement for males 51–70 years is 800 mg.
Reprinted with permission from *Dietary Reference Intakes (DRIs). Estimated Average Requirements,* Food and Nutrition Board, Institute of Medicine, 2011, by the National Academy of Sciences, Courtesy of the National Academies Press, Washington, D.C.

daily caloric intake is derived from protein, protein requirements should be met. Several protein supplements are available commercially and may be useful additives to the older person's diet.

Although the ability to absorb calcium decreases with age, calcium is still required in the diet to maintain a healthy musculoskeletal system, as well as to promote the proper functioning of the body's blood clotting mechanisms. Older adults may benefit from calcium supplements, but they should discuss their use with their physicians to ensure that other medical problems do not contraindicate them. In addition, caution is needed to avoid excess calcium consumption (see discussion under *Nutritional Supplements*). A good intake of vitamin D and magnesium facilitates calcium absorption.

It is recommended that older adults eat at least five servings of fruits and vegetables daily. Unfortunately, only about one third of older adults consume the recommended amounts (Baker, 2007). The nurse can discuss with older adults the importance of consuming adequate fruits and vegetables and make suggestions on the variety of ways that they can be consumed (e.g., in smoothies or mixed in yogurt or gelatin).

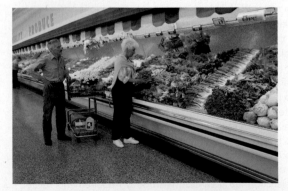

FIGURE 14-1 ■ Although they usually need to ingest fewer calories than younger persons, older adults' diets must include a high quality of nutrients.

MyPlate for Older Adults

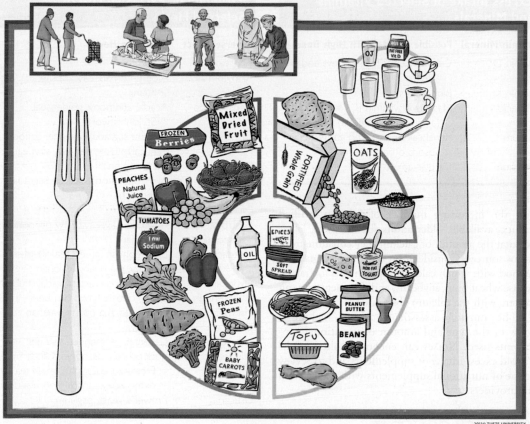

2011© TUFTS UNIVERSITY

FIGURE 14-2 ■ Modified MyPlate for Older Adults. (Available at http://www.nutrition.tufts.edu/research/myplate-older-adults)

Researchers at the U.S. Department of Agriculture (USDA) Human Nutrition Research Center on Aging (HNRCA) at Tufts University have offered a modification to the USDA's MyPlate to more accurately reflect the dietary needs of persons over age 70 years (Fig. 14-2; Tufts, 2012). This replaces the Modified MyPyramid for Older Adults and provides examples of foods that are consistent with the federal government's 2010 Dietary Guidelines for Americans. These guidelines limit foods high in trans and saturated fats, salt, and added sugars. They emphasize whole grains and foods with high levels of vitamins and minerals per serving.

POINT TO PONDER

How do you see your diet affecting your body, mind, and spirit and vice versa? Are there patterns that need to be changed, and, if so, how?

Nutritional Supplements

Today, more than half of all adults take nutritional supplements on a daily basis. Vitamin and mineral requirements for older adults are undetermined and, presently, the RDAs for the general adult population need to be applied to the older age group. Although not a panacea, nutritional supplements can compensate for inadequate intake of nutrients and deficiencies resulting from diseases and medication effects. Niacin, riboflavin, thiamine, and vitamins B_6, C, and D are the most common nutrients found to be deficient in older adults. However, caution is needed because vitamins, minerals, and herbs, particularly in high doses, can produce adverse effects (Tables 14-3 and 14-4) and interact with many medications (Table 14-5).

For example, excess calcium consumption (i.e., in excess of 2,000 mg/day) can lead to problems such as kidney stones. If calcium supplements are used, no more than 500 mg should be taken at any one time because larger amounts are not absorbed as well.

TABLE 14-3 Risks Associated With Excess Intake of Selected Vitamins and Minerals

Vitamin/Mineral	Possible Effects With High Doses
Vitamin D	Calcium deposits in kidneys and arteries
Vitamin K	Blood clots
Folic acid	Masking of vitamin B$_{12}$ deficiency (a cause of dementia)
Calcium	Renal calculi; impaired ability to absorb other minerals
Potassium	Cardiac arrest

With the increasing number of calcium-fortified products available, older adults should check labels and total the amount of calcium they consume from various sources. Consideration must also be given to the food with which calcium supplements are taken, because wheat bran, soybeans, and other legumes can interfere with the calcium absorption.

The nursing assessment should include a review of the type and amount of nutritional supplements used. Nurses can encourage older adults to avoid excess intake of supplements and to review the use of nutritional supplements with their health care providers.

KEY CONCEPT

Vitamin, mineral, and herbal supplements can be beneficial, but caution is needed to avoid adverse consequences from their misuse.

Special Needs of Women

Heart disease, cancer, and osteoporosis are among the nutrition-related conditions to which older women

TABLE 14-4 Adverse Effects of Extended or Excessive Use of Selected Herbs

Adverse Effect	Causative Herbs
Anorexia	Green tea
Arrhythmias	Aloe (internal), cascara sagrada, ma huang
Constipation	Acacia, agrimony, goldenseal, St. John's wort
Diarrhea	Cascara sagrada, cayenne, daffodil, eucalyptus, green tea, soybean
Eczema	Garlic, onion
Edema	Aloe, buckthorn, cascara sagrada, rhubarb
Fever	Echinacea
Gastrointestinal discomfort	Cayenne, kavakava, saw palmetto, valerian
Headache	Black cohosh, green tea, lily-of-the-valley, ma huang, valerian
Hypokalemia	Buckthorn, cascara sagrada, rhubarb
Hypotension	Black cohosh, hawthorn berry
Insomnia	Green tea, ma huang, valerian
Jaundice	Kavakava
Liver damage	Cayenne, germander, uva-ursi
Nausea/vomiting	Black cohosh, celandine, daffodil, Echinacea, eucalyptus, green tea, lily-of-the-valley, sandalwood, uva-ursi
Urticaria	Brewer's yeast, psyllium
Vertigo	Green tea

are susceptible. Attention to dietary requirements and reduction of diet-related risks can reduce some of these problems.

From 64 to 74 years of age, the rate of heart disease among women equals that of men. The reduction of fat intake to 30% kcal or less (70 g in an

TABLE 14-5 Herb–Drug Interactions

Herb	Drug	Effect of Interaction
Aloe barbadensis	Cardiac glycosides	Increased effects of drug
	Corticosteroids	Increased potassium loss
	Thiazide diuretics	Increased potassium loss
Cascara sagrada	Thiazide diuretics	Increased potassium loss
Feverfew	Salicylates	Increased antithrombotic effect
	Warfarin sodium	Increased antithrombotic effect
Ginkgo biloba	Antithrombotic drugs	Increased antithrombotic effect
Kavakava	Central nervous system depressants	Increased sedation
White willow	Salicylates	Increased antithrombotic effect

1,800-cal diet) can be beneficial in reducing the risk of heart disease in older women. Research is attempting to disclose the role of low-fat intake in reduced risk of breast cancer, which could support another benefit to limiting fat intake. Alcohol consumption also has a role in breast cancer; the daily intake of 40 g or more of alcohol has been linked to an increased risk of breast cancer (40 g of alcohol equals 30 oz of beer or 3 oz of 100-proof whiskey). Thus, reducing alcohol intake is advisable.

Nearly all women are affected by some degree of osteoporosis by the time they reach their seventh decade of life. The risk of bone loss is increased by estrogen reduction, obesity, inactivity, smoking, and the excessive consumption of caffeine and alcohol. The risk of fracture from brittle bones and the complications that follow warrant consideration to prevent bone loss by controlling risks. Postmenopausal women should have a daily calcium intake of at least 1,000 mg. Calcium from carbonate and citrate is the most common form of calcium supplement. Calcium carbonate, the most cost-effective form, should be taken with a meal at doses of not more than 500 mg at one time to ensure optimal absorption (Straub, 2007).

HYDRATION NEEDS OF OLDER ADULTS

With age, intracellular fluid is lost, resulting in decreased total body fluids. Whereas water comprises approximately 60% of body weight in younger adults, it constitutes 50% or less of body weight in older adults. This reduces the margin of safety for any fluid loss; a reduced fluid intake or increased loss that would be only a minor problem in a younger person could be life-threatening to an older person. The Institute of Medicine recommends fluid intake for men over the age of 50 years of 3.7 L/day and for women of the same age group 2.7 L/day (equivalent to 11 to 15 glasses containing 8 oz). Some health conditions may require less fluid intake. Nurses should evaluate older adults for factors that can cause them to consume less fluid, such as:

- age-related reductions in thirst sensations
- fear of incontinence (physical condition and lack of toileting opportunities)
- lack of accessible fluids
- inability to obtain or drink fluids independently
- lack of motivation
- altered mood or cognition
- nausea, vomiting, and gastrointestinal distress

When such factors are present or there is any suspicion regarding the adequacy of fluid intake, fluid intake and output should be recorded and monitored (see Nursing Diagnosis Highlight: Deficient Fluid Volume).

NURSING DIAGNOSIS HIGHLIGHT

DEFICIENT FLUID VOLUME

Overview

Deficient fluid volume refers to a state of dehydration in which intracellular, extracellular, or vascular fluid is less than that required by the body. This condition can be indicated by increased output, reduced intake, concentrated urine, weight loss, hypotension, increased pulse, poorer skin turgor, dry skin and mucous membranes, increased body temperature, weakness, and elevated serum creatinine, blood urea nitrogen, and hematocrit.

Causative or contributing factors

Vomiting, diarrhea, polyuria, excessive drainage, profuse perspiration, increased metabolic rate, insufficient intake due to physical or mental limitation, inaccessible fluids, medications (e.g., diuretics, laxatives, sedatives).

Goal

The patient possesses an intake and output balance within 200 mL and has cause of problem identified and corrected.

Interventions

- Perform a comprehensive assessment to identify underlying cause of fluid volume deficit; obtain treatment for underlying cause as appropriate.
- Maintain a strict record of intake and output.
- Closely monitor vital signs, urine specific gravity, skin turgor, mental status.
- Monitor patient's weight daily until problem is corrected.
- Encourage fluids, at least 3.7 L/day for men and 2.7 L/day for women during a 24-hour period unless contraindicated; offer foods that are high in fluid content (e.g., gelatin, sherbets, soup); keep fluids easily accessible.
- Consult with physician regarding need for intravenous fluid replacement; if prescribed, monitor carefully because of high risk of overhydration in elderly persons.
- Assist with or provide good oral hygiene.
- Identify persons at high risk for dehydration and closely monitor their intake and output.

Fluid restriction not only predisposes older adults to infection, constipation, and decreased bladder distensibility but also can lead to serious fluid and electrolyte imbalances. Dehydration, a life-threatening condition to older persons because of their already reduced amount of body fluid, is demonstrated by dry, inelastic skin; dry, brown tongue; sunken cheeks; concentrated urine; blood urea value elevated above 60 mg/dL; and, in some cases, confusion.

At the other extreme, older adults are also more sensitive to overhydration caused by decreased cardiovascular and renal function. Overhydration is a consideration if intravenous fluids are needed therapeutically.

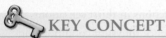

KEY CONCEPT

The age-related decline in body fluids reduces the margin of safety when insufficient fluid is consumed or extra fluid is lost.

PROMOTION OF ORAL HEALTH

Pain-free, intact gums and teeth will promote the ingestion of a wider variety of food. The ability to meet nutritional requirements in old age is influenced by basic dental care throughout one's lifetime. Poor dental care, environmental influences, inappropriate nutrition, and changes in gingival tissue commonly contribute to severe tooth loss in older persons. After the third decade of life, periodontal disease becomes the first cause of tooth loss; by 70 years of age, most people lose all their teeth. Growing numbers of aging adults are preserving their teeth as they grow older; however, without attention to the prevention of periodontal disease, they, too, could face their senior years without their natural teeth. In addition to teaching methods to prevent periodontal disease, nurses must ensure that older adults and their caregivers understand the signs of this condition so that they can seek help in a timely manner. Signs of periodontal disease include:

■ bleeding gums, particularly when teeth are brushed
■ red, swollen, painful gums
■ pus at gum line when pressure is exerted
■ chronic bad breath
■ loosening of teeth from gum line

The use of a toothbrush is more effective than swabs or other soft devices in improving gingival tissues and removing soft debris from the teeth. Lemon-glycerin swabs dry the oral mucosa and contribute to tooth enamel erosion. Mouthwashes with high alcohol content can be too harsh for older mouths; diluting a commercial mouthwash with water (half and half) is recommended. Care should be taken not to traumatize the tissues when performing oral hygiene because they are more sensitive, fragile, and prone to irritation in older adults. Loose teeth should be extracted to prevent them from being aspirated and causing a lung abscess.

Obviously, a lifetime of poor dental care cannot be reversed. Geriatric dental problems need to be prevented early in a person's life. Although the specialty of geriatric dentistry has grown, many persons do not have access to this service or the financial means to avail themselves of this care. Through education, nurses can make the public aware of the importance of good, regular dental care and oral hygiene at all ages and inform patients that aging alone does not necessitate the loss of teeth.

Many older adults believe that having dentures eliminates the need for dental care. Nurses must correct this misconception and encourage continued dental care for the individual with dentures. Lesions, infections, and other diseases can be detected by the dentist and corrected to prevent serious complications from developing. Changes in tissue structure may affect the fit of the dental appliances, which then require readjustment. Poorly fitting dentures need not always be replaced; sometimes they can be lined to ensure a proper fit. Nurses can explain this to older adults, who may resist correction because of concern for the expense involved. Most importantly, dental appliances should be used and not kept in a pocket or dresser drawer! Wearing dental appliances allows proper chewing, encouraging older people to introduce a wider variety of foods into their diets.

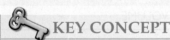

KEY CONCEPT

Dental problems can affect virtually every system of the body; therefore, they must be identified and corrected promptly.

THREATS TO GOOD NUTRITION

Indigestion and Food Intolerance

Indigestion and food intolerance are common among older people because of decreased stomach motility, less gastric secretion, and a slower gastric emptying time. Older persons frequently attempt to manage these problems by using antacids or limiting food intake, but both strategies potentially predispose them to other risks. Other means for managing these problems should be explored. For example, the nurse can suggest eating several small meals rather than three large ones. This not only provides a smaller amount of food to be digested at one time but also helps to maintain a more stable blood glucose level throughout the day. Avoiding or limiting fried foods may be helpful, since it is easier to digest broiled, boiled, or baked food. When food intolerance exists, the person can eliminate specific foods from the diet. Often, older adults need help identifying problem foods, particularly if they have included those foods in their diets throughout their entire lives. Sitting in a high Fowler position while eating and for 30 minutes after meals is helpful as it increases the size of the abdominal and thoracic cavities, provides more room for the stomach, and facilitates swallowing and digestion. Finally, ensuring adequate fluid intake and activity promotes the motility of food through the digestive tract.

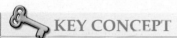

KEY CONCEPT

Self-imposed dietary restrictions and misuse of antacids to manage indigestion can create a new set of problems for older adults.

Anorexia

Anorexia can be related to a variety of conditions, including medication side effects, inactivity, physical illness, or age-related changes, such as decreased taste and smell sensations, reduced production of the hormone leptin, and gastric changes that cause satiation with smaller volumes of food intake. In the older adults particularly, losses and stresses (e.g., death of loved ones, loneliness, financial worries, and living with effects of chronic conditions) could cause anxiety and depression that could affect appetite.

The initial step in managing this problem is to identify its cause. Depending on the cause, treatment could consist of a high-calorie diet, referral to social programs, tube feeding, hyperalimentation, psychiatric therapy, or medications. Some stimulation to the appetite can be achieved through the use of certain herbs, such as ginger root, ginseng, gotu kola, and peppermint. Intake, output, and weight should be monitored; weight loss greater than 5% within a 1-month period and 10% within a 6-month period is considered significant and requires evaluation.

Dysphagia

The incidence of dysphagia increases with age and can take several forms, such as difficulty moving food from the mouth to the esophagus (transfer dysphagia), down the esophagus (transport dysphagia), or from the esophagus into the stomach (delivery dysphagia). Neurologic conditions, such as a stroke, can cause dysphagia, although most cases result from gastroesophageal reflux disease.

A careful assessment that identifies specific swallowing problems is useful in planning the best interventions for the person experiencing dysphagia. Factors to consider include onset, types of foods that present the most problem (solids or liquids), consistent or periodic occurrence, and other symptoms and related complications (e.g., aspiration or weight loss). A referral to a speech pathologist is beneficial in evaluating the problem and developing an individualized care plan.

Although specific interventions will be used to address an individual's needs, some general measures prove useful for all persons with dysphagia, such as having the person sit upright whenever food or fluid is being consumed; allowing sufficient time for eating; ensuring there is no residual food in the mouth before feeding additional food; placing small portions in the mouth; discouraging the person from talking while eating; keeping a suction machine readily available; and monitoring intake, output, and weight. Often, thickened liquids or mechanically altered foods may prove beneficial. Tilting the head to a side and placing food on a particular part of the tongue may be recommended, as may correction of an underlying problem, such as obesity or removal of a structural obstruction.

Constipation

Constipation is a common problem among older persons because of slower peristalsis, inactivity, side effects of drugs, and a tendency toward less fiber and fluid in the diet. If food intake is reduced to relieve discomfort, nutritional status can be threatened. Laxatives, another relief measure, can result in diarrhea, leading to dehydration; if oil-based laxatives are used, fat-soluble vitamins (e.g., A, D, K, and F) can be drained from the body, leading to vitamin deficiencies.

Nurses must recognize constipation as a frequent problem for older adults and encourage preventive measures. Plenty of fluids, fruits, vegetables, and activity is advisable, as is regular and adequate time allowance for a bowel movement. Activity promotes peristalsis and should be encouraged. Fiber is important but must be used with care. Excessive fiber intake can cause bowel obstruction, diarrhea, or the formation of bezoars, which are dense masses of seeds, skins, and other fiber-containing components of plants that form in the stomach (Steinberg & Eitan, 2003). The lower gastric acidity contributes to bezoar development, which is demonstrated by nausea, vomiting, fullness, abdominal pain, and diarrhea. Senna is an effective natural laxative that can be consumed in tablet or tea form. Often, individuals are aware that certain foods (e.g., bananas, prunes, carrots, or oatmeal) facilitate bowel elimination; these should be incorporated into the diet on a regular basis. Laxatives should be considered only after other measures have proved unsuccessful and, when necessary, should be used with great care.

Malnutrition

Because malnutrition is a potential and serious threat to older people, it should be closely monitored. The factors contributing to this problem include decreased taste and smell sensations, reduced mastication capability, slower peristalsis, decreased hunger contractions, reduced gastric acid secretion, less absorption of nutrients because of reduced intestinal blood flow, and a decrease in cells of the intestinal absorbing surface. The effects of medications can contribute to malnutrition (Box 14-1), reinforcing the significance of using nonpharmacologic means to address health conditions when possible.

| BOX 14-1 | Nutritional Risks Associated With Selected Medications |

Anemia
  Colchicine
  Indomethacin
  Methyldopa
  Nitrofurantoin
  Nonsteroidal anti-inflammatory drugs
  Oxyphenbutazone
  Phenylbutazone
  Sulfonamides
Anorexia
  Aminosalicylic acid
  Cardiac glycosides
  Central nervous system stimulants
  Propranolol
  Pyrazinamide
Constipation
  Aluminum hydroxide
  Calcium carbonate
  Cimetidine
  Codeine
  Narcotics
  Nonsteroidal anti-inflammatory drugs
  Sedatives—hypnotics
Diarrhea
  Ampicillin
  Ascorbic acid
  Cardiac glycosides
  Cimetidine
  Laxatives
  Magnesium-based preparations
  Neomycin
  Nonsteroidal anti-inflammatory drugs
  Penicillins
  Tetracyclines
Fluid and electrolyte disturbances
  Corticosteroids
  Diuretics
  Estrogens
  Laxatives
  Prednisone
Gastrointestinal upset
  Aspirin

  Colchicine
  Corticosteroids
  Erythromycin
  Estradiol
  Estrogens
  Fenoprofen
  Ibuprofen
  Indomethacin
  Naproxen
  Nonsteroidal anti-inflammatory drugs
  Oxyphenbutazone
  Phenylbutazone
  Probenecid
  Tetracycline
  Tolmetin
Nausea/vomiting
  Allopurinol
  Antibiotics
  Anticancer drugs
  Anticholinesterases
  Anticonvulsants
  Antidysrhythmics
  Antihistamines
  Antihypertensives
  Cardiac glycosides
  Chloral hydrate
  Codeine
  Colchicine
  Diuretics
  Ibuprofen
  Levodopa
  Naproxen
  Narcotics
  Nonsteroidal anti-inflammatory drugs
  Potassium
  Probenecid
  Propranolol
  Reserpine
  Tamoxifen
  Thiamine
  Tolmetin
  Vasodilators

Socioeconomic factors contributing to malnutrition also must be considered, along with lifelong eating patterns (e.g., history of skipping breakfast or high consumption of "junk foods").

The appearance of older people can be misleading and delay the detection of a malnourished state. Some of the clinical signs of malnutrition include:

- weight loss greater than 5% in the past month or 10% in the past 6 months
- weight 10% below or 20% above ideal range
- serum albumin level lower than 3.5 g/100 ml.
- hemoglobin level below 12 g/dL
- hematocrit value below 35%

Other problems can indicate malnutrition, such as delirium, depression, visual disturbances, dermatitis, hair loss, pallor, delayed wound healing, lethargy, and fatigue. It is crucial that nurses use keen assessment skills to recognize early malnourishment in older adults and encourage good nutritional practices to prevent its occurrence.

ADDRESSING NUTRITIONAL STATUS AND HYDRATION IN OLDER ADULTS

A wide range of physical, mental, and socioeconomic factors affect nutritional status in later life. Because these factors can change, regular nutritional assessment is necessary. Effective nutritional assessment involves collaboration among a physician, nurse, nutritionist, and social worker. Assessment Guide 14-1 describes the basic components of the nutritional assessment.

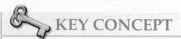

KEY CONCEPT

A variety of physical, psychological, and socioeconomic factors influence nutritional status.

Specific interventions discussed in this chapter can help address threats to good nutrition and hydration. In addition, it is important to consider that, often, a minor service link can enhance an older adult's nutritional status. In addressing the nutritional needs of older adults, the nurse must consider a wide range of services, including the Supplemental Nutrition Assistance Program, formerly known as food stamps, Meals on Wheels, shopping and meal preparation assistance through volunteer organizations, home health aides for feeding assistance, congregate eating programs, and nutritional and psychological counseling.

In addition to the physiological considerations, the social and cultural aspects of food are important to consider. To many people, the preparation, serving, and consumption of food signify a caring act. Social connection with others and celebrations typically involve food. Appreciation is often expressed through the gift of an edible treat. Encouraging friends and family to bring special treats to older persons who are in the hospital or nursing home and assisting them in engaging in celebrations are beneficial acts. For example, in a nursing home setting, nursing staff can assist a resident's family in finding a private area in the facility in which they can host a family luncheon to celebrate a special event.

The nurse must also consider cultural variables affecting nutrition. Ethnic and religious factors can influence food selection and preparation and eating patterns and practices. In some cultures, specific foods are seen as having healing benefit. For example, some Asian Americans believe that health is a balance of yin and yang and may select certain hot or cold foods to restore balance. An understanding of unique cultural factors affecting dietary practices is essential to individualized care.

ASSESSMENT GUIDE 14-1
NUTRITIONAL STATUS

HISTORY

- Review health history and medical record for evidence of diagnoses or conditions that can alter the purchase, preparation, ingestion, digestion, absorption, or excretion of foods.
- Review medications for those that can affect appetite and nutritional state.
- Review the type and amount of any nutritional supplements used.
- Ask the patient to describe his or her diet, meal pattern, food preferences, and restrictions.
- Request that the patient keep a diary of all food intake for a week.

PHYSICAL EXAMINATION

- Inspect hair. Hair loss or brittleness can be associated with malnutrition.
- Inspect skin. Note persistent "goose bumps" (vitamin B_6 deficiency); pallor (anemia); purpura (vitamin C deficiency); brownish pigmentation (niacin deficiency); red scaly areas in folds around eyes and between nose and corner of mouth (riboflavin deficiency); dermatitis (zinc deficiency); and fungal infections (hyperglycemia).
- Test skin turgor. Skin turgor, although poor in many older adults, tends to be best in the areas over the forehead and sternum; therefore, these are preferred areas to test.
- Note muscle tone, strength, and movement. Muscle weakness can be associated with vitamin and mineral deficiencies.
- Inspect eyes. Ask about changes in vision, night vision problems (vitamin A deficiency). Note the patient's percentile rank.
- Inspect oral cavity. Note dryness (dehydration), lesions, condition of tongue, breath odor, condition of teeth or dentures.
- Ask about signs and symptoms: sore tongue, indigestion, diarrhea, constipation, food distaste,

weakness, muscle cramps, burning sensations, dizziness, drowsiness, bone pain, sore joints, recurrent boils, dyspnea, dysphagia, anorexia, appetite changes.
- Observe person drinking or eating for difficulties.

Biochemical Evaluation

- Obtain blood sample for screening of total iron binding capacity, transferrin saturation, protein, albumin, hemoglobin, hematocrit, electrolytes, vitamins, prothrombin time.
- Obtain urine sample for screening of specific gravity.

Anthropometric Measurement

- Measure and ask about changes in height and weight. Use age-adjusted weight chart for evaluating weight. Note weight losses of 5% within the past 1 month and 10% with the past 6 months.
- Determine triceps skinfold measurement (TSM). To do so, grasp a fold of skin and subcutaneous fat halfway between the shoulder and elbow and measure with a caliper. Note the patient's percentile rank.
- Measure the midarm circumference (MC) with a tape measure (using centimeters) and use this to calculate midarm muscle circumference (MMC) with the formula:

$$MMC \text{ (cm)} = MC \text{ (cm)} - (0.314 \times TSM \text{ [mm]})$$

The standard MMC is 25.3 cm for men and 23.2 cm for women. MMC below 90% of the standard is considered undernutrition; below 60% is considered protein-calorie malnutrition.

PSYCHOLOGICAL EXAMINATION

- Test cognitive function.
- Note alterations in mood, behavior, cognition, level of consciousness. Be alert to signs of depression (can be associated with deficiencies of vitamin B_6, magnesium, or niacin).
- Ask about changes in mood or cognition

BRINGING RESEARCH TO LIFE

PROFILE OF NURSING HOME RESIDENTS WITH DEMENTIA WHO REQUIRE ASSISTANCE WITH MOUTH CARE

Jablonski, R. A., Kolanowski, A. M., & Litaker, M. (2011). Geriatric Nursing, 32(6), 439–449.

This study described the demographic, functional, and behavioral profile of nursing home residents with dementia who needed verbal or physical assistance with mouth care. Participants were nursing home residents with moderate to severe cognitive impairment. Researchers conducted chart reviews, activities of daily living assessments, resident interviews, and family interviews and, over a 5-day period, videotaped times when behavioral symptoms were most prevalent.

Findings revealed that residents with higher levels of formal education and overall functional capacity were more likely to require verbal support to perform mouth care. They were more adept than those with lower cognitive levels at understanding directions and processing verbal cues; they also had significantly higher scores for the personality trait of openness, which could have made them more willing to accept direction.

The group requiring physical assistance with mouth care were more passive when interacting with people and engaging in activities and had fewer language and executive function skills. Given their lack of intellectual executive function, they tended to benefit from an intervention known as chaining, in which the caregiver initiates the action and then the resident takes over with some assistance as needed.

This study demonstrated the usefulness in assessing specific cognitive domains, such as language and executive function, to determine the strategies (e.g., verbal guidance, starting task and allowing resident to take it over, and performing task for resident) that would be most appropriate for mouth care for older persons with dementia.

PRACTICE REALITIES

Nurse Timms recently has begun working in a nursing home. On the unit in which he is assigned, he notices that mouth care is not given. Although some of the residents have teeth that are in poor condition and dentures that fit poorly, there is no plan for dental care.

During a staff meeting Mr. Timms asked about plans for dental care for the residents. The staff responded, "These people don't have the money to visit a dentist, plus, the nearest dentist is nearly an hour away." The physician says that if a resident has a dental complaint a referral to a dentist will be written, but otherwise, it is a waste of time and money.

Mr. Timms is not content accepting this but as a new employee doesn't want to cause conflict with the team.

What actions could Mr. Timms take?

CRITICAL THINKING EXERCISES

1. List the various physical, mental, and socioeconomic requisites for good nutritional intake.

2. What topics could be included in an oral health education program for older adults?

3. How have the media and advertisements influenced the use of dietary supplements? What can nurses do to assist older adults in separating fact from myth regarding the claims made by manufacturers and distributors of dietary supplements?

4. Describe factors that can negatively influence dietary intake for older adults in a nursing home, a hospital, and at home.

5. Describe the components of a comprehensive nutritional assessment.

RESOURCES

American Dental Association
http://www.ada.org

Academy of Nutrition and Dietetics
http://www.eatright.org

Food and Nutrition Information Center
www.nal.usda.gov/fnic

Mini Nutritional Assessment
http://mna-elderly.com

National Institute of Dental and Craniofacial Research
www.nidcr.nih.gov

Overeaters Anonymous
http://www.overeaters.org

REFERENCES

Baker, H. (2007). Nutrition in the elderly: An overview. *Geriatrics, 62*(7), 28–31.

Dahm, C. C., Keogh, R. H., Spencer, E. A., Greenwood, D. C., Ket, T. J., Fentiman, I. S., Rodwell Bingham, S. A., et al. (2010). Dietary fiber and colorectal cancer risk: A nested case-controlled study using food diaries. *Journal of the National Cancer Institute, 102*(9), 614–626.

Du, H., Van Der, A. D., Boshuizen, H. C., Forouhi, N. G., Wareham, N. J., Halkjaer, J., Feskens, E. J., et al. (2010). Dietary fiber and subsequent changes in body weight and waist circumference in European men and women. *Journal of Clinical Nutrition, 91*(2), 329–226.

Hopping, B. N., Erber, E., Grandinetti, A., Verheus, M., Kolonel, L. N., & Maskarinec, G. (2010). Dietary fiber, magnesium, and glycemic load alter risk of type 2 diabetes in a multiethnic cohort in Hawaii. *Journal of Nutrition, 140*(1), 68–74.

Steinberg, J. M., & Eitan, A. (2003). Prickly pear fruit bezoar presenting as rectal perforation in an elderly patient. *International Journal of Colorectal Disease, 18*(4), 5–7.

Straub, D. A. (2007). Calcium supplementation in clinical practice: A review of forms, doses, and indications. *Nutrition in Clinical Practice, 22*(3), 286–296.

Tufts University, 2012. My Plate for Older Adults. Retrieved May 15, 2012, from http://www.nutrition.tufts.edu/research/myplate-older-adults.

RECOMMENDED READINGS

Recommended Readings associated with this chapter can be found on the web site that accompanies the book. Visit http://thepoint.lww.com/Eliopoulos8e to access the recommended readings and other additional resources associated with this chapter.

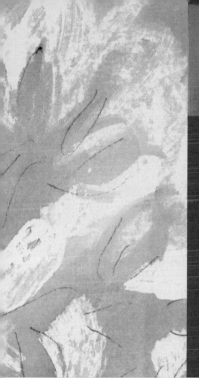

CHAPTER 15

Rest and Sleep

CHAPTER OUTLINE

LEARNING OBJECTIVES

After reading this chapter, you should be able to:

1. Explain differences between younger and older adults in sleep stages and cycles.

2. Describe factors that may disturb sleep in older adults

3. Describe pharmacologic and nonpharmacologic means to promote sleep.

4. Discuss the importance of pain control for promoting rest and sleep.

TERMS TO KNOW

Insomnia: inability to fall sleep, difficulty staying asleep, or premature waking

Nocturnal myoclonus: condition characterized by at least five leg jerks or movements per hour during sleep

Phase advance: falling asleep earlier in the evening and awakening earlier in the morning

Restless leg syndrome: neurological disorder characterized by an uncontrollable urge to move the legs when one lies down

Sleep apnea: disorder in which at least five episodes of cessation of breathing, lasting at least 10 seconds, occur per hour of sleep, accompanied by daytime sleepiness

Sleep latency: delay in the onset of sleep

All human beings must retreat from activity and stimulation to renew their reserves. Several periods of relaxation throughout the day and a block of sleep help promote a healthy pattern of rest. The fact that a person spends nearly one third of his or her lifetime sleeping and resting underscores the significance of these activities. Sleep is often a mirror into our state of health and well-being in that we may be restless and unable to obtain sufficient sleep in the presence of pain, stress, or impaired bodily functions. It also is a factor that affects

NURSING DIAGNOSIS

TABLE 15-1 Aging and Risks to the Ability to Achieve Rest

Causes or Contributing Factors	Nursing Diagnosis
Increased awakening during sleep; sleep stages III and IV less prominent	Disturbed Sleep Pattern related to less prominent sleep stages
Increased incidence of nocturia	Disturbed Sleep Pattern related to nocturia
Altered perception of night environment, resulting from visual and hearing deficits	Anxiety and Fear related to difficulty in falling asleep
Increased incidence of muscle cramps during resting states	Acute Pain related to muscle cramps

health and well-being, as inadequate quality or quantity of sleep is associated with risks to physical and mental health.

POINT TO PONDER

What are your unique sleep and rest requirements, and how well do you meet them? What do you notice about your physical and emotional states when you have had inadequate sleep and rest?

Changes that occur with aging and conditions experienced in later years can interfere with the ability to achieve adequate sleep and rest (Nursing Diagnosis Table 15-1). Astute assessment is necessary to ensure that older adults fulfill sleep and rest requirements and to identify obstacles for which intervention is warranted.

AGE-RELATED CHANGES IN SLEEP

Insomnia, daytime sleepiness, and napping are all highly prevalent among the older adults. In most cases, these experiences result from age-related changes in circadian sleep–wake cycles, sleep architecture (stages), sleep efficiency, and sleep quality (Ancoli-Israel & Martin, 2006).

Circadian Sleep–Wake Cycles

Older adults are more likely to fall asleep earlier in the evening and awaken earlier in the morning, a behavior referred to as *phase advance* (Ancoli-Israel & Martin, 2006). The quantity of sleep does not

change, but the hours in which it occurs may. This change can prove frustrating for older adults who find themselves nodding off during evening activities and wide awake in the early morning hours when everyone else is asleep. In addition, daytime naps may be needed to compensate for reductions in nighttime sleep. Adjusting schedules to accommodate the altered biorhythms could prove useful. Increasing natural light is also useful in pushing the circadian rhythm toward a later hour of sleep.

Sleep Stages

For sleep to be most restful, the person experiences a series of sleep stages. Changes in the amount of time spent in each stage occur with aging (Table 15-2). Reductions in non-rapid eye movement stage sleep and rapid eye movement (REM) stage sleep begin to occur after midlife. Older people sleep less soundly, shift in and out of stage I sleep to a greater degree than younger adults, and spend more time in stages I and II sleep. They have a decline in the proportion of time spent in the deeper stages III and IV sleep.

Sleep Efficiency and Quality

Sleep latency, a delay in the onset of sleep, is more prevalent with advancing age. Beginning in midlife, people become more sensitive to noise while they are sleeping and are awakened by noises that may not cause a reaction in younger adults. Likewise, older individuals are more likely than the young to be awakened by having lights turned on and having changes in room temperature. It is important to consider these factors when caring for older adults in institutional settings. If the sleeping area is noisy, a white noise generator that produces soothing sounds that mask other noises could prove useful. Some people find that a radio achieves the same effect.

KEY CONCEPT

Nurses need to be aware that older adults can be easily awakened by noise and lighting associated with caregiving and other staff activities during the night.

SLEEP DISTURBANCES

Approximately half of the adult population complains of sleep disorders, with the major complaint being insomnia. The nurse can assess for sleep disturbances in the older adult by using a self-rating tool such as the Pittsburgh Sleep Quality Index (see Resources at the end of this chapter). In addition to insomnia, leg movements, sleep apnea, medical conditions, and drugs can disturb sleep in older adults.

TABLE 15-2	Stages of Sleep and Differences in Older Adulthood	

Stage	Characteristics	Differences in Older Adulthood
I	Begins nodding off Can be easily awakened If undisturbed, will reach next stage in a few minutes	More time spent in this stage, most likely due to frequent awakening; increased number of arousals and shifts into non–rapid eye movement (REM) sleep
II	Deeper stage of relaxation reached Some eye movement noted through closed lids Can be easily awakened	No significant change, although older adult may spend more time in this stage
III	Early phase of deep sleep Reduced temperature and heart rate Muscles relaxed More difficult to be awakened	Decreased
IV	Deep sleep and relaxation All body functions reduced Considerable stimulation needed to be awakened Insufficient stage IV sleep can cause emotional dysfunction	Decreased
REM	REM occurs Increased vital signs (sometimes irregular) Will enter REM sleep approximately once every 90 minutes of stage IV sleep Insufficient REM sleep can cause emotional dysfunction, including psychosis	Decreased due to reduced amount of sleep time in general[a]

[a]Certain drugs can also decrease REM sleep, including alcohol, barbiturates, and phenothiazine derivatives.

Insomnia

Insomnia consists of difficulty falling or staying asleep and/or premature waking. It can be difficult to get a fair estimate of the problem because insomnia can have various meanings. People may report that they have insomnia because they awaken at 5 AM, have difficulty falling asleep, do not sleep soundly, or travel to the bathroom several times during the night. This reinforces the importance of recognizing insomnia as a symptom and thoroughly assessing for factors that contribute to disrupted sleep. Insomnia can be a short-term (transient) problem associated with a changed environment, illness, added stress, or anxiety. Chronic insomnia (i.e., insomnia lasting 3 or more weeks) can be related to physical or mental illnesses, environmental factors, substance abuse, or medications. Sedatives may be unnecessary if the underlying cause of insomnia can be addressed.

Nocturnal Myoclonus and Restless Leg Syndrome

Jerking leg movements during sleep can cause awakenings during the night. One such cause of this is known as nocturnal myoclonus, a condition characterized by at least five leg jerks or movements per hour during sleep. Nocturnal myoclonus is associated with the use of tricyclic antidepressants and chronic renal failure.

Restless leg syndrome, a neurological condition characterized by an uncontrollable urge to move the legs, increases in incidence and severity with age. People with restless leg syndrome may describe the sensations with terms such as "uncomfortable," "electrical," "itching," "pins and needles," "pulling," "creepy-crawly," and "painful." Moving the legs brings relief of the sensations but also interferes with sleep. It can be caused by iron deficiency anemia, uremia, Parkinson's disease, rheumatoid arthritis, diabetes, or neurological lesions; it is believed to be associated with alterations in dopamine and iron metabolism. Antidepressants, antihistamines, antipsychotics, alcohol, caffeine, hypoglycemia, and simple and refined carbohydrates can contribute to this syndrome. Dehydration worsens symptoms; drinking a glass of water may relieve symptoms for some individuals, as can massage and the application of heat or cold.

Although the long-term effectiveness in older adults has not been sufficiently studied, both nocturnal myoclonus and restless leg syndrome are treated with dopaminergic drugs, benzodiazepines, opioids, anticonvulsants, adrenergics, and iron supplements.

Sleep Apnea

Sleep apnea is a significant disorder in which at least five episodes of cessation of breathing, lasting at least 10 seconds, occur per hour of sleep, accompanied by daytime sleepiness. It is characterized by snoring and sudden awakening and gasping for air. The prevalence is three times greater in men than in women and higher in persons who are overweight or obese.

This disorder can be caused by a defect in the central nervous system that affects the diaphragm (central sleep apnea), a blockage in the upper airway that interferes with normal air flow (obstructive sleep apnea), or a combination of both (mixed). Snoring usually accompanies the obstructive type. The interruption of sleep can result in daytime fatigue and sleepiness; nurses should assess for sleep apnea when these symptoms are present.

Sleep disorder clinics and other resources can assist in evaluating the disorder and determining the best treatment plan, which could consist of weight reduction, medications, continuous positive airway pressure, and/or surgery to remove obstructions or realign bite.

Sleeping in a supine position should be avoided because it allows the tongue to fall back and block the airway. Alcohol and other drugs with depressant effects can aggravate the problem by decreasing respiratory drive and relaxing throat muscles. Patients need to be cautioned about driving and using machinery if daytime drowsiness is present.

Medical Conditions That Affect Sleep

Health conditions, particularly chronic diseases, can interfere with sleep by producing symptoms such as nocturia, incontinence, pain, orthopnea, apnea, muscle cramps, and tremors. Cardiovascular conditions that produce nocturnal cardiac ischemia can interfere with sleep due to the dyspnea and transient angina that occur. Fluctuating blood glucose levels can interfere with the sleep of persons who have diabetes. Gastric pain can awaken persons with gastroesophageal reflux disease. Chronic obstructive pulmonary disease and other respiratory conditions can disrupt sleep with coughing and dyspnea. Musculoskeletal conditions can cause pain. People with dementia have minimal stage II and REM sleep, no stage IV sleep, and frequent arousals from sleep. Depression and other emotional disturbances can alter sleep.

Because medical conditions can affect sleep, it is important to consider that changes in sleep patterns may indicate signs of other undetected problems in older persons. Although early morning rising is not unusual for older adults, a sudden change to earlier awakening or insomnia may be symptomatic of an emotional disturbance or alcohol abuse. Sleep disturbances also may arise from cardiac or respiratory problems, which produce difficulties, such as orthopnea and pain related to poor peripheral circulation. Restlessness and confusion during the night may indicate an adverse reaction to a sedative. Nocturnal frequency may be a clue to the presence of diabetes. It is important to assess both the quality and quantity of sleep.

Drugs That Affect Sleep

Like medical conditions, medications used to treat those conditions can affect sleep. Older adults experiencing sleep problems should identify and review their medications with their physicians. Examples of drugs that can interrupt sleep include anticholinergics, antidepressants, antihypertensives (centrally acting ones), benzodiazepines, β-blockers, diuretics, levodopa, steroids, theophylline, and thyroid preparations. Hypnotics interfere with REM and deep sleep stages and can cause daytime drowsiness (due to their extended half-lives in older people), thereby creating difficulties in falling asleep for the patient.

Examples of specific drugs that affect sleep include diphenhydramine HCl (Benadryl capsules); nicotine (NicoDerm Nicotine Transdermal System); fluoxetine HCl (Prozac); theophylline (Theo-X Extended-Release tablets); and alprazolam (Xanax). Many of the top nonprescription sleep aids contain diphenhydramine (Benadryl) as a primary ingredient; because Benadryl carries a high risk of anticholinergic side effects in older adults, these should be avoided.

Sleep can be interrupted by nightmares caused by drugs, particularly those that affect neurotransmitters. These include some antianxiety drugs, antidepressants, antihistamines, β-blockers, analgesics, antiparkinson drugs, sedatives, smoking cessation aids, statins, and drugs used in the treatment of dementia. If the patient reports having nightmares, a review of medications could prove useful.

Caffeine and alcohol can also negatively affect sleep. Eliminating caffeine and alcohol is advisable if sleep disorders are present. Nurses can educate older adults about the caffeine content of food and beverages.

Other Factors Affecting Sleep

An apartment located on a busy street, a snoring spouse, an excessively warm room, and bright hallway lights of a nursing home are among the examples of environmental factors that can interfere with sleep. Adjusting to a new environment, as can occur when one relocates to an assisted living community or the home of a child, can affect sleep. Caffeine and alcohol consumption can impair the ability to fall asleep and achieve a satisfying quality of sleep. Pain and other symptoms (e.g., dyspnea when supine) can cause problems falling and staying asleep, as can an uncomfortable mattress. Exploring these issues when sleep problems are present is an important part of the sleep assessment.

PROMOTING REST AND SLEEP IN OLDER ADULTS

Every assessment needs to include a sleep history which includes:

- review of time spent in sleep and naps, quality of sleep
- medication review
- bedtime routines
- presence of sleep disturbances, if present:
  - length of time present
  - characteristics (e.g., falling asleep, staying asleep, and early awakening)
  - type of bedding and sleep environment
  - food and fluid consumed several hours prior to bedtime
  - medications used to address sleep disturbances
  - factors interfering with sleep (e.g., pain, voiding, and nightmares)
  - effects (e.g., daytime drowsiness, irritability, and fatigue)
  - management

When an older adult is experiencing a disturbed sleep pattern, the nurse plays an important role in identifying ways to improve sleep (see Nursing Diagnosis Highlight: Disturbed Sleep Pattern). Plans may involve pharmacologic and nonpharmacologic measures to promote sleep and measures to control pain.

Pharmacologic Measures to Promote Sleep

Older adults often have difficulty falling asleep. Unfortunately, frequently the first means used to encourage sleep is the administration of a sedative. Sedatives must be used with the utmost care. Barbiturates are general depressants, especially to the central nervous system, and they can significantly depress some vital body functions, lowering basal metabolic rate more than it already is and decreasing blood pressure, mental activity, and peristalsis to the extent that other problems may develop. These serious effects, combined with a greater susceptibility to adverse reactions, warrant that barbiturates be used with extreme caution. Non-barbiturate sedatives also create problems and should be used only when absolutely necessary. Because of the prolonged half-life of medications in older persons, the effects

of sedatives may exist into the daytime and result in confusion and sluggishness. Sometimes these symptoms are treated with medications, further complicating the situation. Occasionally, sleeping medications will reverse the normal sleep rhythm. All sedatives may decrease body movements during sleep and predispose the older person to the many complications of reduced mobility.

Nonpharmacologic Measures to Promote Sleep

Alternatives to sedatives should be used to induce sleep whenever possible. The nurse may assess the older person's rest and activity schedules, sleep environment, and diet to identify possible interventions.

Activity and Rest Schedules

The person's activity schedule should first be evaluated. Satisfying, regular activity promotes rest and relaxation (Fig. 15-1). If a person has been inactive in a bed or wheelchair all day, most likely he or she will not be sleepy at bedtime. Including more stimulation and activity during the day may be a solution.

Greater amounts of rest are required by older people and should be interspersed with periods of activity throughout the day. Many older adults focus all their activity in the early part of the day so that they will have the evening free. For instance, the early morning hours may be used for household cleaning, marketing, club meetings, gardening, cooking, and laundering; the evening hours may then be spent watching television, reading, or sewing. This pattern may be an outgrowth of

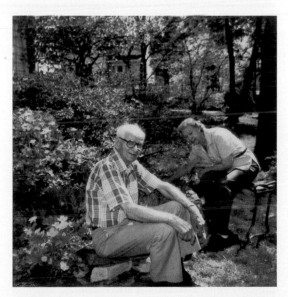

FIGURE 15-1 ■ Daytime activity promotes nighttime sleep.

NURSING DIAGNOSIS HIGHLIGHT

DISTURBED SLEEP PATTERN

Overview

A sleep pattern disturbance exists when the quantity or quality of sleep causes disruption to daily function. This disturbance can be displayed by problems falling or staying asleep, nighttime sleep of less than 4 hours, daytime drowsiness, frequent yawning, lack of energy or motivation to engage in activities, dark circles under eyes, weakness, and disturbances in mood or cognition.

Causative or contributing factors

Age-related decrease in stage IV sleep, nocturia, muscle cramps, orthopnea, dyspnea, angina, poor peripheral circulation, cough, incontinence, diarrhea, insufficient activity or exercise, immobility, pain, new environment, depression, confusion, anxiety, medications (e.g., antidepressants, antihypertensives, tranquilizers), noise, interruptions, high caffeine consumption.

Goals

The patient will:
- obtain 5 to 8 hours of sleep daily
- be free from symptoms and signs associated with sleep pattern disturbance

Interventions

- Assess sleep pattern. Ask the patient about number, length, and quality of naps; activity pattern; bedtime; quality of sleep; awakening time; symptoms and interruptions of sleep. Attempt to identify and correct factors associated with sleep disturbance.
- Increase daytime activity; limit naps, reduce caffeine.
- Consult with physician regarding eliminating medications that are known to disrupt sleep.
- Maintain bedroom temperature between 70°F (21°C) and 75°F (24°C); control interruptions; provide a night-light.
- Assist patient with toileting at bedtime. Be aware that renal circulation improves when one lies down; therefore, the patient may need to toilet shortly after going to bed.
- Use measures that are known to stimulate sleep, such as soft music, television, drinking warm milk.
- Offer back rubs, evening care, and other comfort measures to relax the patient and induce sleep.
- Instruct patient in measures to improve sleep.
- If sedatives are necessary, use those that are least disruptive to sleep cycle and monitor 24-hour effects from the drug.
- Reduce the potential for injury by having bed in lowest position, using side rails, providing night-light, adjusting lighting so that patient does not have to travel from dark bedroom to bright bathroom, encouraging patient to ask for assistance with transferring and ambulating as needed.
- Record or have patient record sleep pattern (e.g., time to bed, time when asleep, times awakened during the night, signs and symptoms during sleep, rising time, self-assessment of restfulness).

---

decades of employment, whereby one worked during the day and relaxed in the evening. Older people need insight into the advantages of pacing activities throughout the entire day and providing ample periods for rest and naps between activities. The nurse may find it useful to review the older person's daily activities hour by hour and assist in developing patterns that more equally distribute activity and rest throughout the day.

Furthermore, the amount of time allotted for sleep must be evaluated. One should not expect the older person who goes to bed at 8 PM to be able to sleep until 8 AM the following day.

Environment

Exposure to sunlight during the day can facilitate sleep at night. A warm bath at bedtime can promote muscle relaxation and encourage sleep, as can a back rub, a comfortable position, and the alleviation of pain or discomfort. A quiet environment

at a temperature preferred by the individual should be provided. Flannel sheets and electric blankets can promote comfort and relaxation; electric blankets should be used to preheat the bed and should be turned off when the individual enters the bed to reduce the health hazards associated with electromagnetic fields.

Food and Supplements

Foods high in carbohydrates tend to raise the level of serotonin in the brain, which could have a sedating effect; therefore, a protein and carbohydrate snack at bedtime may encourage sleep. Valerian root tea or herbal tincture consumed 45 minutes before bedtime can also facilitate sleep. The supplement melatonin (a synthetic form of the hormone that is naturally stimulated by darkness) has gained popularity for improving the quality of sleep in adults of all ages by correcting imbalances in the body's circadian rhythm. Because melatonin

CONSIDER THIS CASE

Mr. and Mrs. E, both 83 years of age, live alone in a busy, high-crime area of a large city. Mr. E has a mild dementia but is able to function well with his wife's assistance and supervision. Over the past year, however, he has had significant changes in his sleep pattern in which he awakens several times during the night to use the bathroom and sleeps most of the day. He has a tendency to drink caffeinated sodas when he awakens if his wife doesn't stop him, so she often will get out of bed when he does to make sure he drinks caffeine-free liquids. Mrs. E's frequent awakening with her husband compounds a long-term problem she has had with getting out of bed when she hears any street sound to assure no one is breaking into their home. Mrs. E is not comfortable napping during the day and tends to feel tired most of the time.

THINK CRITICALLY

- What risks do their sleep patterns present for Mr. and Mrs. E?
- What recommendations would you have for this couple?

---

supplements may interact with immunosuppressants, antidepressants, antipsychotics, warfarin, and other medications, it is wise for the pharmacist and physician to review the safety of using melatonin in combination with medications.

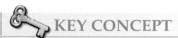
KEY CONCEPT

Regular exercise, exposure to sunlight during the day, and non-caffeinated herbal teas at bedtime are three measures to help older adults fall asleep naturally.

Stress Management

Stress is a normal part of life, but it can interfere with rest and sleep. Most individuals confront a variety of physical and emotional stressors daily, such as temperature changes, pollutants, viruses, injury, interpersonal conflicts, time pressures, fear, bad news, and unpleasant or difficult tasks. Many real or perceived threats to our physical, emotional, and social well-being and balance can create stress. Demands and activity levels are not necessarily correlated with stress; for example, a busy schedule or numerous responsibilities to juggle may be less stressful than a boring, monotonous existence.

Regardless of the source of the stress, the body reacts by stimulating the sympathetic nervous system. This causes stimulation of the pituitary gland, the release of adrenocorticotropic hormone, and an increase in the body's adrenaline supply.

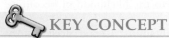
KEY CONCEPT

Unrelieved chronic stress can lead to heart disease, hypertension, cerebrovascular accident, ulcers, and other health disorders.

It is important, therefore, to prevent chronic stress from developing. The key to stress control is not avoiding stress, but managing it by learning compensatory measures. Some of these measures are outlined as follows:

- *Respond to stress in a healthy manner.* Good nutrition, rest, exercise, and other sound health practices strengthen the body's ability to confront stress. When in a stressful situation, adherence to these principles continues to be important. It is beneficial to learn to remain calm when faced with stress; reacting in an unhealthy manner worsens the situation.

- *Manage lifestyle.* Little in the lives of most people would bring the world to a halt if not completed at a certain time or in a specific manner. Things should be put in perspective; for example, what difference will it really make if the clothes are not washed today or if one is 10 minutes late? Whenever possible, anticipate the consequences of a situation so that the stress of an unpredictable situation can be reduced.

- *Relax.* Be it a good book, swimming, weaving, travel, music, or wood carving, find something in which to get absorbed so that there is some respite from life's demands. Yoga, meditation, qigong, guided imagery, and relaxation exercises can be effective. Also, herbs can be of benefit, including chamomile and lavender to promote relaxation and American ginseng to protect the body from the ill effects of stress.

- *Pray.* People of faith look to a higher power with whom they can share and understand life's burdens. The "unloading" of one's problems during prayer can also be a rest-inducing activity in that it clears the mind of the day's stresses. Furthermore, the repeated words or rituals associated with prayer can offer the same therapeutic benefits as meditation and relaxation exercises.

POINT TO PONDER

What are the three major stresses in your life? What are you doing to minimize their negative effects? What more could you be doing to control stress in your life?

Pain Control

The presence of pain can threaten the ability of older adults to obtain adequate rest and sleep. Although the results of studies regarding the effects of aging on pain sensitivity are inconclusive, the prevalence of chronic pain–causing conditions, such as osteoarthritis and postherpetic neuralgia, is high among older adults. Not only can pain interfere with sleep, but it can also reduce activity levels, depress mood, and result in other factors that can affect sleep and rest patterns.

Identifying the cause of pain is the essential first step to controlling it. Undiagnosed medical conditions can be the source of the problem, but so can psychological factors, poor positioning, and adverse drug reactions. A comprehensive assessment is crucial. Consideration should be given to factors that precipitate, aggravate, and relieve pain. Nurses can assist patients in self-evaluating pain with the use of rating scales that use numbers or diagrams to indicate severity of pain (see Chapter 16).

Because of the risks associated with drugs, nonpharmacologic measures to control pain should be attempted whenever possible. Among these measures are proper positioning, diversional activities, guided imagery, biofeedback, yoga, massage, therapeutic touch, acupuncture, and magnet therapy. If nonpharmacologic means of pain relief are ineffective and drugs are necessary, it is advisable to begin with the weakest type and dosage of analgesic and gradually increase as necessary. See Chapter 16 for more information on pain management.

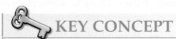

KEY CONCEPT

Massages, warm soaks, relaxation exercises, guided imagery, and diversion can provide effective relief of many types of pain.

BRINGING RESEARCH TO LIFE

SLEEP-DISORDERED BREATHING, HYPOXIA, AND RISK OF MILD COGNITIVE IMPAIRMENT AND DEMENTIA IN OLDER WOMEN

Yaffe, K., Laffan, A. M., Harrison, S. L., Redline, S., Spira, A. P., Ensrud, K. E., Stone, K. L., et al. (2011). Journal of the American Medical Association, 306(6), 613–619.

This study examined the relationship between sleep and cognition. The researchers identified 298 women who did not have cognitive impairments or dementia. Four years after the initial screening, sleep specialists went to the subjects' homes and monitored the women as they slept. Specialized equipment measured brain activity, heart rhythm, leg movements, breathing, and blood oxygen. The presence of sleep apnea was able to be tracked with the equipment.

One year later (5 years after the initial cognitive screening), the women were given tests to measure cognitive abilities, memory, and verbal fluency. The records of women whose tests suggested the presence of cognitive impairment were reviewed by clinical experts to confirm the diagnosis. It was found that women with sleep apnea were almost twice as likely to become cognitively impaired. Although the researchers could not conclude that sleep apnea causes dementia, the findings suggest that spending a large portion of sleep time in a state of hypoxia, as occurs with sleep apnea, contributes to the likelihood of becoming cognitively impaired.

This study demonstrates the importance of nurses obtaining a good sleep history and identifying signs of sleep apnea in older adults. Identifying sleep apnea and assisting in obtaining treatment for this condition could prevent or delay the onset of cognitive impairment in older adults.

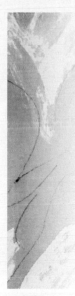

PRACTICE REALITIES

One of the hospital's units is dedicated to people who are out of immediate crisis but in need of close observation and treatment for several weeks. It is not uncommon for vital signs to be checked and treatments performed at any time around the clock. The busyness of the unit resembles an intensive care unit.

The nurses have noted that older patients in particular have difficulty sleeping, display high levels of fatigue during the day, and often experience delirium. They believe interruptions to sleep are a major contributing factor.

What can the nurses do to assist older patients in obtaining adequate rest and sleep while still attending to their critical care needs?

CRITICAL THINKING EXERCISES

1. What nonpharmacologic measures can be incorporated into an older adult's lifestyle to facilitate sleep?

2. What stresses do older adults face that are different from those encountered by other age groups?

RESOURCES

American Sleep Apnea Association
http://www.sleepapnea.org

Hartford Institute of Geriatric Nursing
Try This: Best Practices in Nursing Care to Older Adults, The Pittsburgh Sleep Quality Index
http://www.nursingcenter.com/prodev/ce_article.asp?tid=790064

National Sleep Foundation
http://www.sleepfoundation.org

Restless Leg Syndrome Foundation
http://www.rls.org

REFERENCE

Ancoli-Israel, S., & Martin, J. L. (2006). Insomnia and daytime napping in older adults. *Journal of Clinical Sleep Medicine, 15*(2), 333–342.

RECOMMENDED READINGS

Recommended Readings associated with this chapter can be found on the web site that accompanies the book. Visit **http://thepoint.lww.com/Eliopoulos8e** to access the recommended readings and other additional resources associated with this chapter.

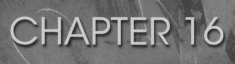

Comfort and Pain Management

LEARNING OBJECTIVES

After reading this chapter, you should be able to:

1. Define comfort.
2. Describe the characteristics and effects of pain in older adults.
3. Describe the components of a comprehensive pain assessment.
4. Outline components of a pain management plan, including complementary therapies, dietary changes, medications, and comforting strategies.

TERMS TO KNOW

Acute pain: abrupt onset and lasting a short time

Neuropathic pain: occurs from an abnormal processing of sensory stimuli by the central or peripheral nervous system

Nociceptive pain: arises from mechanical, thermal, or chemical noxious stimuli; can be somatic or visceral

Persistent pain: chronic pain that has been present for 3 months or longer

COMFORT

Comfort is a relative term. To some people it can mean sufficient control of pain to capture a few hours of rest; other individuals may view comfort as freedom from physical and mental stress; and still others may consider luxurious, pampered living synonymous with comfort. The word comfort is derived from the Latin word *confortare*, which means to strengthen greatly.

Webster's Dictionary offers definitions that include "to relieve from distress, lessen misery, have freedom from pain and worry, calm, and inspire with hope." From a holistic perspective, comfort can be viewed as a sense of physical, emotional, social, and spiritual peace and well-being.

Comfort tends to be a state often taken for granted until it is threatened. People coast along without pain or distress, not giving much thought to the comfort they are experiencing. But then something happens—unrelenting gastric pain develops, joints ache while doing routine tasks, a suspicious lump is found in a breast—and the comfort cart is upset. Unfortunately, with advancing age, the incidence of factors that can threaten comfort increases.

PAIN: A COMPLEX PHENOMENON

Pain is the greatest threat to comfort. A definition of pain that was accepted for decades describes pain as "an unpleasant sensory and emotional experience associated with actual or potential tissue damage" (American Pain Society, 2003; International Association for the Study of Pain, 2012). It is now accepted that pain is subjective and relies on the patient's perception and report (International Association for the Study of Pain, 2012).

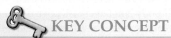

KEY CONCEPT

Pain is referred to as the fifth vital sign because it is such an important indicator of an individual's health status.

PREVALENCE OF PAIN IN OLDER ADULTS

Pain is highly prevalent in the older population, with a majority experiencing some degree of pain on a daily basis (Horgas, Elliott, & Marsiske, 2009).

The impact of pain is far-reaching and is increasingly prevalent with advancing age. The National Center for Health Statistics (2006) reports that:

- One in four adults reports suffering a daylong bout of pain in the past month.
- Three fifths of adults 65 years and older said they had experienced pain that lasted for 1 year or more.
- Low back pain is among the most common complaints, along with migraine or severe headache and joint pain, aching, or stiffness. The knee is the joint that causes the most pain according to the report. (Interestingly, knee

replacement surgeries have risen dramatically for people over age 65 years.)

- Reports of severe joint pain increased with age, and women reported severely painful joints more often than men.

It may be difficult to determine the accuracy of the reported prevalence of pain in older persons. On one hand, older adults may underreport pain because they do not want to be viewed as complainers, lack the funds to seek treatment, or erroneously believe that pain is a normal part of being old. On the other hand, pain could be overreported by some older people who see reporting this symptom as an effective means to get the attention of family members and health care professionals. These possibilities reinforce the importance of exploring pain during every assessment and reviewing the relationship of other factors (physical, emotional, socioeconomic, and spiritual) to this symptom.

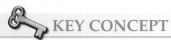

KEY CONCEPT

The complex phenomenon of pain is a stressor to physical, emotional, and spiritual well-being.

Types of Pain

There are several ways in which pain is classified. One classification is by the pathophysiological mechanism that causes it. The two main types that arise from tissue damage are nociceptive pain and neuropathic pain. *Nociceptive pain* arises from mechanical, thermal, or chemical noxious stimuli to the A-delta and C afferent nociceptors. These nociceptors are found in fasciae, muscles, joints, and other deep structures, and their activation causes a transduction of painful stimuli along the primary afferent fiber of the dorsal horn of the spinal column. Neurotransmitters (e.g., somatostatin, cholecystokinin, and substance P) carry the pain signal through secondary neurons to the brain where the signal is interpreted. Common forms of nociceptive pain include:

- Somatic pain: characteristic of pain in the bone and soft tissue masses. The pain is well localized and described as throbbing or aching.
- Visceral pain: associated with disorders that can cause generalized or referred pain. The pain is described as deep and aching.

Neuropathic pain occurs from an abnormal processing of sensory stimuli by the central or peripheral nervous system and is associated with diabetic neuropathies, postherpetic neuralgias, and other insults to the nervous system. The pain is sharp, stabbing, tingling, or burning, with a sudden onset of high intensity. It can last a few seconds or linger for a longer period.

Pain is also described according to its onset and duration. *Acute pain* has an abrupt onset, can be severe, but lasts only a short time; it usually is responsive to analgesics and other pain management approaches. *Persistent or chronic pain* is that which has been present for 3 months or longer and can be of mild to severe intensity. *Acute pain* has the potential to develop into persistent pain.

Pain Perception

The role of age in pain perception is unclear. Results of studies examining the effects of aging on pain sensitivity vary according to the type of pain. There is some evidence of a reduced sensitivity for thermal pain with advancing age (Gagliese & Katz, 2003; Lariviere, Goffaux, Marchand, & Julien, 2007). Research on aging and mechanical pain threshold has been minimal, although the limited studies that have been done indicate a decreased sensitivity to mechanical pain in older people (Pickering, Jourdan, Eschalier, & Dubray, 2002). Studies have not revealed an age effect for electrical pain thresholds. Furthermore, understanding the effects of aging on the experience of pain is complicated by the chronic diseases that are common in late life. For example, it could be that older adults do not have reduced pain sensitivity but rather experience a decreased transmission of signals associated with diseased tissues. Much remains to be learned about the relationship of aging and pain perception.

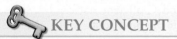

KEY CONCEPT

Research is inconclusive concerning the role of aging on pain perception and tolerance; therefore, the nurse must try to assess and understand each patient's unique pain experience.

Effects of Unrelieved Pain

Unrelieved pain can lead to many complications for older adults. For example, if movement causes pain, the person may limit mobility and, consequently, develop pressure ulcers, pneumonia, and constipation. The individual experiencing pain may have a poor appetite or lack the motivation to eat and drink properly; malnutrition and dehydration can result. The experience of chronic or unrelenting pain can cause a person to become depressed, hopeless, and spiritually distressed. To provide adequate relief from pain and reduce the risk of complications, effective pain management is essential.

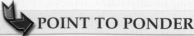

POINT TO PONDER

Reflect on the worst pain you have experienced. How did that affect your activities, relationships, and outlook?

PAIN ASSESSMENT

Effective pain management begins with qualitative and quantitative assessment of this symptom. Inquiries into the presence of pain are an essential component of every assessment. When patients indicate that they experience pain, nurses can ask them to describe it through the use of questions similar to those shown in Assessment Guide 16-1. Questions that facilitate descriptive rather than yes-or-no answers offer better insights into the pain experience. If medications are used for pain management, ask specific questions about the type, dosage, frequency, and effectiveness. The more detailed the pain history, the better the likelihood of developing an effective pain management plan.

Physical examination offers additional insights into patients' pain. Painful areas identified during the interview should be examined for discoloration, swelling, trigger points, and other signs. The nurse notes sensitivity to touch and restricted movement to the area, along with body language indicative of pain (e.g., grimacing, favoring a side, or rubbing an area).

Ongoing assessment is essential to determine the status of the pain and effectiveness of interventions.

Patients with cognitive impairments present special challenges to pain assessment. These individuals may not have the ability to interpret or report their symptoms; therefore, a greater burden falls on the nurse to adequately identify and assess pain. Box 16-1 lists signs that could indicate pain in persons who are cognitively impaired. That patients with cognitive impairments do not offer specific complaints does not mean they are free from pain. When the nurse identifies a patient's unique manifestations of pain, he or she should ensure they are well documented in the health record for future reference in assessment.

Cultural factors must also be considered during the pain assessment. In some cultures, people may be socialized to tolerate pain without expression, whereas in other groups, dramatic expression of pain may be the norm. Likewise, some men may have been raised with the belief that "real men don't admit to pain" and not acknowledge the severity of their discomfort. These factors support that the nurse must be thorough and astute when assessing pain.

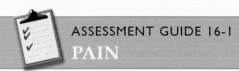

ASSESSMENT GUIDE 16-1
PAIN

MEDICAL HISTORY

- Acute conditions
- Chronic conditions
- Surgeries
- Medications
- Significant recent events (e.g., relocation, death of spouse, fall)

GENERAL OBSERVATIONS

- Grimacing, crying, moaning, clutching fists
- Limitations of movement
- Favoring or rubbing of specific body part
- Discoloration
- Swelling

INTERVIEW

- Where is the pain located? Does it stay in one place or travel to other locations?
- What does it feel like? Stabbing? Throbbing? Aching? Dull? Sharp?
- On a scale of 0 to 10, with 0 being no pain and 10 being unbearable pain, how would you rate it as typically being? How would you rate it when it is at its best? At its worst?
- How frequently does it occur? Several times a day? Daily? A few times a week? Every few weeks?

- How long does it last? A few seconds? A few hours? All day?
- Is the pain related to any medical problems, injuries, or unusual events?
- What factors seem to bring it on?
- What factors worsen it? Activity? Weather? Stress?
- Is it worse at certain times of the day?
- What helps to relieve the pain? Medications? Positions? Special treatments?
- If medications are used, what are they, what is their dosage, how are they taken, and what effects do they produce?
- Are any complementary or alternative therapies used? If so, what, how, and with what results?
- How does the pain affect your life? sleep? appetite? activity? socialization? self-care? home responsibilities? relationships?

PHYSICAL EXAMINATION

- Range of motion
- Sensitivity to touch, guarding
- Temperature of affected area as compared with adjacent areas
- Weakness, numbness
- Swelling
- Bruises, cuts
- Inflammation

BOX 16-1 | Signs That Could Indicate Pain in Persons With Cognitive Impairments

Grimacing
Crying, moaning
Increased vital signs
Perspiration
Increased pacing, wandering
Aggressive behaviors
Hitting, banging on objects
Splinting or guarding body part
Agitation
Poorer function
Change in sleep pattern
Change in appetite or intake
Decreased socialization

A variety of pain assessment instruments provide standardized methods for objectively evaluating pain such as the following:

- *Numeric rating scale.* This commonly used tool asks the patient to rate pain on a scale from 1 to 10, with 1 representing minimal pain and 10 the worst pain imaginable. The scale can be difficult for older adults who have trouble thinking in abstract terms and has been found unreliable in persons who are cognitively impaired (Ferrell, Ferrell, & Rivera, 1995).

- *Visual analog scale.* This simple but effective pain assessment tool uses a horizontal line with "no pain" on the left end and "pain as bad as it can possibly be" on the right end (Carr, Jacox, & Chapman, 1992). The patient indicates where his or her pain falls on the scale. A modified version of this tool uses faces, with 0 being a smile and 6 being a crying grimace.

- *McGill Pain Questionnaire.* This popular and widely used tool contains 78 words categorized into 20 groups, a drawing of the body, and a Present Pain Intensity scale (Melzack & Katz, 2001). This tool is effective for use with persons who are either cognitively normal or impaired (Ferrell et al., 1995). Its length and reliance on reading or hearing the items can pose problems with some individuals.

Barriers to using standardized tools must be considered. Patients need to receive clear instructions and have an opportunity to practice using the tool. Using the same tool consistently facilitates the collection of data that are comparable and meaningful.

The fact that patients have not complained about pain does not guarantee its absence in their lives. Approximately 25% of pain sufferers do not inform their physicians about their pain and another 43.2% informed their physicians when there was at least moderate interference with their activities and sleep (Watkins, Wollan, Melton, & Yawn, 2006). The reality that many people attempt to live with pain reinforces the importance of nurses inquiring about this symptom with routine assessments.

AN INTEGRATIVE APPROACH TO PAIN MANAGEMENT

Nurses can be influential in guiding the development of a pain management plan that is individualized and comprehensive. Before implementing symptomatic treatment, underlying causes for the pain need to be identified and corrected as possible. Goals set the foundation for the interventions planned and need to be realistic, specific, and achievable, for example:

- reduce pain level from 9 to ≤5 within the next 5 days
- obtain at least 5 hours of sleep without interruptions from pain
- independently bathe and dress without restrictions from pain within the next week

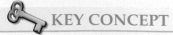 **KEY CONCEPT**

In addition to medical problems, poor positioning or posture, inactivity, emotional issues, and adverse drug reactions could be at the root of new or worsened pain. Improving these underlying factors is the first step in pain management.

Even if the underlying causes for pain cannot be identified or corrected, nurses can still plan interventions to manage what may be chronic pain (Nursing Diagnosis Highlight: Chronic Pain).

Common components of pain management plans include complementary therapies, dietary changes, medications, and comforting nursing care.

Complementary Therapies

Although medications have a significant role in pain management, they should not be the only approach used. Increasingly, therapies that once were considered "alternative" or "unorthodox" are being used as complementary approaches to pain management as part of effective integrative care. Using this vision for added options to address pain, possible interventions that could be used in a comprehensive pain management program include:

- *Acupressure:* use of pressure over points along meridians (what in traditional Chinese medicine are believed to be invisible channels of energy [qi] running through the body) to unblock energy flow and restore or promote the balance of qi
- *Acupuncture:* placement of needles under the skin at acupoints along meridians to unblock energy flow and restore or promote the balance of qi
- *Aromatherapy:* branch of herbal medicine that uses scents from the essential oils of plants to create physiological and emotional effects (e.g., use of lavender, geranium, rose, and sandalwood scents to calm)
- *Biofeedback:* process of teaching people to bring specific bodily functions under voluntary control
- *Chiropractic:* use of manipulation or adjustment of the spine and joints to correct misalignments that can be causing dysfunction and pain
- *Electrical stimulation:* use of electrical currents administered to the skin and muscles via electrodes placed on the painful part of the body
- *Exercises:* gentle stretching and range of motion exercises
- *Guided imagery:* suggesting images that can create specific reactions in body
- *Heat and cold therapies:* use of hot or cold pads, packs, dips (e.g., paraffin), baths, massage, or environments (e.g., sauna)
- *Herbal medicine:* use of plants for therapeutic benefit (Box 16-2)
- *Homeopathic remedies:* use of dilute forms of biological material (plant, animal, or mineral) that produce symptoms similar to that caused by the disease or condition
- *Hypnosis:* guiding person into trancelike state in which increased receptivity to suggestion is possible
- *Massage:* manipulation of soft tissue by using rubbing, kneading, rolling, pressing, slapping,

| BOX 16-2 | **Herbs Used for Pain Management** |

Because many herbs can interact with medications, the nurse should consult with an herb-knowledgeable professional before suggesting the use of any herb. Herbs commonly used to help manage pain include the following:

- *Capsaicin/capsicum (chili pepper oil):* used topically for joint and nerve pain; relief provided within a few days
- *Devil's claw:* effective for inflammatory-related pain; taken orally in dried or extract form; can take several weeks to work

- *Feverfew:* beneficial for prevention of migraines; used orally; best to take in capsule or extract form because plant leaves can be highly irritating to the mouth
- *Ginger:* reduces inflammation and nausea
- *Turmeric:* useful with inflammatory conditions
- *Valerian:* relaxes muscles; has a mild sedative effect
- *White willow:* relieves inflammation and general pain

and tapping movements (called bodywork when combined with deep tissue manipulation, movement awareness, and energy balancing)

- *Meditation:* using deep relaxation to calm the body and mind and focus on the present
- *Naturopathy:* use of proper nutrition, pure water, fresh air, exercise, rest, and other natural means
- *Osteopathy:* branch of physical medicine that uses physical therapy, joint manipulation, and postural correction
- *Prayer:* petition to God or other divine power through direct or intercessory praying

- *Progressive relaxation:* series of exercises that help the body achieve a state of deep relaxation
- *Supplements:* use of specific nutritional products (e.g., B-complex vitamins to enhance function of nervous system; bromelain, fish oil, ginger, turmeric, and devil's claw to reduce inflammation; topical capsaicin to block pain signal; feverfew and vitamin B_2 to reduce migraines)
- *Touch:* Therapeutic Touch and Healing Touch are forms of energy healing in which the caregiver places hands over various parts of the patient's body to manipulate the patient's energy field (Box 16-3)

NURSING DIAGNOSIS HIGHLIGHT

CHRONIC PAIN

Overview
Persistent (chronic) pain is a state in which the uncomfortable sensation of pain is not time limited and must be managed on a long-term basis.

Causative or contributing factors
Arthritis, shingles, terminal cancer, phantom limb, depression, ineffectiveness of analgesic

Goal
The patient will experience a reduction in or elimination of pain and safely use effective pain relief measures

Interventions
- Perform a comprehensive assessment to assist in identifying the underlying cause and nature of pain. Review pain relief measures used and their effectiveness.

- If patient currently is not using one, instruct in the use of a scale for self-assessment of pain.
- Teach patient and/or caregivers pain control measures such as guided imagery, self-hypnosis, biofeedback, yoga.
- Discuss benefits of acupuncture, chiropractic, homeopathy, herbs, and other complementary therapies with health care providers and refer accordingly.
- Assure analgesics are used properly.
- Control environmental stimuli that may affect pain (e.g., loud noise, bright lights, and extreme temperatures).
- Use music therapeutically for relaxation.
- Refer to resources for pain management, such as the American Pain Society and National Chronic Pain Outreach Association.
- Monitor level of pain and continued effectiveness of pain relief measures.

BOX 16-3   The Use of Touch for Comfort

Touch has been a means of providing comfort since the earliest of times. In addition to its therapeutic benefits, physical contact through the act of touch conveys caring and warmth, which promotes emotional comfort and well-being. A variety of modalities use some form of touch to promote comfort that nurses can learn; these include:

ACUPRESSURE

A major therapy within traditional Chinese medicine that has existed for over 2,000 years, acupressure uses the application of pressure to specific points on the body. It is based on the belief that there are invisible channels throughout the body called meridians, through which energy (qi) flows. It is believed that illness and symptoms develop when the flow of energy becomes blocked or imbalanced. Placing pressure on the points that correspond to the part of the body experiencing discomfort can bring relief. For example, placing pressure for a few minutes on the depressions at the base of the skull about two inches from the middle of the neck can offer relief from headache pain.

MASSAGE

Massage is widely used as a means to promote comfort and relaxation. It consists of the manipulation of soft tissue by rubbing, kneading, rolling, pressing, slapping, and tapping movements. In addition to back rubs, hand and foot massages can promote relaxation, rest, and comfort.

TOUCH THERAPIES

Therapeutic touch (TT) and Healing Touch (HT) are popular complementary therapies used by nurses to relieve pain, reduce anxiety, and enhance immune function. TT became popular in nursing in the 1970s with the work and research of Delores Krieger who advanced the theory that people are energy fields and that obstructed energy could be responsible for unhealthy states. By drawing on the universal field of energy and transferring this energy to the patient, the patient's own inner resources for healing could be mobilized. Although the word touch is used in its title, TT actually involves minimal physical contact. Instead, the nurse passes his or her hands over the client's body to assess the energy field and mobilizes areas in which energy is blocked by directing energies to that area.

HT is an offshoot of TT that incorporates additional healing approaches to the basic ones of TT to open energy blockages, seal energy leaks, and rebalance the energy field. There is a six-level educational program for HT.

For more information on these therapies, see related associations listed under Resources.

- *Yoga:* discipline that combines breathing exercises, meditation, and specific postures (asanas) to aid in achieving sense of balance and health

POINT TO PONDER

What methods, other than medications, do you use to manage pain? What facilitates or limits your use of complementary and alternative pain management approaches?

Nurses need to be knowledgeable about the uses and contraindications of various therapies to be able to offer guidance to patients. Also, nurses should be familiar with the licensing requirements for various complementary and alternative practitioners and assist patients in locating qualified therapists. Education and counseling are important to ensure patients make informed choices about their therapists.

Dietary Changes

Diet can influence inflammation and its pain, particularly arthritic pain that is common in the older population. Arachidonic acid is a primary precursor in the synthesis of omega-6 to proinflammatory eicosanoids. Therefore, eliminating foods that contain arachidonic acid or that are converted into arachidonic acid can be beneficial to persons who suffer from inflammatory conditions. Foods to consider avoiding include animal products, high-fat dairy products, egg yolks, beef fat, safflower, corn, sunflower, soybean, and peanut oils. White flour, sugars, and "junk foods" also are believed to contribute to inflammation.

A deficiency of B-complex vitamins can contribute to pain caused by damaged or misfiring nerves. Consuming green leafy vegetables can provide B-complex vitamins, along with chemicals that enhance serotonin.

In addition, some foods can reduce or protect against inflammation. Foods rich in omega-3 fatty acids can reduce inflammation; these include cold water fish (e.g., salmon, tuna, sardines, mackerel, and halibut) and their oils, flaxseed and flaxseed oil, canola oils, walnuts, pumpkin seeds, and omega-3 enhanced eggs. Antioxidants offer protection against inflammation, and chief among them are flavonoids. Flavonoids inhibit enzymes that synthesize eicosanoids, thereby interfering with the inflammatory process. Sources of flavonoids include red, purple, and blue fruits, such as berries and their juices; black or green tea; red wine; chocolate; and cocoa. Fresh pineapple also is considered helpful in reducing inflammation. The herbs garlic, ginger, and turmeric (the main ingredient in curry powder) also are believed to have anti-inflammatory effects.

Medication

Using medications to manage pain in older adults can be complicated because of the high number of drugs this age group consumes and unique pharmacokinetics and pharmacodynamics (see Chapter 18). The risk of adverse effects is higher than in younger age groups, but this should not deter analgesic use in older adults. Rather, analgesics need to be used appropriately and monitored closely.

If nonpharmacologic means of pain relief are ineffective and drugs are necessary, it is advisable to begin with the weakest type and dosage of analgesic and gradually increase as necessary. Trials of nonopioids should be used before resorting to opioids. Adjuvant drugs (e.g., tricyclic antidepressants, anticonvulsants, antihistamines, and caffeine) can be useful in the control of nonmalignant pain or in combination with opioid drugs.

Narcotics should be used discriminately in older persons because of the high risk of delirium, falls, decreased respirations, and other side effects. Administering a nonnarcotic analgesic with the narcotic could decrease the amount of narcotic that is needed. Analgesics should be administered regularly to maintain a constant blood level; fear of addiction should not be a factor in appropriately using analgesics to assist patients in achieving relief.

Acetaminophen is the most commonly used drug for mild to moderate pain relief in older people, followed by nonsteroidal anti-inflammatory drugs (NSAIDs), with ibuprofen the most used of this drug group. Before advancing to an opioid analgesic, the patient should try a different NSAID. For moderate to severe pain, opioids of choice include codeine, oxycodone, and hydrocodone; these are available in combination with nonopioids to enhance benefits from the additive effect. Morphine and fentanyl patches are used for severe pain.

Propoxyphene is contraindicated for older adults, because it does not offer any added benefits but has the potential for central nervous system (CNS) and cardiac toxicity. Pentazocine is another drug that should not be used by older persons because of its high risk of causing delirium, seizures, and cardiac and CNS toxicity.

Nurses should closely observe responses to medications to determine if the drug and its schedule of administration are appropriate. Around-the-clock dosing or the use of sustained-release drugs is useful in the management of continuous pain. If at all possible, medications should be administered on a schedule to prevent pain, rather than treat it after it develops.

Regular reevaluation of patients' response to medications is essential. Medications may change in their effectiveness over time, necessitating a change in the prescription. Also, side effects and adverse reactions can develop with drugs that have been used for a long time without incident.

Comforting

Heavy assignments, fast-paced schedules, and pressures to complete tasks are common experiences for nurses in today's health care system. In the midst of all the *doing* that is demanded, the significance of *being* with patients can be minimized. However, comforting and healing occur through the time spent being with patients.

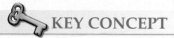
KEY CONCEPT

Healing is not synonymous with being cured. Rather, it implies living in harmony and peace with a health condition.

Granted, the quantity of time nurses have available to spend with patients is limited, but the quality of that time is significant to comforting and healing (Fig. 16-1). Quality time with patients that fosters comforting is reflected by:

- *Giving the patient undivided attention regardless of the length of the interaction.* One method for achieving this is to pause before coming in contact with the patient, take a deep breath, and mentally affirm that you are going to focus on the patient during the time you are together. Sometimes it is helpful to visualize a basket that you are leaving the burdens and tasks of the day in as you enter the patient's room or home.

- *Listening attentively.* Encourage the patient to speak and demonstrate interest through body language and feedback. Feeling that he or she is not heard adds to the patient's discomfort.

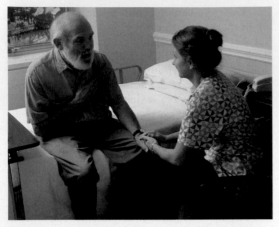

FIGURE 16-1 ■ The quality of time nurses spend with patients is significant to comforting and healing. Spending quality time involves giving patients undivided attention, regardless of the length of the interaction.

■ *Explaining.* Describe procedures, changes, and progress. Do not assume that a patient understands a routine procedure.

■ *Touching.* Gently rubbing the patient's shoulders, massaging the feet, or holding a hand offers a caring, comforting connection.

■ *Perceiving.* Watch for signs that could indicate distress, such as sighing, tear-filled eyes, and flat affect. Validate your observations and inquire about their cause (e.g., "Mrs. Haines, you seem a little distracted today. Is there something you'd like to talk about?"). As tempting as it may be to ignore a problem that is not verbalized, this would not be a healing approach.

 POINT TO PONDER

Have you ever been tempted to ignore a problem that you suspect but that the person hasn't verbalized? What were your motives for doing this?

Assuring patients' comfort is a dynamic process (Fig. 16-2) that requires reevaluation and readjustment as needs and status change. It requires sensitivity by nurses to patients' cues of distress and a commitment to alleviate suffering. It affords an opportunity for nurses to demonstrate the healing art of their profession.

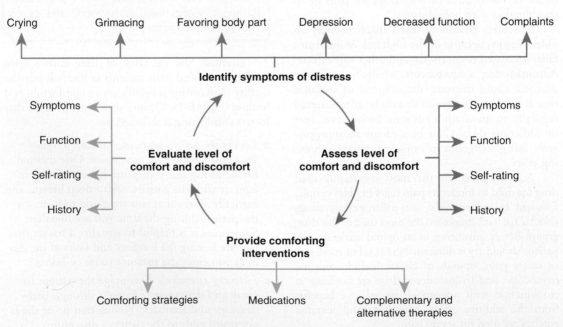

FIGURE 16-2 ■ Pain and comforting cycle.

BRINGING RESEARCH TO LIFE

PAIN ASSESSMENT IN PEOPLE WITH INTELLECTUAL OR DEVELOPMENTAL DISABILITIES

Baldridge, K. H., & Andrasik, F. (2010). American Journal of Nursing, 110(12), 28–37.

Research has shown that people with intellectual or developmental disabilities experience significant rates of acute and chronic pain yet they are often undertreated or not treated at all. Believing that health care professionals either lacked proper skills to assess pain in these populations or did not recognize nonverbal expressions of pain, the authors searched the literature for relevant clinical studies on the issue of pain in people with intellectual or developmental disabilities. They found few studies and reported on those they did find.

Studies have shown that people with intellectual or developmental disabilities can demonstrate self-injurious behaviors (e.g., head banging, hitting self, and throwing self into hard object) when in pain, along with behavioral problems. Communication, daily living skills, socialization, and motor skills could be adversely affected. Caregivers who were familiar with a person's behavior could be reliable reporters of pain in people with intellectual or developmental disabilities; however, family members and other caregivers who were less familiar with the person's behavior and expression of pain may be unreliable in reporting the symptom.

Existing pain assessment tools for people with intellectual or developmental disabilities vary in their reliability and validity and usually have to be adapted for individual use. Additional research related to these tools is needed.

People with cognitive impairments and developmental disabilities suffer from the same types of pain-causing conditions as other individuals; however, they may not be able to adequately communicate their pain. To compensate for this deficit, nurses need to utilize special approaches to assure pain is identified. The lack of the report of pain in people with intellectual or developmental disabilities should not be interpreted as the absence of pain. Nurses should remember that in addition to the objective tools and signs used for pain assessment, learning about the individual and using creative approaches could prove useful.

PRACTICE REALITIES

Eighty-two-year-old Mr. Petro lives in the community with his wife who has dementia. He is very dedicated to his wife and does an outstanding job caring for her and managing the household.

You are aware that Mr. Petro has osteoarthritis and have noticed that he grimaces and displays other signs of pain when he moves. When asked about his symptoms, he admits to having significant pain and says he isn't using any medications as he needs to be alert for his wife. "If it's a choice between being too zonked out on drugs and being mentally and physically sharp," he comments, "I need to go with being sharp." He shows prescriptions for analgesics that he hasn't filled and seems adamant about not using medications.

What could be done to help Mr. Petro address his need for pain management?

CRITICAL THINKING EXERCISES

1. How does society reinforce symptomatic treatment of pain rather than correction of the underlying problem?
2. Develop an integrative care plan for the management of an older adult who experiences chronic arthritis pain.
3. Why could prayer offer relief to someone who is suffering physically and emotionally?
4. Describe possible reasons that reimbursement is provided for medical procedures for pain relief rather than for comforting strategies that nurses could provide.

RESOURCES

American Academy of Pain Management
http://www.aapainmanage.org

American Chronic Pain Association
http://www.theacpa.org

American Massage Therapy Association
www.amtamassage.org

American Pain Society
http://www.ampainsoc.org

Healing Touch International, Inc.
www.healingtouch.net

Massage Bodywork Resource Center
www.massageresource.com

**Nurse Healers and Professional Associates
(Therapeutic Touch)**
www.therapeutic-touch.org

REFERENCES

American Pain Society. (2003). *Principles of analgesic use in the treatment of acute pain and cancer pain.* Glenview, IL: American Pain Society.

Carr, D.B., Jacox, A.K., Chapman, C.R., Ferrel, B., Fields, H.L., Heidrich, G., et al. (1992). *Acute pain management: Operative or medical procedures and trauma. Clinical Practice Guideline No. 1* (AHCPR Publication No. 92-0032). Rockville, MD: AHCPR, Public Health Service, US Department of Health and Human Services.

Ferrell, B. A., Ferrell, B.R., & Rivera, L. (1995). Pain in cognitively impaired nursing home patients. *Pain and Symptom Management, 10*(8):591–598.

Gagliese, L., & Katz, J. (2003). Age differences in postoperative pain are scale dependent: A comparison of measures

of pain intensity and quality in younger and older surgical patients. *Pain, 103*(1), 11–20.

Horgas, A. L., Elliott, A. F., & Marsiske, M. (2009). Pain assessment in persons with dementia. Relationship between self-report and behavioral observation. *Journal of the American Geriatrics Society, 57*(1), 126–132.

International Association for the Study of Pain (2012). Pain terms. Retrieved July 12, 2012 from http://www.iasp-pain.org/AM/Template.cfm?Section=Pain_Definitions&Template=/CM/HTMLDisplay.cfm&ContentID=1728

Lariviere, M., Goffaux, P., Marchand, S., & Julien, N. (2007). Changes in pain perception and descending inhibitory controls start at middle age in healthy adults. *Clinical Journal of Pain, 23*(6), 506–510.

Melzack, R., & Katz, J. (2001). The McGill Pain Questionnaire: Appraisal and current status. In D. Turk & R. Melzack (Eds.), *Handbook on pain assessment* (2nd ed., pp. 35–52). New York, NY: Guilford.

National Center for Health Statistics. (2006). National Center for Health Statistics Report: Health, United States, 2006, Special Feature on Pain. Accessed July 12, 2012 from http://www.cdc.gov/nchs/pressroom/06facts/hus06.htm

Pickering, G., Jourdan, D., Eschalier, A., & Dubray, C. (2002). Impact of age, gender and cognitive functioning on pain perception. *Gerontology, 48,* 112–118.

Watkins, E, Wollan, PC, Melton, LJ, & Yawn, BP. (2006). Silent pain sufferers. *Mayo Clinic Proceedings, 81*(2):167–171.

RECOMMENDED READINGS

Recommended Readings associated with this chapter can be found on the web site that accompanies the book. Visit **http://thepoint.lww.com/Eliopoulos8e** to access the recommended readings and other additional resources associated with this chapter.

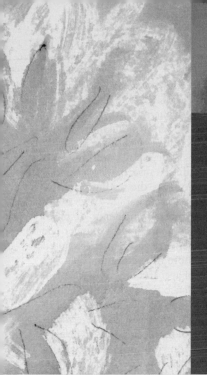

CHAPTER 17

Safety

LEARNING OBJECTIVES

After reading this chapter, you should be able to:

1. Describe the effects of aging on safety.
2. Discuss the significance of the environment to physical and psychological health and well-being.
3. List the impact of age-related changes on the function and safety of the environment.
4. Describe adjustments that can be made to the environment to promote safety and function of older persons.
5. Identify bathroom hazards and ways to minimize them.
6. Discuss the effect of the environment on psychosocial health.
7. List factors that contribute to falls in older adults.
8. List measures to reduce older persons' intrinsic risks to safety and well-being.
9. Discuss unique safety risks of individuals with functional impairments.

CHAPTER OUTLINE

TERMS TO KNOW

Injury: an act that results in harm

Macroenvironment: elements in the larger world that affect groups of people or entire populations

Microenvironment: the immediate surroundings with which a person closely interacts

Restraint: anything that restricts movement; can be physical or chemical

Throughout life, human beings confront threats to their lives and well-being, such as acts of nature, pollutants, communicable diseases, accidents, and crime. Normally, adults take preventive action to avoid these hazards and, should they occur, attempt to control them to minimize their impact. Older persons face the same hazards as any adult, but their risks are compounded by age-related factors that reduce their capacity to protect themselves from and increase their vulnerability to safety hazards. Gerontological nurses need to identify safety risks when assessing older adults and provide interventions to address existing and potential threats to safety, life, and well-being.

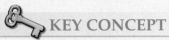

KEY CONCEPT

Age-related changes can reduce the capacity of older adults to protect themselves from injury and increase their vulnerability to safety hazards.

AGING AND RISKS TO SAFETY

The injury rate for older adults falls in the midrange for all age groups, with 196 per 1,000 persons injured among those aged 65 years and older (Department of Commerce, 2010). Older women have a higher rate of injuries than any adult female age group, whereas the rate among men declines through adult years. The death rate from accidents is significant among the older population, with 45, 106, and 287 deaths from injury per 100,000 people in those aged 65 to 74, 75 to 84, and 85 years and older, respectively (Census Bureau, 2012). Accidents rank as the sixth leading cause of death for older adults, with falls leading the cause of injury-related deaths.

Age-related changes, altered antigen–antibody response (see Chapter 29), and the high prevalence of chronic disease cause older persons to be highly susceptible to infections. Pneumonia and influenza rank as the fourth leading cause of death in this age group, and pneumonia is the leading cause of infection-related death (see Chapter 31). Older adults have a threefold greater incidence of nosocomial pneumonia as compared with younger age groups; older adults experience gastroenteritis caused by *Salmonella* species more frequently than persons younger than 65 years of age; and urinary tract infections increase in prevalence with age. Older adults account for more than half of all reported cases of tetanus, endocarditis, cholelithiasis, and diverticulitis. Atypical symptomatology often results in delayed diagnosis of infection, contributing to older adults' higher mortality rate from infections; for instance, older persons are more likely to die from appendicitis than younger persons due to the altered presentation of symptoms delaying diagnosis.

Altered pharmacokinetics, self-administration problems, and the high volume of drugs consumed by older individuals can also lead to considerable risks to safety. Risks include adverse effects and accidents resulting from effects such as drowsiness or dizziness. It is estimated that 5% to 30% of geriatric admissions to hospitals are associated with inappropriate drug administration.

Nursing Diagnosis Table 17-1 lists the various age-related factors that can pose risks to the safety and well-being of older adults and potential nursing problems associated with these risks.

NURSING DIAGNOSIS

TABLE 17-1 Aging and Risks to Safety

Causes or Contributing Factors	Nursing Diagnosis
Decrease in intracellular fluid	Deficient Fluid Volume related to easier development of dehydration
Loss of subcutaneous tissue; less natural insulation; lower basal metabolic rate	Risk of Injury and Risk of Acute Confusion related to hypothermia
Decreased efficiency of heart	Activity Intolerance related to alterations (decrease) in cardiac output
Reduced strength and elasticity of respiratory muscles; decreased lung expansion; inefficient cough response; less ciliary activity	Risk of Infection related to reduced ability to expel accumulated or foreign matter from lungs
Reduced oxygen use under stress	Risk of Ineffective Peripheral Tissue Perfusion and Risk of Ineffective Cerebral Tissue Perfusion related to changes in cardiovascular response to stress
Poor condition of teeth	Risk of Infection related to dental disease or aspirated tooth particles

Weak gag reflex	Risk of Infection related to aspiration
Altered taste sensation	Imbalanced Nutrition: More Than Body Requirements of salt or sweets related to taste deficit
Reduction in filtration of wastes by kidneys	Risk of Injury related to ineffective elimination of wastes from bloodstream
Higher prevalence of urinary retention	Risk of Infection related to stasis of urine
More alkaline vaginal secretions	Risk of Infection related to inadequate acid environment to inhibit bacterial growth
Decreased muscle strength	Risk of Injury related to reduced muscle strength
Demineralization of bone	Risk of Injury and Impaired Physical Mobility related to increased tendency of bones to fracture
Delayed response and reaction time	Risk of Injury related to inability to respond in timely manner
Poor vision and hearing	Risk of Injury and Impaired Home Maintenance related to misperception of environment
Reduced lacrimal secretions	Risk of Injury and Risk of Infection related to decreased ability to protect cornea
Distorted depth perception	Risk of Injury related to decreased ability to judge changes in level of walking surface
Increased threshold for pain and touch	Risk of Injury, Risk of Infection, and Impaired Skin Integrity related to less ability to sense problems, such as pain and pressure
Less elasticity and more dryness and fragility of skin	Impaired Skin Integrity and Risk of Infection related to easier skin breakdown
Poor short-term memory	Risk of Injury and Noncompliance related to inability to recall medication administration, treatments
High prevalence of polypharmacy	Ineffective Health Maintenance and Risk of Injury related to combining drugs inappropriately, drug interactions, and side effects

IMPORTANCE OF THE ENVIRONMENT TO HEALTH AND WELLNESS

The environment can be considered as consisting of two parts, the microenvironment and the macroenvironment. The microenvironment refers to our immediate surroundings with which we closely interact (e.g., furnishings, wall coverings, lighting, room temperature, and room sounds). The macroenvironment consists of the elements in the larger world that affect groups of people or even entire populations (e.g., the weather, pollution, traffic, and natural resources). Because the microenvironment can be more easily manipulated and realizes more immediate benefits, it is the focus of this discussion.

Ideally, the environment provides more than shelter; it should promote continued development, stimulation, and satisfaction to enhance our psychological well-being. This is particularly important for older adults, many of whom spend considerable time in their homes or in a bedroom of a facility. To achieve the fullest satisfaction from their microenvironments, older adults must have various levels of needs met within their surroundings. This can be exemplified by comparing environmental needs with the basic human needs postulated by Maslow (Table 17-2). Similar to Maslow's theory, it can be hypothesized that higher level satisfaction from the environment cannot be achieved unless lower level needs are fulfilled. This may explain why some older individuals have the following priorities and problems:

- They do not think installing a free smoke detector is important when there are rodents in their apartment.
- They refuse to have their house remodeled because it will make them look too affluent in a high-crime neighborhood and be a target for burglary.
- They remain socially isolated rather than invite guests to a house perceived as shabby.

TABLE 17-2 Environmental Needs Based on Maslow's Hierarchy

Basic Human Needs	Environmental Needs
Self-actualization	A space that promotes the realization of all potential, inspiring objects, beautiful grounds, relaxation aids
Self-esteem	A home one can feel pride in having, elegant decor, status symbols
Trust	A niche in which one can feel confident, control over lifestyle, consistent layout/furnishings/temperature/lighting
Love	A place one derives pleasure from being, familiar and comfortable furniture, favorite objects, attractive
Security	A haven from external threats, ability to safeguard personal possessions, adequate lighting, locks, smoke detectors, alarms
Physiological needs	A shelter in which to live, adequate ventilation, room temperature about 75°F (24°C), functioning utilities and appliances, pest control

■ They are unwilling to engage in creative arts and crafts if they are adjusting to a new and unfamiliar residence.

Nurses must be realistic in their assessment of the environment to determine which levels of needs are being addressed and to plan measures to promote the fulfillment of higher level needs.

 POINT TO PONDER

What aspects of your home environment contribute to the fulfillment of the higher level needs based on Maslow's hierarchy?

IMPACT OF AGING ON ENVIRONMENTAL SAFETY AND FUNCTION

Previous chapters have described some of the changes experienced with aging. These, along with limitations imposed by highly prevalent chronic diseases, create special environmental problems for older people, such as those listed in Table 17-3.

Of course, specific disabilities accompany various diseases and create unique environmental problems, as is witnessed with a person who is cognitively impaired.

TABLE 17-3 Potential Environmental Impact of Various Physical Limitations

Limitation	Potential Environmental Impact
Presbyopia	Decreased ability to focus and visualize near objects
Cornea less translucent, transmits less light	More external light needed to produce adequate image on retina
Decreased opacity of sclera, allows more light to enter eye	Colors more washed out, more contrast required
Yellowing of lens	Distorted color vision, particularly for browns, beiges, blues, greens, violets
Senile cataracts cloud lens	Glare more bothersome
Macular degeneration	Vision more difficult, more magnification needed
Senile miosis, pupil size decreased, less light reaches retina	Slower light-to-dark accommodation
Decreased visual field	Peripheral vision narrower
Presbycusis	Distortion of normal sounds
Dependency on hearing aid	Amplification of all environmental sounds
Reduced olfaction	Odors, smoke, gas leaks difficult to detect
Less discriminating touch sensation	Less stimulation from textures
Less body insulation, lower body temperature	More sensitivity to lower environmental temperatures
Slower nerve conduction	Slower response to stimuli, less ability to regain balance
Decreased muscle tone and strength	Increased difficulty rising from a seated position, fatigue easier, less elevation of toes during ambulation, shuffling gait

Stiff joints	Difficulty climbing stairs, manipulating knobs and handles
Urinary frequency, nocturia	Frequent need for easily accessible bathroom
Shortness of breath, easily fatigued	Stairs, long hallways difficult to negotiate
Poor short-term memory	Forget to lock doors, turn off appliances
High use of medications, causing hypotension, dizziness	Increased risk of falls

Based on common limitations found among older people, most older adults need an environment that is safe, functional, comfortable, personal, and normalizing and that compensates for their limitations. Creating such an environment requires considering lighting, temperature, colors, scents, floor coverings, furniture, sensory stimulation, noise control, bathroom hazards, and psychosocial factors. Box 17-1 provides a checklist for assessing basic standards for the older adult's environment.

BOX 17-1 | Environmental Assessment Checklist

Standard	YES	NO	COMMENTS
Smoke detector			
Telephone			
Fire extinguisher			
Vented heating system			
Minimal clutter			
Functioning refrigerator			
Proper food storage			
Adequately lighted hallways and stairways			
Handrails on stairs			
Floor surface even, easy to clean, requiring no wax, free of loose scatter rugs and deep-pile carpets			
Doorways unobstructed, painted a contrasting color from wall			
Bathtub or shower with nonslip surface, safety rails, no electrical outlets nearby			
Hot water temperature less than 110°F (43°C)			
Windows screened, easy to reach and open			
Ample number of safe electrical outlets, probably 3 feet higher than level of floor for easy reach, not overloaded			
Safe stove with burner control on front			
Shelves within easy reach, sturdy			
Faucet handles easy to operate, clearly marked hot and cold			
Proper storage of medications, absence of outdated prescriptions			

For wheelchair use:
- Doorways and hallways clear and wide enough for passage
- Ramps or elevator
- Bathroom layout to provide maneuvering
- Sinks, furniture low enough to reach

Lighting

Light has a more profound effect than simply illuminating an area for better visibility. For example, light affects the following:

- *Function.* An individual may be more mobile and participate in more activities in a brightly lit area, whereas a person in a dim room may be more sedate.
- *Orientation.* An individual may lose the perspective of time in a room that is constantly lit or darkened for long periods. For example, persons exposed to the bright lighting in intensive care units for several days often cannot determine if it is day or night. A person who awakens in a pitch-dark room may be disoriented for a few seconds.
- *Mood and behavior.* Blinking psychedelic lights cause a different reaction from candlelight. In restaurants, customers are quieter and eat more slowly with soft, low illumination levels than with harsh, high ones.

Several diffuse lighting sources rather than a few bright ones are best in areas used by older adults. Fluorescent lights are the most bothersome because of eye strain and glare. The use of fluorescent lighting for economic reasons actually may not be cost-effective; although less expensive to operate, they have higher maintenance costs. Sunlight can be filtered by sheer curtains. The nurse should assess the environment for glare, paying particular attention to light bouncing off shining floors and furniture. Evaluate lighting from a seated position because insufficient lighting, shadows, glare, and other problems can appear differently from chair or bed level than from a standing position.

Nightlights help facilitate orientation during the night and provide visibility to locate light switches or lamps for nighttime mobility. A soft red light can be useful at night in the bedroom to improve night vision.

Exposure to natural light during the normal 24-hour dark–light cycle helps to maintain body rhythms, which, in turn, influence body temperature, sleep cycles, hormone production, and other functions. When the sleep–wake cycle is interrupted, the body's internal rhythms can be disrupted. This factor warrants consideration in hospital and nursing home settings, where areas may be lit around the clock to facilitate staff activities; darkening areas at night can assist in maintaining normal body rhythms. Nurses should also consider the lack of exposure to natural sunlight often experienced by institutionalized or homebound ill older individuals. Consideration should be given to taking these individuals outdoors, when possible, and opening windows to allow natural sunlight to enter.

Temperature

It has been known from Galen's time in 160 AD that hot and cold temperatures affect human beings. Research has shown that a direct correlation exists between body temperature and performance (Cheung, 2007). Tactile sensitivity, vigilance performance, and psychomotor tasks become impaired in temperatures below 55°F (13°C).

Because older adults have lower normal body temperatures and decreased amounts of natural insulation, they are especially sensitive to lower temperatures (Fig. 17-1); thus, maintaining adequate environmental temperature is significant. The recommended room temperature for an older person should not be lower than 75°F (24°C). The older the person is, the narrower the range of temperatures tolerated without adverse reactions. Room temperatures less than 70°F (21°C) can lead to hypothermia in older adults.

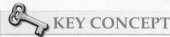

KEY CONCEPT

Older adults are sensitive to lower environmental temperatures because of their lower body temperature and decreased amount of natural insulation.

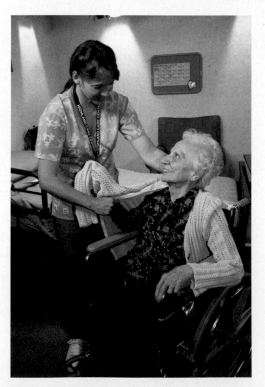

FIGURE 17-1 ■ Because older adults are especially sensitive to lower temperatures, controlling the environmental temperature is important. Additional layers of clothing may also be needed.

Although not as significant a problem as hypothermia, hyperthermia can also create difficulty for older persons, who are more susceptible to its ill effects than younger adults. Brain damage can result from temperatures exceeding 106°F (41°C). Even in geographic areas that do not experience excessively high temperatures, consideration must be given to the temperature of rooms or homes in which doors and windows are not opened and no air conditioning is present. Persons with diabetes or cerebral atherosclerosis are at high risk for becoming hyperthermic.

Colors

There is much debate concerning the best environmental color scheme for older people. Colors such as red, yellow, and white can be stimulating and increase pulse, blood pressure, and appetite, whereas blue, brown, and earth tones can be relaxing. Orange can stimulate appetite, whereas violet has the opposite effect. Green is considered the master healer color and gives a sense of well-being. Black and gray can be depressing. Although certain colors are associated with certain effects, experiences with colors play a significant part in individual reactions to and meanings inferred from various colors. Because individual response can vary, it may be best to focus on the use of colors to enhance function and, whenever possible, on the personal preference of the room's resident. Contrasting colors are helpful in defining doors, stairs, and level changes within an area. When the desire is to not draw attention to an area (e.g., a storage closet), walls should be a similar color or within the same color family. Certain colors may be used to define different areas; for example, bedrooms may be blue and green, eating and activity areas orange and red, and lounge areas gray and beige.

Patterned wall and floor coverings can add appeal to the environment; however, wavy patterns and diagonal lines can cause a sensation of dizziness and could worsen the confusion of persons with cognitive impairments. Using a simple pattern or a mural on one wall of the room can be effective and pleasing.

Scents

Scents have been used for aesthetic and medicinal purposes from the earliest of times. Although the use of perfumes and colognes is hardly new, the therapeutic use of scents, aromatherapy (or phytomedicine), has become popular in the United States only recently. However, it is a commonly used extension of orthodox medicine in countries such as Germany and France.

Involving more than just the smelling of pleasant fragrances, aromatherapy is the therapeutic use of essential oils. Essential oils are highly volatile droplets made by plants and stored in their veins, glands, or sacs; when they are released (by crushing or breaking

open the plant), the aroma is released along with them. When the chemicals within the essential oils are inhaled, they are carried to the olfactory bulb, stimulating nerve impulses that travel to the limbic system of the brain for processing. An organ called the amygdala is housed in the limbic system and stores memories associated with different scents. In some cases, the memories can be dormant for many years.

Essential oils can also be absorbed through the skin through baths, compresses, or rubbing or massaging them onto the skin surface. Like topical medications, these oils are absorbed and produce physiologic effects.

Floor Coverings

Carpeting is an effective sound absorber, and for most people it represents warmth, comfort, and a homelike atmosphere. There even has been speculation that the use of carpeting in institutional settings can reduce the number of fractures associated with falls. However, carpeting does create problems, which include the following:

- *Static electricity and cling.* Many older persons have a shuffling gait and incomplete toe lift during ambulation; this can produce uncomfortable static electricity, and the clinging of slippers and shoe soles to the carpeting could cause falls.
- *Difficult wheelchair mobility.* The more plush the carpet is, the more difficult it becomes to roll wheels on its surface.
- *Cleaning.* Spills are more difficult to clean on a carpeted surface; even with washable surfaces, discoloration can result.
- *Odors.* Cigarette smoke and other odors can cling to carpeting, creating unpleasant odors that last. Urine, vomitus, and other substances demand special deodorizing efforts that may not prove effective.
- *Pests.* The undersurface of carpeting provides a wonderful environment in which cockroaches, moths, fleas, and other pests can reside.

To derive some of the benefits of carpeting, carpeting may be applied to some of the wall surface rather than the floor. This can provide a noise buffer, textural variation, and a decor with fewer housekeeping and maintenance problems than floor carpeting.

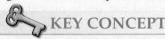 **KEY CONCEPT**

Carpeting a portion of the wall can provide a buffer for noise and offer a variation in room decor.

Scattered and area rugs provide an ideal source for falls and should not be used. Tiled floor covering should be laid on a wood foundation rather than directly on a cement surface for better insulation and cushion. Bold designs can cause dizziness and confusion in ambulation; a single solid color is preferable. A nonglare surface is essential for older adults. Floor treatments that create a nonslip surface are particularly useful in bathrooms, kitchens, and areas leading from outside doors.

Furniture

Furnishings should be appealing, functional, and comfortable. A firm chair with arm rests provides support and assistance in rising from or lowering into the seat; low, sinking cushions are difficult for older people to use. Chairs should also be of an appropriate height to allow the individual's feet to rest flat on the floor with no pressure behind the knees. Rockers provide relaxation and some exercise to older people. Love seats are preferable to larger sofas because no one risks being seated in the center without arm rests for assistance.

Upholstery for all furniture should be easy to clean, so leather and vinyl coverings are more useful than cloth. Upholstery should be fire resistant, with a firm surface without buttons or seams in areas that come in contact with the body. Rather than the back, seat, and arm rest being one connecting unit, open space where these sections meet allows for ventilation and easier cleaning. Recliners can promote relaxation and provide a means for leg elevation, but they should not require strenuous effort to change positions.

Tables, bookcases, and other furniture should be sturdy and able to withstand weight from persons leaning for support. If table lamps are used, bolting them to the table surface can prevent their being knocked over in an attempt to locate them in the dark. Foot stools, candlestick tables, plant stands, and other small pieces of furniture would be best placed in low-traveled areas, if they are present at all. Furniture and clutter should not obstruct the path from the bedroom to the bathroom.

Drawers should be checked for ease of use. Sanding and waxing the corners and slides can facilitate their movement. In hanging mirrors, the height and function of the user must be considered; obviously, persons confined to wheelchairs will need a lower level than their ambulatory counterparts.

Individuals with cognitive impairments need a particularly simple environment. Furniture should look like furniture and not pieces of sculpture. The use of furniture should be clear. Placement of a commode chair next to a sitting chair can be confusing and result in the improper use of both.

Sensory Stimulation

By making thoughtful choices and capitalizing on the objects and activities of daily life, much can be done to create an environment that is pleasing and stimulating to the senses. Some suggestions are:

- textured wall surfaces
- soft blankets and spreads
- differently shaped and textured objects to hold (e.g., a round sheepskin-covered throw pillow and a square tweed-covered one)
- murals, pictures, sculptures, and wall hangings
- plants and freshly cut flowers
- coffee brewing, food cooking, perfumes, and oils
- birds to listen to and animals to pet
- soft music

Different areas in the person's living space can be created for different sensory experiences. The appetite of nursing home residents could be much improved if, within their own dining area, they could smell the aroma of their coffee brewing or bread toasting rather than just having the finished product placed on a tray before them.

For bed-bound persons or those with limited opportunity for sensory stimulation, special efforts are necessary. In addition to the suggestions given, one could regularly change the wall hangings in their rooms. Many libraries and museums will loan artwork free of charge. Collaboration with a local school can yield unique art for the older person and meaningful art projects for the students. A "sensory stimulation box" that contains objects of different textures, shapes, colors, and fragrances could provide an activity.

Noise Control

Sound produces a variety of physiologic and emotional effects. Many of the sounds we take for granted—television, traffic noise, conversation from an adjoining room, appliance motors, leaking faucets, and paging systems—can create difficulties for the older person. Many older adults already experience some hearing limitation as a result of presbycusis and need to be especially attentive to compensate for this deficit.

Environmental sounds compete with the sounds that older adults want or need to hear, such as a telephone conversation or the evening news, resulting in poor hearing and frustration. Unwanted, disharmonic, or chronic noise can be a stressor and cause physical and emotional symptoms.

Ideally, noise control begins with the design of the building. Careful landscaping and walls can buffer outdoor noise. Acoustical ceilings, drapes, and carpeting—also useful on walls—are helpful, as is attention to appliance and equipment maintenance. Radios and televisions should not be playing when no one is listening; if one person needs a louder volume, earphones for that individual can prevent others from being exposed to high volumes. In institutional settings, individual pocket pagers are less disruptive than intercoms and paging systems.

Bathroom Hazards

Many accidental injuries occur in the bathroom and can be avoided with common sense and inexpensive measures. Particular attention should be paid to the following aspects:

- *Lighting.* A small light should be on in the bathroom at all times. Because urinary frequency and nocturia are common, older adults use the bathroom often and can benefit from the increased visibility. Constant lighting is especially helpful if the switch is located outside the bathroom, so that the individual does not have to enter a dark area and then search for a switch.

- *Floor surface.* Towels, hair dryers, and other items should not be left on the bathroom floor, and throw rugs should not be used. For older people, falls are dangerous under any circumstance, but the high likelihood of falling and striking one's head on the hard surface of a tub or toilet increases the potential seriousness of the fall. Leaks should be corrected to avoid creating slippery floors, which are another cause of falls.

- *Faucets.* Lever-shaped faucet handles are easier to use than round ones or those that must have pressure exerted on them. Older people can risk falling or burning themselves by releasing too much hot water as they struggle to turn a faucet handle. This problem supports the need to control hot water temperature centrally. Color coding the faucet handles makes differentiation of hot and cold easier than small letters alone.

- *Tubs and shower stalls.* Nonslip surfaces are essential for tubs and shower floors. Grab bars on the wall and safety rails attached to the side of the tub offer support during transfers and a source of stabilization when bathing (Fig. 17-2). A shower or bath seat offers a place to sit when showering and, for tub bathers, a resting point when lifting to transfer out of the tub. Because a drop in blood pressure may follow bathing, it may be beneficial to have a seat alongside the tub to enable the bather to rest when drying.

- *Toilets.* Grab bars or support frames aid in the difficult task of sitting down and rising from a toilet seat. Because the low height of toilet seats makes them difficult for many older people to use, a raised seat attachment could prove useful.

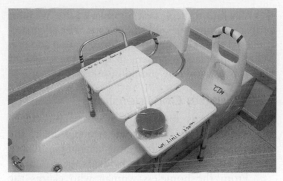

FIGURE 17-2 ■ Safety features in this shower include grab bars, safety rails, shower seat, and transfer seat.

- *Electrical appliances.* The use of electric heaters, hair dryers, and radios in the bathroom produces a considerable safety risk. Even healthy, agile persons can accidentally slip and pull an electrical appliance into the tub with them.

Medical supply stores and health care equipment suppliers offer a variety of devices that can make the bathroom and other living areas safer and more functional. Sometimes less expensive replicas can be homemade and be equally effective. It is much wiser to invest in and use these assistive devices to prevent an injury than to wait until an injury occurs.

Fire Hazards

Older adults have a risk of burn injuries as a result of common hazards in the home. Kitchen fires often result when unattended pots with boiling liquids become dry, because the person has forgotten them. Older individuals can aid in preventing these fires by staying in the kitchen while cooking, setting a timer to remind them to check the pot, or using a microwave to heat liquids.

Careless disposal of matches or cigarette butts, falling asleep holding a cigarette, and clothing or linens catching fire while a cigarette is being lit are potential risks to older smokers. Older smokers need to be cautioned about these risks. Restricting smoking to specific locations and times of the day can aid in reducing the risks.

For those older adults who rely on space heaters, inspection of the heater is beneficial in assuring its safety. Space heaters should have an automatic shut-off mechanism to prevent fire if the heater is knocked over or falls and intact electrical cords. They should be used with an appropriate electrical outlet (i.e., one that is not overloaded).

Fireplaces may provide warmth and a cozy atmosphere, but can also cause fires. Wood burning fireplaces need cleaning to prevent chimney blockage;

this may be a difficult task for older adults. Without proper cleaning, fire and smoke cannot be adequately vented and can result in smoke inhalation and fire. When a fireplace is present in the home, questions about its use and care should be asked.

Psychosocial Considerations

Physical objects form only a partial picture of the environment. The human elements make the picture complete. Feelings and behavior influence and are influenced by the individual's surroundings.

From the homeless woman who claims the same department store alcove as her resting place each night to the nursing home resident who forbids anyone to open her bedside cabinet, most people want a space to define as their own. This territoriality is natural and common; many of us would become uncomfortable with a visitor to our office sifting through the papers on our desk, a house guest looking through our closets, or a stranger snuggling close to us on a subway when the rest of the seats are empty. The annoyance we feel at having someone looking into our window, peering over a privacy fence into our yard, playing music loudly enough to be heard in our home, or staring at us demonstrates that our personal space and privacy can be invaded without direct physical contact.

To the dependent, ill, older person, privacy and personal space are no less important, but they may be more difficult to achieve. In an institutional setting, staff and other patients may make uninvited contact with a person's territory and self at any time, ranging from the confused resident who wanders into others' rooms to staff members who lift blankets to check if the bed is dry. Even in the home, well-intentioned relatives may not think twice about discarding or moving personal possessions in the name of housekeeping or entering a bathroom unannounced just to ensure that all is well. The more dependent and ill individuals are, the more personal space and privacy may be invaded. Unfortunately, for these individuals who have experienced multiple losses and a shrinking social world, the regulation of privacy and personal space may be one of the few controls they can exercise. It is important that caregivers realize and respect this need through several basic measures:

- Define specific areas and possessions that are the individual's (e.g., this side of the room; this room in the house; this chair, bed, or closet).

- Provide privacy areas for periods of solitude. If a private room is not available, arrange furniture to achieve maximum privacy (e.g., beds on different sides of the room facing different directions, use of bookshelves and plants as room dividers).

- Request permission to enter personal space. Imagine an invisible circle of about 5 to 10 feet around the person and ask before coming into it: "May I sit your new roommate next to you?" "Is it all right to come in?" "May I clean the inside of your closet?"

- Allow maximum control over one's space.

KEY CONCEPT

It is important for the nurse to recognize the older adult's need for personal space. Regulation of personal space and privacy may be among the few existing controls that can be exercised by persons who have experienced multiple losses and a shrinking social world.

Components of the environment can facilitate or discourage mental and social activity. Clocks, calendars, and newspapers promote orientation and knowledge of current events. Easily accessible books and magazines challenge the mind and expand horizons. Games and hobbies can offer stimulation and an alternative to watching television. The placement of chairs in clusters or in busy but not heavily trafficked areas is conducive to interaction and involvement with a larger world.

Although fewer than 5% of older adults reside in nursing homes, approximately 25% of older persons will spend some time in such a facility during their last years of life. Nursing homes are not reflections of normal homelike environments; adjustment to them can be difficult. Familiar surroundings are replaced with new and strange sights, sounds, odors, and people. Cues that triggered memory and function are gone, and new ones must be mastered at a time when reserves are low. Relatives and neighbors who gave love and understanding are replaced with people who know only that person before them now and who have many tasks to be done. The individual who is experiencing this may have a variety of reactions, such as:

- depression over the loss of health, personal possessions, and independence

- regression because of the inability to manage the stress at hand

- humiliation by having to request basic necessities and minor desires, such as toileting, a cup of tea, or a cigarette

- anger at the loss of control and freedom

Nursing homes cannot offer the same satisfaction as the person's own home, but the institutional environment can be enhanced through:

- an attractive decor
- inclusion of the individual's personal possessions
- respect for privacy and personal territory
- recognition of the individuality of the resident
- allowance of maximum control over activities and decision making
- environmental modifications to compensate for deficits

The human environment will be more important to the nursing home resident than the physical surroundings. Superior interior decoration and lovely color schemes mean little when respect, individuality, and sensitivity are absent.

THE PROBLEM OF FALLS WATCH&LEARN

One of the significant concerns about safety in later life relates to the incidence of falls. Studies have indicated that one third of persons aged 75 years and older experience a fall each year and half of these experience multiple falls (Centers for Disease Control and Prevention [CDC], 2004, 2007). The consequences of falls are serious; 20% of the hospital and 40% of the nursing home admissions of older adults are related to falls (Sterling, O'Connor, & Bonadies, 2001). Even if no physical injury occurs, fall victims may develop a fear of falling again (i.e., postfall syndrome) and reduce their activities as a result; this can lead to unnecessary dependency, loss of function, decreased socialization, and a poor quality of life.

Risks and Prevention

Many factors contribute to the high incidence of falls in older adults (Box 17-2). Common risk factors include the following:

- *Age-related changes*: reduced visual capacity; problems differentiating shades of the same color, particularly blues, greens, and violets; cataracts; poor vision at night and in dimly lit areas; less foot and toe lift during stepping; altered center of gravity leading to balance being lost more easily; slower responses; urinary frequency

---

BOX 17-2   **Risk Factors for Falls**

AGE-RELATED FACTORS

History of falls
Female aged 75 years and older
Impaired vision
Gait disturbance
Postural hypotension

HEALTH CONDITIONS OR FUNCTIONAL IMPAIRMENTS

Physical disability
Incontinence, nocturia
Delirium, dementia
Mood disturbance
Dizziness
Weakness
Fatigue
Ataxia
Paralysis
Edema
Use of cane, walker, wheelchair, crutch, or brace
Use of restraint
Presence of IV, indwelling catheter
Unstable cardiac condition
Neurologic disease
Parkinsonism

Transient ischemic attack
Cerebrovascular accident
Diabetes mellitus
Peripheral vascular disease
Orthopedic disease
Foot problems
Multiple diagnoses

MEDICATIONS

Antidepressants
Antihypertensives
Antipsychotics
Diuretics
Sedatives
Tranquilizers
Multiple medications

ENVIRONMENTAL FACTORS

Newly admitted to hospital/nursing home
Unfamiliar environment
Highly polished floors
Inadequate environmental lighting
Absence of railings, grab bars
Poor environmental design
Clutter, equipment

- *Improper use of mobility aids*: using canes, walkers, wheelchairs without being prescribed, properly fitted, or instructed in safe use; not using brakes during transfers
- *Medications*: particularly those that can cause dizziness, drowsiness, orthostatic hypotension, and incontinence, such as antihypertensives, sedatives, antipsychotics, diuretics
- *Unsafe clothing*: poor-fitting shoes and socks, long robes or pants legs
- *Disease-related symptoms*: postural hypotension, incontinence, reduced cerebral blood flow, edema, dizziness, weakness, fatigue, brittle bones, paralysis, ataxia, mood disturbances, confusion
- *Environmental hazards*: wet surfaces, waxed floors, objects on floor, poor lighting
- *Caregiver-related factors*: improper use of restraints and bedrails, delays in responding to requests, unsafe practices, poor supervision of problem behaviors

A history of falls can predict an individual's risk of future falls; therefore, nurses should carefully assess persons who have experienced a fall or even a minor stumble to identify factors that may increase their risk of this problem. Interventions should be planned accordingly.

Caution is needed to address the risk of falls associated with postural hypotension. This is a common problem that causes dizziness when older adults first stand after awakening. On awakening, older adults should spend several minutes resting in bed and stretching their muscles, followed by several more minutes of sitting on the side of the bed before rising to a standing position. The orthostatic effect of rising to a standing position after bathing, coupled with the dilation of peripheral vessels from the warm bath water, also leads to fainting and falls. Rubber mats or nonslip strips, a bath seat, and resting before rising are essential measures in the bathtub.

Health care facilities can find it beneficial to have an active program to prevent falls that incorporates some of the interventions described in the Nursing Diagnosis Highlight: Risk for Injury. Regular, careful inspection of the environment and prompt correction of environmental hazards (e.g., leaks, cracks in walkways, and broken bed rails) are essential (see Box 17-1). An evaluation of risk of falling should be incorporated into the assessment of each older client. The Hendrich II Fall Risk Model is a short tool that aids in assessing fall risk (see Resources

at the end of this chapter). Staff should orient older clients to new environments and reinforce safe practices, such as using bed rails, braking wheelchairs and stretchers during transfers, and promptly cleaning spills.

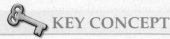

KEY CONCEPT

A program to prevent falls is essential to settings that provide services to older adults.

Some falls will occur despite the best preventive measures. Caregivers should assess the fall victim and keep him or her immobile until a full examination for injury is done. Skin breaks or discoloration, swelling, bleeding, asymmetry of extremities, lengthening of a limb, and pain are among the findings to note. Medical examination and x-rays are warranted for even the slightest suspicion of a fracture or other serious injury. Fractures often are not readily apparent immediately after the fall; it may be only when the person attempts to resume normal activity that the injured bone becomes misaligned. Also, areas other than the direct point of impact may be injured in the fall; for instance, a person may have fallen on the knee, but the force of the fall may have placed enough stress on the hip to fracture the femur. Careful examination and observation can aid in the prompt diagnosis of injury and introduction of appropriate treatment.

In addition to physical injury resulting from a fall, older adults may experience psychological trauma. Falls can cause an older adult to feel vulnerable and fearful of losing independence. Unnecessary restriction of activity may result. Patients may share this information during the assessment when asked about falls; further, possible signs could indicate a fear of falling, such as excess caution in changing positions and ambulating, unnecessarily restricting mobility, grabbing furniture or a wall while walking or transferring, or apparent anxiety when ambulating. It can be useful to offer suggestions for preventing falls (e.g., wearing safe shoes, keeping areas well lighted, holding on to rails when climbing stairs, and avoiding climbing ladders) while encouraging maximum activity.

Risks Associated With Restraints

Throughout most of the 20th century, restraints were widely used in health care settings under the belief that they would prevent falls, promote

NURSING DIAGNOSIS HIGHLIGHT

RISK OF INJURY

Overview

Many older persons are limited in their ability to protect themselves from hazards to their health and well-being. Indications that this diagnosis exists can be manifested through a history of frequent falls or accidents, the presence of an unsafe environment, adverse drug reactions, infections, frequent hospitalizations, and altered mood or cognition.

Causative or contributing factors

Age-related changes, health problems, weak or immobile state, sensory deficits, improperly fitted or used mobility aids, unsafe use of medications, unsafe environment, altered mood or cognitive function.

Goal

The patient is free from injury.

Interventions

- Assess risk of injury to patient (e.g., falls risk, activities of daily living and impaired activities of daily living function, mental status, gait, medication use, nutritional status, environment, knowledge of injury prevention practices).
- Identify patients at high risk for injury and plan measures to reduce their specific risks.
- Orient patients to new environments.
- Encourage patients to wear prescribed eyeglasses, hearing aids, and prosthetic devices.
- Ensure patients use canes, walkers, and wheelchairs properly and only when prescribed.

- Avoid the use of physical or chemical restraints unless assessed to be absolutely necessary; use proper procedures to ensure safety when they are used.
- Advise patients to change positions slowly, holding on to a stable object as they do.
- Keep floors free from litter and clutter.
- Provide good lighting in all areas used by patient.
- Store cleaning solutions and other poisonous substances in a safe area.
- Encourage patients to use handrails and grab bars.
- Assist patients as needed with transfers.
- Review medications used for continued need, effectiveness, appropriateness of dosage; instruct patients in safe medication use.
- Be sure patients wear well-fitted, low-heeled shoes and robes and pants of an appropriate length.
- Promptly detect and obtain treatment for changes in physical or mental health status.
- Review home environment for safety risks and assist patient in obtaining assistance in eliminating risks (e.g., low cost home improvements, housekeeping aid, or senior housing).
- If safety risks are associated with insufficient finances (inability to purchase prescriptions, heating oil, or home repairs), refer patient to social service agency to explore possibility of obtaining assistance.

---

patients' compliance with treatments, and aid in managing behavioral symptoms. This practice was generally unchallenged until the 1990s, when studies began to emerge suggesting that restraints contribute to serious injuries and worsen cognitive function (Capezuit, Strumpf, Evans, Grisso, & Maslin, 1998). Since then, the combination of research-based clinical evidence, clinical enlightenment, advocacy groups' efforts, and changed standards and regulations concerning restraints has contributed to a significant reduction in restraint use (Squillace, Remsburg, Bercovitz, Rosenoff, & Branden, 2007).

Restraints consist of anything that restricts freedom of movement. They can consist of physical restraints, such as seat belts, vests, wrist ties, "geri-chairs," bilateral full-length side rails, and chemical restraints, which are drugs given

solely for the purpose of discipline or staff convenience.

Applying physical restraints to an already agitated person increases his or her fear and worsens behavioral symptoms. This hardly reflects caring, compassionate practice. In addition, restraints can lead to serious complications, including aspiration, circulatory obstruction, cardiac stress, skin tears and ulcers, anorexia, dehydration, constipation, incontinence, fractures, and dislocations.

 POINT TO PONDER

How do you think you would react if you entered a hospital or nursing home room in which your loved one was being cared and found that person struggling to be freed from applied restraints?

Evidence now exists that the use of physical restraints can be significantly reduced without increasing staffing or injuries (Strumpf, Evans, & Bourbonniere, 2001). Therefore, nonuse of physical and chemical restraints is a standard that gerontological nurses should promote in all clinical settings. A thorough assessment is beneficial in identifying factors that contribute to agitation and other negative behaviors; these factors could include visual deficits, impaired hearing, unrelieved pain, delirium, dyspnea, excess sensory stimulation, and lack of familiarity with a new environment. Addressing the specific factor contributing to the behavior could calm the patient and eliminate the need for restraints. When behaviors cannot be modified, alternatives to restraints can be considered, such as:

- placing patient in a room near the nursing station in which close observation and frequent contact are facilitated
- one-to-one supervision and companionship (often, family members and volunteers can provide this)
- use of electronic devices that alert staff when the patient attempts to get out of bed or leaves a designated area
- repositioning, soothing communication, touch, and other comfort measures
- frequent reality orientation and reassurance
- diversional activities

Close observation and documentation of patients' responses to restraints and alternatives to restraints are essential.

INTERVENTIONS TO REDUCE INTRINSIC RISKS TO SAFETY

When a fall, injury, or other problem occurs, older adults take longer to recover and risk significantly more complications; thus, the key word in safety is *prevention*. Because of intrinsic risk factors often present in older adults, additional preventive measures are needed beyond those practices that promote safety for persons of any age. A variety of practical methods, most of which are inexpensive, promote safety and should be considered in the care of older adults. These measures not only aid in avoiding injury and illness but also can increase self-care capacity.

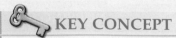

KEY CONCEPT

Prevention is important because older adults require more time to recover from injuries and suffer more complications.

Reducing Hydration and Nutrition Risks

Adequate fluid intake can be difficult for older adults, particularly if they are depressed, demented, or physically incapable of maintaining good fluid and food intake. Thirst perception declines with age, causing older persons to be less aware of their fluid needs. Sometimes a self-imposed fluid restriction is a means of managing urinary frequency; in other situations the mental capacity to respond to the thirst sensation may be lacking. The result is insufficient fluid intake, which causes the body's already reduced tissue fluid reserves to be tapped. Unless contraindicated, older adults should ingest at least 1,500 mL of fluid each day. Many sources other than plain water can provide this requirement, including soft drinks, coffee, juices, Jello, ices, and fresh citrus fruits.

Poor oral health, gastrointestinal symptoms, altered cognition, depression, and dependency on others for food can lead to poor food intake. Even healthy older people may have difficulty ingesting a proper diet because of factors such as limited funds, problems in shopping for food, and lack of motivation to prepare healthy meals. The fatigue, weakness, dizziness, and other symptoms associated with a poor nutritional status can predispose older adults to accidents and illness. An appropriate quality and quantity of food intake can increase the body's resistance to such problems. See Chapter 14 for more specific information about hydration and nutritional needs.

Addressing Risks Associated With Sensory Deficits

Changes in vision that occur with aging can pose threats to safety. Most people older than 40 years require corrective lenses for vision. The visual capacity of older adults can change frequently enough that regular evaluation of vision and the effectiveness of prescribed lenses is warranted. Annual eye examinations are helpful not only in ensuring the appropriateness of corrective lenses but also in detecting, in a timely fashion, the many eye disorders that increase in prevalence with age.

To compensate for reduced peripheral vision, affected individuals should be approached from the front rather than from the back or side, and furniture and frequently used items should be arranged in full view. Altered depth perception may hamper the ability of the aged to detect changes in levels; this may be alleviated by providing good lighting, eliminating clutter on stairways, using contrasting colors on stairs, and providing signals to indicate when a change in level is being approached. The filtering of low-tone colors is an important consideration when decorating areas for older adults; bright reds, oranges, and yellows and contrasting colors on doors and windows can be appealing and helpful. Difficulty in differentiating between low-tone colors should be considered if urine testing is being taught to older diabetics because these tests often require color differentiation. Cleaning solutions, medications, and other materials should be labeled in large letters to prevent accidents or errors.

Hearing deficits also pose a safety risk, as directions and warnings can be missed or misinterpreted. Audiometric evaluation should be obtained for persons with hearing impairments to determine possible corrective measures and the benefit of hearing aids. Older persons should be advised not to purchase a hearing aid without an evaluation and prescription for their specific needs.

Explanations and directions for diagnostic tests, medication administration, or other therapeutic measures should be explained in written, as well as verbal, form. Hearing impaired individuals should live close to someone with adequate hearing, who can alert them when fire alarms or other warnings are sounded. Specially trained dogs for the hearing impaired, similar to seeing-eye dogs, may prove useful; local hearing and speech associations can provide information on this and other resources.

Vision and hearing limitations of older adults produce difficulties for care providers who need to communicate necessary questions, warnings, or directions during the night. Whispering to avoid awakening other sleeping individuals may be missed by the older person who has a reduced ability to hear or whose hearing aid is removed, and lip reading is difficult in dimly lit bedrooms. Focusing a flashlight on the lips of the speaker can help the individual read lips, and cupping the hands over the ear and speaking directly into it can aid hearing. A stethoscope also can be used to amplify conversation by placing the earpieces into the individual's ear and speaking into the bell portion. It is a good idea to explain these procedures during the day so that the patient will understand your actions during the night.

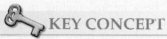 **KEY CONCEPT**

Conversation with a hearing impaired individual during the night can be facilitated by placing the earpieces of a stethoscope into the impaired person's ears and speaking into the bell or diaphragm.

Other sensory deficits, although more subtle, can predispose older adults to serious risks. A decreased sense of smell can cause older adults to miss warning odors and prevent differentiating between harmful and harmless substances. Because older adults may not be able to detect a gas odor before gas intoxication occurs, electric stoves may be better options than gas stoves. The loss of taste receptors may cause older adults to use excessive amounts of salt and sugar in their diets, which is a possible health hazard. Reduced tactile sensation to pressure from shoes, dentures, or unchanged positions can lead to skin breakdown, and the inability to differentiate between temperatures can cause burns. Nurses should plan careful observation, education, and environmental modifications to compensate for specific deficits.

Addressing Risks Associated With Mobility Limitations

Slower response and reaction times may be safety hazards. Older pedestrians may misjudge their ability to cross streets as traffic lights change, and older drivers may not be able to react quickly enough to avoid accidents; if family members are not available to escort and transport these individuals, assistance may be obtained through local social service agencies. Slower movement and poor coordination subject older adults to falls and other accidents; loose rugs, slippery floors, clutter, and poorly fitting slippers and shoes should be eliminated. Because poor judgment, denial, or lack of awareness of their limitations may prevent them from protecting themselves, older people should be advised not to take risks, such as climbing ladders or sitting on ledges to wash windows.

Monitoring Body Temperature

Temperature fluctuations can be hazardous to older individuals. The normal body temperature of many older persons is lower than that found in younger persons (e.g., temperatures as low as 97°F [36°C] can be a normal finding in older adults). Temperature elevation indicating a health problem can be missed if one is not aware of the person's baseline norm. For instance, a 99°F (37°C) temperature may not be alarming to the caregiver; however, if it is 2°F above the individual's norm, an infection may be present and, if undiscovered, can lead to complications. In addition to having an undetected, untreated, underlying problem, an unrecognized temperature elevation places an added burden on the heart. For every 1°F elevation, the heart rate increases approximately 10 beats/min—a stress that older hearts do not tolerate well. At the other extreme, hypothermia develops more easily in older people and can cause serious complications and death.

Preventing Infection

Because the risk of developing infections is considerably greater in older persons than in younger adults, avoiding situations that contribute to infection is necessary. Contact with persons who have known or suspected infections should be avoided, as should crowds (e.g., in shopping malls, classrooms, and movie theaters) during flu season.

Vaccines should be kept up-to-date. The Centers for Disease Control and Prevention recommends that persons aged over 65 years, nursing home residents, and persons who have close contact with either of these groups be vaccinated against influenza annually. Pneumococcal vaccines, administered once in a lifetime, and tetanus vaccines every 10 years should also be current. In addition to avoiding external sources of infection, older adults must be careful to ensure they do not create situations that predispose them to infection, such as immobility, malnutrition, and poor hygiene. Of course, good infection control practices are a must for preventing iatrogenic infections in older persons who receive services from health care providers.

Some evidence suggests that the herbs Echinacea, goldenseal, and garlic can help prevent infection and that ginseng can assist with infection prevention by protecting the body from the ill effects of stress. See Chapter 29 for more information on promoting immunologic health.

Suggesting Sensible Clothing

Shoes that are too large, offer poor support, or have high heels can lead to falls, as can loose hosiery and robes or pants legs that drag on the floor. Garters and tight-fitting shoes or garments can obstruct circulation. Hats and scarves can decrease the visual field. Clothing that is practical, properly fitting, and conducive to activity is advisable.

Using Medications Cautiously

The high number of drugs consumed by older adults and the differences in the pharmacokinetics in the aged can lead to serious adverse effects. Drugs should be prescribed only when necessary and after nonpharmacologic measures of treatment have proved ineffective. Older adults and their caregivers should be taught the proper use, side effects, and interactions of all drugs they are taking and be advised in the discrete use of over-the-counter drugs. (See Chapter 18 for more information on drugs.)

Avoiding Crime

Older adults are particularly vulnerable to criminals who view them as ready targets. In addition to being victims of actual crimes, older adults often are so fearful of potentially becoming victims of crime that they may be reluctant to leave their homes. Reasonable discretion should be used in traveling alone or at night and in opening doors to strangers. Likewise, older people should use caution in negotiating contracts and seek the advice of family members or professionals as needed. Gerontological nurses may want to identify crime prevention programs offered in the community by law enforcement agencies, faith communities, senior centers, and other groups; if such programs are not available, nurses can assist in their development.

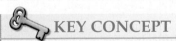 KEY CONCEPT

Older adults are particularly vulnerable to purse snatchings, burglaries, and scams by con artists.

Promoting Safe Driving

Older adults drive an estimated 84 billion miles annually. Although when examined as a group, drivers over age 60 years have lower accident rates than persons under age 30 years, accident rates begin to skyrocket after age 75 years. After age 85 years, older drivers are involved in four times the number of accidents on a mile-per-mile basis as persons aged 50 to 59 years, and when they are involved in accidents, they are 15 times more likely to die than drivers in their forties (Carr, 2000; Insurance Institute for Highway Safety, 2006; National Highway Traffic Safety Administration, Department of Transportation, 2006; Shallenbarger, 2012). The Insurance Institute for Highway Safety attributes the higher rates of deadly accidents to the fact that older adults tend to avoid freeway driving where crashes per mile are lower; in addition, older persons are more frail and less likely to survive the injuries sustained (Shallenbarger, 2012).

Nurses should assist older drivers in identifying risks to safe driving (e.g., poor vision, use of medications that reduce alertness, and slower reflexes) and encourage them to evaluate their continued ability to drive safely. They also should educate older adults about the reality that driving is a complex skill requiring rapid cognitive and psychomotor responses and that age-related changes (e.g., reduced peripheral vision, sensitivity to glare, and slower response and reaction times) can affect responses, even in the absence of diseases and medications. Rather than cease driving altogether, some older adults may find it useful to restrict their driving to daylight hours, noncongested areas, and good weather. Local chapters of the Automobile Association of America, the American Association of Retired Persons, and senior citizen groups can be contacted for safe driving classes that could be offered to older adults. If such programs do not exist in the community, the gerontological nurse could stimulate interest and assist in developing programs as a means of advocating for the safety of older drivers.

POINT TO PONDER

Many people take calculated risks, such as exceeding the speed limit, practicing unsafe sex, abusing drugs, and failing to perform regular breast self-examinations. What risks do you take and why do you do so? What can you do to change this behavior?

Promoting Early Detection of Problems

The early identification and correction of health problems helps minimize risks to safety. Regular professional assessment is important; however, self-evaluation by older adults can be equally beneficial because they will recognize changes or abnormalities in themselves that signal problems. Nurses can teach older adults how to perform the following measures:

- take their own temperature and pulse (do not assume that everyone knows the right way to use and read a thermometer or palpate a pulse)
- listen to their own lungs with a stethoscope (they may not be able to diagnose the sounds they hear, but they will be able to recognize a new or changed sound)
- observe changes in their own sputum, urine, and feces that could indicate problems
- identify the effectiveness, side effects, and adverse reactions of their medications
- recognize symptoms that should warrant professional evaluation

Confusion, disorientation, poor judgment, and decreased memory handicap older adults' ability to protect themselves from hazards to their health and well-being. When these symptoms occur, they are not to be taken lightly or accepted as normal. Often, the root of the problem can be a reversible disorder, such as hypotension, hypoglycemia, or infection. A thorough assessment is crucial to selecting the appropriate treatment modality and correcting the problem before complications occur.

KEY CONCEPT

Changes, problems, and difficulties older adults mention should be investigated, because they can be indicators of serious conditions.

A review of the individual's behaviors and function can pinpoint potential safety risks. Examples of situations to note include:

- smoking in bed
- incontinence
- inappropriate use of a walker or other mobility aid
- dizziness resulting from a new medication
- driving a car with poor vision
- cashing Social Security checks in a high-crime area
- having an active pet that is constantly underfoot

Nurses can identify these risks by observing and asking about routine activities, responsibilities, and typical tasks performed. Steps to correct potential problems should be taken before an incident occurs.

Addressing Risks Associated With Functional Impairment

A particularly high risk to safety exists when persons are functionally impaired, such as in Alzheimer's disease. Cognitively impaired individuals may not understand the significance of symptoms, may lack the capability to avoid hazards, and may be unable to communicate needs and problems to others. Examples of specific impairments that could heighten safety risks include significant memory deficits, disorientation, dementia, delirium, depression, deafness, low vision, aphasia, and paralysis.

When such conditions exist, an assessment should be made to determine how activities of daily living (e.g., food preparation, telephone use, medication administration, laundry, and housekeeping) are affected. Interventions are then planned to address specific problems and can include:

- referring the individual to occupational therapists, audiologists, ophthalmologists, psychiatrists, and other specialists for evaluation of the existing condition and prescription of appropriate treatment

- providing assistive devices and mobility aids and instruction in their use

- helping the person to prepare and label drugs for unit dose administration; develop a triggering and recording system for drug administration

- arranging for telephone reassurance, home health aid, home-delivered meals, housekeeper, emergency alarm system, or other community resources to assist the impaired person

- instructing and supporting family caregivers as they supervise and care for the impaired individual

- modifying the individual's environment to reduce hazards and promote function

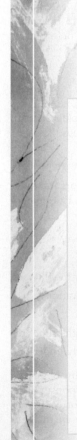

BRINGING RESEARCH TO LIFE

DEVELOPING A SELF-REPORTED TOOL ON FALL RISK BASED ON TOILETING RESPONSES ON IN-HOSPITAL FALLS

Ko, A., Nguyen, H. V., Chan, L., Shen, Q., Ding, X. M., Chan, D. L., Clemson, L., et al. (2012). Geriatric Nursing, 33(1), 9–16.

During an 8-month period, the researchers assessed older hospital patients for the risk of falls using the standard STRATIFY fall screening tool and a two-item self-reported questionnaire developed for this study. The participants were then followed to determine the occurrence of falls. The researchers believed that in-hospital fall risk screening tools could be more useful if they were based on patients' judgment.

The items on the two-item questionnaire on self-toileting behaviors asked patients what they would do if they needed to go to the toilet and if they were worried about falling on their way to the toilet. There was no relationship between how patients responded to the two questions and their incidence of falling; however, patients whose answers could not be interpreted had a higher risk of falling, believed to be attributed to confusion. Patients who were assessed to be at high risk for falls on the STRATIFY scale were 9.5 times more likely to fall than those who were found to be at low risk.

One of the possible conclusions that could be drawn from this study is that persons who are cognitively competent are more cautious and reduce their risk of falling. This study supported the association between cognitive impairment and falls that has been shown in other studies. The use of a self-reported tool could prove to be a means to quickly identify patients at risk for falls in that those who had difficulty providing responses may have cognitive impairments that make them a high-risk group.

Evidence of impaired cognitive function at admission or the development of a delirium during a hospital stay increases the risk of falls and warrants nursing interventions to reduce this risk.

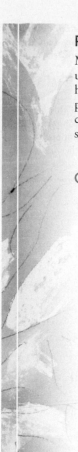

PRACTICE REALITIES

Mrs. Dean is an 85-year-old nursing home resident. She has good cognitive function but an unsteady gait due to the effects of a past stroke and generalized weakness. Although she has had physical therapy and knows how to use a walker, Mrs. Dean has fallen a few times in the past several months. Although the falls have only resulted in bruises, Mrs. Dean's daughter is concerned that her mother is going to fall and sustain a serious fracture so she asks the nursing staff to have Mrs. Dean use a wheelchair and not ambulate.

What is the best action for the staff to take?

CRITICAL THINKING EXERCISES

1. Explain how Maslow's theory of low-level needs having to be fulfilled before one can concentrate on the fulfillment of high-level needs relates to satisfaction from one's environment.

2. What lighting, color selection, and decorations would be most therapeutic for the following areas used by older persons?
   - bedroom
   - recreation room
   - dining room

3. List at least six hazards for older adults in the average bathroom.

4. What measures can be taken to humanize an institutional environment?

5. Describe the safety risks that could result from the following health problems: hypertension, arthritis, right-sided weakness, and Alzheimer's disease.

6. What changes could be made to the average home to make it user friendly and safe for older adults?

7. What content could be included in a program to educate older adults about actions they can take to avoid accidents and injuries?

RESOURCES

AAA Foundation for Traffic Safety Senior Driver Website
http://seniordriving.aaa.com

Hartford Institute for Geriatric Nursing
Try This: Best Practices in Nursing Care to Older Adults Issue 8, Fall Risk Assessment: Hendrich II Fall Risk Model
http://consultgerirn.org/uploads/File/trythis/try_this_8.pdf

REFERENCES

Capezuit, E., Strumpf, N., Evans, L. K., Grisso, J. A., & Maslin, G. (1998). The relationship between physical restraint removal and falls and injuries among nursing home residents. *Journal of Gerontology, 53A*, M47–M52.

Carr, D. B. (2000). The older adult driver. *American Family Physician, 50*(1), 141–150.

Centers for Disease Control and Prevention. (2004). *Web-based Injury Statistics Query and Reporting System (WISQARS)* [database online]. National Center for Injury Prevention and Control, Centers for Disease Control and Prevention (producer). Retrieved August 1, 2007 from http://www.cdc.gov/ncipc/wisqars

Centers for Disease Control and Prevention. (2007), *Falls in nursing homes,* National Center for Injury Prevention and Control, Centers for Disease Control and Prevention. Retrieved October 7, 2012 from http://www.cdc.gov/ncipc/factsheets/nursing.htm

Cheung, S. S. (2007). Neuropsychological determinants of exercise tolerance in the heat. *Progressive Brain Research, 165*, 45–60.

Insurance Institute for Highway Safety. (2006). *Fatality facts, older people.* Arlington, VA: Insurance Institute for Highway Safety. Retrieved October 7, 2012 from http://www.iihs.org/research/fatality.aspx?topicName=Olderpeople

National Highway Traffic Safety Administration, Department of Transportation. (2006). *Traffic safety facts 2005: Older population.* Washington, DC: National Highway Traffic Safety Administration, Department of Transportation. Retrieved August 1, 2007 from http://www-nrd.nhtsa.dot.gov/Pubs/TSF2005.PDF

Shallenbarger, S. (2012). Safer over 70: drivers keep the keys. *Wall Street Journal, February 29, 2012*, D3.

Squillace, M. R., Remsburg, R. E., Bercovitz, A., Rosenoff, E., & Branden, L. (2007). An introduction to the National Nursing Assistant Survey. Washington, DC: National Center for Health Statistics. *Vital Health Statistics, 1*(44), 1–54.

Sterling, D. A., O'Connor, J. A., & Bonadies, J. (2001). Geriatric falls: Injury severity is high and disproportionate to mechanism. *Journal of Trauma-Injury, Infection and Critical Care, 50*(1), 116–119.

Strumpf, N., Evans, L., & Bourbonniere, M. (2001). Restraints. In M. Mezey (Ed.), *The encyclopedia of elder care* (pp. 567–569). New York, NY: Springer.

U.S. Census Bureau, Statistical Abstract of the U.S. (2012). *Death and death rates by leading causes of death and age.* Retrieved from http://www.census.gov/compendia/statab/2012/tables/12s0122.pdf

U.S. Department of Commerce. (2010). *Statistical abstract of the United States.* Washington, DC: Bureau of the Census. Retrieved from www.census.gov/compendia/statab

RECOMMENDED READINGS

Recommended Readings associated with this chapter can be found on the web site that accompanies the book. Visit **http://thepoint.lww.com/Eliopoulos8e** to access the recommended readings and other additional resources associated with this chapter.

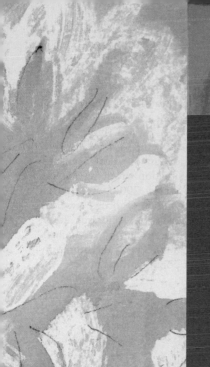

CHAPTER 18

Safe Medication Use

LEARNING OBJECTIVES

After reading this chapter, you should be able to:

1. Describe the unique aspects of drug pharmacokinetics and pharmacodynamics in older people.

2. List measures to promote safe drug use.

3. Describe alternatives to medications.

4. Identify proper uses and risks associated with common drug groups used with older adults.

TERMS TO KNOW

Beers criteria: originally developed by a group headed by Dr. Mark H. Beers, listing of drugs that carry high risks for older adults and criteria for potentially inappropriate medication use in older adults

Biological half-life: the time necessary for half of a drug to be excreted from the body

Pharmacokinetics: refers to the absorption, distribution, metabolism, and excretion of drugs

Pharmacodynamics: refers to the biologic and therapeutic effects of drugs at the site of action or on the target organ

Polypharmacy: use of multiple medications

When caring for older adults, it is important for the nurse to understand special considerations for medication use in the older population. Drugs act differently in older adults than in younger adults and require careful dosage adjustment and monitoring. Older adults are also more likely than other populations to take more than one medication regularly, increasing the risk of interactions and adverse reactions. To minimize the risks associated with drug therapy and ensure that medications do not create more problems than they solve, close supervision and adherence to sound principles of safe drug use are essential in gerontological nursing.

EFFECTS OF AGING ON MEDICATION USE

Medication use in older adults presents special challenges because of the number of drugs commonly used, age-related changes that affect drug pharmacokinetics and pharmacotherapeutics, and an increased risk of adverse reactions (Fig. 18-1).

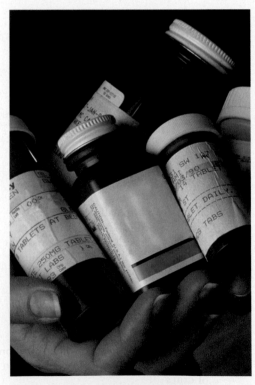

FIGURE 18-1 ■ The high prevalence of drugs consumed by older people and the complexity of drug dynamics in old age require gerontological nurses to evaluate regularly the continued need, appropriateness of dosage, and intended and adverse effects of every drug given to older individuals.

Polypharmacy and Interactions

The high prevalence of health conditions in the older population causes this group to use a large number and variety of medications. Drug use by older adults has been steadily increasing every year; most older people use at least one drug regularly, with the more typical situation involving the use of several drugs daily (Skufca, 2007). Researchers have found that the number of drugs used by older persons increases with age (Gorard, 2006; Kaufman, Kelly, Rosenberg, Anderson, & Mitchell, 2002; Page & Ruscin, 2007). The most commonly used drugs by the older population include:

- cardiovascular agents
- antihypertensives
- analgesics
- antiarthritic agents
- sedatives
- tranquilizers
- laxatives
- antacids

The drugs on this list can cause adverse effects (e.g., confusion, dizziness, falls, and fluid and electrolyte imbalances) that threaten older people's quality of life. Furthermore, when taken together, some of these drugs can interact and cause serious adverse effects (Table 18-1).

Taking more than one drug also increases the risk of drug–food interactions (Table 18-2). With the increasing use of herbal remedies, drug–herb interactions and adverse effects of herbs may also occur (Table 18-3). When caring for older adults, particularly those taking more than one medication, it is important for nurses to monitor for signs of possible interactions.

 POINT TO PONDER

How often do you rely on medications to curb appetite, promote sleep, stimulate bowel elimination, or manage a headache or some other symptom? Why do you choose to use medications rather than address the underlying cause or use a natural means to correct the problem? How can you change this?

Altered Pharmacokinetics

Pharmacokinetics refers to the absorption, distribution, metabolism, and excretion of drugs.

TABLE 18-1 Interactions Among Popular Drug Groups

	Antacids	Antianxiety	Anticoagulants	Antidiabetics	Antidepressants	Antihypertensives	Anti-inflammatory	Antipsychotics	Digitalis preparations	Laxatives	Salicylates	Sedatives	Thiazide Diuretics	Tricyclic Antidepressants
Antacids			↓					↓	↓					
Antianxiety			↑			↑								
Anticoagulants (oral)				↑										
Antidiabetics														
Antidepressants	↑	↑				↓						↑		
Antihypertensives				↑								↑	↑	
Anti-inflammatory				↑	↑									
Antipsychotics												↑		
Digitalis Preparations														
Laxatives									↓					
Sedatives		↑												
Thiazide Diuretics			↓	↑							↓			
Tricyclic Antidepressants	↑	↑				↓						↑		

Arrows indicate the effect of drugs listed in the left-hand column on those listed across the top.

TABLE 18-2 Examples of Food and Drug Interactions

Drug	Potential Interactions
Acetaminophen	Accumulation to toxic level if more than 500 mg vitamin C supplements are ingested daily
Allopurinol	Impairs iron absorption, leading to iron deficiency anemia
	Combined with alcohol or simple carbohydrates can increase blood uric acid level
Aluminum antacids	Depletes phosphate and calcium
	Decreases absorption of vitamins A, C, and D and magnesium, thiamine, folacin, and iron
Antihistamines	Ingestion of large amounts of alkaline foods (e.g., milk, cream, almonds, alcohol) can prolong action
Aspirin	Can cause iron deficiency anemia as a result of gastrointestinal bleeding
	Causes vitamin C deficiency (12+ aspirin tablets daily)
	Causes thiamine deficiency
Calcium carbonate antacids	Cause deficiencies of phosphate, folacin, iron, thiamine
Calcium supplements	Combined with large doses of vitamin D can cause hypercalcemia
	Absorption decreased by foods rich in oxalate (e.g., spinach, rhubarb, celery, peanuts), phytic acid (e.g., oatmeal and other grain cereals), phosphorous (chocolate, dried beans, dried fruit, peanut butter)
Chlorpromazine HCl	Large amounts of alkaline foods can delay excretion
	Can increase blood cholesterol
Cimetidine	Reduces iron absorption

(Continues)

TABLE 18-2 **Examples of Food and Drug Interactions** (Continued)

Drug	Potential Interactions
Clonidine HCl	Effectiveness reduced by tyramine-rich foods (e.g., chicken and beef livers, bananas, sour cream, meat tenderizers, salami, yeast, chocolate)
	Can cause sodium and fluid retention
Colchicine	Effectiveness decreased by caffeine
	Some herbal teas contain phenylbutazone, which can increase blood uric acid and decrease effectiveness of antigout drugs
Dicumarol	Effectiveness reduced by foods rich in vitamin K (e.g., cabbage, broccoli, asparagus, spinach, turnip greens)
Digitalis	Can cause deficiencies of thiamine, magnesium, and zinc
	Calcium supplements increase the risk of toxicity
Estrogen	Hastens breakdown of vitamin C
Ferrous supplements	Absorption decreased by antacids, increased by vitamin C
Furosemide	Increases excretion of calcium, magnesium, potassium, and zinc
Hydralazine	Can cause vitamin B_6 deficiency
Levodopa	Effectiveness reduced by high-protein diet
	Can cause deficiencies of potassium, folacin, and vitamins B_6 and B_{12}
Magnesium antacids	Can deplete phosphate and calcium
Magnesium-based laxatives	30 mL contains nearly four times the average daily intake of magnesium; toxicity can result
Mineral oil	Decreases absorption of vitamins A, D, and K
Phenobarbital	Increases breakdown of vitamins D and K
	Impairs absorption of vitamins B_6 and B_{12} and folic acid
Phenylbutazone	Inhibits absorption of iodine
Phenytoin	Increases breakdown of vitamins D and K
	Reduces absorption of folacin
Potassium supplements	Absorption decreased by dairy products
	Impairs absorption of vitamin B_{12}
Probenecid	Effectiveness decreased by coffee, tea, or cola
Spironolactone	Increases excretion of calcium
	Decreases excretion of potassium leading to potassium toxicity
Theophylline	Effectiveness reduced by high-carbohydrate diet
Thiazides	Increases excretion of calcium, potassium, magnesium, zinc
	Can decrease blood glucose level
Thioridazine	Excretion delayed by high-alkaline diet
Warfarin	Effectiveness reduced by large amounts of vitamin K in diet

TABLE 18-3 **Potential Adverse Effects and Drug Interactions of Selected Herbs**

Herb	Potential Adverse Effects and Drug Interactions
Aloe	Allergic dermatitis; increases effects of cardiac glycosides; increases potassium loss when taken with corticosteroids or thiazide diuretics
Angelica	Rash when the person is exposed to sunlight; can interact with calcium channel blockers
Balm	Interferes with thyroid-stimulating hormone
Barberry	Drastic reductions in blood pressure, heart rate, and respirations with large doses
Bayberry	Edema, elevation of blood pressure; contraindicated in persons with history of cancer
Black cohosh	Depression of cardiac function leading to bradycardia and hypotension; estrogen-like properties can cause abnormal coagulation and liver dysfunction; can interact with estrogen
Bloodroot	Bradycardia, arrhythmia, impaired vision, thirst

Cascara sagrada	Severe intestinal cramps
Celery	Hypokalemia with long-term use
Chaparral	Liver damage
Coltsfoot	Liver toxicity, fever
Comfrey	Liver toxicity
Dandelion	Hypokalemia with long-term use
Ephedra (ma huang)	Elevation of blood pressure and heart rate, insomnia, dizziness, anxiety; can interact with ephedrine
Feverfew	Interference with coagulation; when taken orally can cause mouth ulcers, loss of taste sensation, swelling of oral cavity; increases anticoagulation effects of aspirin and warfarin sodium
Garlic	Anticoagulation effect, hypotension, increases effects of antidiabetic agents
Ginkgo biloba	Anticoagulation effect, irritability, restlessness, insomnia, nausea, vomiting, diarrhea; increases effects of anticoagulants
Ginseng	Elevation of blood pressure, insomnia ·
Goldenseal	Vasoconstriction
Hawthorne	Dramatic reductions in blood pressure
Hops	Drowsiness, increased effects of sedatives and tranquilizers
Licorice	Edema, hypertension, hypokalemia, and hypernatremia with long-term use
Mistletoe	Bradycardia; potentially fatal
Parsley	Hypokalemia with long-term use
Red clover	Estrogen-like effects, contraindicated in persons with estrogen-dependent cancer
Rhubarb	Severe abdominal cramps, diarrhea
Senna	Can increase effects of digoxin
St. John's wort	Acts as monoamine oxidase inhibitor; hypertension, photosensitivity, nausea, vomiting

Absorption

Generally, older people have fewer problems in the area of drug absorption than with distribution, metabolism, and excretion of drugs. However, a variety of factors can alter drug absorption, such as:

- *Route of administration.* Drugs given intramuscularly, subcutaneously, orally, or rectally are not absorbed as efficiently as drugs that are inhaled, applied topically, or instilled intravenously.

- *Concentration and solubility of drug.* Drugs that are highly soluble (e.g., aqueous solutions) and in higher concentrations are absorbed with greater speed than less soluble and less concentrated drugs.

- *Diseases and symptoms.* Although once considered outcomes of aging because they are commonly present, decreased intracellular fluid, increased gastric pH, decreased gastric blood flow and motility, reduced cardiac output and circulation, and slower metabolism can slow drug absorption and are more the result of underlying disease states than normal age-related changes. Conditions such as diabetes mellitus and hypokalemia can increase the absorption of drugs, whereas pain and mucosal edema will slow absorption.

Although nurses can do little to improve many of the underlying factors responsible for altered drug absorption, they can use measures to maximize the absorption of drugs. Exercise stimulates circulation and aids in absorption. Properly used heat and massage likewise increase blood flow at the absorption site. Preventing fluid volume deficit, hypothermia, and hypotension is beneficial in facilitating absorption. Preparations that neutralize gastric secretions should be avoided if a low gastric pH is required for drug absorption. The nurse should monitor for interactions discussed previously that may affect drug absorption. Consideration should also be given to using the most effective administration route for the drug.

Distribution

Although it is difficult to predict with certainty how drug distribution will differ among older adults, changes in circulation, membrane permeability, body temperature, and tissue structure can modify this process. For example, adipose tissue increases compared with lean body mass in older persons, especially in women; therefore, drugs stored in adipose tissue (i.e., lipid-soluble drugs) will have increased tissue concentrations, decreased plasma concentrations, and a longer duration in the body. Decreased cardiac output can raise the plasma levels of drugs while reducing their deposition in reservoirs; this is particularly apparent with water-soluble drugs. Reduced serum albumin levels can be problematic if several protein-bound drugs are consumed and compete for the same protein molecules; the unbound drug concentrations increase and the effectiveness of the drugs will be threatened. Highly protein-bound drugs that may compete at protein-binding sites and displace each other include acetazolamide, amitriptyline, cefazolin, chlordiazepoxide, chlorpromazine, cloxacillin, digitoxin, furosemide, hydralazine, nortriptyline, phenylbutazone, phenytoin, propranolol, rifampin, salicylates, spironolactone, sulfisoxazole, and warfarin. When monitoring the blood levels of medications, it is also important to evaluate the serum albumin level. For instance, raising the dosage of phenytoin because the blood level is low can lead to toxicity if the serum albumin is also low.

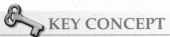

KEY CONCEPT

When several drugs are taken concurrently, protein-bound drugs may not achieve desired results because of ineffective binding to reduced protein molecules.

Conditions such as dehydration and hypoalbuminemia decrease drug distribution and result in higher drug levels in the plasma. When these conditions exist, lower dosage levels may be necessary.

Metabolism, Detoxification, and Excretion

Conditions such as dehydration, hyperthermia, immobility, and liver disease can decrease the metabolism of drugs. As a consequence, drugs can accumulate to toxic levels and cause serious adverse reactions. Careful monitoring is essential. Along this line, the extended biological half-life of many of the drugs consumed by older adults warrants close evaluation of drug clearance. Estimated creatinine clearance must be calculated based on the age, weight, and serum creatinine level of the individual because serum creatinine levels alone may not reflect a reduced creatinine clearance level.

In advanced age, there may be a reduced secretion of some enzymes, which interferes with the metabolism of drugs that require enzymatic activity. Most important, the detoxification and conjugation of drugs may be significantly reduced, so that the drug stays in the bloodstream longer. Some evidence indicates larger drug concentrations at administration sites in older persons.

The renal system is primarily responsible for the body's excretory functions, and among its activities is the excretion of drugs. Drugs follow a path through the kidneys similar to that of most constituents of urine. After systemic circulation, the drug filters through the walls of glomerular capillaries into the Bowman capsule. The drug continues down the tubule, where substances beneficial to the body will be reabsorbed into the bloodstream through proximal convoluted tubules and where waste substances excreted through the urine flow into the pelvis of the kidney. Capillaries surrounding the tubules reabsorb the filtered blood and join to form the renal vein. It is estimated that to promote this filtration process almost 10 times more blood circulates through the kidneys than through similarly sized body organs. The reduced efficiency of body organs with advanced age affects the kidneys as well, complicating drug excretion in older adults. Nephron units are decreased in number, and many of the remaining ones can be nonfunctional in older individuals. The glomerular filtration rate and tubular reabsorption are reduced. Decreasing cardiac function contributes to the almost 50% reduction in blood flow to the kidneys. The implications of reduced kidney efficiency are important. Drugs are not as quickly filtered from the bloodstream and are present in the body longer. The biological half-life, or the time necessary for half of the drug to be excreted, can increase as much as 40% and increase the risk of adverse drug reactions. Drugs that have a likelihood of accumulating because of an increased biological half-life include antibiotics, barbiturates, cimetidine, digoxin, and salicylate.

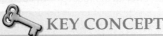

KEY CONCEPT

The extended biological half-life of drugs in older adults increases the risk of adverse reactions.

The liver also has many important functions that influence drug detoxification and excretion. Carbohydrate metabolism in the liver converts glucose into glycogen and releases it into the bloodstream when needed. Protein metabolism in the parenchymal cells of the liver is responsible for the loss of the amine groups from amino acids, which aid in the formation of new plasma proteins, such as prothrombin and fibrinogen, as well as in the conversion of some poisonous nitrogenous by-products into nontoxic substances such as vitamin B_{12}. Also important is the liver's formation of bile, which breaks down fats through enzymatic action and removes substances such as bilirubin from the blood. The liver decreases in size and function with age, and hepatic blood flow declines by 45% between the ages of 25 and 65 years. This could affect the metabolism of some drugs, such as antibiotics, cimetidine, chlordiazepoxide, digoxin, lithium, meperidine, nortriptyline, and quinidine.

Altered Pharmacodynamics

Pharmacodynamics refers to the biologic and therapeutic effects of drugs at the site of action or on the target organ. Information on pharmacodynamics in the older population has been limited but is growing as increased research is done in this area. At this point, some of the known differences in older adults' responses to drugs include increased myocardial sensitivity to anesthesias and increased central nervous system (CNS) receptor sensitivity to narcotics, alcohol, and bromides.

Increased Risk of Adverse Reactions

The risk of adverse reactions to drugs is so high in older people that some geropharmacologists suggest that any symptom in an older adult be suspected as being related to a drug until proven otherwise (Patel, 2003). The following are some general factors to remember in regard to adverse reactions:

- The signs and symptoms of an adverse reaction to a given drug may differ in older persons.
- A prolonged time may be required for an adverse reaction to become apparent in older adults.
- An adverse reaction to a drug may be demonstrated even after the drug has been discontinued.
- Adverse reactions can develop suddenly, even with a drug that has been used over a long period of time without problems.

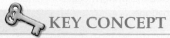

KEY CONCEPT

The risk of adverse drug reactions is high in older adults because of age-related differences in pharmacokinetics and pharmacodynamics.

Varying degrees of mental dysfunction often are early symptoms of adverse reactions to commonly prescribed medications for older adults, such as codeine, digitalis, methyldopa, phenobarbital, L-dopa, diazepam (Valium), and various diuretics. Any medication that can promote hypoglycemia, acidosis, fluid and electrolyte imbalances, temperature elevations, increased intracranial pressure, and reduced cerebral circulation also can produce mental disturbances. Even the most subtle changes in mental status could be linked to a medication and should be reviewed with a physician. Older adults easily may become victims of drug-induced cognitive dysfunction. Unfortunately, mental and behavioral dysfunction in older adults is sometimes treated symptomatically (i.e., with medications but without full exploration of

the etiology). This approach will not correct a drug-related problem and can predispose the individual to additional complications from the new drug.

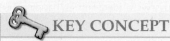

KEY CONCEPT

Nurses should ensure that drug-induced cognitive and behavioral problems are not treated with additional drugs.

PROMOTING THE SAFE USE OF DRUGS

Avoiding Potentially Inappropriate Drugs: Beers Criteria

In 1991, Dr. Mark H. Beers et al. published a paper that identified drugs that carry high risks for older adults (Beers, Ouslander, Rollingher, Reuben, & Beck, 1991). This work was developed further to provide criteria for potentially inappropriate medication use in older adults (Beers, 1997; Fick et al., 2003; The American Geriatrics Society 2012 Beers Criteria Update Expert Panel, 2012). These criteria included drugs that were inappropriate to use in general (Box 18-1) and drugs that were inappropriate to use in the presence of specific conditions (Table 18-4). Some of the major drugs of concern include anticholinergics, tricyclic antidepressants (TCAs), antipsychotics, barbiturates (except when used as anticonvulsants), and benzodiazepines. These criteria have been widely accepted in geriatric care circles as a means to reduce both adverse drug effects and drug costs. In fact, in 1999, the Centers for Medicare and Medicaid Services adopted the criteria for use in nursing home surveys and later the Joint Commission also adopted the criteria as a potential sentinel event in hospitals.

Reviewing Necessity and Effectiveness of Prescribed Drugs

The scope of drug use and significant adverse reactions that can result necessitate that gerontological nurses ensure drugs are used selectively and cautiously. Nurses should review all prescription and nonprescription medications used by patients and ask themselves these questions:

- *Why is the drug ordered?* Consider whether the drug is really needed. Perhaps warm milk and a back rub could eliminate the need for the sedative; maybe the patient had a bowel movement this morning and now does not need the laxative. The medication may be used because it has been prescribed for years and no one has considered its discontinuation.

BOX 18-1   Inappropriate Drugs to Use in Older Adults

The following drugs were identified as having a high risk of adverse reactions in older adults:

First-generation antihistamines (as single agent or as part of combination products): brompheniramine, carbinoxamine, chlorpheniramine, clemastine, cyproheptadine, dexbrompheniramine, dexchlorpheniramine, diphenhydramine (oral), doxylamine, hydroxyzine, promethazine, triprolidine

Antiparkinson agents: benztropine (oral), trihexyphenidyl

Antispasmodics: belladonna alkaloids, clidinium-chlordiazepoxide, dicyclomine, hyoscyamine, propantheline, scopolamine

Antithrombotics: dipyridamole (oral short acting), ticlopidine

Anti-infective: nitrofurantoin

Cardiovascular: disopyramide; dronedarone, digoxin (>0.125 mg/day), nifedipine (immediate release), spironolactone (>25 mg/day)

Alpha1 blockers: doxazosin, prazosin, terazosin

Alpha-blockers, central: clonidine, guanabenz, guanfacine, methyldopa, reserpine (>0.1 mg/day)

Antiarrhythmic drugs (Class Ia, Ic, III): amiodarone, dofetilide, dronedarone, flecainide, ibutilide, procainamide, propafenone, quinidine, sotalol

Central Nervous System:

Tertiary tricyclic antidepressants, alone or in combination: amitriptyline, chlordiazepoxide-amitriptyline, clomipramine, doxepin (>6 mg/day), imipramine, perphenazine-amitriptyline, trimipramine

Antipsychotics, first (conventional) and second (atypical) generation: mesoridazine, thioridazine

Barbiturates: amobarbital, butabarbital, butalbital, mephobarbital, pentobarbital, phenobarbital, secobarbital

Benzodiazepines: *Short and intermediate acting:* alprazolam, estazolam, lorazepam, oxazepam, temazepam, triazolam; *Long acting:* clorazepate, chlordiazepoxide, chlordiazepoxide-amitriptyline, clidinium-chlordiazepoxide, clonazepam, diazepam, flurazepam, quazepam

Chloral hydrate

Meprobamate

Nonbenzodiazepine hypnotics: eszopiclone, zolpidem, zaleplon

Ergot mesylates: isoxsuprine

Endocrine: Androgens: methyltestosterone, testosterone; desiccated thyroid; estrogens with or without progestins; growth hormone; insulin, sliding scale; megestrol; Sulfonylureas (long duration): chlorpropamide, glyburide

Gastrointestinal: metoclopramide; mineral oil, given orally; trimethobenzamide

Pain Medications:

Meperidine

Non–cyclooxygenase-selective nonsteroidal anti-inflammatory drugs, oral: aspirin (>325 mg/day), diclofenac, diflunisal, etodolac, fenoprofen, ibuprofen, ketoprofen, meclofenamate, mefenamic acid, meloxicam, nabumetone, naproxen, oxaprozin, piroxicam, sulindac, tolmetin

Indomethacin, ketorolac, includes parenteral

Pentazocine

Skeletal muscle relaxants: carisoprodol, chlorzoxazone, cyclobenzaprine, metaxalone, methocarbamol, orphenadrine

Adopted from The American Geriatrics Society 2012 Beers Criteria Update Expert Panel. (2012). The American Geriatrics Society Updated Beers Criteria for potentially inappropriate medication use in older adults, Table 2. 2012 American Geriatrics Society Beers Criteria for potentially inappropriate medication use in older adults. *Journal of the American Geriatrics Society, 60*(4), 616–631.

■ *Is the smallest possible dosage ordered?* Older adults usually require lower dosages of most medications because of the delayed time for excretion of the substance. Larger dosages increase the risk of adverse reactions.

■ *Is the patient allergic to the drug?* Sometimes the physician may overlook a known allergy, or perhaps the patient neglected to share an allergy problem with the physician. The nurse may be aware of a patient's sensitivities to certain drugs.

Consideration must also be given to new signs that could indicate a reaction to a drug that has been used for a long period without trouble.

■ *Can this drug interact with other drugs, herbs, or nutritional supplements that are being used?* It is useful to review resource material to identify potential interactions—they are too numerous for anyone to commit to memory!

■ *Are there any special instructions accompanying the drug's administration?* Some drugs should be

TABLE 18-4	Inappropriate Drugs to Use in Older Adults in the Presence of Specific Diagnoses or Condition
A High Potential for Adverse Reactions Exists in Patients With:	**When the Patient Is Taking:**
Anorexia, malnutrition	Central nervous system (CNS) stimulants
Arrhythmias	Tricyclic antidepressants
Bladder flow obstructions	Anticholinergics and antihistamines, gastrointestinal antispasmodics, muscle relaxants, oxybutynin, flavoxate, anticholinergics, antidepressants, decongestants, and tolterodine
Blood clotting disorders or are using anticoagulants	Aspirin, nonsteroidal anti-inflammatory drugs (NSAIDs), dipyridamole, ticlopidine, clopidogrel
Cognitive impairment	Barbiturates, anticholinergics, antispasmodics, muscle relaxants, CNS stimulants
Chronic obstructive pulmonary disorder	Long-acting benzodiazepines, beta-blockers
Depression	Benzodiazepines (long-term use), sympatholytic agents
Gastric or duodenal ulcers	NSAIDs and aspirin
Heart failure	Disopyramide and high sodium–containing drugs
Hypertension	Phenylpropanolamine HCl
Insomnia	Decongestants, theophylline, methylphenidate, monoamine oxidase inhibitors, amphetamines
Parkinson disease	Metoclopramide, conventional antipsychotics, tacrine
Seizures	Clozapine, chlorpromazine, thioridazine, thiothixene
Seizure disorder	Bupropion
Stress incontinence	Alpha-blockers, anticholinergics, tricyclic antidepressants, long-acting benzodiazepines
Syncope, falls	Short- to intermediate-acting benzodiazepines, tricyclic antidepressants

Source: The American Geriatrics Society 2012 Beers Criteria Update Expert Panel. (2012). The American Geriatrics Society Updated Beers Criteria for potentially inappropriate medication use in older adults, Table 3. 2012 American Geriatrics Society Beers Criteria for potentially inappropriate medication use in older adults due to drug–disease or drug–syndrome interactions that may exacerbate the disease or syndrome. *Journal of the American Geriatrics Society, 60*(4), 616–631.

given on an empty stomach, others with a meal. Certain times of the day may be better for drugs to be given than others.

■ *Is the most effective route of administration being used?* A person who cannot swallow a large tablet may do better with a liquid form. Suppositories that are expelled because of ineffective melting or oral drugs that are vomited obviously will not have the therapeutic effect of the drug given in a different manner.

Nurses must go through a mental checklist of these questions when administering medications and teach older persons who are responsible for their own medication administration, as well as their caregivers, to do the same.

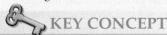

KEY CONCEPT

Regular review of a drug's ongoing necessity and effectiveness is essential.

Promoting Safe and Effective Administration

The most common way to administer drugs is orally. Oral medications in the form of tablets, capsules, liquids, powders, elixirs, spirits, emulsions, mixtures, and magmas are used either for their direct action on the mucous membrane of the digestive tract (e.g., antacids) or for their systemic effects (e.g., antibiotics and tranquilizers). Although oral administration is simple, certain problems can interfere with the process. Dry mucous membranes of the oral cavity, common in older individuals, can prevent capsules and tablets from being swallowed. If they are then expelled from the mouth, there is no therapeutic value; if they dissolve in the mouth, they can irritate the mucous membrane. Proper oral hygiene, ample fluids for assistance with swallowing and mobility, proper positioning, and examining the oral cavity after administration will ensure that the patient receives the full benefit of the medicine during its travel through the gastrointestinal (GI) system. Some older people may not even be aware that a tablet is stuck to the roof of their dentures or under their tongue.

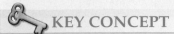

KEY CONCEPT

To ensure that oral medications achieve full benefit, encourage good oral hygiene, ample fluids, and proper positioning to facilitate swallowing.

Because enteric-coated and sustained-release tablets should not be crushed, the nurse should consult with a physician for an alternative form of the drug if a tablet is too large to be swallowed. As a rule, capsules are not to be broken open and mixed. Medications are put into capsule form so that unpleasant tastes will be masked or the coating will dissolve when it comes into contact with specific GI secretions. Some vitamin, mineral, and electrolyte preparations are bitter, and even more so for older persons, whose taste buds for sweetness are lost long before those for sourness and bitterness. Combining the medication with foods and drinks such as applesauce and juices can make them more palatable and prevent gastric irritation, although there may be a problem if the full amount of medicated food is not ingested. Individuals should be informed that the food or drink they are ingesting contains a medication. Oral hygiene after the administration of oral drugs prevents an unpleasant aftertaste.

Drugs prescribed in suppository form for local or systemic action are inserted into various body cavities and act by melting from body heat or dissolving in body fluids. Because circulation to the lower bowel and vagina is decreased and the body temperature is lower in many older individuals, a prolonged period may be required for the suppository to melt. If no alternative route can be used and the suppository form must be given, a special effort must be made to ensure that the suppository is not expelled.

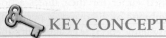

KEY CONCEPT

Lower body temperature and decreased circulation to the lower bowel and vagina can prolong the time required for suppositories to melt.

Intramuscular and subcutaneous administration of drugs is necessary when immediate results are sought or when other routes cannot be used, either because of the nature of the drug or the status of the individual. The upper, outer quadrant of the buttocks is the best site for intramuscular injections. Frequently, the older person will bleed or ooze after the injection because of decreased tissue elasticity; a small pressure bandage may be helpful.

Alternating the injection site will help to reduce discomfort. Medication should not be injected into an immobile limb because the inactivity of the limb will reduce the rate of absorption. For a person receiving frequent injections, the nurse should check for signs of infection at the injection site; reduced subcutaneous sensation in older persons or absence of sensation, as that experienced with a stroke, may prevent the person from being aware of a complication at the injection site.

Occasionally, intravenous administration of drugs is necessary. In addition to observing the effects of the medication, the nurse needs to be alert to the amount of fluid in which the drug is administered. Declining cardiac and renal function make older people more susceptible not only to dehydration but also to overhydration. The nurse must closely monitor for signs of circulatory overload, including elevated blood pressure, increased respirations, coughing, shortness of breath, and symptoms associated with pulmonary edema. Intake and output balance, body weight, and specific gravity are useful to monitor. Of course, the nurse should also monitor older patients for complications associated with intravenous therapy in any age group, for example, infiltration, air embolism, thrombophlebitis, and pyrogenic reactions. Decreased sensation may mask any of these potential complications, emphasizing the necessity for close nursing observation.

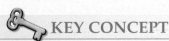

KEY CONCEPT

Older adults are at risk for circulatory overload during intravenous drug therapy; close monitoring is essential.

Providing Patient Teaching

Because so many older people are responsible for self-medication, nurses should promote self-care capacity in this area. The nurse should assess a patient's risk for medication errors (Box 18-2) and plan interventions to minimize those risks. Some of the factors that could interfere with safe drug administration include:

- *Functional limitations:* Impairments in the person's ability to perform activities of daily living or instrumental activities of daily living could create challenges in the ability to administer medications. These problems could include the inability to travel to a pharmacy to have a prescription filled, problems removing lids from medication containers, difficulty pouring the drugs or obtaining fluids to take with them, and impaired swallowing.

BOX 18-2 Risk Factors for Medication Errors

- Use of multiple medications
- Cognitive impairment
- Hearing deficits
- Arthritic or weak hands
- History of noncompliance with medical care
- Lack of knowledge regarding medications
- Limited finances
- Illiteracy
- Lack of support system
- History of inappropriate self-medication
- Presence of expired or borrowed medications in home

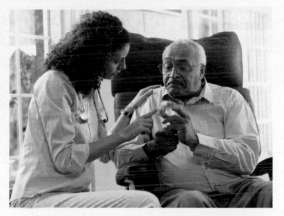

FIGURE 18-2 ■ The nurse teaches the older adult about his medications to promote safe self-care.

■ *Cognitive limitations:* Older adults could have impairments that prevent them from remembering to take the medications; forgetting that they did take the medication and retaking them; and confusing medications, dosage, or schedule.

■ *Educational limitations:* Persons with limited education may have difficulty reading and understanding instructions and labels.

■ *Sensory limitations:* Hearing deficits can cause instructions to be missed or misunderstood. Poor vision can prevent labels and instructions from being adequately seen.

■ *Financial limitations:* Limited funds could cause the older person to not fill prescriptions, skip dosages, or use an old prescription or someone else's similar medication.

■ *Choice:* Some individuals may make a conscious decision to not take their medications due to dislike of the effects, poor motivation, preference to use funds for other purposes, or denial of their condition.

A detailed description, both verbal and written, should be given to older people and their caregivers, outlining the drug's name, dosage schedule, route of administration, action, special precautions, incompatible foods or drugs, and adverse reactions (Fig. 18-2). A color-coded dosage schedule can assist persons who have visual deficits or who are illiterate. Medication labels with large print and caps that can be easily removed by weak or arthritic hands should be provided. During every patient–nurse visit, the nurse should review the patient's medication schedule and new symptoms. A variety of potential medication errors can be prevented or corrected by close monitoring. Some of the classic self-medication errors include incorrect dosage, noncompliance arising from misunderstanding, discontinuation or unnecessary continuation of drugs without medical advice, and the use of medications prescribed for previous illnesses. Box 18-3 describes guidelines to use in teaching older adults about safe drug use.

Monitoring Laboratory Values

Blood tests often are done to determine the blood levels of certain medications and to assess if the drug is achieving the desired result. This monitoring is especially important for older adults as their body functions can change over time, thereby altering the metabolism and excretion of medications. In addition, drugs can behave differently in older persons. Lack of adherence to administration schedules can also be determined through laboratory testing.

Nurses should consult with the physician and pharmacist as to the type and frequency of blood work necessary for specific medications. For community-based older adults, it is important to assure they can travel to the site of laboratory testing; limited mobility, unavailability of help to transport or escort them, lack of funds, and poor memory could interfere with obtaining the necessary testing.

ALTERNATIVES TO DRUGS

Older adults have many health conditions for which drugs can prove helpful. However, drugs can produce serious adverse effects that can result in greater threats to older persons than their primary health conditions. It is crucial that drugs be used cautiously and that the benefits and risks of drugs be weighed to ensure they result in more good than harm.

Sometimes lifestyle changes can improve conditions and eliminate the need for medications. These can include diet modifications; regular exercise; effective stress management techniques; and regular schedules for sleep, rest, and elimination.

BOX 18-3 **Tips for Safe Drug Use: Teaching Tool**

- Keep a current list of all of the following that you use:
  - prescription drugs
  - over-the-counter drugs
  - vitamins, minerals, and other nutritional supplements
  - herbal and homeopathic remedies
  - and show this to your health care providers
- For each drug, herb, homeopathic remedy, or nutritional supplement that you use, know (and, if possible, have this information written down) the:
  - dosage
  - administration schedule
  - administration instructions (take on full or empty stomach, take only if symptom is present, discontinue after x days)
  - purpose
  - usual side effects
  - adverse effects that you should bring to the attention of your health care provider
  - precautions (when you should not take it; interactions with food, other drugs, or substances)
  - storage instructions
  - where purchased/obtained

- Learn as much as you can about the drugs you are taking by reading the literature that comes with the drug and consumer drug reference books that are available at your local library or bookstore.
- Recognize that your drug dosage may be different from someone else's dosage who is taking the same drug.
- Be aware that you can develop adverse effects to drugs that you have taken for years without problems. Review your symptoms with your health care provider.
- Try to reduce the drugs you are using. Discuss with your health care provider improvements in your symptoms or other changes that could cause a drug to no longer be needed.
- Periodically review your drug dosages with your health care provider to see if any changes in your body's function could lead to reduced dosages.
- Try to manage new symptoms naturally rather than with drugs.
- Do not take new drugs without consulting your health care provider.

Alternative and complementary therapies provide new avenues for treating health conditions. These therapies have grown in acceptance and popularity among consumers and can offer effective and safe approaches to managing health conditions. Often, alternative therapies can replace the need for drugs or enable lower dosages of drugs to be used. It is crucial for nurses to be aware of the uses, limitations, precautions, and possible adverse reactions associated with alternative therapies so that they can help older adults be informed consumers.

 POINT TO PONDER

How can you envision using alternative and complementary therapies as substitutes for or adjuncts to drug therapy in your practice? What obstacles could you face in attempting to integrate these therapies into your practice and what could you do to overcome them?

REVIEW OF SELECTED DRUGS

The remainder of this chapter reviews major drug groups and the main concerns related to their use in the older population. This section is not intended to be an all-inclusive drug review; readers are advised to consult with current drug references and pharmacists for comprehensive information.

Analgesics

With the high prevalence of pain among older adults, analgesics are widely used. Of the analgesics, the nonsteroidal anti-inflammatory drug (NSAID) aspirin is particularly popular because of its effectiveness and low cost. Older adults are especially sensitive to the effects of aspirin and more likely to experience side effects. Of the various side effects of aspirin, GI bleeding is one of the most serious. When iron deficiency anemia is detected in older persons, it is important to inquire about aspirin consumption, which could be related to GI bleeding. Using buffered or enteric-coated aspirin preparations and avoiding taking aspirin on an empty stomach are helpful measures in preventing GI irritation and bleeding. Insomnia can occur when patients are using caffeine-containing aspirin products (e.g., Anacin, Butalbital Compound, Cope, Fiorinal, and Stanback Powder), so it is important to inquire about the specific brand of aspirin when collecting drug information from a patient. Occasionally disturbances of the CNS develop when persons with decreased renal function use aspirin. Aspirin suppositories can cause irritation of the rectum. Symptoms related to this include changes in mental status, dizziness, tinnitus, and deafness. When patients are on low-sodium diets, consideration must be given to their aspirin intake as a large intake of sodium salicylate (as could occur with patients taking aspirin regularly for arthritis) can contribute a significant amount of sodium to the diet.

Acetaminophen is another popular analgesic among older people with mild to moderate pain. Despite its relative lack of anti-inflammatory activity, it often is recommended for the initial treatment of osteoarthritis. The total daily dose should not exceed 4,000 mg as high doses taken long term can cause irreversible hepatic necrosis. Liver enzymes can be elevated with long-term use at lower doses. Acetaminophen doses should be adjusted for patients with altered liver function. As with aspirin and caffeine products, acetaminophen products that contain caffeine or pseudoephedrine hydrochloride (e.g., Dristan Cold No Drowsiness Formula Maximum Strength Caplets, Excedrin Aspirin-Free Caplets, Sine-Off Maximum Strength No Drowsiness Formula Caplets, and Sinutab) can cause insomnia. Acetaminophen can cause false results with some blood glucose tests; inquiry should be made about the new use of the drug when new alterations in blood glucose levels are discovered. Patients with renal or liver disease have a high risk of serious side effects when using acetaminophen.

Short-acting opioids (codeine, fentanyl, meperidine, morphine, and oxycodone) are used for mild to moderate pain and typically would be tried before long-acting opioids (fentanyl, morphine sustained release, and oxycodone sustained release) are initiated. Opioids should be used with caution in older adults due to an increased risk of adverse effects, especially respiratory depression. Common adverse effects of these drugs include constipation, nausea, vomiting, sedation, lethargy, weakness, risk of falls, confusion, and dependency. Because older adults are more likely to suffer from prostatic hypertrophy or obstruction and age-related renal function impairments, they are at risk for experiencing opioid-induced urinary retention. Meperidine is the least preferred opioid because it is excreted by the kidney; because older adults are more likely to have decreased renal function, the risk of toxic reactions to this drug is high.

Nursing guidelines for older adults taking analgesics include the following:

- Assess the symptom of pain carefully for its underlying cause. Improving or eliminating the cause of the pain may make the use of an analgesic unnecessary.
- Explore nonpharmacologic means to manage pain, such as relaxation exercises, massages, warm soaks, and diversional activities.
- If nonpharmacological means of pain control are unsuccessful, begin with the weakest type and dose of analgesic and gradually increase so that the patient's response can be evaluated.
- Administer analgesics regularly to maintain a constant blood level.
- Observe for signs of infection other than fever in patients who are taking aspirin or acetaminophen as the antipyretic effect of these drugs can mask fevers associated with infection.
- Because bleeding and delayed clotting times can result from long-term aspirin use, observe for signs of anemia, bleeding, and altered hemoglobin and prothrombin time (PT).
- Note signs of salicylate toxicity, which include dizziness, vomiting, tinnitus, hearing loss, sweating, fever, confusion, burning in the mouth and throat, convulsions, and coma.
- Observe for hypoglycemic reactions, which can occur when persons with diabetes combine aspirin with sulfonylureas.
- Use narcotics very carefully in older adults.
- If there has been a known or suspected overdose of any drug from this group, refer the patient for emergency help at once, even if no symptoms are present. Signs of poisoning may not appear for several days, although liver damage may be occurring.
- Be alert to interactions:
  - Aspirin can increase the effects of oral anticoagulants, oral antidiabetic agents, cortisone-like drugs, penicillins, and phenytoin
  - Aspirin can decrease the effects of probenecid, spironolactone, and sulfinpyrazone
  - Aspirin's effects can be increased by large doses of vitamin C and decreased by antacids, phenobarbital, propranolol, and reserpine
  - Acetaminophen's effects can be decreased by phenobarbital
  - Narcotic analgesics can increase the effects of antidepressants, sedatives, tranquilizers, and other analgesics
  - The effects of narcotics can be increased by antidepressants and phenothiazines; nitrates can increase the action of meperidine
  - Meperidine can decrease the effects of eye drops used for the treatment of glaucoma

Antacids

Decreased gastric acid secretion and increased intolerance to fatty and fried foods make indigestion a common occurrence in late life and antacids popular drugs. It is important, however, that nurses assess the reason for antacid use. What patients believe to be indigestion actually could be gastric cancer or ulcer; also, cardiac disorders can present with atypical symptoms that resemble indigestion. Chronic antacid use could warrant the need for a diagnostic evaluation.

The availability and widespread use of antacids can cause some individuals to minimize the seriousness of these drugs. Antacids are drugs and they do interact with other medications. Sodium bicarbonate– and magnesium-containing antacids can cause fluid and electrolyte imbalances by promoting diarrhea; sodium bicarbonate can cause hypernatremia and metabolic acidosis; calcium carbonate can lead to hypercalcemia; prolonged use of aluminum hydroxide can cause hyperphosphatemia; and long-term use of calcium-based antacids can lead to constipation and renal problems. Therefore, it is important to use these drugs carefully and only when needed.

Nursing guidelines for older adults taking antacids include the following:

- During assessments, ask specifically about the use of antacids. Some patients may not consider over-the-counter antacid medications of concern and may omit them when reporting their medication histories.

- Ensure that patients who have used antacids frequently or over a long period of time have been evaluated for the underlying cause of their problem.

- Avoid administering other medications within 2 hours of administration of an antacid, unless otherwise ordered, to prevent the antacid from interfering with drug absorption.

- Monitor bowel elimination. Constipation can result from the use of aluminum hydroxide and calcium antacids; diarrhea can occur when magnesium hydroxide combinations are used.

- Advise patients who are on sodium-restricted diets to avoid using sodium bicarbonate as an antacid.

- Be alert to interactions:
  - Aluminum hydroxide can increase the effects of meperidine and pseudoephedrine
  - Magnesium hydroxide can increase the effects of dicumarol
  - Most antacids can decrease the effects of barbiturates, chlorpromazine, digoxin, iron preparations, isoniazid, oral anticoagulants, penicillin, phenytoin, phenylbutazone, salicylates, sulfonamides, tetracycline, and vitamins A and C

Antibiotics

Age-related changes in the immune system and the high prevalence of disease processes cause older adults to be highly susceptible to infections. Antibiotics can play a role in treating these infections; however, excessive use of antibiotics has contributed to the emergence and spread of antibiotic-resistant bacteria. Penicillin resistance in *Streptococcus pneumoniae* has increased significantly, as has resistance to macrolides, doxycycline, trimethoprim–sulfamethoxazole, and second- and third-generation cephalosporins. Antibiotic-resistant *S. pneumoniae* is of serious concern because this pathogen is the leading cause of community-acquired bacterial pneumonia, bacterial meningitis, and bacterial sinusitis. Oral thrush, colitis, and vaginitis are common secondary infections from antibiotic therapy that can cause discomfort and a new set of problems. Further, adverse reactions to antibiotics occur more frequently in older adults than in other age groups. With the serious consequences, antibiotic therapy must be used selectively and cautiously.

Any antibiotic can cause diarrhea, nausea, vomiting, anorexia, and allergic reactions. Parenteral vancomycin and aminoglycosides (e.g., amikacin, gentamicin, and tobramycin) require close monitoring due to the risk of causing hearing loss and renal failure; renal function tests should be done regularly during the use of these medications. Fluoroquinolones (e.g., ciprofloxacin and moxifloxacin) increase the risk of hypo- and hyperglycemia in older adults and can cause prolonged QTc intervals; this group of antibiotics is not used in patients with known prolonged QTc intervals or who are receiving certain antiarrhythmic agents. Cephalosporins can cause false results with urine testing for glucose.

Nursing guidelines for older adults taking antibiotics include the following:

- Ensure that cultures are obtained when an infection is suspected or present; different antibiotics are effective for different infections.

- Administer antibiotics on a regular schedule to maintain a constant blood level. Reinforce to patients that they should not skip doses. Consider developing a medication chart or calendar to assist the older patient in remembering to administer the drugs.

- Observe for signs of superinfections, which can develop with long-term use of antibiotics.

- Be alert to interactions:
  - Penicillins are protein-bound drugs. When taken with other highly protein-bound drugs

(e.g., aspirin, phenytoin, valproate, aripiprazole, buspirone, and clozapine) the effects of penicillin can be reduced, and penicillin, in turn, can reduce the effects of other protein-bound drugs

- The effects of ampicillin and carbenicillin can be decreased by antacids, chloramphenicol, erythromycin, and tetracycline
- The effects of doxycycline can be decreased by aluminum-, calcium-, or magnesium-based laxatives, antacids, iron preparations, phenobarbital, and alcohol
- The effects of sulfisoxazole can be increased by aspirin, oxyphenbutazone, probenecid, sulfinpyrazone, and para-aminosalicylic acid. Sulfisoxazole can increase the effects of alcohol, oral anticoagulants, oral antidiabetic agents, methotrexate, and phenytoin
- Probenecid delays the excretion of most antibiotics, with the risk that their levels will accumulate in the blood and increase the side effects

Anticoagulants

Anticoagulants are effective in preventing both arterial and venous thrombosis and are often prescribed for patients with a history of thromboembolic disorders, heart attacks, strokes, and coronary disorders, as well as for prophylaxis for patients who have had hip surgery and mitral valve replacement. Although beneficial, anticoagulants have a narrow treatment range and carry a higher risk of bleeding in older persons.

Usually, heparin is prescribed for rapid anticoagulation, followed by warfarin (coumarin) for long-term use. Neither of these drugs dissolves existing clots, but rather prevents the formation of new ones. Heparin is known to block the eosinophilic response to adrenocorticotropic hormone and insulin. Osteoporosis and spontaneous fractures are a risk to persons who have used heparin for a long time.

Nursing guidelines for older adults taking anticoagulants include the following:

- Ensure that patients using anticoagulants have their PT/international normalization ratio (INR) monitored; discuss the recommended frequency with the physician.
- Age-adjusted dosages may be prescribed; consult with the physician.
- Administer anticoagulants at the same time each day to maintain a constant blood level.
- Observe for signs of bleeding; teach patients to observe for these signs.

- Educate patients about the need to be careful about diet. A large intake of vitamin K–rich foods (asparagus, bacon, beef liver, cabbage, fish, cauliflower, and green leafy vegetables) can reduce the effectiveness of anticoagulants. Mango and papaya can increase INR. High doses of vitamin E can increase bleeding risk.
- Advise patients to refrain from taking herbal products until they have reviewed them with their health care provider. Many herbs interact with anticoagulants.
- Keep vitamin K readily available as an antidote when patients are receiving anticoagulants.
- Advise patients to avoid using aspirin as it can interfere with platelet aggregation and cause bleeding. Three grams or more of salicylates—a level that could be reached by persons who use aspirin for arthritic pain—is sufficient to cause hemorrhage in older adults.
- Be alert to interactions:
  - Anticoagulants can increase the effects of oral hypoglycemic agents and phenytoin and decrease the effects of cyclosporine and phenytoin
  - The effects of anticoagulants can be increased by acetaminophen, allopurinol, alteplase, amprenavir, androgens, aspirin and some other NSAIDs, azithromycin, bismuth subsalicylate, some calcium channel blockers, capsaicin, broad spectrum antibiotics, chlorpromazine, colchicine, ethacrynic acid, mineral oil, phenylbutazone, phenytoin, probenecid, reserpine, thyroxine, tolbutamide, and TCAs
  - The effects of anticoagulants can be decreased by antacids, antithyroid agents, barbiturates, carbamazepine, chlorpromazine, cholestyramine, estrogens, rifampin, thiazide diuretics, and vitamin K
  - Heparin's effects can be partially reduced by digoxin, antihistamines, nicotine, and tetracyclines

Anticonvulsants

Seizures in older adults can result from a history of epilepsy, injury, hypoglycemia, infections, electrolyte imbalance, or drug reactions. Treating many of these conditions can eliminate the seizures and the need for anticonvulsant drugs; this reinforces the importance of a comprehensive assessment and diagnostic testing to identify the precise cause.

Anticonvulsants can be used singularly or in combination to sustain a blood level that will control seizures with the fewest side effects. Older people have a higher risk of toxicity from anticonvulsants, necessitating that they be used cautiously. Carbamazepine, lamotrigine, valproate, and gabapentin are preferred over phenobarbital and phenytoin for treating older patients with epilepsy.

In addition to seizures, anticonvulsants can be prescribed for the treatment of bipolar disorders, schizoaffective disorders, chronic neuropathic pain, prevention of migraines, and other conditions.

Nursing guidelines for older adults taking anticonvulsants include the following:

- Observe for and inquire about possible side effects of these drugs, including change in bowel habits, abnormal bruising, bleeding, pallor, weakness, jaundice, muscle and joint pain, nausea, vomiting, anorexia, dizziness (increasing the risk of falls), blurred vision, diplopia, confusion, agitation, slurred speech, hallucinations, arrhythmias, hypotension, sleep disturbances, tinnitus, urinary retention, and glycosuria.

- As these drugs can depress psychomotor activity, ensure patients have adequate physical activity.

- Ensure periodic evaluations of blood levels are done for drugs for which this is required and/or available (e.g., carbamazepine, phenytoin, phenobarbital, primidone, and valproic acid).

- Be aware that these drugs can worsen any existing liver or kidney disease.

- Anticonvulsants should not be discontinued abruptly. Advise patients to check with their physicians before discontinuing these drugs.

- Advise patients to avoid grapefruit and grapefruit juice when taking these drugs as grapefruit increases the risk of toxicity.

- Monitor closely patients with existing glaucoma, coronary artery disease, or prostate disease. Anticonvulsants can aggravate these conditions.

- Note that some anticonvulsants can cause photosensitivity.

- Be alert to interactions:

  • Anticonvulsants can increase the effects of analgesics, antihistamines, propranolol, sedatives, and tranquilizers

  • Anticonvulsants can decrease the effects of cortisone and anticoagulants

  • The CNS depressant effects can be increased and the anticonvulsant effects decreased when some anticonvulsants are used with TCAs

  • Anticonvulsants and digitalis preparations taken concurrently significantly increase the risk of toxicity from both drugs

Antidiabetic (Hypoglycemic) Drugs

Antidiabetic drugs require careful dosage adjustment based on the individual's weight, diet, and activity level. Drugs in this group fall under insulin and sulfonylureas. The self-injection of insulin can be a challenge for some older adults, particularly those with arthritic hands, poor vision, or cognitive impairment. Ongoing assessment of the ability of older adults and their family caregivers to manage injections is essential. People who still are producing some degree of insulin may take sulfonylureas. Examples include chlorpropamide, glimepiride, glipizide, glyburide, tolazamide, and tolbutamide; metformin is not recommended for persons over age 80 years due to the risk of metabolic acidosis.

Chlorpropamide and glyburide are not drugs of choice for older adults because they have a long half-life and increase the risk of serious hypoglycemia.

Hypoglycemia is a more probable and serious problem for older diabetics than ketosis. Some of the classic signs of hypoglycemia may not be present in older adults; confusion and slurred speech may give the first clue of this complication.

See Chapter 27 for more information about the care of the patient who has diabetes. Nursing guidelines for older adults taking antidiabetic drugs include the following:

- Teach individuals with diabetes and their caregivers about the proper use and storage of medications and recognition of hypo- and hyperglycemia. Reinforce that all insulin or oral antidiabetic drugs are not interchangeable (i.e., different drugs have different potency, onset, and duration).

- Ensure that people with diabetes wear or carry identification to alert others of their diagnosis in the event they are found unconscious or confused.

- For patients using insulin, examine injection sites regularly. Local redness, swelling, pain, and nodule development at the injection site can indicate insulin allergy. A sunken area at the infection site can be caused by atrophy and hypertrophy associated with insulin lipodystrophy—a harmless although unattractive condition.

- Report conditions that could alter antidiabetic drug requirements, such as fever, severe trauma, prolonged diarrhea or vomiting, altered thyroid function, or heart, kidney, or liver disease.

- Advise patients to avoid drinking alcohol as this can lead to a significant drop in blood sugar.

- Be alert to interactions:

  • The effects of antidiabetic drugs can be increased by alcohol, oral anticoagulants, cimetidine, isoniazid, phenylbutazone, ranitidine, sulfinpyrazone, and large doses of salicylates

- The effects of antidiabetic drugs can be decreased by chlorpromazine, cortisone-like drugs, furosemide, phenytoin, thiazide diuretics, thyroid preparations, and cough and cold medications
- Antidiabetic drugs can increase the effects of anticoagulants

Antihypertensive Drugs

Good circulation becomes increasingly difficult to achieve in later life because of reduced elasticity of peripheral vessels and the accumulation of deposits in the lumen of vessels. To compensate for increased peripheral resistance, systolic blood pressure may rise. Likewise, diastolic blood pressure may increase in response to an age-related reduction in cardiac output. Although these increases in blood pressure may compensate for changes that could interfere with adequate circulation, they create new associated risks when blood pressure enters a level considered hypertensive (>140 mm Hg systolic and/or >90 mm Hg diastolic).

Because diuretics blunt the sodium- and water-retaining effects of many other antihypertensive drugs such as beta-blockers, they are the most commonly used medication in combination antihypertensive agents. Diuretics cause blood vessels to dilate and help the kidneys eliminate salt and water, thereby decreasing fluid volume throughout the body and lowering blood pressure. Beta-blockers stop the effects of the sympathetic division, the part of the nervous system that can rapidly respond to stress by increasing blood pressure. Examples include acebutolol, atenolol, betaxolol, bisoprolol, carteolol, metoprolol, nadolol, penbutolol, pindolol, propranolol, and timolol. Side effects of beta-blockers can include dizziness, fainting, bronchospasm, bradycardia, heart failure, possible masking of low blood sugar levels, impaired peripheral circulation, insomnia, fatigue, shortness of breath, depression, Raynaud's phenomenon, vivid dreams, hallucinations, sexual dysfunction, and, with some beta-blockers, an increased triglyceride level.

Angiotensin-converting enzyme (ACE) inhibitors (e.g., lisinopril) are well tolerated antihypertensive drugs and are popular initial agents in the treatment of hypertension. They dilate arterioles by preventing the formation of angiotensin II, which causes arterioles to constrict and block the action of ACE, which converts angiotensin I to angiotensin II. Examples include benazepril, captopril, enalapril, fosinopril, lisinopril, moexipril, perindopril, quinapril,

ramipril, and trandolapril. Cough is a common side effect of this drug. In patients for whom ACE inhibitor and diuretic combinations are indicated but not tolerated, angiotensin II receptor antagonist (e.g., losartan) and diuretic combinations may be used.

Calcium channel blockers cause arterioles to dilate by a completely different mechanism. Examples include amlodipine, diltiazem (sustained release only), felodipine, isradipine, nicardipine, nifedipine (sustained release only), nisoldipine, and verapamil. Side effects of these drugs include headache, dizziness, flushing, fluid retention, problems in the heart's electrical conduction system (including heart block), bradycardia, heart failure, enlarged gums, and constipation. ACE inhibitors and calcium channel blockers may be prescribed in combination to lower blood pressure, as may other combinations.

Alpha-blockers (doxazosin, prazosin, and terazosin) and angiotensin II blockers (candesartan, eprosartan, irbesartan, losartan, telmisartan, and valsartan) are among the other drugs that could be prescribed for hypertension management.

Nursing guidelines for older adults taking antihypertensive drugs include the following:

- Assess blood pressure carefully. Obtain readings with the patient in lying, sitting, and standing positions.
- Help patients in learning and using nonpharmacologic measures to reduce blood pressure, such as weight reduction, restriction of sodium and alcohol intake, moderate aerobic exercise, and stress management techniques.
- Monitor patients closely when therapy is initiated. Some antihypertensives can cause significant hypotension initially. Advise patients to change positions slowly to prevent falls. If diuretics are prescribed, monitor for diuretic-induced dehydration.
- Ensure that patients obtain laboratory work as ordered. Monitoring of serum potassium is especially important when patients are receiving ACE inhibitors with potassium or potassium-sparing diuretics.
- Monitor patients for side effects.
- Reinforce to patients the importance of adhering to treatment even when symptoms are absent.
- Some antihypertensives should not be abruptly discontinued. Advise patients to check with their physicians before discontinuing these drugs.
- Be alert to interactions:
  - Antihypertensive drugs can increase the effects of barbiturates, insulin, oral antidiabetic drugs, sedatives, and thiazide diuretics

- The effects of antihypertensives can be decreased by amphetamines, antacids, antihistamines, salicylates, and TCAs
- Verapamil can increase the blood digoxin level.
- The effects of propranolol can be increased by cimetidine, ciprofloxacin, and diuretics
- Grapefruit juice can affect the bioavailability and alter the effects of calcium channel blockers
- Individual drugs have specific interactions; carefully review drug literature to learn about them

Nonsteroidal Anti-inflammatory Drugs

The high prevalence of arthritis in the older population contributes to the wide use of NSAIDs. These drugs are effective in relieving mild to moderate pain and inflammation; however, they usually are not used unless lower risk analgesics (e.g., acetaminophen) have failed to be beneficial. Examples of NSAIDs include diclofenac, diflunisal, flurbiprofen, indomethacin, meclofenamate, naproxen, piroxicam, salicylates, and tolmetin.

Cyclooxygenase-II (COX-2) inhibitors are a new class of NSAIDs introduced in 1998 that were believed to have the advantage of causing less gastric irritation. They are called COX-2 inhibitors because they block an enzyme called cyclooxygenase, which is believed to trigger pain and inflammation in the body. In 2005, a Food and Drug Administration (FDA) advisory committee concluded that COX-2 inhibitors increase the risk of heart attacks and strokes. However, the FDA agreed to allow some of these drugs (celecoxib [Celebrex]) to be sold because, for many people, the benefits of the drugs outweighed the cardiovascular risks. When patients are taking celecoxib, careful monitoring is necessary. Side effects to observe for include swelling of the face, fingers, hands, and lower legs; severe stomach pain; and signs of bleeding. People who are allergic to sulfa drugs may have allergic reactions to celecoxib.

Oxyphenbutazone and phenylbutazone, although effective within days after therapy is initiated, are extremely potent drugs and carry a high risk of adverse effects for older adults. They should not be used in patients with blood disorders, dementia, GI ulcers, glaucoma, or cardiac, renal, liver, or thyroid disease. Long-term therapy is discouraged.

Any NSAID can cause or worsen renal failure, raise blood pressure, and exacerbate heart failure. Nursing guidelines for older adults taking NSAIDs include the following:

- NSAIDs have a narrowed therapeutic window, and toxic levels accumulate much easier and at lower doses in older adults. Closely observe for

and ask about side effects, such as GI symptoms, impaired hearing, and indications of CNS disturbances. Be aware that older adults are at higher risk of developing delirium as a side effect to these drugs.

- Ensure blood evaluations are done regularly.
- Administer these drugs with food or a glass of milk, unless contraindicated, to reduce GI irritation.
- If patients are using aspirin for cardioprotective effects and are started on an NSAID, review this with the physician or pharmacist as some NSAIDs (e.g., ibuprofen) can reduce the cardiac benefit of aspirin.
- Prolonged use of indomethacin, meclofenamate, piroxicam, and tolmetin can cause CNS effects (e.g., headache, dizziness, drowsiness, and confusion). When reviewing patients' drugs, note if these drugs have been used for an extended time and review this with the physician and pharmacist.
- Be alert to interactions:
  - NSAIDs can increase the effects of oral anticoagulants, insulin, oral antidiabetic drugs, cyclosporine, lithium, penicillin, phenytoin, and sulfa drugs; they can decrease the effects of diuretics and beta-blockers
  - When celecoxib is used with aspirin, lithium, or fluconazole, there is an increased risk of serious side effects
  - Oxyphenbutazone can decrease the effects of digitoxin

Cholesterol-Lowering Drugs

Increasing numbers of aging individuals are alert to the risks associated with elevated levels of low-density lipoprotein (LDL) cholesterol. Direct-to-consumer marketing of cholesterol-lowering drugs has also increased the awareness of this problem. The result has been a growing use of cholesterol-lowering drugs. These drugs have shown benefit in reducing cardiovascular events and mortality in older adults.

The main goal in lowering cholesterol is to lower LDL and raise high-density lipoprotein (HDL). Treatment goals are individualized, based on the unique profile of the individual patient. Often, prior to initiating therapy, other interventions are used (e.g., eating a heart-healthy diet, exercise programs, and weight reduction). Cholesterol-lowering drugs include statins, niacin, bile acid resins, fibric acid derivatives, and cholesterol absorption inhibitors.

Statins (HMG-CoA reductase inhibitors), usually the first line of treatment, block the production of cholesterol in the liver. Examples include rosuvastatin (Crestor), atorvastatin (Lipitor), fluvastatin (Lescol), lovastatin (Mevacor), pravastatin (Pravachol), and simvastatin (Zocor). There also are combination statins, such as Advicor, a combination of a statin and niacin, and Caduet, a combination of a statin (atorvastatin) and the antihypertensive amlodipine (Norvasc). As these drugs can impair liver function, liver function tests should be done prior to initiating therapy and at regular intervals thereafter. Muscle pain is an important symptom to note in patients using statins as these drugs can cause myopathy and the breakdown of skeletal muscle, which can precipitate renal failure.

Niacin, or nicotinic acid, is a B complex vitamin that—in addition to being available in the diet—can be prescribed at high dosages to lower LDL and raise HDL cholesterol. Examples include Niacor, Niaspan, and Slo-Niacin. The main side effects are flushing, itching, tingling, and headache; aspirin can reduce many of these symptoms. Niacin can interfere with glucose control and aggravate diabetes. It also can exacerbate gallbladder disease and gout.

Bile acid resins work inside the intestine, where they bind to bile and prevent it from being reabsorbed into the circulatory system. Examples include cholestyramine (Questran and Questran Light), colestipol (Colestid), and colesevelam (WelChol). The most common side effects are constipation, gas, and upset stomach. These drugs can interact with diuretics, beta-blockers, corticosteroids, thyroid hormones, digoxin, valproic acid, NSAIDs, sulfonylureas, and warfarin; consult with the physician and pharmacists as to the length of time to wait between the administration of these drugs and bile acid resins.

Fibric acid derivatives, although their mechanism of action is not fully clear, are thought to enhance the breakdown of triglyceride-rich particles, decrease the secretion of certain lipoproteins, and induce the synthesis of HDL. Examples include fenofibrate (Tricor), gemfibrozil (Lopid), and fenofibrate (Lofibra). Liver function tests and complete blood count should be evaluated prior to initiating therapy and on a regular basis thereafter.

Cholesterol absorption inhibitors work by inhibiting the absorption of cholesterol in the intestines. Vytorin is a newer drug that is a combination of ezetimibe (Zetia) and the statin simvastatin.

Nursing guidelines for older adults taking cholesterol-lowering drugs include the following:

- Assist patients in implementing dietary and lifestyle modifications to help reduce cholesterol levels.
- Ensure that patients receive liver functions and other necessary tests as ordered.

- Monitor for interactions and follow precautions for each category of cholesterol-lowering drugs as discussed above.

Cognitive Enhancing Drugs

With nearly 5 million people suffering from dementia and approximately 30 million having some type of memory disorder, there has been increasing development of drugs to improve cognitive functions. These drugs include:

- *Cholinesterase inhibitors:* donepezil (Aricept), galantamine (Razadyne), rivastigmine tartrate (Exelon), and tacrine (Cognex).
- *NMDA receptor antagonists:* memantine (Namenda).

These drugs can cause many side effects, including nausea; vomiting; diarrhea; anorexia; weight loss; urinary frequency; muscle cramps; joint pain, swelling, or stiffness; fatigue; drowsiness; headache; dizziness; nervousness; depression; confusion; changes in behavior; abnormal dreams; difficulty falling asleep or staying asleep; discoloration or bruising of the skin; and red, scaling, itchy skin.

Nursing guidelines for older adults taking cognitive enhancing drugs include the following:

- Evaluate patients' mental status, cognition, and activities of daily living prior to initiation of therapy and periodically thereafter during prolonged treatment. Monitor for signs and symptoms of GI bleed. Ensure that patients using tacrine have regular liver function tests.
- Recommend that patients on these drugs be reevaluated as their underlying disorder progresses.
- Cholinesterase inhibitors can affect cardiac conduction in patients with existing conduction disorders or who are using medications that affect the heart rate. Review potential risks with the physician and pharmacist.
- Avoid abrupt discontinuation of these drugs. Advise patients to check with their physicians before discontinuing these drugs.
- Instruct patients that tacrine is best taken on an empty stomach, and galantamine is best taken with food.
- Be alert to interactions with anticholinergics, aspirin (high doses used for arthritis), cholinergic drugs, cholinesterase inhibitors, long-term use of NSAIDs, carbamazepine, dexamethasone, phenobarbital, phenytoin, and rifampin.

Digoxin

Digitalis preparations are used in the treatment of congestive heart failure, atrial flutter or fibrillation, supraventricular tachycardia, and extrasystoles to increase the force of myocardial contraction through direct action on the heart muscle. The resulting improvement in circulation helps to reduce edema, as well.

Daily doses in older adults ordinarily should not exceed 0.125 mg except if used to control atrial arrhythmia and ventricular rate. Digoxin should be used with caution in patients with impaired renal function.

Nursing guidelines for older adults taking digoxin include the following:

- Check and/or instruct patients and their caregivers to check pulse for rate, rhythm, and regularity prior to administering digoxin.

- The usual biological half-life of these drugs can be extended in older adults, increasing their risk of digitalis toxicity. Signs of toxicity include bradycardia, diarrhea, anorexia, nausea, vomiting, abdominal pain, delirium, agitation, hallucinations, headache, restlessness, insomnia, nightmares, aphasia, ataxia, muscle weakness and pain, cardiac arrhythmias, and high serum drug levels (although *toxicity can occur in the presence of normal serum levels*). Promptly report any signs of possible toxicity.

- Hypokalemia makes patients more susceptible to toxicity. Ensure that patients consume potassium-rich foods and that serum potassium is evaluated regularly.

- Older adults can present signs of toxicity with normal plasma levels of the drug. Be certain to monitor for signs.

- Be alert to interactions:
  - The effects of digoxin can be increased by alprazolam, amphotericin, benzodiazepines, carvedilol, cyclosporine, erythromycin, ethacrynic acid, fluoxetine, guanethidine, ibuprofen, indomethacin, phenytoin, propranolol, quinidine, tetracyclines, tolbutamide, trazodone, trimethoprim, verapamil, and some other drugs
  - The effects of digoxin can be decreased by antacids, cholestyramine, kaolin-pectin, laxatives, neomycin, phenobarbital, phenylbutazone, and rifampin
  - The risk of toxicity is increased with digitalis preparations taken with cortisone, diuretics, parenteral calcium reserpine, and thyroid preparations

Diuretics

Diuretics are used in the treatment of a variety of cardiovascular disorders such as hypertension and congestive heart failure. There are several major types that work in different ways:

- *Thiazides:* inhibit sodium reabsorption in the cortical diluting site of the ascending loop of Henle and increase the excretion of chloride and potassium. Examples include chlorothiazide, hydrochlorothiazide, and metolazone.

- *Loop diuretics:* inhibit reabsorption of sodium and chloride at the proximal portion of the ascending loop of Henle. Examples include bumetanide, ethacrynic acid, and furosemide.

- *Potassium-sparing diuretics:* antagonize aldosterone in the distal tubule, causing water and sodium, but not potassium, to be excreted. Examples include amiloride, spironolactone, and triamterene.

Under normal circumstances, older adults are at high risk for developing fluid and electrolyte imbalances; diuretic therapy increases this risk considerably. Special attention must be paid to recognizing signs of imbalances early and correcting them promptly.

Nursing guidelines for older adults taking diuretics include the following:

- Plan an administration schedule that interferes least with the patient's schedule. Morning administration is usually preferable.

- Monitor intake and output, and assure adequate fluids are consumed.

- Teach patients and their caregivers to recognize and promptly report signs of fluid and electrolyte imbalance: dry oral cavity, confusion, thirst, weakness, lethargy, drowsiness, restlessness, muscle cramps, muscular fatigue, hypotension, reduced urinary output, slow pulse, and GI disturbances.

- Because postural hypotension can occur from the use of these drops, careful attention should be paid to preventing falls.

- Observe for signs of latent diabetes, which sometimes can be manifested during thiazide diuretic therapy.

- Monitor hearing in patients receiving loop diuretics as these drugs can cause transient ototoxicity.

- Diuretics can worsen existing liver disease, renal disease, gout, and pancreatitis and raise blood glucose in diabetics. Monitor patients with these conditions carefully.

- Ensure serum electrolytes, glucose, and blood urea nitrogen are evaluated periodically.

- Be alert to interactions:
  - Diuretics can increase the effects of antihypertensives and decrease the effects of allopurinol, digoxin, oral anticoagulants, antidiabetic agents, and probenecid
  - The effects of diuretics can be increased by analgesics and barbiturates; diuretics' effects can be decreased by cholestyramine and large quantities of aspirin (administer these drugs at least 1 hour before)

Laxatives

Age-related reduction in peristalsis and the tendency of many older adults to be less active, consume low-fiber diets, and take medications that are constipating cause constipation to be a common problem. Nonpharmacologic measures to promote bowel elimination should be used before resorting to the use of laxatives. When laxatives are necessary, they should be selectively chosen and used. Laxatives differ in their function:

- *Bulk formers* (e.g., methylcellulose) absorb fluid in the intestines and create extra bulk, which distends the intestines and increases peristalsis. They usually take 12 to 24 hours to take effect. Bulk formers need to be mixed with large amounts of water. These compounds should not be used when there is any indication of intestinal obstruction.
- *Stool softeners* (e.g., docusate sodium) collect fluid in the stool, which makes the mass softer and easier to move. They do not affect peristalsis; they take effect in 24 to 48 hours.
- *Hyperosmolars* (e.g., glycerin) pull fluid into the colon, causing bowel distension that increases peristalsis. These take effect within 1 to 3 hours; they are contraindicated when there is the risk of fecal impaction.
- *Stimulants* (e.g., cascara sagrada) irritate the smooth muscle of the intestines and pull fluid into the colon, causing peristalsis. They take effect in 6 to 10 hours. Stimulants can cause intestinal cramps and excessive fluid evacuation.
- *Lubricants* (e.g., mineral oil) coat fecal material to facilitate its passage. They take effect in 6 to 8 hours. These compounds are not recommended for older adults.

Nursing guidelines for older adults taking laxatives include the following:

- Recognizing that it is a common geriatric risk, assist older adults in preventing constipation.

- When patients complain of constipation, assess carefully before suggesting or administering a laxative.
- Reinforce to older adults and their caregivers that laxatives, although popular, are drugs and can cause side effects and interact with other drugs.
- Teach patients that good fluid intake must accompany the use of bulk-forming laxatives and stool softeners to prevent the accumulation of stool leading to bowel obstruction.
- Be alert to interactions:
  - Laxatives can reduce the effectiveness of many oral medications by increasing the speed of their passage through the GI system
  - Chronic use of mineral oil can deplete the body's fat-soluble vitamins (vitamins A, D, E, and K)

Psychoactive Drugs

Antianxiety Drugs (Anxiolytics)

Financial worries, deaths, crime, illness, and many of the other problems commonly faced by older adults give legitimate cause for anxiety. Financial aid, counseling, self-care instruction, and other interventions can yield better long-term results in treating situational anxiety than a medication alone, and these measures may also prevent additional problems from arising as a result of adverse drug reactions. According to the Diagnostic and Statistical Manual of Mental Disorders (American Psychiatric Association, 2013), antianxiety medications should only be used when there is generalized anxiety disorder, panic disorder, anxiety that accompanies another psychiatric disorder, sleep disorder, significant anxiety in response to a situational trigger, or delirium, dementia, and other cognitive disorders with associated behaviors that are well documented, persistent, not due to preventable or correctable reasons, and create such distress or dysfunction to make the person a risk to self or others.

When they are deemed necessary, benzodiazepines are common antianxiety drugs used in older persons. The CNS depressants can include short-acting benzodiazepines (e.g., alprazolam, estazolam, lorazepam, oxazepam, and temazepam) and long-acting benzodiazepines (e.g., chlordiazepoxide, clonazepam, diazepam, flurazepam, and quazepam). Older adults are more likely to experience side effects, which could include dizziness, unsteady gait, drowsiness, slurred speech, and confusion. Although less common, other side effects could include abdominal or stomach cramps, increased heart rate, increased perspiration, sensitivity to light, seizures, and hallucinations. Some patients experience insomnia, irritability, and nervousness after they discontinue taking these drugs. As benzodiazepines are on the Beers list of inappropriate drugs for older adults, they need to be used with utmost care and usually only until the slower acting medications have begun to act.

Meprobamate, diphenhydramine, and hydroxyzine are not advised for use with older adults. Patients who have used meprobamate for a long period of time can become physically and psychologically dependent on the drug and need to be weaned from it slowly.

Nursing guidelines for older adults taking anxiolytics include the following:

- Ensure that approaches other than medications have been attempted prior to having an antianxiety drug prescribed. Even if these measures were tried and ineffective previously, they should be tried again.

- Advise patients to change positions slowly and to avoid operating a car or machinery that requires mental alertness and fast responses.

- Instruct patients to incorporate foods in the diet that can promote bowel elimination as these drugs can be constipating. Monitor bowel elimination.

- Monitor nutritional status and weight to assure food intake is not jeopardized by possible lethargy or GI upset.

- Advise caution in grapefruit consumption; this fruit can increase the concentration of these drugs.

- Advise patients that several days of administration may be necessary before clinical effects from the medication are noted and that the effects could continue several days after the drug is discontinued.

- Avoid alcohol when these drugs are used and limit caffeine.

- Be alert to interactions:
  - Antianxiety drugs can increase the effects of anticonvulsants, antihypertensives, oral anticoagulants, and other CNS depressants
  - The effects of antianxiety drugs can be increased by TCAs
  - Diazepam can increase the effects of digoxin and phenytoin, leading to toxicity; diazepam can decrease the effects of levodopa

Antidepressants

The incidence of depression increases with age, contributing to it being the major psychiatric diagnosis in older adults. Depression may be a problem that some older adults have struggled with throughout their lives or a new symptom in response to life circumstances that they now face.

There are several different classes of antidepressants available, including alpha-adrenoceptors (e.g., mirtazapine), dopamine reuptake blocking compounds (e.g., bupropion), monoamine oxidase inhibitors, serotonin antagonists (5-hydroxytryptamine-2 receptor; e.g., nefazodone and trazodone), selective serotonin–norepinephrine reuptake inhibitors (e.g., duloxetine and venlafaxine), selective serotonin reuptake inhibitors (SSRIs; e.g., citalopram, escitalopram, fluoxetine, fluvoxamine, paroxetine, and sertraline), and TCAs. Of these, the SSRIs tend to be well tolerated and effective in older adults and typically do not cause cardiotoxicity, orthostatic hypotension, or anticholinergic effects that often are experienced with TCAs. Citalopram, sertraline, and escitalopram have fewer drug–drug interactions. Although popular, TCAs have side effects that can pose risks to older adults, such as anticholinergic effects, orthostatic hypotension, and arrhythmias, especially in patients with cardiovascular disease.

Nursing guidelines for older adults taking antidepressants include the following:

- Assess factors contributing to depression. In some situations, obtaining financial aid, receiving grief counseling, joining a group, and other actions can improve the cause of the depression and reduce or eliminate the need for drugs.

- Explore the use of other therapies in addition to antidepressants to improve mood.

- Ensure that the lowest effective dosage of the drug is used to reduce the risk of adverse effects.

- Advise patients that several weeks of therapy commonly is required before improvement is noted.

- Monitor the plasma level of the drug. Be aware that dosage adjustment may be needed.

- Observe for, ask about, and report side effects, including diaphoresis, urinary retention, indigestion, constipation, hypotension, blurred vision, difficulty voiding, increased appetite, weight gain, photosensitivity, and fluctuating blood glucose levels.

- The dizziness, drowsiness, and confusion that can occur in older adults can increase the risk of falls, so special precautions are needed.

- Dryness of the mouth can be an uncomfortable side effect of these drugs. Advise patients to use sugarless mints, ice chips, or a saliva substitute to improve this symptom. Monitor oral health closely because dry mouth increases the risk of dental disease.

■ Some antidepressants need to be discontinued gradually. Advise patients not to abruptly stop taking the drugs.

■ Observe patients for a worsening of depression symptoms or suicidal thinking or behavior; bring these findings to the physician's attention immediately.

■ Be alert to interactions:

• Antidepressants can increase the effects of anticoagulants, atropine-like drugs, antihistamines, sedatives, tranquilizers, narcotics, and levodopa

• Antidepressants can decrease the effects of clonidine, phenytoin, and various antihypertensives

• The effects of antidepressants can be increased by alcohol and thiazide diuretics

• Bupropion can increase the risk of seizures

Antipsychotics

Antipsychotic medications are commonly used to treat older adults with delirium, agitation, and psychosis due to Alzheimer's disease and schizophrenia. The effectiveness of antipsychotics in controlling symptoms has enabled many individuals to improve their quality of life and function; however, these drugs can have profound adverse effects, necessitating careful prescription and close monitoring.

There are two major classes of antipsychotic drugs:

■ *First-generation (conventional/typical) agents:*

• chlorpromazine (Thorazine)

• fluphenazine (Prolixin)

• haloperidol (Haldol)

• loxapine (Loxitane)

• molindone (Moban)

• perphenazine (Trilafon)

• pimozide (Orap)

• thioridazine (Mellaril)

• thiothixene (Navane)

• trifluoperazine (Stelazine)

■ *Second-generation (atypical) agents:*

• aripiprazole (Abilify)

• clozapine (Clozaril)

• fluoxetine and olanzapine (Symbyax)

• olanzapine (Zyprexa)

• paliperidone (Invega)

• quetiapine (Seroquel)

• risperidone (Risperdal)

• ziprasidone (Geodon)

Because they were viewed as having a lower risk of adverse effects and greater tolerability, the atypical antipsychotics have largely replaced the conventional/typical agents. However, the atypical antipsychotics have been found to have their own set of side effects that are of concern in geriatric care, such as postural hypotension, sedation, and falls. The FDA has determined that the treatment of behavioral disorders in older patients with dementia with atypical or second-generation antipsychotic medications is associated with increased cerebrovascular adverse events and mortality and issued a black box warning for these drugs (U.S. Food and Drug Administration, 2005). These drugs should only be used for the treatment of schizophrenia and not for behavioral disturbances associated with dementias.

The serious risks associated with these drugs and the paucity of clinical trials with psychotropic medications in the older population in general and in patients with dementia in particular (Jeste et al., 2007) demand that nonpharmacologic interventions be used before initiating drug therapy. Nonpharmacologic interventions can include addressing factors that contribute to symptoms, environmental modifications, behavioral interventions, and treatment of other conditions.

Nursing guidelines for older adults taking antipsychotics include the following:

■ Ensure that patients receive a thorough physical and mental health evaluation before any antipsychotic drug is prescribed.

■ Whenever possible, attempt to use other interventions to address symptoms prior to using antipsychotics.

■ Antipsychotics should be used for the treatment of specific disorders and not as a means of managing behavior. Using antipsychotics to control behaviors alone can be viewed as chemically restraining patients.

■ Drugs have a longer biological half-life in older adults; assure the lowest possible dosage is initially used.

■ Older adults are more sensitive to the *anticholinergic effects* of these medications: dry mouth, constipation, urinary retention, blurred vision, insomnia, restlessness, fever, confusion, disorientation, hallucinations, agitation, and picking behavior. They also are at greater risk for developing *extrapyramidal* symptoms: tardive dyskinesia, parkinsonism, akinesia, dystonia. Observe and report these symptoms promptly.

■ Patients taking antipsychotics are at high risk for falls due to the hypotensive and sedative effects. Implement fall prevention measures for these individuals.

■ Constipation is a common side effect of antipsychotics. Advise patients to include fiber and other foods in diet that promote regular bowel movement and monitor bowel elimination.

■ Men with prostatic hypertrophy may develop urinary hesitance and retention when using antipsychotics. Advise patients and caregivers to monitor urinary symptoms and report changes promptly.

■ Gradual weaning rather than abrupt withdrawal from these drugs is recommended.

■ Response to these drugs can vary in older adults, necessitating close monitoring.

■ Be alert to interactions:

• The effects of antipsychotics can be reduced by anticholinergic drugs, phenytoin, and antacids

• Antipsychotics can increase the effects of sedatives and antihypertensives and decrease the effects of levodopa

• Alcohol can increase the sedative action and depressant effects of these drugs on brain function

Sedatives/Hypnotics

Hypnotics and sedatives often are prescribed for older adults for the treatment of insomnia, nocturnal restlessness, anxiety, confusion, and related disorders. The dose will determine if the same drug will have a hypnotic or sedative effect.

Generally, chloral hydrate, diphenhydramine, flurazepam, hydroxyzine, quazepam, and triazolam are not drugs of choice for older adults for the management of insomnia (McSpadden & Yale, 2006).

Because tolerance to sedatives can develop after prolonged use, continued evaluation of effectiveness is necessary. It is not unusual for restlessness, insomnia, and nightmares to occur after sedatives are discontinued.

Nursing guidelines for older adults taking sedatives/hypnotics include the following:

■ Before these drugs are used, evaluate factors contributing to insomnia. Adjusting environmental lighting or temperature, controlling noise, eliminating caffeine, increasing physical activity, relieving pain, giving a back rub, and controlling symptoms of diseases can improve sleep and eliminate the need for a sedative.

■ Carefully monitor patients who are using sedatives as they are at higher risk for falls and fractures.

■ Be alert to interactions:

• Sedatives and hypnotics can increase the effects of oral anticoagulants, antihistamines, and analgesics and decrease the effects of cortisone and cortisone-like drugs

• The effects of sedatives and hypnotics can be increased by alcohol, antihistamines, and phenothiazines

There are other groups of drugs that older adults can use. It is advantageous to learn about drugs before administering them, understand the impact specific drugs can have on older adults, teach older adults how to use individual drugs safely, and regularly monitor for side effects and adverse reactions.

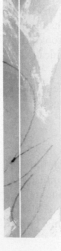

BRINGING RESEARCH TO LIFE

MEDICATION BELIEFS AND ANTIHYPERTENSIVE ADHERENCE AMONG OLDER ADULTS: A PILOT STUDY

Ruppar, T. M., Dobbels, F., & DeGeest, S. (2012). Geriatric Nursing, 33(2), 89–95.

Many older adults require antihypertensive therapy to reduce their risk of heart attacks, strokes, heart failure, and renal disease; however, medication adherence tends to be low in this population. As beliefs are predictors of behavior, this study sought to explore this area. In the past, most studies that have explored the relationship between medication beliefs and medication adherence have used self-reported data, which is believed to underestimate adherence problems; in addition, few have focused on medication beliefs of older adults with hypertension. This study used the Beliefs About Medicines Questionnaire to measure beliefs and electronic monitoring to measure adherence.

Participants had to be aged 60 years or older, have a self-reported diagnosis of hypertension, be taking an antihypertensive that they self-administered, be cognitively intact, and be able to read and write in English. The selected participants had a median age of 74 years, 79% were female, 79% were Caucasian, 58% had some college education with another 27% having completed high school, and their self-reported years with hypertension ranged from 9 months to 50 years.

The findings supported those of previous studies in that older adults with negative beliefs about medications had greater adherence problems. Their concerns centered on medication dependency, long-term effects, and lifestyle disruptions.

This study demonstrates the importance of assessing patients' understanding and beliefs about the impact of their medications, both at the time of initial prescription and periodically thereafter. Misconceptions about the effects of medications need to be identified and clarified and explanations provided of the risks and benefits of medications

PRACTICE REALITIES

Mrs. Hemmings, an 83-year-old who lives alone in the community, is a patient of a medical practice where, unless an acute situation arises, she usually is seen by her physician every 6 months. She has six different prescription drugs, which she takes for hypertension, glaucoma, and osteoporosis.

On her visit to the medical office today, when her vital signs are taken by the nurse, her blood pressure is found to be 190/165. When the physician enters and takes her blood pressure again 15 minutes later, it is found to be 180/160. The physician asks if she has been taking her antihypertensive medication and diuretic, and she indicates she has. "In fact," Mrs. Hemmings says, "I'm running to the bathroom all night long to urinate."

The physician changes Mrs. Hemmings' antihypertensive to a more potent drug and leaves the room.

What should have been done differently prior to the new medication being prescribed? What could the nurse do to assist Mrs. Hemmings in this situation?

CRITICAL THINKING EXERCISES

1. List age-related changes that affect the way in which drugs behave in older persons.

2. What key points would you include in a program to educate senior citizens about safe drug use?

3. What interventions could you employ to aid an older adult who has poor memory to safely administer medications?

4. Review the major drug groups and identify those that address problems that could potentially be managed with nonpharmacologic means.

REFERENCES

American Psychiatric Association. (2013). *Diagnostic and statistical manual of mental disorders* (5th ed.). Washington, DC: Author.

Beers, M. H. (1997). Explicit criteria for determining potentially inappropriate medication use by the elderly. *Archives of Internal Medicine, 157,* 1531–1536.

Beers, M. H., Ouslander, J. G., Rollingher, J., Reuben, D. B., & Beck, J. C. (1991). Explicit criteria for determining inappropriate medication use in nursing home residents. *Archives of Internal Medicine, 151,* 1825–1832.

Fick, D. M., Cooper, J. W., Wade, W. E., Waller, J. L. Maclean, J. R., & Beers, M. H. (2003). Updating the Beers criteria for potentially inappropriate medication use in older adults. Results of a U.S. consensus panel of experts. *Archives of Internal Medicine, 163*(22), 2716–2724.

Gorard, D. A. (2006). Escalating polypharmacy. *QJM, 99*(11), 797–800.

Jeste, D. V., Blazer, D., Casey, D., Meeks, T. Salzman, C., Schneider, L., Yaffe, K., et al. (2007). ACNP White Paper: Update on use of antipsychotic drugs in elderly persons with dementia. *Neuropsychopharmacology, 18,* 1–14. Retrieved August 1, 2012 from http://www.neuropsychopharmacology.org

Kaufman, D. W., Kelly, J. P., Rosenberg, L., Anderson, T. E., & Mitchell, A. A. (2002). Recent patterns of medication use in the ambulatory adult population of the United States: The Slone survey. *Journal of the American Medical Association, 287*(3), 337–344.

McSpadden, C. S., & Yale, S. (2006). *Unnecessary medications in the elderly. A guide to improving therapeutic outcomes* (pp. 7–28). Miamisburg, OH: MED-PASS Inc.

Page, R. L., II, & Ruscin, J. M. (2007). The risk of adverse drug events and hospital-related morbidity and mortality among older adults with potentially inappropriate medication use. *American Journal of Geriatric Pharmacotherapy, 4*(4), 297–305.

Patel, R. B. (2003). Polypharmacy and the elderly. *Journal of Infusion Nursing, 26*(3), 166–169.

Skufca, L. (2007). *Are Americans age 45+ using drugs wisely: A 2006 study research report.* Washington, DC: AARP.

The American Geriatrics Society 2012 Beers Criteria Update Expert Panel. (2012). The American Geriatrics Society Updated Beers Criteria for potentially inappropriate medication use in older adults. *Journal of the American Geriatrics Society, 60*(4), 616–631.

U.S. Food and Drug Administration. (2005). FDA public health advisory: Deaths from antipsychotics in elderly patients with behavioral disturbances. Retrieved October 7, 2012 from http://www.fda.gov/Drugs/DrugSafety/Postmarket DrugSafetyInformationforPatientsandProviders/Drug SafetyInformationforHeathcareProfessionals/Public HealthAdvisories/ucm053171.htm

RECOMMENDED READINGS

Recommended Readings associated with this chapter can be found on the web site that accompanies the book. Visit **http://thepoint.lww.com/Eliopoulos8e** to access the recommended readings and other additional resources associated with this chapter.

UNIT 5

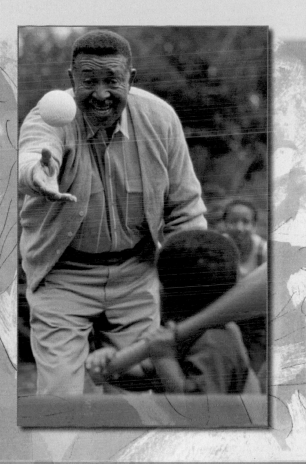

Facilitating Physiological Balance

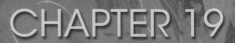

Respiration

LEARNING OBJECTIVES

After reading this chapter, you should be able to:

1. List the impact of age-related changes on respiratory health.

2. Describe measures to promote respiratory health in older adults.

3. Discuss the risks, symptoms, and care considerations associated with selected respiratory illnesses.

4. Describe interventions that can aid in preventing complications and promoting self-care in older persons with respiratory conditions.

TERMS TO KNOW

Chronic obstructive pulmonary disease (COPD): group of diseases including asthma, chronic bronchitis, and emphysema

Elastic recoil: lungs' ability to expand and contract

Kyphosis: curvature of the spine causing bowing out of upper spine

Total lung capacity: maximum volume that lungs can expand during fullest inspiration

Vital capacity: maximum amount of air that can be expelled following maximum inspiration

Respiratory health is vital to the older person's ability to maintain a physically, mentally, and socially active life. It can make the difference between a person maximizing opportunities to live life to the fullest and being too fatigued and uncomfortable to leave the confines of home. A lifetime of insults to the respiratory system from smoking, pollution, and infection takes its toll in old age, making respiratory disease a leading cause of disability and the fourth leading cause of death in persons over 70 years of age. However, positive health practices to promote effective breathing can benefit respiratory health at any age and minimize limitations imposed by problems.

EFFECTS OF AGING ON RESPIRATORY HEALTH

The effects of aging create a situation in which respiratory problems can develop more easily and be more difficult to manage. Changes in the respiratory system are noted in upper airway passages. The nose experiences connective tissue changes that reduce support and can cause nasal septal deviations that interfere with the passage of air. Reduced secretions from the submucosal gland cause the mucus in the nasopharynx to be thicker and harder to expel; this also can cause a chronic tickle in the throat and coughing. Although it may appear to be a relatively minor consideration, hair in the nostrils becomes thicker with age and may readily accumulate a greater amount of dust and dirt particles during inspiration. Unless these particles are removed and the nasal passage is kept patent, there may be an interference with the normal inspiration of air. Blowing the nose and mild manipulation with a tissue may adequately rid the nostrils of these particles. When particles are difficult to remove, a cotton-tipped applicator moistened with warm water or saline solution may help loosen them. Caution should be taken not to insert the cotton-tipped applicator too far into the nose because trauma can easily result. Any nasal obstruction not easily removed should be brought to the physician's attention.

The trachea stiffens due to calcification of its cartilage. Coughing is reduced due to a blunting of the laryngeal and coughing reflexes.

The lungs become smaller in size and weight with age. Various connective tissues responsible for respiration and ventilation are weaker. The elastic recoil of the lungs during expiration is decreased because of less elastic collagen and elastin, and expiration requires the active use of accessory muscles. Alveoli are less elastic, develop fibrous tissue, and contain fewer functional capillaries. The loss of skeletal muscle strength in the thorax and diaphragm, combined with the loss of resilient force that holds the thorax in a slightly contracted position, contributes to the slight kyphosis and barrel chest seen in many older adults. The net effect of these changes is a reduction in vital capacity and an increase in residual volume—in other words, less air exchange and more air and secretions remaining in the lungs.

Further, age-related changes external to the respiratory system can affect respiratory health in significant ways. A reduction in body fluid and reduced fluid intake can cause drier mucous membranes, impeding the removal of mucus and leading to the development of mucous plugs and infection. Altered pain sensations can cause signals of respiratory problems to be unnoticed or mistaken for non-respiratory disorders. Different norms for body temperature can cause fever to present at an atypically lower level, potentially being missed and allowing respiratory infections to progress without timely treatment. Loose or brittle teeth can dislodge or break, leading to lung abscesses and infections from the aspiration of tooth fragments. Relaxed sphincters and slower gastric motility further contribute to the risk of aspiration. Impaired mobility, inactivity, and side effects from the numerous medications used by the older population can decrease respiratory function, promote infection, interfere with early detection, and complicate treatment of respiratory problems. Nursing Diagnosis Table 19-1 lists respiratory risks associated with aging. Astute assessment is essential to reducing the morbidity and mortality associated with these conditions (Assessment Guide 19-1).

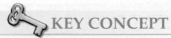

KEY CONCEPT

Pieces of brittle teeth can break off, be aspirated, and cause respiratory problems. This reinforces the importance of good oral health and dental care in late life.

RESPIRATORY HEALTH PROMOTION

The high risk of developing respiratory disorders that every older person faces warrants the incorporation of preventive measures into all care plans. Infection prevention is an important component. In addition to the precautions any adult would take, older persons need to be particularly attentive to obtaining influenza and pneumonia vaccines and avoiding exposure to individuals who have respiratory infections (see Chapter 30 for discussion of influenza and pneumonia).

Also, in addition to basic health practices, special attention to promoting respiratory activity is important. Nurses should teach all older adults to do deep breathing exercises several times daily (Fig. 19-1). Keeping in mind that full expiration is more difficult than inspiration for older individuals, these exercises should emphasize an inspiratory–expiratory ratio of 1:3. To help make these exercises routine, link them with other routines, such

NURSING DIAGNOSIS

TABLE 19-1   Aging and Risks to Adequate Respiration

Causes or Contributing Factors	Nursing Diagnosis
Reduced elastic recoil of lungs during expiration	Impaired Gas Exchange Ineffective Breathing Pattern
Increase in residual capacity	Ineffective Breathing Pattern
Decrease in maximum breathing capacity	Ineffective Airway Clearance
Hyperinflation of lung apices and underinflation of lung bases	Impaired Gas Exchange
Reduced number and elasticity of alveoli	Activity Intolerance related to decreased respiratory efficiency
Calcification of tracheal and laryngeal cartilage	Ineffective Airway Clearance
Decrease in vital capacity	Risk of Infection
Reduced ciliary activity	
Increased diameter of bronchioles and alveolar ducts	
Loss of skeletal muscle strength in thorax and diaphragm	
Increased rigidity of thoracic muscles and ribs	
Increased diameter of anteroposterior chest	
Less efficient cough response	

ASSESSMENT GUIDE 19-1

RESPIRATORY FUNCTION

GENERAL OBSERVATIONS

Much can be determined regarding the status of the respiratory system through careful observation of the following:

- *Color:* Coloring of the face, neck, limbs, and nail beds can be indicative of respiratory status. Ruddy, pink complexions often occur with emphysema and are associated with hypoxia, which is caused by a high carbon dioxide level in the blood that inhibits involuntary neurotransmission from the pons to the diaphragm for inspiration. In the presence of chronic bronchitis, patients can have a blue or gray discoloration caused by the lack of oxygen binding to the hemoglobin.
- *Chest structure and posture:* The anteroposterior chest diameter increases with age—significantly so in the presence of chronic obstructive pulmonary disease (COPD). Note abnormal spinal curvatures (e.g., kyphosis, scoliosis, and lordosis).
- *Breathing pattern:* Observe the chest for symmetrical expansion during respirations, as well as the depth, rate, rhythm, and length of respirations. Decreased expansion of the chest can be caused by pain,

fractured ribs, pulmonary emboli, pleural effusion, or pleurisy. Ask the patient to change positions, walk, and cough to see if these activities result in any changes.

INTERVIEW

Some older persons may give unreliable accounts of their past respiratory symptoms or have grown so accustomed to living with their symptoms that they do not consider them unusual. Specific questions can assist in revealing disorders, such as the following:

- "Do you ever have wheezing, chest pain, or a heavy feeling in your chest?"
- "How often do you get colds? Do you get colds that keep returning? How do you treat them?"
- "How far can you walk? How many steps can you climb before getting short of breath?"
- "Do you have any breathing problems when the weather gets cold or hot?"
- "How many pillows do you sleep on? Do breathing problems (e.g., coughing and shortness of breath) ever awaken you from sleep?"

- "How much do you cough during the day? During each hour? Can you control it?"

- "Do you bring up sputum, phlegm, or mucus when you cough? How much? What color? Is it the consistency of water, egg white, or jelly?"

- "How do you manage respiratory problems? How often do you use cough syrups, cold capsules, inhalers, vapors, rubs, or ointments?"

- "Did you ever smoke? If so, for how long and when and why did you stop? How many cigarettes or cigars do you smoke daily? Do people you live with or spend a lot of time with smoke?"

- "What kind of jobs have you had over your lifetime? Any in factories or chemical plants?"

- "Do you live or have you lived near factories, fields, or high-traffic areas?"

More specific questions increase the likelihood of obtaining a full and accurate history of factors related to respiratory health. Ascertain and document the dates of influenza and pneumonia vaccines as well.

PHYSICAL EXAMINATION

- Palpate the posterior chest to evaluate the depth of respirations, degree of chest movement, and presence of masses or pain. Normally there is bilateral movement during respirations and reduced expansion of the base of the lungs. Tactile fremitus is usually best felt in the upper lobes; increased fremitus in the lower lobes occurs with pneumonia and masses. COPD and pneumothorax can cause a lack of fremitus in the upper lobes.

- Percussion of the lungs should produce a resonant sound. Auscultation of the lungs should reflect normal bronchial, vesicular, and bronchovesicular breath sounds; crackles, rhonchi, and wheezes are abnormal findings.

Review assessment data for actual and potential nursing diagnoses that can be used in guiding the care plan.

---

as before meals or every time the person sits down to watch the news. Even healthy, active people can benefit from including these exercises in their daily activities. Yoga is another practice that can aid in respiration.

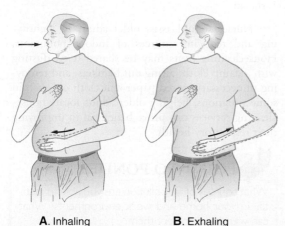

A. Inhaling   **B.** Exhaling

FIGURE 19-1 ■ Breathing exercises should emphasize forced expiration. (**A**) With one hand on the stomach (below the ribs) and the other over the middle anterior chest, the patient should inhale to the count of one. The hand over the stomach should move outwardly as the diaphragm and stomach move downward; the hand over the chest should not move. (**B**) Expire air to the count of three. The hand over the stomach should be pulled closer to the body as the diaphragm and stomach move upward; the hand over the chest should not move.

POINT TO PONDER

Take a few minutes to slow down, close your eyes, and do deep breathing exercises. What effects did this have on your body, mind, and spirit? How could these exercises benefit you if you did them several times throughout the day?

Because smoking is the most important factor contributing to respiratory disease, smoking cessation is an important health promotion measure. Many older smokers started their habit at a time when the full effects of smoking were not realized and smoking was considered fashionable, sociable, and sophisticated. Although smokers may be aware of the health hazards associated with smoking, it is an extremely difficult habit to break.

Smoking has significant effects on the respiratory system, including bronchoconstriction, early airway closure, reduced ciliary action, inflammation of the mucosa, and increased mucous secretions and coughing. The effects on respiratory health may initially be so subtle and gradual that they are not realized. Unfortunately, by the time signs and symptoms become apparent, considerable damage to the respiratory system may have occurred, compounding age-related changes to the system. Smokers have twice the incidence of lung cancer, a higher incidence of all respiratory diseases, and more complications with respiratory problems and commonly suffer from productive coughs, shortness of breath, and reduced breathing capacity. Nicotine can interact with medications, as well. Although maximum benefit is obtained by not starting to smoke in the first place or quitting early in life, smoking cessation is beneficial at any age. Local chapters of the American Lung Association, health departments, clinics, and commercial agencies offer a wide range of smoking cessation approaches that may be useful.

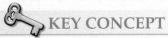

KEY CONCEPT

The use of tobacco in any form carries an increased risk of health problems.

Immobility is a major threat to pulmonary health, and older adults frequently experience conditions that decrease their mobility. Preventing fractures, pain, weakness, depression, and other problems that could decrease mobility is an essential goal. Older adults, their family members, and caregivers all need to be educated about the multiple risks associated with immobility. It may be tempting for the older person to reduce activity or for caring family members to encourage that person to rest on days when arthritis or other discomforts are bothersome, unless it is understood that by doing so, more discomfort and disability can result. When immobility is unavoidable, hourly turning, coughing, and deep breathing will promote respiratory activity; blow bottles and similar equipment can also be beneficial. Persons who are chair-bound may need the same attention to respiratory activity as the bed-bound to ensure their lungs are fully expanded.

Older persons should be advised against treating respiratory problems themselves. Many over-the-counter cold and cough remedies can have serious effects in older adults and can interact with other medications being taken. These drugs can also mask symptoms of serious problems, thereby delaying diagnosis and treatment. Older adults should know that a cold lasting more than 1 week may not be a cold at all, but something more serious that requires medical attention.

It is important to review all medications used by older persons for their impact on respiration. Decreased respirations or rapid, shallow breathing can be caused by many of the drugs commonly prescribed for geriatric conditions; these drugs include analgesics, antidepressants, antihistamines, antiparkinson agents, synthetic antispasmodics, sedatives, and tranquilizers. As always, alternatives to drugs should be used whenever possible.

Environmental factors also influence respiratory health. Indirect room ventilation is best for older people who are more susceptible to drafts; fibrosis, which is common in older people, can be aggravated by chilling and drafts. Considerable attention has been paid to pollutants such as ozone, carbon monoxide, and nitrogen oxide that reduce the quality of the air we breathe outdoors. However, indoor air pollution can affect respiratory health as well. Synthetic or plastic building materials can emit gas; spores, animal dander, mites, pollen, plaster, bacteria, and viruses can be present in household dust; and cigarette smoke can add carbon monoxide and cadmium to indoor air. Conscious choices to minimize exposure to air pollution in the places where we reside, work, and play can help alleviate some of the stress to our respiratory systems. Furthermore, the quality of indoor air can be improved by:

- installing and maintaining air filters in heating and air-conditioning systems
- vacuuming regularly (preferably using a central vacuum system or a water-trap vacuum that prevents dust from returning to the room)
- damp-dusting furnishings
- discouraging cigarette smoking
- opening windows to air out rooms
- maintaining green houseplants to help detoxify the air

Nurses should assist older adults in identifying and reducing sources of indoor pollutants. Housecleaning hints may be shared (e.g., dusting with a damp cloth, airing out blankets, and removing unnecessary stored paper and cloth objects); in some situations, helping older adults locate housecleaning services can prove beneficial to improving their respiratory health.

POINT TO PONDER

What sources of air pollution are you able to identify in your home and work environments? What can you do to correct them?

Finally, often overlooked in the prevention of respiratory problems is the significance of a healthy oral cavity. Infections of the oral cavity can lead to respiratory infections or can decrease appetite and facilitate a generally poor health status. As noted, teeth can break or dislodge, leading to lung abscesses, infections, and aspirated tooth fragments. Respiratory infections may decline when loose or diseased teeth are removed.

Some considerations for promoting effective breathing can be found in the Nursing Diagnosis Highlight: Ineffective Breathing Pattern.

SELECTED RESPIRATORY CONDITIONS

Chronic Obstructive Pulmonary Disease

Chronic obstructive pulmonary disease (COPD) represents a group of diseases including a form of asthma, chronic bronchitis, and emphysema. The incidence of COPD is higher in women and in smokers.

Asthma

Some older persons are affected with asthma throughout their lives; others develop it during old age. Its symptoms and management in older adulthood do not differ much from those in other age groups. Because of the added stress that asthma places on the heart, however, older asthmatics have a high risk of developing complications such as bronchiectasis and cardiac problems. They also have higher rates of mortality from this condition. The nurse should help detect causative factors (e.g., emotions, mouth breathing, and chronic respiratory infections) and educate the patient regarding early recognition of and prompt attention to an asthma attack when it does occur.

Careful assessment of the older asthmatic patient's use of aerosol nebulizers is advisable. Due to the difficulty some older people have in properly using inhalers, a spacer or holding chamber may be helpful to allow the inhalant medication to penetrate deep into the lungs. These systems consist of aerochambers that trap the medication or holding chambers that collapse and inflate during inhalation and expiration. Specific instructions are provided with each system. It is beneficial for the nurse to review the use of these devices as part of every assessment of patients who use them.

Precautions to avoid adverse drug effects are important. Overuse of sympathomimetic bronchodilating nebulizers creates a risk of cardiac arrhythmias leading to sudden death. Cromolyn sodium is one of the least toxic respiratory drugs that can be used, although several weeks of therapy may be necessary for benefits to be realized. Some of the new steroid inhalants are effective and carry a lower risk of systemic absorption and adverse reactions than older steroids.

Chronic Bronchitis

Many older persons demonstrate a persistent, productive cough; wheezing; recurrent respiratory infections; and shortness of breath caused by chronic bronchitis. These symptoms may develop gradually, sometimes taking years for the full impact of the disease to be realized, when, because of bronchospasm, patients notice increased difficulty breathing in cold and damp weather. The condition results from recurrent inflammation and mucus production in the bronchial tubes, which, over time, produce blockage and scarring that

---

NURSING DIAGNOSIS HIGHLIGHT

INEFFECTIVE BREATHING PATTERN

Overview

In late life there is a high prevalence of conditions that limit the ability to adequately inflate the lungs or rid them of sufficient amounts of carbon dioxide. Signs such as confusion, dyspnea, shortness of breath, abnormal arterial blood gases, cyanosis, pursed lip breathing, retraction of respiratory muscles during breathing, and shallow respirations could be associated with this diagnosis.

Causative or contributing factors

Weakness, fatigue, pain, paralysis, immobility, altered mental status, and respiratory or musculoskeletal disease.

Goal

The patient displays an effective breathing pattern, is free from signs of ineffective breathing, and possesses normal arterial blood gases.

Interventions

- Instruct patient in breathing exercises (see Fig. 19-1).
- Control symptoms (e.g., pain) that could threaten effective respirations.
- Raise head of bed at least 30° when patient is lying down, unless contraindicated.
- Instruct patient to turn, cough, and deep breathe at least once every 2 hours.
- Monitor rate, depth, and rhythm of respirations; coloring; coughing pattern; blood gases; and mental status.

restricts airflow. Individuals with chronic bronchitis experience more frequent respiratory infections and greater difficulty managing them. Episodes of hypoxia begin to occur because mucus obstructs the bronchial tree and causes carbon dioxide retention. As the disease progresses, emphysema may develop and death may occur from obstruction.

Management of chronic bronchitis, aimed at removing bronchial secretions and preventing obstruction of the airway, is similar for all age groups. Older patients may need special encouragement to maintain good fluid intake and to expectorate secretions. The nurse can be most effective in preventing the development of chronic bronchitis by discouraging chronic respiratory irritation, such as from smoking, and by helping older adults prevent respiratory infections.

POINT TO PONDER

Smoking-related respiratory diseases have an impact not only on the affected individual but also on society in terms of health care costs. What do you think about the costs to society that result from an individual's personal decision to smoke? What incentives could be used by society to discourage this behavior?

Emphysema

Emphysema occurs with increasing incidence in the older population. Factors causing this destructive disease include chronic bronchitis, chronic irritation from dusts or certain air pollutants, and morphologic changes in the lungs, which include distension of the alveolar sacs, rupture of the alveolar walls, and destruction of the alveolar capillary bed. Cigarette smoking also plays a major role in the development of emphysema. The symptoms are slow in onset and initially may resemble age-related changes in the respiratory system, causing many patients to experience delayed identification and treatment of this disease. Gradually, increased dyspnea is experienced, which is not relieved by sitting upright as it may have been in the past. A chronic cough develops. As more effort is required for breathing and hypoxia occurs, fatigue, anorexia, weight loss, and weakness are demonstrated. Recurrent respiratory infections, malnutrition, congestive heart failure, and cardiac arrhythmias are among the more life-threatening complications older adults can experience from emphysema.

Treatment usually includes postural drainage, bronchodilators, the avoidance of stressful situations, and breathing exercises, which are an important part of patient education. Cigarette smoking should definitely be stopped. The older patient may have insufficient energy to consume adequate food and fluid; nurses need to assess for this and arrange for dietary interventions that can facilitate intake (e.g., frequent small feedings and high-protein supplements). If oxygen is used, it must be done with extreme caution and close supervision. It must be remembered that for these patients, a low oxygen level rather than a high carbon dioxide level stimulates respiration. The older patient with emphysema is a high-risk candidate for the development of carbon dioxide narcosis. Respiratory infections should be prevented, and any that do occur, regardless of how minor they may seem, should be promptly reported to the physician. Sedatives, hypnotics, and narcotics may be contraindicated because the patient will be more sensitive to these drugs. It may be useful to consult with patients' physicians regarding the possibility of lung volume reduction surgery (a procedure in which the most severely diseased portions of the lung are removed to allow remaining tissues and respiratory muscles to work better).

Patients with emphysema need a great deal of education and support to be able to manage this disease. Adjusting to the presence of a serious chronic disease requiring special care or even a lifestyle change may be difficult. The patient must learn to pace activities, avoid extremely cold weather, administer medications correctly, and recognize symptoms of infection. Nursing Care Plan 19-1 outlines a sample care plan for the patient with COPD.

KEY CONCEPT

Asthma, chronic bronchitis, and emphysema are grouped in the category of chronic obstructive pulmonary disease because of their common outcome of obstructing airflow.

Lung Cancer

Most lung cancer now occurs in patients older than 65 years. The generational patterns in smoking prevalence are a large factor responsible for this, although improved diagnostic tools and greater numbers of people surviving to advanced years certainly play a role in the high incidence of lung cancer in older adults. Lung cancer occurs more frequently in men, although the rate among women is rising. The incidence and mortality rate from lung cancer are highest among black individuals as compared with white, Hispanic, and Asian populations (Centers for Disease Control and Prevention, 2012). Cigarette smokers have twice

NURSING CARE PLAN 19-1

THE OLDER ADULT WITH CHRONIC OBSTRUCTIVE PULMONARY DISEASE

Nursing Diagnoses: Impaired Gas Exchange related to chronic tissue hypoxia; Risk of Infection related to pooling of secretions in the lungs

Goal	Nursing Actions
The patient maintains a patent airway; the patient expectorates secretions from lungs	■ Teach breathing exercises to increase inspiratory to expiratory ratio using the following guidelines: • slowly inhale to the count of 5 • lean forward (30–40°) and slowly exhale to the count of 10; use pursed lip breathing for expiration • repeat several times, breathing slowly and rhythmically ■ Teach abdominal breathing to assist with expiration using the following guidelines: *In a lying position* • Place a book or small pillow on the abdomen • Push out the abdomen during inspiration; observe the book or pillow rise • Exhale slowly through pursed lips while pulling in the abdomen *In a sitting position* • Hold a book or small pillow against the abdomen • Push out the abdomen against the book or pillow during inspiration • Lean forward, exhale slowly through pursed lips and pull in the abdomen, pressing the book or pillow against the abdomen ■ Instruct patient to cough and breathe deeply at least once every 8 hours. Coughing can be stimulated by deep expiration and could be planned following breathing exercises. ■ Perform postural drainage exercises as ordered; allow rest periods between position changes and be careful to avoid forceful pounding as older adults with brittle bones could experience a fracture. ■ If antibiotics are prescribed, ensure that they are administered on time to maintain a constant blood level. ■ Control contact with persons who have signs of respiratory infection. ■ Note signs of respiratory infection and promptly report to the physician. ■ Maintain a stable room temperature of 75°F. ■ If oxygen is prescribed, administer with caution and close observation to prevent carbon dioxide narcosis (see Fig. 19-2). ■ Ensure that influenza and pneumococcal vaccines have been administered, unless contraindicated.

Nursing Diagnosis: Activity Intolerance related to chronic hypoxia

Goal	Nursing Actions
The patient performs activities of daily living (ADLs) without becoming fatigued or experiencing respiratory symptoms	■ Determine impact of respiratory symptoms on ADLs, identify actual or potential deficits in engaging in ADLs, and provide assistance to compensate for deficits or interventions to increase self-care ability. ■ Schedule rest periods between activities. ■ Identify factors that contribute to activity intolerance (e.g., interruptions to sleep due to coughing and lack of knowledge of ways to schedule activities to preserve energy) and control or improve as possible.

(Continues)

NURSING CARE PLAN 19-1 (Continued)

- Gradually increase activity level; monitor vital signs and discontinue activity if the following occur:
  - decrease in respiratory rate
  - decrease in pulse rate
  - lack of increase in systolic pressure
  - 15 mm Hg increase in diastolic pressure
  - confusion
  - vertigo
  - pain
  - respiratory distress
- Consult with dietician regarding nutritional intake to support activity.

the incidence as nonsmokers. A high incidence also occurs among individuals who are chronically exposed to agents such as asbestos, coal gas, radioactive dusts, and chromates. This emphasizes the importance of obtaining thorough information regarding a patient's occupational history as part of the nursing assessment. Although conclusive evidence is unavailable, some association has been reported between the presence of lung scars, such as those resulting from tuberculosis and pneumonitis, and lung cancer.

 KEY CONCEPT

Chronic exposure to cigarette smoke, asbestos, coal gas, radon gas, and air pollutants contributes to the development of lung cancer.

The individual may have lung cancer long before any symptoms develop. Thus, people at high risk should be screened regularly. Dyspnea, coughing, chest pain, fatigue, anorexia, wheezing, and recurrent upper respiratory infections are part of the symptoms seen as the disease progresses. Diagnosis is confirmed through chest roentgenogram, sputum cytology, bronchoscopy, and biopsy. Treatment may consist of surgery, chemotherapy, or radiotherapy, requiring the same type of nursing care as that for patients of any age with this diagnosis.

Lung Abscess

A lung abscess may result from pneumonia, tuberculosis, a malignancy, or trauma to the lung. Aspiration of foreign material can also cause a lung abscess; this may be a particular risk to aged persons who have decreased pharyn-

geal reflexes. Symptoms, which resemble those of many other respiratory problems, include anorexia, weight loss, fatigue, temperature elevation, and a chronic cough. Sputum production may occur, but this is not always demonstrated in older persons.

Diagnosis and management are the same as that for other age groups. Modifications for postural drainage, an important component of the treatment, are discussed later in this chapter. Because protein can be lost through the sputum, a high-protein, high-calorie diet should be encouraged to maintain and improve the nutritional status of the older patient.

GENERAL NURSING CONSIDERATIONS FOR RESPIRATORY CONDITIONS

Recognizing Symptoms

Older adults should be advised to seek medical attention promptly if any sign of a respiratory infection develops (see Chapter 30). Frequently, older people do not experience chest pain associated with pneumonia to the same degree as younger adults do, and their normally lower body temperature can cause an atypical appearance of fever (i.e., at lower levels than would occur for younger persons). Thus, by the time symptoms are visible to others, pneumonia can be in an advanced stage.

The nurse should teach older persons to report changes in the character of sputum, which could be associated with certain disease processes. For example, the sputum is tenacious, translucent, and grayish white with COPD; it is purulent and foul smelling with a lung abscess or bronchiectasis; and it is red and frothy with pulmonary edema and left-sided heart failure.

Preventing Complications

Once respiratory diseases have developed, close monitoring of the patient's status is required to minimize disability and prevent mortality. Close nursing observation can prevent and detect respiratory complications and should include checking the following:

- respiratory rate and volume
- pulse (e.g., a sudden increase can indicate hypoxia)
- blood pressure (e.g., elevations can occur with chronic hypoxia)
- temperature (e.g., not only to detect infection but also to prevent stress on the cardiovascular and respiratory systems as they attempt to meet the body's increased oxygen demands imposed by an elevated temperature)
- neck veins (e.g., for distension)
- patency of airway
- coughing (e.g., frequency, depth, and productivity)
- quality of secretions
- mental status

ENSURING SAFE OXYGEN ADMINISTRATION

Oxygen therapy should be used prudently to treat respiratory disorders in older adults. COPD or chronic high levels of oxygen (from oxygen therapy) can contribute to a person retaining a higher amount of carbon dioxide in his or her lungs; carbon dioxide retention increases the risk of developing the serious complication of carbon dioxide narcosis during oxygen therapy (Fig. 19-2). The nurse should monitor blood gases and observe the patient for symptoms of carbon dioxide narcosis, which include confusion, muscle twitching, visual defects, profuse perspiration, hypotension, progressive degrees of circulatory failure, and cerebral depression, which may be displayed as increased sleeping or a deep comatose state.

Because inappropriate oxygen administration can have serious consequences for older persons, nurses must strictly adhere to proper procedures when it is used. The nurse should check the gauge frequently to ensure that it is set at the prescribed level and check the oxygen flow for any interruption or blockage from an empty tank, kinked tubing, or other problems. The nurse should evaluate and recommend the method of administration that will be most effective for the individual patient. Older patients who breathe by

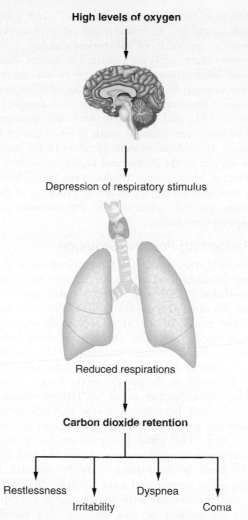

High levels of oxygen

↓

Depression of respiratory stimulus

↓

Reduced respirations

↓

Carbon dioxide retention

Restlessness   Dyspnea
       Irritability   Coma

FIGURE 19-2 ■ Oxygen must be administered to older people carefully. Chronic high levels of oxygen can depress the respiratory stimulus in the brain, thereby reducing respiration and promoting carbon dioxide retention.

mouth or have poor control in keeping their lips sealed most of the time may not receive the full benefit of a nasal cannula. An emaciated person whose facial structure does not allow for a tight seal of a face mask may lose a significant portion of oxygen through leakage. A patient who is insecure and anxious inside an oxygen tent may spend oxygen for emotional stress and not gain full therapeutic benefit. The patient's nasal passages should be regularly cleaned to maintain patency. Indications of insufficient oxygenation must be closely monitored; some older persons will not become cyanotic when hypoxic, so the nurse must evaluate other signs.

With increasing numbers of patients being discharged from hospitals on oxygen for home use and with the realization that many older people lack capabilities, knowledge, and caregiver support, realistic appraisals of the patient's ability to use home oxygen safely are crucial. The patient should have information reinforced and receive supervision through home health agencies or other community resources until the patient or caregiver is comfortable and competent with this treatment. The home environment needs to be evaluated for safety. Consideration must be given to the impact of oxygen on the patient and family's total lifestyle; whether home oxygen results in the family having a new lease on life or becoming prisoners in their home can be influenced by the assistance and support they receive.

Performing Postural Drainage

Postural drainage is often prescribed for removing bronchial secretions in certain respiratory conditions. The basic steps for this procedure are the same as those for other adults, with some slight modifications. If aerosol medications are prescribed, the nurse administers them before the postural drainage procedure. The position for postural drainage depends on the individual patient and on the portion of the lung involved. The older patient needs to change positions slowly and be allowed a few minutes to rest between position changes to adjust to the new position. The usual last position for postural drainage—lying face down across the bed with the head at floor level—may be stressful for the older person and have adverse effects. The nurse can consult with the physician regarding the advisability of this position and possible alterations to meet the needs of the individual patient. Cupping and vibration facilitate drainage of secretions; however, old tissues and bones

are more fragile and may be injured more easily. The procedure should be discontinued immediately if dyspnea, palpitation, chest pain, diaphoresis, apprehension, or any other sign of distress occurs. Thorough oral hygiene and a period of rest should follow postural drainage. Documentation of the tolerance of the procedure and the amount and characteristic of the mucus drained is essential.

Promoting Productive Coughing

Coughing to remove secretions is important in the management of respiratory problems; however, nonproductive coughing may be a useless expenditure of energy and stressful to the older patient. Various measures can be used to promote productive coughing. Hard candy and other sweets increase secretions, thereby helping to make the cough productive. The breathing exercises discussed earlier can also be beneficial. A variety of humidifiers can be obtained without prescription for home use; the nurse needs to teach the patient the correct, safe use of such an apparatus. Expectorants also may be prescribed to loosen secretions and make coughing more productive. A basic, although extremely significant, measure to reinforce is good fluid intake. Patients should be advised to use paper tissues, not cloth handkerchiefs, for sputum expectoration. Frequent handwashing and oral hygiene are essential and have many physical and psychological benefits.

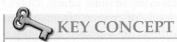

KEY CONCEPT

Nonproductive coughing can be a useless expenditure of energy and can be stressful to an older adult.

CONSIDER THIS CASE

Seventy-nine-year-old Mr. B, who has chronic obstructive pulmonary disease, lives at home with his 80-year-old wife, who has Alzheimer's disease. Mrs. B is able to ambulate and perform activities of daily living with guidance from Mr. B; however, Mrs. B displays poor judgment and requires close supervision. Recently, Mr. B was hospitalized for pneumonia and discharged with home oxygen. His wife, who stayed with a friend during Mr. B's hospitalization, has returned home. Mr. B desires to care for his wife at home but finds his energy reserves are low and has difficulty tracing her steps throughout the house while attached to his oxygen. The couple desperately wants to stay in their home but have no family in the area and receive only limited assistance from friends and neighbors.

THINK CRITICALLY

▪ What are the risks faced by this couple and how can they be minimized?
▪ What assistance could be provided to the couple?

Using Complementary Therapies

Some herbs are believed to affect respiratory health. Mullein, marshmallow, and slippery elm have mucus-secreting effects and can soothe irritated respiratory linings. Lobelia, coltsfoot, and sanguinaria have been used as expectorants. Aromatherapy using eucalyptus, pine, lavender, and lemon may prove useful. Prior to introducing any herbal remedy, the nurse must research for possible interactions with medications the patient is using and discuss with the physician.

Hot, spicy foods (e.g., garlic, onion, and chili peppers) are recommended to open air passages, whereas mucus-forming foods, such as dairy products and processed foods, are ill advised. Vitamins A, C, E, and B_6; zinc; and proteolytic enzymes are suggested as dietary supplements.

Acupuncture, under a trained therapist, is used for the management of asthma, emphysema, and hay fever. Acupressure is being used with some benefit by persons with asthma, bronchitis, and emphysema. Yoga can promote deep breathing and good oxygenation of tissues. Rolfing (a technique using pressure applied with the fingers, knuckles, and elbows to release fascial adhesions and realign the body into balance) and massage can free the rib cage and improve breathing.

Growing numbers of Americans are using complementary therapies for the prevention and management of respiratory conditions. Although the efficacy of these methods may not be fully established, nurses should keep an open mind; if the therapy does no harm and is believed by the individual to be of benefit, positive outcomes could be achieved by combining complementary with conventional treatments.

Promoting Self-Care

Bronchodilators may be prescribed in inhaler form for the treatment of bronchial asthma and other conditions causing bronchospasm, such as chronic bronchitis or emphysema. Effective use of these devices depends on the ability of the individual to manipulate the apparatus and coordinate the spray with inhalation—areas that can be problematic for older persons with slower responses, poorer coordination, arthritic joints, or general weakness. Before an inhaler is prescribed, the ability of the patient to use it correctly must be assessed. Respiratory therapists can be of assistance in recommending devices that can assist patients in overcoming specific obstacles to using inhalers. If the patient is able to manage the skills required for use, instructions and precautions should be reviewed in-depth. The patient and caregivers must understand the serious cardiac effects of excessive use. Normally, one or two inhalations are sufficient to relieve symptoms for 4 hours. To ensure that the inhaler does not become empty unexpectedly and leave the person without medication when needed, the fullness of the inhaler should be evaluated periodically by placing it in a bowl of water. When full, the inhaler will sink; when empty, it will float—varying levels in between indicate partial levels of fullness.

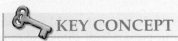

KEY CONCEPT

The effective use of inhalers requires the ability of the user to manipulate the apparatus and coordinate the spray with inhalation—tasks that may be difficult for some older persons.

Not long ago, patients on ventilator support were found in intensive care units of acute hospitals. Today, growing numbers of ventilator-dependent persons are being managed at home or in long-term care facilities. Each ventilator has unique features, and nurses should seek the guidance of a respiratory care specialist to ensure a thorough understanding and correct use of the equipment. Whether in their own homes or in an institutional setting, these patients need strong multidisciplinary support to assist with the complex web of physical, emotional, and social care needs they may present. Nurses can play a significant role in providing a realistic assessment of the abilities of patients and family caregivers to manage ventilator-related care. It makes little sense to use a ventilator to save a patient's life and then threaten that life by sending the person home with a family who cannot meet care needs. Special attention also must be paid to the quality of life of the ventilator-dependent patient; counseling, sensory stimulation, expressive therapies, and other resources should be used.

Providing Encouragement

Respiratory problems are frightening and produce anxiety. Patients with these conditions require psychological support and reassurance, especially during periods of dyspnea. Patients need a complete understanding of their disease and its management to help reduce their anxiety. Repeated encouragement may be required to assist the patient in meeting the demands of a chronic disease. Some patients may find it necessary to spend most of their time indoors to avoid the extremes of hot and cold weather; some may have to learn to transport oxygen with them as they travel outside their homes; some may need to move to a different climate for relief. These changes in lifestyle may have a significant impact on their total lives. As with any persons having chronic diseases, patients with respiratory problems can benefit from being assisted to live the fullest life possible with their conditions, rather than become prisoners to them.

DEPRESSION AND SLEEP DISTURBANCE IN PATIENTS WITH CHRONIC OBSTRUCTIVE PULMONARY DISEASE

Lee, H., Kim, I., Lim, Y., Jung, H. Y., & Park, H. (2011). Geriatric Nursing, 32(6), 408–417.

This descriptive study was done to identify the relationship of sleep disturbances to depression in persons with chronic obstructive pulmonary disease (COPD). Patients with the diagnosis of COPD were recruited from three hospitals. Their mean age was 66 years and 40.5% were between the ages of 70 and 80 years. Eighty-eight percent were men and most participants were married.

A validated tool (Center for Epidemiologic Studies Depression Scale) was used to measure depression, and the COPD and Asthma Sleep Impact Scale of Pokrzywinski et al., was used to measure sleep disturbance related to respiratory symptoms. Physical activity and self-efficacy were also measured using validated tools.

Higher levels of anxiety and depression were found among individuals with sleep disturbances. There was no relationship to depression and the study participants' economic status, pulmonary function, and body mass index. Little was learned about the overall effects of the sleep disturbance; however, just a single night of disturbed sleep was found to decrease pulmonary function measurably.

The findings support the importance of screening for sleep disturbances in individuals who have COPD. When signs of depression are noted in persons with COPD (e.g., sad mood, poor attention to self-care, low motivation to engage in care activities, and noncompliance) or a worsening of pulmonary symptoms occurs, a careful assessment of sleep quantity and quality should be done. As nurses have close relationships with patients and address comprehensive needs, they are the ideal health care professional to identify this problem and assist patients in preventing additional problems.

PRACTICE REALITIES

Mrs. O'Day was discharged from the hospital and you are scheduled to visit her every 3 days for the next 2 weeks to assist in the care of her abdominal incision. She has had a history of recurrent respiratory infections and regularly uses over-the-counter antihistamines for what she has described as "allergies."

Upon your first home visit you find Mr. and Mrs. O'Day, both 76 years old, living with their six cats. The house appears dirty and cluttered, and a strong urine odor from the pets permeates the entire home. Cat hair is on all the upholstered furniture and carpeting.

During the entire visit various cats climb on and off Mrs. O'Day's lap, and she experiences an episode of sneezing and running nose.

You ask her if she has considered that her allergy problem could be related to her cats and she responds, "They probably have something to do with it, but they are my babies and I'm a sucker when a stray shows up needing a home. I couldn't think of parting with them." Mr. O'Day supports his wife's position, stating that "I'm guilty of being a cat lover too."

How could you address the health issues related to the cats while respecting the O'Days' desire to have cats in their household?

CRITICAL THINKING EXERCISES

1. What self-imposed and environmentally imposed risks to younger adults can contribute to the development of respiratory conditions in later life?

2. In what ways can age-related changes affect the development, recognition, and management of respiratory conditions?

3. What key points would you include in an educational program for the promotion of respiratory health in senior citizens?

4. Describe the precautions that must be taken when oxygen is administered to older adults.

RESOURCES

American Lung Association
http://www.lungusa.org

Asthma and Allergy Foundation of America
http://www.aafa.org

National Heart, Lung, and Blood Institute Information Center
http://www.nhlbi.nih.gov

Office on Smoking and Health, Centers for Disease Control and Prevention
http://www.cdc.gov/tobacco

REFERENCE

Centers for Disease Control and Prevention. (2012). *Lung cancer rates by race and ethnicity*. Retrieved July 12, 2012 from http://www.cdc.gov/cancer/lung/statistics/race.htm

RECOMMENDED READINGS

Recommended Readings associated with this chapter can be found on the web site that accompanies the book. Visit **http://thepoint.lww.com/Eliopoulos8e** to access the recommended readings and other additional resources associated with this chapter.

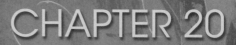

CHAPTER 20

Circulation

LEARNING OBJECTIVES

After reading this chapter, you should be able to:

1. Describe the effects of aging on cardiovascular health and circulation.

2. List factors that promote cardiovascular health.

3. Identify unique features of common cardiovascular diseases in older adults.

4. Describe nursing actions to assist patients with cardiovascular conditions.

TERMS TO KNOW

Arrhythmia: abnormal heart rate or rhythm

Atherosclerosis: hardening and narrowing of arteries due to plaque buildup in vessel walls

Homans' sign: pain when the affected leg is dorsiflexed, usually associated with deep phlebitis of the leg

Hypertension: consistent blood pressure reading of ≥140 systolic and ≥90 diastolic

Physical deconditioning: decline in cardiovascular function due to physical inactivity

Postural hypotension: decline in systolic blood pressure of 20 mm Hg or more after rising and standing for 1 minute

Improved technology for early diagnosis and treatment, along with increased public awareness of the importance of proper nutrition, exercise, and smoking cessation, has resulted in a decline in heart disease in the population as a whole. It is anticipated that future generations will experience fewer deaths and disabilities associated with cardiovascular diseases. Unfortunately, today's older population carries the insults of many years of inadequate preventive, diagnostic, and treatment practices, which cause them to experience cardiovascular disease as the major reason of disability and death. These compound some of the effects that aging has on the cardiovascular system. With the high prevalence of cardiovascular conditions in older adults, it is crucial that actions be planned to prevent and address some of the potential nursing problems related to circulation.

EFFECTS OF AGING ON CARDIOVASCULAR HEALTH

With age, heart valves increase in thickness and rigidity due to sclerosis and fibrosis. The aorta becomes dilated, a slight ventricular hypertrophy develops, and there is thickening of the left ventricular wall. Myocardial muscle is less efficient and loses some of its contractile strength, causing a reduction in cardiac output when the demands on the heart are increased. More time is required for the cycle of diastolic filling and systolic emptying to be completed. Calcification and reduced elasticity of vessels occur, and older hearts are less sensitive to baroreceptor regulation of blood pressure. These changes typically are gradual and become most apparent when the older adult is faced with an unusual physiological stress, such as heightened activity or an infection.

Good tissue health depends on adequate tissue perfusion (i.e., circulation to and from a body part). To ensure good tissue perfusion, arterial blood pressure must remain within a normal range. Unfortunately, older adults are more likely to suffer from conditions that can alter tissue perfusion, such as the following:

- *cardiovascular disease:* arteriosclerotic heart disease, hypertension, congestive heart failure (CHF), and varicosities
- *diseases:* diabetes mellitus, cancer, and renal failure
- *blood dyscrasias:* anemia, thrombus, and transfusion reactions
- *hypotension:* arising from anaphylactic shock, hypovolemia, hypoglycemia, hyperglycemia, and orthostatic hypotension
- *medication side effects:* antihypertensives, vasodilators, diuretics, and antipsychotics
- *other conditions:* edema, inflammation, prolonged immobility, hypothermia, and malnutrition

Nursing Diagnosis Table 20-1 identifies diagnoses associated with age-related risks to circulation. The nurse can assess the adequacy of tissue circulation in older adults by reviewing the individual's health history, evaluating vital signs, inspecting the body, and noting signs or symptoms. Box 20-1 lists indications of ineffective tissue perfusion.

CARDIOVASCULAR HEALTH PROMOTION

Many of the alterations in the cardiovascular system can be modified by lifestyle and diet; therefore, the prevention of cardiovascular problems in all age groups is an important goal for all nurses to consider. By teaching the young and old to identify and lower risk factors related to cardiovascular disease, nurses promote optimum health and function. Important practices to reinforce include eating properly, getting adequate exercise, avoiding cigarette smoke, managing stress, and using proactive interventions when appropriate.

Proper Nutrition

A diet that provides all daily requirements, maintains weight within an ideal range for height and

NURSING DIAGNOSIS

TABLE 20-1 **Aging and Risks to Adequate Circulation**

Causes or Contributing Factors	Nursing Diagnosis
Decreased elasticity of blood vessels	Ineffective Peripheral Tissue Perfusion
Increased resistance of peripheral vessels	Activity Intolerance
Decreased coronary blood flow	Risk of Decreased Cardiac Tissue Perfusion
Reduced proportion of oxygen extracted from arterial blood by tissues	Risk of Decreased Tissue Perfusion
Reduced cardiovascular responsiveness to adrenergic stimulation	Activity Intolerance

BOX 20-1 **Indications of Ineffective Tissue Perfusion**

Hypotension
Tachycardia, decreased pulse quality
Claudication
Edema
Loss of hair on extremities
Tissue necrosis, stasis ulcers
Dyspnea, increased respirations
Pallor, coolness of skin
Cyanosis
Decreased urinary output
Delirium (altered cognition and level of consciousness)
Restlessness
Memory disturbance

age, and controls cholesterol intake is beneficial. Box 20-2 lists some general dietary guidelines for reducing the risk of cardiovascular disease. Some nutritional supplements can also help cardiovascular health (Box 20-3).

Dr. Dean Ornish has promoted a diet that has been shown to be effective not only in preventing but also in reversing heart disease (Ornish, 2005, 2008).

BOX 20-2 **Dietary Guidelines for Reducing the Risk of Cardiovascular Disease**

- Reduce the intake of fried foods, animal fats, and partially hydrogenated fats. Beware of fast foods, which tend to be high in fat and calories.
- Increase the intake of complex carbohydrates and fiber. Use unrefined whole grain products, such as whole wheat, oats and oatmeal, rye, barley, corn, popcorn, brown rice, wild rice, buckwheat, bulgur (cracked wheat), millet, quinoa, and sorghum.
- Maintain caloric intake between ideal ranges. Reduce consumption of nutrient-poor foods.
- Use monounsaturated oils (e.g., canola oil, cold-pressed olive oil) and omega-6 oils (e.g., black currant oil, evening primrose oil).
- Eat fish rich in omega-3 fatty acids (e.g., salmon, trout, and herring) at least twice weekly.
- Reduce intake of red meat, sugar, and highly processed foods.
- Limit alcoholic beverages.

BOX 20-3 **Nutritional Supplements for Cardiovascular Health^a**

Vitamin B$_6$: effective in preventing homocysteine-induced oxidation of cholesterol, which can aid in preventing heart attacks and strokes
Vitamin B$_{12}$: can decrease homocysteine levels
Folic acid: essential for proper metabolism of homocysteine
Vitamin C: helps prevent the formation of oxysterols, maintains integrity of arterial walls
Selenium: reduces platelet aggregation
Magnesium: aids in dilating arteries and facilitating circulation, may prevent calcification of vessels, lowers total cholesterol, raises high-density lipoprotein (HDL) cholesterol, inhibits platelet aggregation
Calcium: may decrease total cholesterol and inhibit platelet aggregation
Chromium: lowers total cholesterol and triglycerides (particularly when combined with niacin), raises HDL cholesterol
Potassium: can aid in reducing reliance on antihypertensives and diuretics
Fish oil: reduces deaths from coronary artery disease, lowers blood pressure

^{a}It is preferable to get necessary vitamins and minerals from the diet, not through supplements.

The Reversal Diet for people who have cardiovascular disease consists of the following:

- less than 10% of calories from fat and very little of those from saturated fat
- high fiber intake
- exclusion of all oils and animal products, except nonfat milk and yogurt
- exclusion of caffeine and other stimulants
- allows, but does not encourage, less than 2 oz of alcohol per day
- no calorie restriction

Ornish's Prevention Diet is intended for persons with a cholesterol level less than 150 or a ratio of total cholesterol to high-density lipoprotein (HDL) cholesterol of less than 3 who have no cardiac disease. It is similar to the Reversal Diet, with the exception that as much as 20% of calories can come from fat. (In addition to dietary modifications, Dr. Ornish's program advocates moderate exercise, increased intimacy, stress reduction, and other healthy practices.)

In recent years, Ornish's diet has been criticized as being too restrictive of fats and contributing to the rise in obesity as people consume excess carbohydrates with the restricted fat intake. Despite the criticism and although many people find the restrictive diet proposed by Ornish to be difficult to follow on a long-term basis, any sustained dietary and lifestyle modification that supports the goals of reduced fats and stimulants, increased dietary fiber and exercise, and effective stress management certainly will move people in the right direction.

 POINT TO PONDER

Does your current diet increase your risk of cardiac disease? If so, what factors could present obstacles to you in changing your dietary pattern to one that is more vegetarian, and what could you do about overcoming these obstacles?

Proper nutrition throughout life is important to prevent hyperlipidemia, which is a significant risk factor in cardiovascular disease. In the past several decades, much has been learned about the significant reduction in cardiovascular and cerebrovascular incidents associated with the reduction of cholesterol levels in middle aged persons. Although there is insufficient research to demonstrate the benefits in persons of advanced age, reducing cholesterol intake is generally a positive practice. (See discussion later in the chapter.) Lifestyle modifications to lower cholesterol can also help people avoid the use of cholesterol medications, which, despite their benefits, can cause side effects, such as muscle pain, weakness, fatigue, erectile dysfunction, memory loss, and burning and tingling in the hands and feet.

Adequate Exercise

Automobiles, elevators, modern appliances, and less physically demanding jobs lead to a more sedentary lifestyle than may be optimally healthy. Related to this may be the practice of being physically inactive during the week and then filling weekends with housecleaning, yard work, and sports activities. A sensible distribution of exercise throughout the week is advisable and is more beneficial to cardiovascular function than are periodic spurts of activity. The lack of physical exercise, known as physical deconditioning, can heighten many of the age-related functional declines that aging people can experience. Fortunately, a slower rate of decline and improved cardiovascular status has been found in middle-aged persons who exercised regularly. Nurses can encourage persons who dislike scheduled

exercise programs to maximize opportunities for exercise during their routine activities (e.g., using stairs instead of an elevator, parking their car on the far end of the lot, or walking to the local newsstand to buy a newspaper instead of having it delivered). Thirty minutes of moderate physical activity at least 5 days per week or 20 minutes of vigorous exercise at least 3 days per week are the recommended levels to reduce the risk of cardiovascular disease.

 KEY CONCEPT

In addition to traditional aerobic, strengthening, and balance exercises, yoga and t'ai chi are good ways to enhance circulation.

Cigarette Smoke Avoidance

Although many smokers are aware of the health risks of cigarettes, breaking the habit is quite difficult, and, for this, people need more than to be told to stop. They require considerable support and assistance, which are often obtainable through smoking cessation programs. Acupuncture has proved helpful to some individuals for smoking cessation. Even if the patient has had repeated failures in attempting to quit, the next try could be successful and should be encouraged. In addition to avoiding cigarette smoking themselves, nurses can instruct people to limit their exposure to the cigarette smoke produced by others, which also can be detrimental.

Stress Management

Stress is a normal part of life. Nurses can teach people to identify the stressors in their lives, their unique reactions to stress, and how they can more effectively manage stress. Relaxation exercises, yoga, meditation, and a variety of other stress-reducing activities can prove beneficial to nearly all persons.

Gerontological nurses understand that it is much easier and more useful to establish good health practices early in life than to change them or deal with their outcomes in old age.

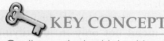 **KEY CONCEPT**

Cardiovascular health in old age begins with positive health practices in younger years.

Proactive Interventions

Research continues to unfold that sheds light on routines that people can establish to promote healthy hearts. An aspirin a day can prove to be a good preventive measure because low-dose aspirin

---

BOX 20-4 **Importance of C-Reactive Protein Screening**

With the awareness that inflammation in the blood-stream can be a cause of myocardial infarction, the American Heart Association and the Centers for Disease Control and Prevention have recommended C-reactive protein (CRP) screening for persons at moderate risk of heart disease (Ridker, 2003). CRP is a marker of inflammation that is a stronger predictor of cardiovascular events than low-density lipoprotein (LDL) cholesterol. Two measures of CRP are suggested, with the lower value or the average being used to determine vascular risk. Because CRP levels are stable over long periods of time, are not affected by food intake, and demonstrate almost no circadian variation, there is no need to obtain fasting blood samples for CRP assessment. The cost of CRP testing is comparable to that of standard cholesterol screening

and may be quite cost-effective in terms of avoiding serious complications and death.

Individuals with CRP levels >3 mg/dL who have LDL cholesterol <130 mg/dL are considered a high-risk group and are advised to follow Adult Treatment Panel (ATP) III lifestyle interventions. People with an elevated CRP and LDL between 130 and 160 mg/dL are at elevated global risk and should be advised to adhere strictly to current ATP treatment guidelines. Those individuals with elevated CRP and LDL levels >160 mg/dL may need to be placed on medications and closely monitored for compliance to their treatment plan.

Significantly elevated levels of CRP could be related to other causes of systemic inflammation, such as lupus or endocarditis; additional diagnostic testing is warranted.

---

has been shown to reduce the risk of heart attack. A daily aspirin dose at 75 to 81 mg is sufficient to provide heart disease prevention benefits, although a dose as low as 30 mg was found to be adequate (Campbell, Smyth, Montalescot, & Steinhubl, 2007). A study of men who consumed alcohol at least 3 or 4 days per week showed a reduction in the risk of myocardial infarction (MI), suggesting that light drinking could be beneficial (Klatsky & Udaltsova, 2007; Leighton & Urquiaga, 2007). Of course, various nutritional supplements are suggested to have a role in cardiovascular health. Although additional insights are needed to fully understand the effects of these types of interventions, at this point it is reasonable to suggest that a daily low-dose aspirin, daily multivitamin supplement, and enjoyment of light alcoholic beverages in moderation could be beneficial to adults of all ages in preventing cardiovascular disease.

For individuals at risk for heart disease, undergoing C-reactive protein screening is another preventive measure (Box 20-4).

A comprehensive assessment of the cardiovascular system is useful not only in identifying signs of disease but also in learning about patients' lifestyle habits that could contribute to cardiovascular disease (Assessment Guide 20-1). During the assessment, the nurse identifies actual and potential problems and develops nursing diagnoses accordingly. Nursing Diagnosis Table 20-2 lists nursing diagnoses related to cardiovascular problems.

CARDIOVASCULAR DISEASE AND WOMEN

With age, the prevalence of cardiovascular disease increases in women, affecting more than one third of women between 45 and 54 years of age and nearly 70% of women 65 years and older. Cardiovascular disease kills 12 times the number of women yearly as breast cancer, yet often is not seen as a significant threat by women. Often women miss signs of cardiovascular disease because the symptoms are less evident than in men; this delay in seeking evaluation can cause the disease to progress to more serious states before diagnosis and treatment are obtained. Women of all ages need to be educated about their risk of cardiovascular disease and measures to promote cardiovascular health. In addition, during routine assessments, women should be asked about symptoms associated with cardiovascular disease to aid in revealing ignored symptoms.

SELECTED CARDIOVASCULAR CONDITIONS

Hypertension

The incidence of hypertension increases with advancing age and is the most prevalent cardiovascular disease of older adults, making it a problem the gerontological nurse commonly encounters. Many older individuals have high blood pressure arising from the vasoconstriction associated with aging, which produces peripheral resistance. Hyperthyroidism, parkinsonism,

ASSESSMENT GUIDE 20-1
CARDIOVASCULAR FUNCTION

Early detection of cardiac problems can be difficult because of the atypical presentation of symptoms, the subtle nature of the progression of cardiac disease, and the ease with which cardiac symptoms can be mistakenly attributed to other health conditions (e.g., indigestion and arthritis). Careful questioning and observation can yield valuable insight into problems that have recently developed or escaped recognition.

Clues to peripheral vascular disorders often can be detected through general contact with patients, who may comment that their feet always feel cold and numb, that they experience burning sensations in the calf, or that they become dizzy on rising. They may ambulate slowly, rub their legs, or kick off their shoes. Varicosities may be noted on the legs. Such observations can be used to introduce discussion of peripheral vascular problems.

GENERAL OBSERVATIONS

Assessment of the cardiovascular system can begin at the moment you see the patient by observing indicators of cardiovascular status. Such observations would note the following:

- *Generalized coloring:* Note pallor, which can accompany cardiovascular disorders.
- *Energy level:* Note fatigue and the amount of activity that can be tolerated.
- *Breathing pattern:* Observe respirations while the patient ambulates, changes position, and speaks. Acute dyspnea warrants prompt medical attention because it can be a symptom of myocardial infarction in older adults.
- *Condition of nails:* Inspect the color, shape, thickness, curvature, and markings in nail beds, which can give insight into problems. Nails may be thick and dry in the presence of cardiovascular disease. Check blanching; circulatory insufficiency can delay the nails' return to pink after blanching. Advanced cardiac disease can cause clubbing of the nails.
- *Status of vessels:* Inspect the vessels on the extremities, head, and neck. Note varicosities, as well as redness on the skin above a vessel.
- *Hair on extremities:* Hair loss can accompany poor circulation.
- *Edema:* Swelling of the ankles and fingers is often indicative of cardiovascular disorders.
- *Mental status:* Inadequate cerebral circulation often manifests itself through confusion; evaluate cognitive function and level of consciousness.

INTERVIEW

The interview should include a review of function, signs, and symptoms. Ask questions pertaining to the following topics.

Symptoms

Inquire regarding the presence of dizziness, light-headedness, edema, cold extremities, palpitations, blackouts, breathing difficulties, coughing, hemoptysis, chest pain, or unusual sensations in the chest, neck, back, or jaws. It is helpful to use specific examples in questions: "Do you ever feel as though there is a vise pressing against your chest?" "Have you ever become sweaty and had trouble breathing while you felt that unusual sensation in your chest?" "Do you find that rings and shoes become tighter as the day goes on?" "Do you ever get the sensation of the room spinning when you rise from lying down?" When symptoms are reported, explore their frequency, duration, and management.

Some patients may be able to relate symptoms to vascular problems. However, others may be unaware that signs such as light-headedness, scaling skin, edema, or discoloration can be associated with peripheral vascular disorders; therefore, asking specific questions is crucial. Elicit information through questions such as the following:

- "Do your arms or legs ever become cold or numb?"
- "Do dark spots or sores ever develop on your legs?"
- "Do your legs get painful or swollen when you walk or stand?"
- "Do you ever have periods of feeling dizzy, light-headed, or confused?"
- "Does one leg ever look larger than the other?"

Changes in Function

Ask the patient if he or she has noted changes in physical or mental function:

- "Do you have difficulty or have you noticed any changes in your ability to walk, work, or take care of yourself?"
- "Do you ever have periods in which your thinking doesn't seem clear?"
- "Have you had to restrict activities or change your lifestyle recently?"

Lifestyle Practices

- "How often do you exercise, for what length of time, and what type of exercises do you do?"
- "What is your pattern of alcohol consumption?"
- "What supplements (vitamin, herbal, and homeopathic) are you using?"
- "Do you do anything to promote health (e.g., take a daily aspirin and follow a special diet)?"

(Continues)

ASSESSMENT GUIDE 20-1 (Continued)
CARDIOVASCULAR FUNCTION

PHYSICAL EXAMINATION

■ Inspect the patient from head to toe, noting areas of irritation or redness over a vessel, distended vessels, edema, and pallor. Blanching of the nail beds gives information about circulation. An examination of the extremities should include palpitation of the pulses and temperature of the extremities and observation of hair distribution on the legs.

■ Assessment of apical and radial pulses should normally reveal a pulse that ranges between 60 and 100 beats/min. Remember that older hearts take longer to recover from stress; thus, tachycardia may be detected as a result of a stress that occurred several hours earlier. If tachycardia is discovered in an older person, reassess in several hours.

■ Assess blood pressure in lying, sitting, and standing positions to determine the presence of postural hypotension (Fig. A); positional drops greater than 20 mm Hg are significant.

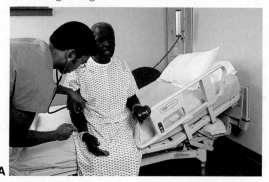

A

■ Auscultate the heart to detect thrills and bruits. Palpate the point of maximal impulse to identify displacement, which can occur with problems such as left ventricular hypertrophy. Measure jugular venous pressure.

■ Palpate pulses bilaterally for condition of the vessel wall, rate, rhythm, quality, contour, and equality at the following sites:

• *Temporal pulse,* the only palpable artery of the head, located anterior to the ear, overlying the temporal bone; normally appears tortuous

• *Brachial pulse* located in the groove between the biceps and triceps; usually palpated if arterial insufficiency is suspected

• *Radial pulse* branching from the brachial artery, the radial artery extends from the forearm to the wrist on the radial side and is palpated on the flexor surface of the wrist laterally

• *Ulnar pulse* also branching from the brachial artery, the ulnar artery extends from the forearm to the wrist on the ulnar side and is palpated on the flexor surface of the wrist medially; usually palpated if arterial insufficiency is suspected

• *Femoral pulse;* the femoral artery is palpated at the inguinal ligament midway between the anterosuperior iliac spine and the pubic tubercle

• *Popliteal pulse* located behind the knee; the popliteal artery is the continuation of the femoral artery. Having the patient flex the knee during palpitation can aid in locating this pulse.

• *Posterior tibial pulse* palpable behind and below the medial malleolus

• *Dorsalis pedis pulse* palpated at the groove between the first two tendons on the medial side of the dorsum of the foot; this and the posterior tibial pulse can be congenitally absent

■ Rate pulses on a scale from 0 to 4:
• 0 = no pulse
• 1 = thready, easily obliterated pulse
• 2 = pulse difficult to palpate and easily obliterated
• 3 = normal pulse
• 4 = strong, bounding pulse, not obliterated with pressure

Often, a stick figure is used to document the quality of pulses at different locations (Fig. B):

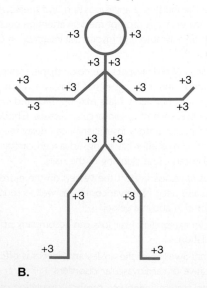

B.

■ While assessing pulses, inspect the vessels for signs of phlebitis. Signs could include redness, tenderness, and edema over a vein. Sometimes, visible signs of inflammation may not be present, and the primary indication that phlebitis exists can be tenderness of the vessel detected through palpation. A positive Homans' sign (i.e., pain when the affected leg is dorsiflexed) can accompany deep phlebitis of the leg.

- Inspect the legs for discoloration, hair loss, edema, scaling skin, pallor, lesions, and tortuous-looking veins.

- Assess skin temperature by touching the skin surface in various areas.

- Assure patient has had recent electrocardiogram and blood screening for cholesterol and C-reactive protein (see Box 20-4).

- Alterations in cerebral circulation can cause disruptions to cognitive function; therefore, a mental status evaluation can provide useful information about circulatory problems.

NURSING DIAGNOSIS

TABLE 20-2 **Nursing Diagnosis Related to Cardiovascular Problems**

Causes or Contributing Factors	Nursing Diagnosis
Insufficient oxygen transport, poor circulation, electrolyte imbalance, bed rest, pain, fatigue, effects of medications, fear of harming self	Activity Intolerance
Change in self-concept, fear of unknown procedures or diagnosis, hospitalization	Anxiety
Bed rest, medications, diet, stress, inactivity, insufficient fluids, pain, hospital environment	Constipation
Bradycardia, tachycardia, congestive heart failure, myocardial infarction, hypertension, cor pulmonale, stress, medications	Ineffective Tissue Perfusion
Vasospasm, occlusion, phlebitis, spasms, diagnostic tests, surgery, poor positioning, exertion	Acute Pain
Separation of patient from family, lack of knowledge	Interrupted Family Processes
Hospitalization, forfeiture of activities, fear of impact	Social Isolation
Patient's illness; financial, physical, and psychological burdens of illness; hospitalization; role changes	Interrupted Family Processes
Change in function, disability, procedures, pain, lack of knowledge	Fear
Ascites, hypovolemia, anorexia	Deficient Fluid Volume
Decreased cardiac output, excess fluid intake, dependent venous pooling/stasis	Excess Fluid Volume
Change in body function or lifestyle, pain	Chronic Low Self-Esteem
Lack of knowledge, loss of independence	Ineffective Health Maintenance
Disability, pain, fatigue	Impaired Home Maintenance
Impaired oxygen transport, invasive procedures, medications	Risk of Infection, Risk of Disuse Syndrome
Poor circulation, fatigue, immobility, pain, medications	Risk of Injury
Unfamiliar diagnostic tests, diagnosis, treatments, diet, ineffective coping, denial	Deficient Knowledge
Pain, fatigue, bed rest, edema, medications	Impaired Physical Mobility
Lack of knowledge or skill, prescribed plan in conflict with beliefs and practices, insufficient funds	Noncompliance
Anorexia, depression, stress, medications, nonacceptance of prescribed diet, anxiety	Imbalanced Nutrition: Less Than Body Requirements
Inability to participate in usual activities, lack of knowledge, hospitalization	Risk of Powerlessness
Immobility, pain, edema, fatigue	Bathing/Dressing/Feeding/Toileting Self-Care Deficit

(Continues)

NURSING DIAGNOSIS (Continued)

TABLE 20-2   Nursing Diagnosis Related to Cardiovascular Problems

Change in body function, new diagnosis, hospitalization, immobility, pain	Disturbed Body Image
Metabolic changes, impaired oxygen transport, medications, immobility, pain, stress, hospital environment	Disturbed Sensory Perception
Pain, fatigue, fear, anxiety, depression, medications, hospitalization, lack of knowledge	Sexual Dysfunction
Edema, immobility, impaired oxygen transport	Impaired Skin Integrity
Impaired oxygen transport, immobility, hospitalization, pain, anxiety, inactivity, medications, depression	Disturbed Sleep Pattern
Metabolic or electrolyte imbalances, medications, anxiety, depression	Risk of Acute Confusion
Decreased cardiac output, myocardial infarction, angina, congestive heart failure, hypertension, vasoconstriction, hypotension, immobility, medications	Risk of Decreased Cardiac Tissue Perfusion, Risk of Ineffective Peripheral Tissue Perfusion
Diuretics, bed rest, hospital environment, anxiety	Impaired Urinary Elimination

Paget's disease, anemia, and thiamine deficiency can also be responsible for hypertension.

Individuals with systolic pressure ≥140 and diastolic pressure ≥90 are considered hypertensive. Some providers take a conservative approach and will not prescribe treatment for hypertension unless the blood pressure exceeds 160 systolic and 90 diastolic. The nurse should carefully assess the patient's blood pressure by checking it several times with the person in standing, sitting, and prone positions. Anxiety, stress, or activity before the blood pressure check should be noted, because these factors may be responsible for a temporary elevation. The anxiety of being examined by a physician or of preparing for and experiencing a visit with a health care provider frequently causes elevated blood pressure in a usually normotensive individual.

Awakening with a dull headache, impaired memory, disorientation, confusion, epistaxis, and a slow tremor may be symptoms of hypertension. The presence of these symptoms with an elevated blood pressure reading usually warrants treatment. Hypertensive older patients are advised to rest, reduce their sodium intake, and, if necessary, reduce their weight. Aggressive antihypertensive therapy is discouraged for older persons because of the risk of a sudden dangerous decrease in blood pressure. Nurses should observe for signs indicating blood pressure that is too low to meet the patient's demands, such as dizziness, confusion, syncope, restlessness, and drowsiness. An elevated blood urea nitrogen level may also be present. These signs should be observed for and communicated to the physician if they appear. In the management of the older hypertensive person, it is a challenge to achieve a blood pressure

level high enough to provide optimum circulation yet low enough to prevent serious related complications.

Controversy still exists as to the proper treatment of hypertension in older patients; therefore, hypertensive older adults may receive a wide range of therapy, rather than antihypertensive drugs alone. Drugs that can be used to treat hypertension include diuretics, beta-blockers, calcium channel blockers, and angiotensin-converting enzyme (ACE) inhibitors. Because they have a higher risk of adverse reactions from antihypertensive drugs, older patients should be assisted in using non-pharmacologic measures to reduce blood pressure whenever possible. Biofeedback, yoga, meditation, and relaxation exercises can prove effective in reducing blood pressure (Yeh, Davis, & Phillips, 2006). In fact, the National Institutes of Health recommended meditation over prescription drugs for mild hypertension (Astin, Shapiro, Eisenberg, & Forys, 2003). Fish oil supplements can reduce blood pressure in hypertensive individuals. Higher whole grain intake was associated with a reduced risk of hypertension in middle-aged and older women, suggesting a potential role for increasing whole grain intake in the primary prevention of hypertension and its cardiovascular complications (Wang et al., 2007). Some herbs have hypotensive effects, including garlic, hawthorn berries, rauwolfia, and periwinkle. Conversely, other herbs such as ginseng and licorice can cause a rise in blood pressure when used regularly. The impact of herbs on blood pressure emphasizes the need to inquire about the use of these products during the assessment.

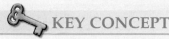

Hypotension

A decline in systolic blood pressure of 20 mm Hg or more after rising and standing for 1 minute is postural hypotension; a similar reduction within 1 hour of eating is postprandial hypotension. Various studies have shown that many older adults experience problems related to postural and postprandial hypotension due to the increased intake of vasoactive medications and concomitant decrease in physiologic function, such as baroreceptor sensitivity (Frishman, Azer, & Sica, 2003). This can be secondary to age-related changes, such as blunting of the baroreflex-mediated heart rate response to hypotensive and hypertensive stimuli and the presence of diseases that affect the heart. Postprandial hypotension can also be related to antihypertensive medications taken before eating and a high carbohydrate intake at meals (the effects can be prevented by drinking a caffeinated beverage after the meal). Hypotension can have serious consequences for older persons, including a high risk of falls, stroke, syncope, and coronary complications.

Congestive Heart Failure

The incidence of CHF increases significantly with age and is a leading cause of hospitalization of older adults. It is a potential complication in older patients with arteriosclerotic heart disease; the successful treatment of older people with MI with thrombolytic agents contributes to the increasing incidence. Coronary artery disease is responsible for most cases of CHF, followed by hypertension; other risk factors that can precipitate CHF in older adults include diabetes mellitus, dyslipidemia, sleep-disordered breathing, albuminuria, anemia, chronic kidney disease, use of illicit drugs, sedentary lifestyle, and psychological stress. This problem is common in older adults because of age-related changes, such as reduced elasticity and lumen size of vessels and rises in blood pressure that interfere with the blood supply to the heart muscle. The decreased cardiac reserves limit the heart's ability to withstand effects of disease or injury.

Symptoms of CHF in older patients include dyspnea on exertion (the most common finding), confusion, insomnia, wandering during the night, agitation, depression, anorexia, nausea, weakness, shortness of breath, orthopnea, wheezing, weight gain, and bilateral ankle edema. On auscultation, moist crackles are heard. The nurse should promptly report to the physician the detection of any of these symptoms.

History and physical examination assist in confirming the diagnosis of CHF. The New York Heart Association has developed four categories of CHF that can be used in classifying the severity of the disease and guiding treatment (NYHA allows use of this classification system without permission):

- *Class 1:* Cardiac disease without physical limitation
- *Class 2:* Symptoms experienced with ordinary physical activity; slight limitations may be evident
- *Class 3:* Symptoms experienced with less than ordinary activities; physical activity significantly limited
- *Class 4:* Symptoms experienced with any activity and during rest; bed rest may be required

Management of CHF in older adults is basically the same as in middle-aged adults, commonly consisting of bed rest, ACE inhibitors, beta-blockers, digitalis, diuretics, and a reduction in sodium intake. The patient may be allowed to sit in a chair next to the bed; usually, complete bed rest is discouraged to avoid the potential development of thrombosis and pulmonary congestion. The nurse should assist the patient into the chair, provide adequate support, and, while the patient is sitting, observe for signs of fatigue and dyspnea and changes in skin color and pulse.

The presence of edema and the poor nutrition of the tissues associated with this disease, along with the more fragile skin of the aged, all predispose the patient to a greater risk of skin breakdown. Regular skin care and frequent changes of positioning are essential. CHF is a frightening, and often recurring, condition requiring a great deal of reassurance and emotional support. Nursing Care Plan 20-1 offers a basic care plan for the older adult with heart failure.

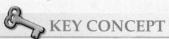

Pulmonary Emboli

The incidence of pulmonary emboli is high in older persons, although detection and diagnosis of it in this age group are challenging. Patients at high

NURSING CARE PLAN 20-1

THE OLDER ADULT WITH HEART FAILURE

Nursing Diagnosis: Activity Intolerance related to decreased cardiac output, pain, dyspnea, fatigue

Goal	Nursing Actions
The patient tolerates light to moderate activity without pain, dyspnea, or dysrhythmias	■ Assess patient's ability to engage in activities of daily living; note presence of symptoms at various levels of activity. ■ Schedule activities to avoid clustering of strenuous activities together (e.g., shower, diagnostic test, physical therapy); plan rest periods before and after activities. ■ Consult with physician to develop plan to gradually increase activity; monitor response and adjust activity accordingly. ■ Administer oxygen as needed and prescribed; use nasal prongs rather than mask, because a mask tends to further increase anxiety and may not achieve an adequate seal against the patient's face. (Be aware that oxygen may be prescribed at lower levels or contraindicated for patients with chronic hypoxia.) ■ Prevent and control pain; be alert to unique manifestations of pain in older adults (e.g., altered mental status, apprehension, changes in functional capacity). ■ Assess vital signs at rest and with activity. Note signs of decreased cardiac output (e.g., drop in blood pressure, increased pulse). ■ Monitor cardiac rhythm as ordered via electrocardiography or telemetry. ■ Administer antidysrhythmic drugs as ordered; monitor response. ■ Note alterations in mental status that could indicate cerebral hypoxia (e.g., confusion, restlessness, decreased level of consciousness, agitation). ■ Provide diversional activities to accommodate level of activity tolerance.

Nursing Diagnosis: Impaired Skin Integrity related to edema and poor tissue nutrition

Goal	Nursing Actions
The patient is free from pressure ulcers and other impairments in skin integrity	■ Assess amount of time patient can remain in position before signs of pressure are apparent; develop individualized turning and repositioning schedule. ■ Use sheepskin, cushions, and other protective devices. ■ Keep skin clean and dry. ■ Ensure patient consumes adequate diet; consult with nutritionist for diet plan as needed.

Nursing Diagnoses: Excess Fluid Volume related to ineffective pumping action of heart; Imbalanced Nutrition: Less Than Body Requirements related to decreased appetite, dyspnea, dietary restrictions, side effects of treatments

Goal	Nursing Actions
The patient maintains fluid and electrolyte balance The patient ingests sufficient nutrients to meet body's metabolic needs without increasing cardiac workload	■ Weigh patient daily (same time of day, same amount of clothing, same scale); record and report changes in weight that exceed 3 lb without relationship to dietary change. ■ Inspect extremities, periorbital areas, and sacrum for edema; assess for jugular venous distension. ■ Elevate and support extremities while patient sits. ■ Apply antiembolism stockings or elastic wraps as ordered; remove for 10 minutes every 8 hours and inspect skin. ■ Ensure patient complies with fluid and sodium restrictions as ordered; educate patient as necessary.

- Record and evaluate intake and output.
- Consult with dietitian regarding dietary restrictions and incorporating patient's preferences into diet.
- Administer diuretics as ordered; observe for signs of related fluid and electrolyte imbalances; educate patient as necessary.
- Monitor specific gravity and laboratory studies (e.g., blood urea nitrogen, creatinine, electrolytes).
- Instruct patient to identify and report symptoms of worsening of condition (e.g., swelling of ankles, loss of appetite, weight gain, shortness of breath).

Nursing Diagnosis: Deficient Knowledge related to lifestyle modifications and caregiving needs associated with congestive heart failure

Goal	Nursing Actions
The patient describes care plan requirements and self-care measures The patient demonstrates maximum self-care	■ Assess learning needs. ■ Consult with multidisciplinary team regarding recommendations pertaining to diet and fluid intake, activity, medications, exercise guidelines, and any precautions. ■ Teach patient how to distribute rest and activity throughout the day to reduce workload of heart. ■ Review symptoms that patient should identify and report, including weight gain of ≥3 lb within a one to several day time period, increased fatigue or weakness, dizziness, fainting or feeling faint, edema, shortness of breath, dyspnea with activities that were previously tolerated, cough, chest pain, abdominal pain or bloating, bleeding, bruising, or vomiting. ■ Refer to community resources as needed (e.g., support groups, healthy cooking classes). ■ Supply with telephone numbers of physician, case manager, and other relevant contacts.

risk for developing this problem are those with a fractured hip, CHF, arrhythmias, and a history of thrombosis. Immobilization and malnourishment, which are frequent problems in the older population, can contribute to pulmonary emboli. Symptoms to observe include confusion, apprehension, increasing dyspnea, slight temperature elevation, pneumonitis, and an elevated sedimentation rate. Older patients may not experience chest pain because of altered pain sensations, or their pain may be attributed to other existing problems. A lung scan or angiography may be done to confirm the diagnosis and establish the location, size, and extent of the problem. Treatment of pulmonary emboli in older adults does not significantly differ from that used for the young.

Coronary Artery Disease

Coronary artery disease is the popularly used phrase for ischemic heart disease. The prevalence of coronary artery disease increases with advanced age, so that some form of this disease exists in most persons 70 years of age or older.

Angina

A symptom of myocardial ischemia, the anginal syndrome presents in an atypical pattern in older adults, making detection difficult. Pain may be diffuse and of a less severe nature than described by younger adults. The first indication of this problem may be a vague discomfort under the sternum, frequently after exertion or a large meal. The type of pain described and the relationship of the onset of pain to a meal may cause the patient and the health professional to attribute this discomfort to indigestion. As this condition progresses, the patient may experience precordial pain radiating down the left arm. Other symptoms can include coughing, syncope, sweating with exertion, and episodes of confusion.

The recurrence of anginal syndromes over many years can result in the formation of small areas of myocardial necrosis and fibrosis. Eventually, diffuse myocardial fibrosis occurs, leading to myocardial weakness and the potential risk of CHF.

Nitroglycerin has been effective in preventing and treating anginal attacks. Older persons are more likely to experience orthostatic hypotension with nitrates resulting from loss of vasomotor and baroreceptor reactivity. Because this drug may cause a drop in blood pressure, lower dosages may be indicated. The nurse cautions the patient to sit or lie down after taking the tablet to prevent fainting episodes and falls. To prevent swallowing the tablet and thus blocking its absorption, patients should not swallow their saliva for several minutes after sublingual administration. Long-acting nitrates are usually not prescribed for older adults.

To prevent anginal syndromes, the nurse teaches and helps the patient to avoid factors that may aggravate this problem, such as cold wind, emotional stress, strenuous activity, anemia, tachycardia, arrhythmias, and hyperthyroidism. Acupuncture has been shown to reduce the frequency and severity of angina attacks in some individuals and is a consideration. Because the pain associated with an MI may be similar to that of angina, patients should be instructed to notify the physician or nurse if pain is not relieved by nitroglycerin. Patients' charts should include factors that precipitate attacks, as well as the nature of the pain and its description by the patient, the method of management, and the usual number of nitroglycerin tablets used to alleviate the attack. Education and support in reducing risk factors complement the plan of care.

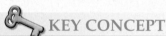

KEY CONCEPT

Some anginal attacks can be prevented by avoiding factors such as cold wind, emotional stress, strenuous activity, anemia, and tachycardia.

Myocardial Infarction

MI is frequently seen in older persons, especially in men with a history of hypertension and arteriosclerosis. The diagnosis of MI can be delayed or missed in older adults because of an atypical set of symptoms and the absence of pain. Symptoms include pain radiating to the left arm, the entire chest, the neck, jaw, and the abdomen; numbness in arms, neck, or back; confusion; moist, pale skin; decreased blood pressure; syncope; shortness of breath; cough; low-grade fever; and an elevated sedimentation rate. Output should be observed because partial or complete anuria may develop as this problem continues. Arrhythmias may occur, progressing to fibrillation and death, if untreated.

The trend in treating MI has been to reduce the amount of time in which the patient is limited to bed rest and to replace complete bed rest with allowing the patient to sit in an armchair next to the bed. The patient should be assisted into the chair with minimal exertion by him or her. Arms should be supported to avoid strain on the heart. Not only does this armchair treatment help to prevent many of the complications associated with immobility, it also prevents pooling of the blood in the pulmonary vessels, thereby decreasing the work of the heart.

Early ambulation following an MI is encouraged. Typically, patients are allowed out of bed within a few days of an uncomplicated MI and are ambulating shortly thereafter. Getting out of bed early can be beneficial for the heart (using a bedpan puts more work on the heart than using a commode), maintains the body's condition, and assists in the prevention of complications associated with immobility.

Thrombolytic therapy is commonly used, and because older persons are more susceptible to cerebral and intestinal bleeding, close nursing observation for signs of bleeding is essential. Nurses should be alert to signs of developing pulmonary edema and CHF, potential complications for the geriatric patient with an MI. These and other observations, such as persistent dyspnea, cyanosis, decreasing blood pressure, rising temperature, and arrhythmias, reflect a problem in the patient's recovery and should be brought to the physician's attention promptly.

Fitness programs have shown to be beneficial for older persons with coronary artery disease in improving cardiac functional capacity, reducing ischemic episodes, decreasing the risk of complications, and promoting a sense of well-being and control over the disease. Walking, swimming, and bicycling are excellent rhythmic, aerobic means of exercise for older adults. Aggressive sports are not necessarily excluded but do present a greater challenge in controlling heart rate during the exercise. All exercise sessions should begin with a 5-minute warm-up and end with a 5- to 10-minute cooldown of low-intensity exercises. Nurses should advise patients to obtain a medical evaluation and exercise test before engaging in a fitness program. Usually, a target heart rate of approximately 70% to 85% of the maximal heart rate is recommended during exercise.

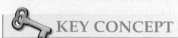

KEY CONCEPT

Fitness programs for older adults with coronary artery disease can improve cardiac functional capacity, reduce ischemic episodes, decrease the risk of complications, and promote a sense of well-being and control over the condition.

Hyperlipidemia

The risk of coronary artery disease associated with elevated total cholesterol increases with age, primarily because of increases in low-density lipoprotein (LDL). In addition to age, older persons may have conditions that can cause lipoprotein disorders, such as uncontrolled diabetes, hypothyroidism, uremia, and nephrotic syndrome, or be using corticosteroids, thiazide diuretics, and other drugs that increase the risk.

Diagnosis

Patient evaluation should include obtaining a full lipid profile rather than just a plasma total cholesterol level. Because cholesterol values can change from day to day, no single laboratory value should be used to classify a patient. Triglyceride levels are sensitive to food; therefore, a definitive screening test requires that the patient fast for 12 hours prior to testing. An HDL level greater than 60 mg/dL is desirable; triglycerides greater than 200 mg/dL are borderline and greater than 240 mg/dL are high. An LDL less than 100 mg/dL is recommended for people with coronary heart disease or diabetes; a level less than 130 mg/dL is advised for persons without coronary heart disease or diabetes who have two or more coronary risk factors; LDL less than 160 mg/dL is desirable for persons without coronary heart disease or diabetes who have one or no risk factors.

If secondary causes of lipoprotein disorders (e.g., diet high in saturated fat or cholesterol, excessive alcohol intake, exogenous estrogen supplementation, poorly controlled diabetes, uremia, and use of beta-blockers or corticosteroids) can be ruled out, a primary or familial lipoprotein disorder may be present. The most common familial lipoproteinemias are transmitted as autosomal dominant traits, so children of older adults affected by this condition need screening and counseling regarding lifestyle practices that can prevent hypercholesterolemia.

Treatment

Dietary changes and exercise are the initial approaches to treating this condition. The American Heart Association's (AHA) step 1 diet is recommended for initial treatment. If the patient is already following a diet similar to the step 1 diet, a step 2 diet will be prescribed. The gerontological nurse should refer patients to a nutritionist for guidance on these diets. As mentioned, the Dean Ornish diet is more restrictive than the AHA diet and has been shown to improve LDL levels. Box 20-5 lists some general dietary guidelines. Other lifestyle practices that

---

BOX 20-5 General Dietary Guidelines for Persons With Hyperlipoprotein Conditions

Reduce intake of egg yolks and organ meats
Increase consumption of soluble fibers (e.g., barley, oats)
Reduce red meat intake and substitute with fish, chicken, and turkey
Substitute olive oil for vegetable oils
Use skim milk and nonfat cottage cheese
Substitute buttermilk for cream toppings
Eat plenty of fresh fruits and vegetables

---

can assist include reducing weight and limiting alcohol intake.

A variety of medications can be used if diet and lifestyle modifications alone do not bring about results. The drugs of first choice for elevated LDL cholesterol are the 3-hydroxy-3-methylglutaryl-coenzyme (HMG-CoA) reductase inhibitors (e.g., atorvastatin, fluvastatin, lovastatin, pravastatin, rosuvastatin, and simvastatin). Also known as statins, this class of drugs is very effective for lowering LDL cholesterol levels and has few immediate short-term side effects. Bile acid sequestrants (cholestyramine and colestipol), nicotinic acid (niacin [Nicolar]), HMG-CoA, fibric acid derivatives (gemfibrozil and clofibrate), and omega-3 fatty acids (fish oils) can also be used.

Some alternative and complementary therapies have also proven beneficial in reducing cholesterol levels, such as water-soluble fiber (oats, guar gum, pectin, and mixed fibers), garlic supplements, green tea, and antioxidant vitamins A, C, and E and beta-carotene.

Arrhythmias

Digitalis toxicity, hypokalemia, acute infections, hemorrhage, anginal syndrome, and coronary insufficiency are some of the many factors that cause an increasing incidence of arrhythmias with age. Of the causes mentioned, digitalis toxicity is the most common. Symptoms associated with arrhythmias include weakness, fatigue, palpitations, confusion, dizziness, hypotension, bradycardia, and syncope.

The basic principles of treatment for arrhythmias do not vary much for older adults. Tranquilizers, antiarrhythmic drugs, digitalis, and potassium supplements are part of the therapy prescribed; cardioversion may also be done. Patient education may be warranted to help the individual modify diet, smoking, drinking, and activity patterns. The nurse should be aware that digitalis toxicity can progress in the absence of clinical signs and with blood levels within a normal range, and that the effects can be evident even 2 weeks after the drug has been discontinued. This reinforces the importance of nursing assessment and monitoring to detect subtle changes and atypical symptoms. Older people have a higher mortality rate from cardiac arrest than other segments of the population, emphasizing the need for close nursing observations and early problem detection to prevent this serious complication.

Peripheral Vascular Disease

Arteriosclerosis

Arteriosclerosis is a common problem among older persons, especially those who have diabetes. Unlike atherosclerosis, which generally affects the large vessels coming from the heart, arteriosclerosis most often affects the smaller vessels farthest from the

heart. Arteriography and radiography can be used to diagnose arteriosclerosis, and oscillometric testing can assess the arterial pulse at different levels. If surface temperature is evaluated as a diagnostic measure, the nurse should keep the patient in a warm, stable room temperature for at least 1 hour before testing. Treatment of arteriosclerosis includes bed rest, warmth, Buerger-Allen exercises (Box 20-6), and vasodilators. Occasionally, a permanent vasodilation effect is achieved by performing a sympathetic ganglionectomy.

Special Problems Associated With Diabetes

Persons with diabetes, who have a high risk of developing peripheral vascular problems and associated complications, commonly display diabetes-associated neuropathies and infections that affect vessels throughout the entire body. Arterial insufficiency can present in several ways. Resting pain may occur as a result of intermittent claudication; arterial pulses may be difficult to find

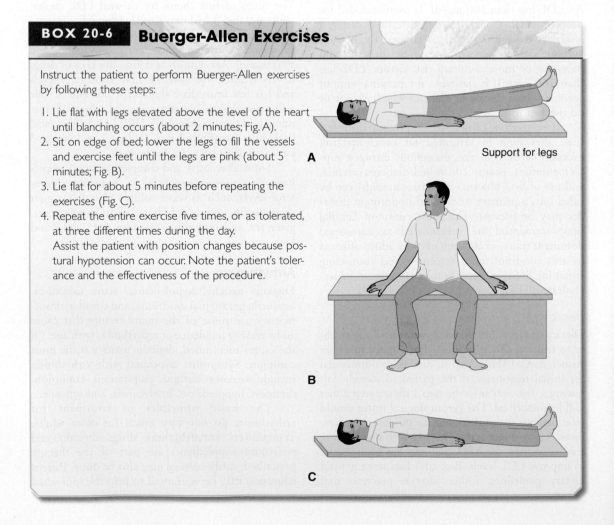

BOX 20-6 **Buerger-Allen Exercises**

Instruct the patient to perform Buerger-Allen exercises by following these steps:

1. Lie flat with legs elevated above the level of the heart until blanching occurs (about 2 minutes; Fig. A).
2. Sit on edge of bed; lower the legs to fill the vessels and exercise feet until the legs are pink (about 5 minutes; Fig. B).
3. Lie flat for about 5 minutes before repeating the exercises (Fig. C).
4. Repeat the entire exercise five times, or as tolerated, at three different times during the day.
   Assist the patient with position changes because postural hypotension can occur. Note the patient's tolerance and the effectiveness of the procedure.

Support for legs

A

B

C

or totally absent; and skin discoloration, ulcerations, and gangrene may be present. Diagnostic measures, similar to those used to determine the degree of arterial insufficiency with other problems, include oscillometry, elevation–dependency tests, and palpation of pulses and skin temperatures at different sites. When surgery is possible, arteriography may be done to establish the exact size and location of the arterial lesion. The treatment selected will depend on the extent of the disease. Walking can promote collateral circulation and may constitute sufficient management if intermittent claudication is the sole problem. Analgesics can provide relief from resting pain.

Because many of today's older adults may have witnessed severe disability and death among others with the disease they have known throughout their lives, they need to be assured that improved methods of medical and surgical management—perhaps not even developed at the time their parents and grandparents had diabetes—increase their chances for a full, independent life.

Aneurysms

In older adults, advanced arteriosclerosis is usually responsible for the development of aneurysms, although they may also result from infection, trauma, syphilis, and other factors. Some aneurysms can be seen by the naked eye and are able to be palpated as a pulsating mass; others can only be detected by radiography. A thrombosis can develop in the aneurysm, leading to an arterial occlusion or rupture of the aneurysm—the most serious complication associated with this problem.

Aneurysms of the abdominal aorta most frequently occur in older people. Patients with a history of arteriosclerotic lesions, angina pectoris, MI, and CHF more commonly develop aneurysms in this area. A pulsating mass, sometimes painful, in the umbilical region is an indication of an abdominal aortic aneurysm. Prompt correction is essential to prevent rupture. Fewer complications and deaths result from surgical intervention before rupture. Among the complications that older adults can develop after surgery for this problem are hemorrhage, MI, cerebrovascular accident, and acute renal insufficiency. The nurse should observe closely for signs of postoperative complications.

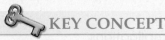
KEY CONCEPT

Abdominal aortic aneurysms are a high risk in persons with a history of arteriosclerotic lesions, angina pectoris, myocardial infarction, and congestive heart failure.

Aneurysms can develop in peripheral arteries, the most common sites being the femoral and popliteal arteries. Peripheral aneurysms can usually be palpated, thus establishing the diagnosis. The most serious complication associated with peripheral aneurysms is the formation of a thrombus, which can occlude the vessel and cause loss of the limb. As with abdominal aortic aneurysms, early treatment reduces the risk of complications and death. The lesion may be resected and the portion of the vessel removed replaced, commonly with a prosthetic material. For certain patients, a lumbar sympathectomy can be performed. The nurse should be aware that these patients can develop a thrombus postoperatively and assist the patient in preventing this complication.

Varicose Veins

Varicosities, a common problem in old age, can be caused by lack of exercise, jobs entailing a great deal of standing, and loss of vessel elasticity and strength associated with the aging process. Varicosities in all ages can be detected by the dilated, tortuous nature of the vein, especially the veins of the lower extremities. The person may experience dull pain and cramping of the legs, sometimes severe enough to interfere with sleep. Dizziness may occur as the patient rises from a lying position because blood is localized in the lower extremities and cerebral circulation is reduced. The effects of the varicosities make the skin more susceptible to trauma and infection, promoting the development of ulcerative lesions, especially in the obese or diabetic patient (Box 20-7).

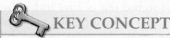
KEY CONCEPT

Persons with varicose veins can experience dizziness when rising from a lying position because blood is localized in the lower extremities and cerebral circulation is reduced.

Treatment of varicose veins is aimed toward reducing venous stasis. The patient elevates and rests the affected limb to promote venous return. Exercise, particularly walking, will also enhance circulation. The nurse should make sure that elastic stockings and bandages are properly used and not constricting and that the patient is informed of the causes of venous status (e.g., prolonged standing, crossing the legs, and wearing constricting clothing) to prevent the development of complications and additional varicosities. Ligation and stripping of the veins require the same principles of nursing care used for other age groups undergoing this surgery.

Topics to Include in Teaching the Patient With a Leg Ulcer

Venous ulcers result from chronic deep vein insufficiency or severe varicosities. The nurse teaches patients with venous ulcers to promote tissue perfusion and prevent complications as follows:

- Use gravity to promote circulation and reduce edema by elevating the lower extremity when sitting and by avoiding prolonged standing, sitting, and crossing the legs.
- Prevent pressure on the ulcer by using an overbed cradle to keep linens from touching the extremity.
- Prevent constriction to circulation by avoiding tight socks or garters.
- Control pain by using an analgesic; taking an analgesic approximately 30 minutes prior to the dressing change can reduce some of the discomfort associated with the procedure.
- Change the dressing as prescribed (if the patient is unable to perform the procedure independently, instruct a caregiver).
- Promote circulation by exercising (e.g., walking, swimming, stationary bicycling, dorsiflexion of the feet).

Venous Thromboembolism

An increasing incidence of venous thromboembolism is found among older adults. Patients who have been restricted to bed rest or have had recent surgery or fractures of a lower extremity are high-risk candidates. Although the veins in the calf muscles are the most frequently seen sites of this problem, it also occurs in the inferior vena cava, iliofemoral segment, and various superficial veins.

The symptoms and signs of venous thromboembolism depend on the vessel involved. The nurse should be alert for edema, warmth over the affected area, and pain in the sole of the foot. Edema may be the primary indication of thromboembolism in the veins of the calf muscle, because discoloration and pain are often absent in aged persons with this problem. If the inferior vena cava is involved, bilateral swelling, aching and cyanosis of the lower extremities, engorgement of the superficial veins, and tenderness along the femoral veins will be present. Similar signs will appear with involvement of the iliofemoral segment, but only on the affected extremity.

The location of the thromboembolism will dictate the treatment used. Elastic stockings or bandages, rest, and elevation of the affected limb may promote venous return. Analgesics may be given to relieve any associated pain. Anticoagulants may be administered, and surgery may be performed as well. The nurse should help the patient to avoid situations that cause straining and to remain comfortable and well hydrated.

GENERAL NURSING CONSIDERATIONS FOR CARDIOVASCULAR CONDITIONS

Prevention

The high incidence and potentially disabling effects of cardiovascular disease demand conscientious actions by gerontological nurses to incorporate preventive measures into their planning and caregiving. Education, counseling, coaching, and rehabilitative/restorative activities facilitate prevention on three levels:

1. *Primary:* to prevent disease from developing in healthy older adults
2. *Secondary:* to strengthen the abilities of persons who are diagnosed with disease to avoid complications and worsening of their conditions and achieve maximum health and function
3. *Tertiary*: to maximize capabilities through rehabilitative and restorative efforts so that the disease doesn't create additional problems

The measures for promoting cardiovascular health described at the beginning of this chapter are advantageous to incorporate into any health promotion plan for older adults.

Keeping the Patient Informed

Basic diagnostic and treatment measures for cardiovascular problems of older adults will not differ greatly from those used with younger patients, and the same nursing measures can be applied. Because of sensory deficits, anxiety, poor memory, or illness, the older patient may not fully comprehend or remember the explanations given for diagnostic and treatment measures. Full explanations with reinforcement are essential. Patients and their families should have the opportunity to ask questions and to discuss their concerns openly. Often procedures that seem relatively minor to the nurse, such as frequent checks of vital signs, may be alarming to the unprepared patient and family.

Preventing Complications

The edema associated with many cardiovascular diseases may promote skin breakdown, especially in older people who typically have more fragile skin. Frequent changes of position are essential.

The body should be supported in proper alignment, and dangling arms and legs off the side of a bed or chair should be avoided. A frequent check of clothing and protective devices can aid in detecting constriction due to increased edema. Protection, padding, and massage of pressure points are beneficial. If the patient is to be on a stretcher, an examining table, or an operating room table for a long time, protective padding placed on pressure points beforehand can provide comfort and prevent skin breakdown. When much edema is present, excessive activity should be avoided because it will increase the circulation of the fluid, with the toxic wastes it contains, and can subject the patient to profound intoxication. Weight and circumferences of extremities and the abdomen should be monitored to provide quantitative data regarding changes in the edematous state.

Accurate observation and documentation of fluid balance are especially important. Within any prescribed fluid restrictions, fluid intake should be encouraged to prevent dehydration and facilitate diuresis; water is effective for this. Fluid loss through any means should be measured; volume, color, odor, and specific gravity of urine should be noted. Intravenous fluids must be monitored carefully, particularly because excessive fluid infusion results in hypervolemia and can subject older adults to the risk of CHF. Intravenous administration of glucose solution could stimulate the increased production of insulin, resulting in a hypoglycemic reaction if this solution is abruptly discontinued without an adequate substitute.

Vital signs must be checked regularly, with close attention to changes. A temperature elevation can reflect an infection or an MI. The body temperature for older individuals may be normally lower than for younger adults; it is important to record the patient's normal temperature when well to have a baseline for comparison. It is advisable to detect and correct temperature elevations promptly because a temperature elevation increases metabolism, thereby increasing the body's requirements for oxygen, and causes the heart to work harder. A decrease in temperature slows metabolism, causing less oxygen consumption and less carbon dioxide production and fewer respirations. A rise in blood pressure is associated with a reduced cardiac output, vasodilation, and lower blood volume. Hypotension can result in insufficient circulation to meet the body's needs; symptoms of confusion and dizziness could indicate insufficient cerebral circulation resulting from a reduced blood pressure. Pulse changes are significant. In addition to cardiac problems, tachycardia could indicate hypoxia caused by an obstructed airway. Bradycardia may be associated with digitalis toxicity.

Oxygen is frequently administered in the treatment of cardiovascular diseases, and in older patients it requires most careful use. The nurse should observe the patient closely for hypoxia. Patients using a nasal cannula may breathe primarily by mouth and reduce oxygen intake. Although a face mask may remedy this problem, it does not guarantee sufficient oxygen inspiration. Older patients may not demonstrate cyanosis as the initial sign of hypoxia; instead, they may be restless, irritable, and dyspneic. These signs also can indicate high oxygen concentrations and consequent carbon dioxide narcosis, a particular risk to older patients receiving oxygen therapy. Blood gas levels will provide data to reveal these problems, and early correction is facilitated by keen nursing observation.

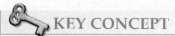

KEY CONCEPT

Instead of demonstrating cyanosis, older adults with hypoxia can become restless, irritable, and dyspneic.

Anorexia may accompany cardiovascular disease, and special nursing assistance may be necessary to help patients meet their nutritional needs. Several smaller meals throughout the entire day rather than a few large ones may compensate for poor appetite and reduce the work of the heart. Favorite foods, served attractively, can be effective. Patients should be encouraged to maintain a regular intake of glucose, the primary source of cardiac energy. Education may be necessary regarding low-sodium, low-cholesterol, and low-calorie diets. Therapeutic dietary modifications should attempt to incorporate ethnic food enjoyed by patients; patients may reject a prescribed special diet if they believe they must forfeit the foods that have been an important component of their lives for decades. It may be necessary to negotiate compromises; a realistic, although imperfect, diet with which patients are satisfied is more likely to be followed than an ideal one that patients cannot accept. The nurse should review foods included in the diets and inform patients of the sodium, cholesterol, and caloric contents of these items. These foods can then be categorized as those that should be eaten "never," "occasionally or not more than once monthly," and "as desired." Patients should learn to read labels of food, beverages, and drugs for sodium content; they must understand that carbonated drinks, certain analgesic preparations, commercial alkalizers, and homemade baking soda mixtures contain sodium.

🔑 KEY CONCEPT

One way to promote dietary compliance is to classify foods for the patient as those that should "never be eaten," "eaten occasionally," or "eaten as desired."

Straining from constipation, enemas, and removal of fecal impactions can cause vagal stimulation, a particularly dangerous situation for patients with cardiovascular disease. Measures to prevent constipation must be an integral part of the care plan for these patients; a stool softener may be prescribed. If bed rest is prescribed, range-of-motion exercises should be performed, because they will cause muscle contractions that compress peripheral veins and thereby facilitate the return of venous blood.

Patients who are weak or who fall asleep while sitting need to have their heads and necks supported to prevent hyperextension or hyperflexion of the neck. All older persons, not only those with cardiovascular disease, can suffer a reduction in cerebral blood flow from the compression of vessels during this hyperextension or hyperflexion. Those with CHF need good positioning and support. A semi-recumbent position with pillows supporting the entire back maintains good body alignment, promotes comfort, and assists in reducing pulmonary congestion. Cardiac strain is reduced by supporting the arms with pillows or armrests. Footboards help prevent foot-drop contracture; patients should be instructed in how to use them for exercising.

If hepatic congestion develops, drugs may detoxify more slowly. Because older adults may already have a slower rate of drug detoxification, nurses must be acutely aware of signs indicating adverse reactions to drugs. Digitalis toxicity particularly should be monitored and could present with a change in mental status, nausea, vomiting, arrhythmias, and a slow pulse. Because hypokalemia sensitizes the heart to the effects of digitalis, prevention through proper diet and the possible use of potassium supplements is advisable.

Promoting Circulation

Because older adults experience age-related changes and a high prevalence of health conditions that heighten their risk of altered tissue perfusion, gerontological nurses should promote interventions that improve tissue circulation to:

- ensure that blood pressure is maintained within an acceptable range (usually under 140 mm Hg systolic and 90 mm Hg diastolic)

- prevent and eliminate sources of pressure on the body

- remind or assist patients to change positions frequently

- prevent pooling of blood in the extremities

- encourage physical activity

- prevent hypothermia and maintain body warmth (particularly of the extremities)

- massage the body unless contraindicated (e.g., in the presence of deep vein thrombosis and pressure ulcer)

- monitor drugs for the side effect of hypotension

- educate to reduce risks (e.g., avoiding excess alcohol ingestion, cigarette smoking, obesity, and inactivity)

- periodically evaluate physical and mental health to identify signs and symptoms of altered tissue perfusion

Nurses can play a significant role in preventing peripheral vascular problems. Health education for persons of all ages should reinforce the importance of exercise in promoting circulation; factors that can interfere with optimal circulation, such as crossing legs and wearing garters, should be reviewed. Weight control can be encouraged because obesity can interfere with venous return. Tobacco use should be discouraged because it may cause arterial spasms. Immobility and hypotension should be prevented to avoid thrombus formation. Figure 20-1 illustrates exercises that may benefit patients with peripheral vascular disease. Yoga and

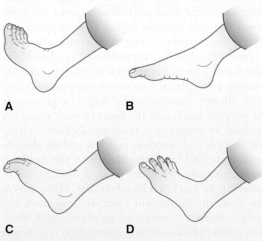

FIGURE 20-1 ■ Foot and toe exercises. **(A)** Foot flexion. **(B)** Foot extension. **(C)** Curling toes. **(D)** Moving toes apart.

t'ai chi can also promote circulation. In addition, Buerger-Allen exercises (see Box 20-6) may be prescribed, and the patient and family members or caregivers will need to learn how they are done correctly and comfortably. Instruction in the correct use of support hose or special elastic stockings is important.

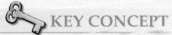

KEY CONCEPT

Circulation can be enhanced by exercise, support hose, and avoidance of obesity, immobility, hypotension, and obstructive clothing.

Providing Foot Care

Persons with peripheral vascular disease must pay special attention to the care of their feet, which should be bathed and inspected daily. To avoid injury, patients should not walk in bare feet. Any foot lesion or discoloration should be promptly brought to the attention of the physician or nurse. These patients are at high risk for developing fungal infections from the moisture produced by normal foot perspiration; it is not unusual for older people to develop fungal infections under their nails, emphasizing the importance of regular, careful nail inspection. If untreated, a simple fungal infection can lead to gangrene and other serious complications. Placing cotton between the toes and removing shoes several times during the day will help keep the feet dry. Shoes should be large enough to avoid any pressure and safe enough to prevent any injuries to the feet; they should be aired after wearing. Laces should not be tied tightly because they can exert pressure on the feet. Colored socks may contain irritating dyes and would be best to avoid; socks should be changed regularly. Although the feet should be kept warm, the direct application of heat to the feet (as with heating pads, hot water bottles, and soaks) can increase the metabolism and circulatory demand, thereby compounding the existing problem.

Managing Problems Associated With Peripheral Vascular Disease

Ischemic foot lesions may be present in patients with peripheral vascular disease. If eschars are present, they should be loosened to allow drainage. Careful debridement is necessary to avoid bleeding and trauma; chemical debriding agents may be useful. Systemic antibiotic agents can be helpful in controlling cellulitis. Topical antibiotics usually are not used because epithelialization must occur before bacterial flora can be destroyed. Analgesics may be administered to relieve associated pain. Good nutrition, particularly an adequate protein intake, and the maintenance of muscle strength and joint motion are essential. Various surgical procedures may be used in treating ischemic foot lesions, including bypass grafts, sympathectomies, and amputations.

Loss of a limb may represent a significant loss of independence to older people, regardless of the reality of the situation. With an altered body image, new roles may be assumed as other roles are forfeited. Patients and their families need opportunities to discuss their fears and concerns. Making them aware of the likelihood of a normal life and the availability of appliances that make ambulation, driving, and other activities possible may help reduce anxieties and promote a smoother adjustment to the amputation. The rehabilitation period can be long for older adults and may necessitate frequent motivation and encouragement by nursing staff.

Promoting Normality

An often unasked question of older patients relates to the impact of their cardiovascular condition on sexual activity. They may be reluctant to inquire because they fear being ridiculed or causing shock that "someone their age would still be interested in sex." They may resign themselves to forfeiting sexual activity under the misconception that they will further harm their hearts; research has demonstrated that patients often place unnecessary restrictions on sexual activities following heart attacks. Nurses should encourage discussion of this subject and introduce the topic if patients seem unable to do so themselves. If there is fear of injuring the heart by resuming sexual activity, the nurse should provide realistic explanations, including when sex can be resumed, how medications can affect sexual function, how to schedule medications for beneficial impact during sexual activity, and sexual positions that produce the least cardiac strain.

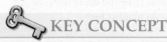

KEY CONCEPT

Nurses should offer patients realistic explanations about the relationship of cardiovascular conditions and sexual function.

Relaxation and rest are both important in the treatment of cardiovascular disease, and it is wise to remember that a patient who is at rest is not necessarily relaxed. The stresses from hospitalization, pain, ignorance, and fear regarding disability; alterations in lifestyle; and potential death can cause the patient to become anxious, confused, and irrational. Reassurance and support are needed, including full explanations of diagnostic tests, hospital or institutional routines, and other activities. The nurse must provide opportunities for patients and their families to discuss questions, concerns, and fears. Realistic explanations of any required restrictions and lifestyle changes should emphasize that patients need not become "cardiac cripples" just because they have a cardiac disease. Most patients can live a normal life and need to be reassured of this. (Refer to the Resources list at the end of the chapter for organizations with resources to help patients live with cardiovascular disorders.)

Integrating Complementary Therapies

The benefits of digitalis (foxglove) in treating heart disease have stimulated interest in the use of other herbs for preventing and treating cardiovascular disorders. One such herb that shows promise is hawthorn berry, which has been found to dilate blood vessels to improve circulation to the heart, relieve spasms of the arterial wall, and produce a hypotensive effect (Mashour, Lin, & Frishman, 2000). Garlic, because it contains antioxidant sulfur compounds, has shown some value in dissolving clots (Fugh-Berman, 2000). Ginger has been shown to lower cholesterol. Patients are wise to discuss the use of medicinal herbs with their health care practitioners and to avoid exceeding recommended dosages.

Some of the nonconventional measures to facilitate deep relaxation and reduce stress can be effective in reversing heart disease. Meditation has been shown to increase blood flow and oxygen consumption (Canter, 2003). Biofeedback, guided imagery, t'ai chi, and yoga have been shown to lower blood pressure and heart rate (Astin et al., 2003). During treatments, acupuncture has lowered blood pressure (Turnbull & Patel, 2007).

Some patients may find yoga beneficial to their circulation because the various asanas (postures) used in yoga increase circulation because of the effects on the endocrine glands and nerve plexuses. Acupressure massage techniques using rubbing, kneading, percussion, and vibration can improve circulation. The herb ginkgo biloba has shown promise as being effective in improving cerebral and peripheral circulation. The future may hold additional noninvasive measures to improve circulation.

Although the full benefits of complementary therapies are in the process of being discovered, these measures are less intrusive and less expensive than conventional treatments and, for the most part, carry minimal risk. Nurses should consider the use of these therapies to prevent heart disease and complement conventional treatments when pathology exists.

CONSIDER THIS CASE

Although 68 years of age, Ms. U continued to carry a full-time teaching load at the university and had no plans of retirement in the foreseeable future. While hiking last week, Ms. U developed chest pain and went to the hospital emergency department for evaluation. She was diagnosed to have a myocardial infarction and, after a brief hospitalization, was sent home on a thrombolytic agent. As she followed a healthy diet and exercised regularly, the cardiologist recommended no other treatment, but did want to see Ms. U at regular intervals. Ms. U now is afraid to resume her physical activities and is contemplating retirement because of "her heart condition."

THINK CRITICALLY

▪ What do you assess to be the issues with Ms. U?
▪ What could you do to assist her?

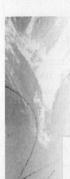

BRINGING RESEARCH TO LIFE

HARMFUL EFFECTS OF NSAIDS AMONG PATIENTS WITH HYPERTENSION AND CORONARY ARTERY DISEASE

Bavry, A. A., Khalign, A., Gong, Y., Handberg, E. M., Cooper-DeHoff, R. M., & Pepine, C. J. (2011). American Journal of Medicine, 124(7), 614–620.

There has been little known about the safety of the chronic use of nonsteroidal anti-inflammatory drugs (NSAIDs) in hypertensive patients with coronary artery disease. To explore this issue, this study followed patients with hypertension and coronary artery disease for a mean

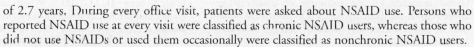

of 2.7 years. During every office visit, patients were asked about NSAID use. Persons who reported NSAID use at every visit were classified as chronic NSAID users, whereas those who did not use NSAIDs or used them occasionally were classified as nonchronic NSAID users.

Chronic NSAID users had a 47% higher risk of death or nonfatal myocardial infarction (MI) or stroke, a 126% increase in cardiovascular deaths, and a 66% increase in total MIs. Based on these findings, the researchers concluded that NSAIDs need to be avoided in persons with hypertension who have coronary artery disease.

As NSAIDs are common over-the-counter medications and often used in the older population, the findings of this study are relevant. Nurses need to include this warning when teaching patients with hypertension and coronary artery disease and specifically ask about NSAID use during every visit with these patients.

PRACTICE REALITIES

You are conducting a blood pressure screening and health education program at a local senior citizen center. One of the participants, a 76-year-old retired single man, is found to have a slightly elevated blood pressure. When you bring this to his attention he acknowledges that he has had a history of this and that his doctor advised him to reduce his sodium intake. "That's fine to say," says the gentleman, "but I don't cook and have a limited income. Most times I eat cheap carryout or snack foods. Even if I could afford fresh fruits, vegetables, and fish they don't sell them at the local convenience store and I don't drive. I just have to make the best of what I've got."

You learn that this man's financial, transportation, and food preparation issues are real as he lives in a basic studio apartment in a poor section of the city.

How could you assist this man?

CRITICAL THINKING EXERCISES

1. How does the lifestyle of the average American contribute to the risk of developing cardiovascular disease with age?
2. List the complications to the general health status of the older adult that can arise as a result of a cardiovascular disorder.
3. Outline general topics you would address when teaching an older individual who is recovering from a myocardial infarction.
4. What measures could you advise young adults to incorporate into their health practices that would promote cardiovascular health in late life?

RESOURCES

American Heart Association
http://www.amhrt.org

Mended Hearts (for patients with heart disease)
http://www.mendedhearts.org

National Amputation Foundation
http://www.nationalamputation.org

National Heart, Lung, and Blood Institute
http://www.nhlbi.nih.gov

REFERENCES

Astin, J. A., Shapiro, S. L., Eisenberg, D. M., & Forys, K. L. (2003). Mind-body medicine: State of the science, implications for practice. *Journal of the American Board Family Practice, 16*(2), 131–147.

Campbell, C. L., Smyth, S., Montalescot, G., & Steinhubl, S. R. (2007). Aspirin dose for the prevention of cardiovascular disease: A systematic review. *Journal of the American Medical Association, 297*(18), 2018–2024.

Canter, P. H. (2003). The therapeutic effects of meditation. *British Medical Journal, 326*(7398), 1049–1050.

Frishman, W. H., Azer, V., & Sica, D. (2003). Drug treatment of orthostatic hypotension and vasovagal syncope. *Heart Disease, 5*(1), 49–64.

Fugh-Berman, A. (2000). Herbs and dietary supplements in the prevention and treatment of cardiovascular disease. *Preventive Cardiology, 3*(1), 24–32.

Klatsky, A. L., & Udaltsova, N. (2007). Alcohol drinking and total mortality risk. *Annals of Epidemiology, 15*(5 Suppl.), S63–S67.

Leighton, F., & Urquiaga, I. (2007). Changes in cardiovascular risk factors associated with wine consumption in intervention studies in humans. *Annals of Epidemiology, 17*(5 Suppl.), S32–S36.

Mashour, N. H., Lin, G. I., & Frishman, W. H. (2000). Herbal medicine for the treatment of cardiovascular disease. In P. B. Fontanarosa (Ed.), *Alternative medicine: An objective assessment* (p. 286). Chicago: American Medical Association.

Ornish, D. (2005). Comparison of diets for weight loss and heart disease risk reduction. *Journal of the American Medical Association, 293*(13), 1589–1590.

Ornish, D. (2008). *Dr. Dean Ornish's program for reversing heart disease.* New York, NY: Ivy Books.

Ridker, P. M. (2003). Clinical application of C-reactive protein for cardiovascular disease detection and prevention. *Circulation, 107*(3), 363–369.

Turnbull, F., & Patel, A. (2007). Acupuncture for blood pressure lowering: Needling the truth. *Circulation, 115*(24), 3048–3049.

Wang, L., Gaziano, J. M., Liu, S., Manson, J. E., Buring, J. E., & Sesso, H. D. (2007). Whole- and refined-grain intakes and the risk of hypertension in women. *American Journal of Clinical Nutrition, 86*(2), 472–479.

Yeh, G. Y., Davis, R. B., & Phillips, R. S. (2006). Use of complementary therapies in patients with cardiovascular disease. *American Journal of Cardiology, 98*(5), 673–680.

RECOMMENDED READINGS

Recommended Readings associated with this chapter can be found on the web site that accompanies the book. Visit **http://thepoint.lww.com/Eliopoulos8e** to access the recommended readings and other additional resources associated with this chapter.

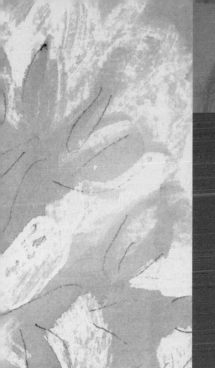

CHAPTER 21

Digestion and Bowel Elimination

CHAPTER OUTLINE

LEARNING OBJECTIVES

After reading this chapter, you should be able to:

1. Describe how aging affects gastrointestinal health.

2. Discuss measures to promote gastrointestinal health in older adults.

3. List symptoms and management of selected gastrointestinal conditions in older adults.

TERMS TO KNOW

Anorexia: lack of appetite

Cholelithiasis: the formation or presence of gallstones in the gallbladder

Diverticulitis: inflammation or infection of the pouches of intestinal mucosa

Dysphagia: difficulty swallowing

Edentulous: without teeth

Esophageal dysphagia: difficulty with the transfer of food down the esophagus

Fecal incontinence: involuntary passage of stool

Flatus: gas

Gingivitis: inflammation of the gums surrounding the teeth

Hiatal hernia: portion of stomach protrudes through opening in diaphragm

Oropharyngeal dysphagia: difficulty transferring food bolus or liquid from the mouth into the pharynx and esophagus

(Continued)

289

Periodontitis: inflammation of the gums extending to the underlying tissues, roots of teeth, and bone

Presbyesophagus: age-related changes to the esophagus causing reduced strength of esophageal contractions and slower transport of food down the esophagus

Digestion and bowel elimination are important functions of the gastrointestinal tract. Significantly fewer older people die from gastrointestinal problems than from diseases of other major body systems; however, these problems often are the source of many complaints and discomforts in this age group. Indigestion, belching, diarrhea, constipation, nausea, vomiting, anorexia, weight gain or loss, and flatulence are among the bothersome problems that increasingly occur, even in the absence of organic cause. Gallbladder disease and various cancers of the gastrointestinal tract increase in incidence in later life. In addition, poor nutrition, medications, emotions, inactivity, and a variety of other factors influence the status of gastrointestinal health.

Usually, older adults are aware of their gastrointestinal discomforts and use various measures to manage symptoms of these problems. In some situations, misinformation can interfere with good gastrointestinal health (e.g., assuming that tooth loss is normal or believing a daily laxative is essential); in other circumstances, self-treatment can delay the diagnosis of pathologies (e.g., using antacids to mask symptoms of stomach cancer). Gerontological nurses play an important role in promoting gastrointestinal health in older adults and intervening when problems are identified.

EFFECTS OF AGING ON GASTROINTESTINAL HEALTH

The gastrointestinal system and accessory structures experience significant changes with age (see Chapter 5). The tongue atrophies, affecting the taste buds and decreasing taste sensations. Changes in taste sensations can also be related to xerostomia (dry mouth), the effects of some medications, diseases, and smoking. Saliva production decreases and swallowing may be more difficult. Presbyesophagus, the degenerative changes in the smooth muscle lining of the lower esophagus, results in weaker esophageal contractions and weakness of the sphincter. As esophageal and stomach motility decrease, food can remain in the upper gastrointestinal system for a longer period of time; as a result, there is a risk of indigestion and aspiration. Decreased elasticity of the stomach reduces the amount of food that the stomach can accommodate at one time. The stomach has a higher pH as a result of the declines in hydrochloric acid and pepsin; this contributes to an increased incidence of gastric irritation in late life. The reduced presence of pepsin can interfere with the absorption of protein, whereas the decrease in hydrochloric acid can interfere with the absorption of calcium, iron, folic acid, and vitamin B_{12}. There are fewer cells on the absorbing surface of the intestinal walls affecting the absorption of dextrose, xylose, calcium, iron, and vitamins B, B_{12}, and D.

Slower peristalsis, inactivity, reduced food and fluid intake, drugs, and a diet low in fiber are responsible for the high incidence of constipation in older individuals. Decreased sensory perception may cause the signal for bowel elimination to go unnoticed, which can promote constipation. There is also a tendency toward incomplete emptying of the bowel with one bowel movement; 30 to 45 minutes after the initial movement, the remainder of the bowel movement may need to occur, and if not heeded, problems may develop.

The structure of the gallbladder and bile ducts is unchanged with age; bile salt synthesis decreases, however, contributing to the risk of gallstone development. The pancreas experiences fibrosis, atrophy, and fatty acid deposits, along with a reduction in pancreatic secretions; this can affect the digestion of fats and contribute to an intolerance for fatty foods. Although liver size decreases with age, liver function remains within normal limits. Hepatic blood flow can be reduced as a result of decreased cardiac output.

GASTROINTESTINAL HEALTH PROMOTION

A variety of gastrointestinal conditions can be avoided by good health practices. Good dental hygiene (Box 21-1) and regular visits to the dentist can prevent disorders that can threaten nutritional intake, general health, comfort, and self-image. The proper quantity and quality of foods can enhance general health and minimize the risk of indigestion and constipation. (See Chapter 14 for more specific information on ways to promote

BOX 21-1   Oral Health Practices for Older Adults

- Brush all tooth surfaces and the tongue at least twice daily with a soft-bristled toothbrush and fluoridated toothpaste. Use an up-and-down brushing motion. If arthritis, weakness, or other problems interfere with the ability to adequately brush teeth, obtain a large-handled, battery-powered, or electric-powered toothbrush.
- Floss between teeth daily. Floss aids are available to compensate for arthritic fingers or other problems that can interfere with flossing.
- If mouthwash is used, avoid those that contain alcohol. (Mouthwash is not a substitute for brushing.)
- Swab sticks (e.g., lemon-glycerin) should be avoided as they dry the oral mucosa and erode tooth enamel.

- Brush the teeth or rinse the mouth after consuming candy or other sweets.
- If dentures are worn, remove them at night and soak them in water. Clean the dentures and the gums of the mouth before replacing the dentures in the mouth.
- If hard candy and gum are desired, use the sugar-free varieties.
- Visit a dentist every 6 months. Less frequent visits are acceptable if a complete set of dentures is worn, but to detect oral diseases, dental evaluation remains important; consult with a dentist as to suggested frequency of visit.

nutritional health.) Knowledge of the relationship of medications to gastrointestinal health is also important.

Natural means to promote bowel elimination is important for older adults to incorporate into their daily routines, including good fluid intake, a diet rich in fruits and vegetables, activity, and the establishment of a regular time for bowel elimination (Fig. 21-1). Dietary fiber intake of 20 to 35 g/day is advisable; however, if fiber intake has been low, the amount should be gradually increased to prevent gas, bloating, diarrhea, and other symptoms. If a person dislikes eating high-fiber foods, these foods can be added to other foods (e.g., adding wheat bran to ground beef or muffins) to mask the taste. Plenty of fluids should accompany increased fiber intake. Because of the tendency for incomplete emptying of the bowel at one time, opportunity should be provided for full emptying and for repeated attempts at subsequent elimination. Sometimes, an older person's request to be taken to the bathroom or to have a bedpan for bowel elimination shortly before a movement occurs is viewed as an unnecessary demand and ignored; it is then wondered why bowel incontinence results. It is useful for older adults to attempt a bowel movement following breakfast, because the morning activity and ingestion of food and fluid following a period of rest stimulate peristalsis.

Astute assessment can reveal problems that patients may have omitted sharing with their health care providers and can identify practices that interfere with good health (Assessment

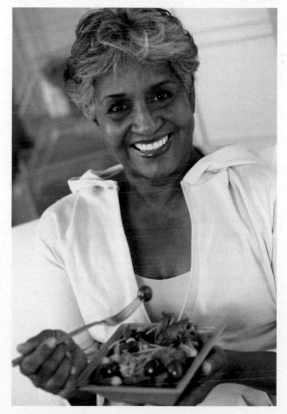

FIGURE 21-1 ■ A diet rich in fruits and vegetables is one natural means to promote bowel elimination.

Guide 21-1). Nursing Diagnosis Table 21-1 lists possible diagnoses related to gastrointestinal problems.

ASSESSMENT GUIDE 21-1
GASTROINTESTINAL FUNCTION

GENERAL OBSERVATIONS

- *General appearance.* Pallor can be associated with blood loss from gastrointestinal bleeding. Weakness and fatigue can be due to malnutrition, fluid and electrolyte imbalances, or bleeding. Note obesity or unusual thinness.

- *Odors.* Unusual breath odors can be associated with disorders. Halitosis can indicate poor oral hygiene practices, disease of the oral cavity or esophagus, lung abscess or infection, liver disease, or uremia.

- *Skin.* Dry skin and skin with poor turgor can indicate dehydration; scaling, itching, discolored skin, or skin eruptions can result from a variety of nutritional deficiencies.

INTERVIEW

Carefully structured questions can reveal hidden problems, particularly in older adults who accept some gastrointestinal symptoms as normal or who have lived with these symptoms for so long that they no longer consider them abnormalities. Questions should review topics such as the following:

- *Status of teeth or dentures.* "When was your last dental exam? How do you care for your teeth or dentures? When did you get your dentures; how do they fit? Do you have any pain, bleeding, or other symptoms?"

- *Taste, appetite.* "Does food taste differently to you than it did in the past? What do you do to make food taste better? How is your appetite; how does it compare to earlier years?"

- *Symptoms.* "Do you ever have a sore mouth, difficulty swallowing, choking, a sense that something has 'gone down the wrong hole,' nausea, vomiting, bleeding from your mouth, blood in your vomitus or stool, pain or burning in your stomach or intestines, diarrhea, constipation, gas, bleeding from your rectum?" Specific questions should be asked to explore each positive response.

- *Weight.* "Have you noticed any recent changes in your weight? Have you been trying to gain or lose weight?"

- *Digestion.* "How often do you have indigestion? What seems to cause it and how is it managed? Is there a sense of fullness or discomfort in the chest after meals? Does regurgitation or belching ever occur?"

- *Elimination.* "How often do you have a bowel movement? Do you have to take special measures to move your bowels? If so, what are they? Do you strain to have a bowel movement? Is there ever blood in your stools or on the toilet tissue? What are the color and consistency of your bowel movements?"

- *Diet.* "Describe what and when you eat in a typical day. Do foods have a different taste to you? Can you shop for and cook meals on your own? Has your eating pattern changed?" *Colorectal screening.* Ask if colorectal screening (e.g., fecal occult blood testing, sigmoidoscopy, and colonoscopy) has been done.

Further questions may be necessary in response to certain problems that emerge through the interview.

PHYSICAL EXAMINATION

Inspection, auscultation, percussion, and palpation aid in validating problems identified through the interview and in detecting undisclosed disorders. A systematic examination of the gastrointestinal system would review the following:

- *Lips.* Note symmetry, color, moisture, and general condition. Because capillaries are abundant in the lips, a bluish discoloration could reflect poor oxygenation. Cracks and fissures can be associated with riboflavin deficiencies, jagged teeth, or poorly fitting dentures.

- *Oral cavity.* With a tongue depressor and flashlight, inspect the mouth. The mucous membrane should be moist and pink. Black persons may have a pigmented mucosa. Excessive dryness of the mucosa or tongue can indicate dehydration. Note lesions or areas of irritation, which could be caused by teeth, dentures, or pathologic conditions. White beads in the oral cavity can be a sign of moniliasis infections and should be cultured. Bleeding and swollen gums are most commonly associated with periodontal disease. Swollen gums also can result from phenytoin therapy or leukemia. Lead poisoning causes a bluish black line along the edge of the gums, but only if teeth are present. Older persons can develop lead poisoning due to occupational exposure or contact within their home environment.

- *Tongue.* Examine the top and bottom surface of the tongue. A coating on the tongue can be associated with poor hygiene or dehydration. A smooth, red tongue occurs with iron, vitamin B_{12}, or niacin deficiencies. Thick, white patches can indicate leukoplakia, which could be precancerous. Give attention to lesions on the tongue that have been present for several weeks because they can be cancerous; they more frequently occur on the bottom surface than on the top of the tongue. Varicosities on the undersurface of the tongue are not unusual findings. Determine if the individual can move the tongue side to side and up and down.

- *Pharynx.* During normal swallowing, the vagus nerve causes the soft palate to rise and block the nasopharynx so that aspiration is prevented. To test this function, press a tongue depressor on the middle of the tongue, but not so far back that gagging results, and ask the patient to say "ah." The soft palate should rise when "ah" is said. If soreness, redness, or white patches are present in the throat, a culture is warranted.

■ *Abdomen.* Have the patient void and then lie supine on a firm surface; inspect the abdomen. Ask about any scars that are present; the patient may have forgotten to mention an appendectomy that occurred 50 years ago. Striae, or stretch marks, are pink or blue if newly developed and silvery white if old; they can result from obesity, ascites, pregnancy, or tumors. Note rashes, indentations, and other findings. Both sides of the abdomen should be symmetrical with no bulging areas. A symmetrical distension most commonly is due to obesity, but can also be associated with ascites or tumors. Central, lower abdominal (i.e., below the umbilicus) distension occurs with bladder distension or tumors of the uterus or ovaries. Central, upper abdominal distension may result from gastric dilation or pancreatic tumors. The abdomen should rise and fall in conjunction with respirations. Peristaltic activity may be observed; sometimes, gently flicking a finger on the abdomen will stimulate peristalsis. With the diaphragm of the stethoscope, bowel sounds can be heard about once every 5 to 15 seconds; they usually are irregular. If no bowel sounds are heard, try stimulating them by flicking a finger on the abdomen. No sounds for at least 5 minutes can indicate the absence of bowel sounds, and medical evaluation would be warranted. Loud, gurgling sounds indicate increased peristaltic activity. Palpation of the abdomen should normally reveal no masses.

■ *Rectum.* Perform a rectal examination with the patient in a standing position, bent over the examination table, or in a left lateral position with the right hip and knee flexed. Inspect the perianal area first. Flaccid skin sacs around the anus are hemorrhoids. Fissures, tumors, inflammation, and poor hygienic practices may be noted. Ask the patient to bear down, which could make additional hemorrhoids or rectal prolapse visible. Ask the patient to bear down again and insert a lubricated gloved finger into the anal canal. Assure the patient that it is normal to feel as if a bowel movement is imminent. The sphincter should tighten around the finger. Masses or other abnormalities along the rectal wall should be noted. A hard mass that prevents full palpation of the rectum may be a fecal impaction. Impactions may or may not be movable. If it is a fecal impaction, fecal material will be found on the glove or a discharge will occur when the examining finger is withdrawn.

■ *Stool.* Obtain a stool specimen; fecal material withdrawn during the rectal examination can give clues to problems. Black, tarry stools can be associated with the ingestion of iron preparations or iron-rich foods or can indicate upper gastrointestinal bleeding; bright-red blood accompanies bleeding from the lower bowel or hemorrhoids; pale, fatty stool can occur with absorption problems; gray or tan stool is caused by obstructive jaundice; and mucus in the stool may result from inflammation.

SELECTED GASTROINTESTINAL CONDITIONS AND RELATED NURSING CONSIDERATIONS

Dry Mouth (Xerostomia)

Saliva serves several important functions, such as lubricating soft tissues, assisting in remineralizing teeth, promoting taste sensations, and helping to control bacteria and fungus in the oral cavity. Reduced saliva, therefore, can have significant consequences.

Dry mouth can result from a variety of factors in addition to age-related slight declines in saliva secretion. Many of the medications used by older persons (e.g., diuretics, antihypertensives, anti-inflammatories, and antidepressants) can affect salivation. Sjögren's syndrome, a disease of the immune system, can reduce salivary gland function and cause severe dryness of the mucous membrane.

Mouth breathing and altered cognition also contribute to this problem.

Persons with dry mouth benefit from frequent oral hygiene, not only because of the comfort obtained but also to reduce the higher risk of dental disease related to dry mouth. Saliva substitutes (e.g., Salivart Synthetic Saliva) are available as gels and rinses; however, sipping water to relieve dryness and stimulating saliva production with hard sugarless candy and gum are effective for many individuals.

Dental Problems

Dental care is important throughout an individual's life. Dental examination can be instrumental in the early detection and prevention of many problems that affect other body systems. Poor condition of teeth can restrict food intake, which can cause constipation and malnourishment (see Chapter

NURSING DIAGNOSIS

TABLE 21-1 **Nursing Diagnoses Related to Gastrointestinal Problems**

Causes or Contributing Factors	Nursing Diagnosis
Anemia, constipation, obesity, vitamin and mineral deficiencies, dehydration	Activity Intolerance
Age-related decreased colonic peristalsis and duller neural impulses for signal to defecate, anorexia, obesity, hemorrhoids, lack of roughage in diet, dehydration, habitual laxative use	Constipation
Medications, peptic ulcer, gastritis, ulcerative colitis, diverticulitis, diabetes, fecal impaction, tube feedings, stress	Diarrhea
Indigestion, constipation, hemorrhoids, flatus	Acute Pain
Uncontrolled diabetes, infection, peritonitis, diarrhea, vomiting, blood loss, insufficient fluid intake, high-solute tube feedings	Deficient Fluid Volume
Diabetes, malnutrition, hemorrhoids	Risk of Infection
Intestinal obstruction, anorexia, nausea, vomiting, poor dental status, altered taste sensations, constipation	Imbalanced Nutrition: Less Than Body Requirements
Altered taste sensations, ethnic preferences, inactivity, lack of motivation to eat well	Imbalanced Nutrition: More Than Body Requirements
Diabetes, cancer, gingivitis, periodontal disease, jagged teeth, poorly fitting dentures, dehydration, malnutrition, dry mouth	Impaired Oral Mucous Membrane

14); it can also detract from appearance, which can affect socialization, and this can result in a poor appetite, which also can lead to malnourishment. Periodontal disease can predispose older adults to systemic infection. Although dental care is important in preventing these problems, financial limitations prevent many older persons from seeking dental attention. Some have the misconception that dentures eliminate the need for regular visits to the dentist; others, like many younger persons, fear the dentist. The nurse should encourage regular dental examination and promote dental care, explaining that serious diseases can be detected by the dentist and helping patients find free or inexpensive dental clinics. Understanding how modern dental techniques minimize pain can alleviate fears. Although older persons may not have had the benefit of fluoridated water or fluoride treatments when younger, topical fluoride treatments are as beneficial to the teeth of older persons as they are to younger teeth. The nurse should instruct patients to inform their dentists about health problems and medications they take to help them determine how procedures need to be modified, what healing rate to expect, and which medications should not be administered.

Dental problems can be caused by altered taste sensation, a poor diet, or a low-budget carbohydrate diet with excessive intake of sweets, which can cause tooth decay. Deficiencies of vitamin B complex and calcium, hormonal imbalances, hyperparathyroidism, diabetes, osteomalacia, Cushing disease, and syphilis can be underlying causes of dental problems, and certain drugs, such as phenytoin, which can cause gingivitis, or antihistamines and antipsychotics, which cause severe dry mouth, can play a part. The aging process itself takes its toll on teeth. Surfaces are commonly worn down from many years of use, varying degrees of root absorption occur, and loss of tooth enamel can increase the risk of irritation to deeper dental tissue. Although benign neoplastic lesions develop more frequently than malignant ones, cancer of the oral cavity, especially in men, increases in incidence with age, as does moniliasis, which is often associated with more serious problems, such as diabetes or leukemia. It should not be assumed that all white lesions found in the mouth are moniliasis; biopsy is important to make sure they are not cancerous. Periodontal disease, which damages the soft tissue surrounding the teeth and supporting bones, has a high incidence among older adults and is a major cause of tooth loss. Dental caries occur less frequently in older people, but they remain a problem.

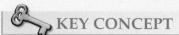

KEY CONCEPT

With age, the teeth experience a wearing down on the surfaces, decrease in the size and volume of pulp, increased brittleness, varying degrees of root absorption, and a loss of enamel.

Good oral hygiene is especially important to older persons, who already may be having problems with anorexia or food distaste. Teeth, gums, and tongue should be brushed regularly using a soft toothbrush, which also can be used in gentle gum massage for people with dentures. Brushing is superior to using swabs, even for the teeth of unconscious patients. Daily flossing of natural teeth should also be performed. Because the buccal mucosa is thinner and less vascular with age, trauma to the oral cavity needs to be avoided. The nurse should notify the dentist and physician of an atonic or atrophic tongue, lesions, mucosa discoloration, loose teeth, soreness, bleeding, or any other problem identified during inspection and care of the oral cavity.

Dysphagia

The incidence of swallowing difficulties increases with age. As swallowing depends on complex mechanisms involving several cranial nerves and the muscles of the mouth, face, pharynx, and esophagus, anything that impacts those structures can cause dysphagia. Gastroesophageal reflux disease (GERD) is a common cause, as are stroke and structural disorders. Dysphagia can be oropharyngeal, characterized by difficulty transferring food bolus or liquid from the mouth into the pharynx and esophagus and more common in persons with neurologic damage, or esophageal, involving difficulty with the transfer of food down the esophagus and more common in persons with motility disorders, sphincter abnormalities, or mechanical obstructions caused by strictures. Symptoms can be mild, such as occasional difficulties swallowing certain types of food, to a complete inability to swallow.

Careful assessment and observation assist in diagnosing the cause of the problem. The nurse should ask patients with dysphagia:

- when the problem began
- what other symptoms accompany the dysphagia (chest pain, nausea, or coughing)
- what types of foods trigger symptoms (e.g., solids or liquids)
- if the problem is intermittent or present with every meal

Observing food intake can offer insights into the nature of the problem. Referral to a speech-language pathologist is essential to developing an effective plan of care.

Prevention of aspiration and promotion of adequate nutritional status are major goals in the care of patients with dysphagia. The nurse should follow the recommendations of the speech-language therapist closely. Often, a soft diet and thickening of liquids are recommended to promote ease of swallowing; however, there are various levels of dietary modification that can be prescribed ranging from pureed to mechanically altered to regular. Patients with dysphagia should eat in an upright position, ingesting small bites in an unhurried manner. Verbal cues may be needed. An easily accessible suction machine is beneficial in the event of choking. It is important to monitor food intake and weight.

Hiatal Hernia

The incidence of hiatal hernia increases with age, affecting about half of people in the United States over age 50 years, and is of greater incidence in older women. There is some thought that the low-fiber diet of Americans contributes to the high prevalence of this condition. The two types of hiatal hernia are sliding (axial) and rolling (paraesophageal). The sliding type is the most common and occurs when a part of the stomach and the junction of the stomach and esophagus slide through the diaphragm. Most patients with GERD have this type of hiatal hernia. In the rolling or paraesophageal type, the fundus and greater curvatures of the stomach roll up through the diaphragm. Heartburn, dysphagia, belching, vomiting, and regurgitation are common symptoms associated with hiatal hernia. These symptoms are especially problematic when the patient is recumbent. Pain (sometimes mistaken for a heart attack) and bleeding also may occur. Diagnosis is confirmed by a barium swallow and esophagoscopy.

Most patients are managed medically. If the patient is obese, weight reduction can minimize the problem. A bland diet may be recommended, as may the use of milk and antacids for symptomatic relief. Several small meals each day rather than three large ones help improve hiatal hernias and may be advantageous to the aged in coping with other age-related gastrointestinal problems. Eating before bedtime should be discouraged. Some patients may find it helpful to sleep in a partly recumbent position. H2 blockers, such as ranitidine, cimetidine, or nizatidine, and proton-pump inhibitors like lansoprazole and omeprazole often are prescribed. Nursing Care Plan 21-1 offers a sample care plan for the patient with hiatal hernia.

NURSING CARE PLAN 21-1

THE OLDER ADULT WITH HIATAL HERNIA

Diagnosis: Acute Pain

Goal	Nursing Actions
The patient is free from discomfort related to hiatal hernia	■ Assist patient in identifying situations that cause discomfort (e.g., bending, bedtime snacking); advise patient to avoid them.
	■ Teach and support low-calorie diet if obesity is a problem.
	■ Advise patient to eat five to six small-portioned meals during the day rather than three large meals; in a hospital or institutional setting, consult with dietician to arrange this meal plan.
	■ Instruct patient to eat meals slowly and to sit upright while eating and for at least 1 hour thereafter.
	■ Discourage consumption of spicy foods, caffeinated beverages, carbonated beverages, and alcohol.
	■ Advise patient to stop smoking if patient has this habit; refer to smoking cessation program as needed.
	■ Advise patient against consuming food for at least 2 hours prior to bedtime or nap.
	■ Instruct patient to avoid heavy lifting, bending, wearing girdles or tight pants, and coughing or sneezing strenuously.
	■ Prevent constipation to avoid straining during bowel movements.
	■ Elevate upper portion of bed by placing blocks under the head of the bed (this is preferable to raising upper portion of mattress due to risk of shearing force).
	■ Administer antacids as prescribed.

Nursing Diagnosis: Imbalanced Nutrition: Less Than Body Requirements

Goal	Nursing Actions
The patient consumes the prescribed diet; the patient is free from abdominal discomfort	■ Consult with nutritionist and physician to develop diet plan appropriate for the patient.
	■ Instruct patient to eat five or six small-portioned meals rather than three large ones.
	■ Identify foods that increase symptoms and instruct patient to omit these from diet; offer foods of equal nutritive value to replace food eliminated from diet if necessary.
	■ Record and monitor weight and dietary intake.

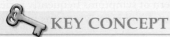

KEY CONCEPT

Several small meals throughout the day, rather than three large ones, not only are beneficial in the management of hiatal hernia but also have advantages for the gastrointestinal health of all older adults.

Esophageal Cancer

Although the incidence has been decreasing, most persons affected by cancer of the esophagus are of advanced age. The most common types are squamous cell carcinoma and adenocarcinoma. This disease commonly strikes between the ages of 50 and 70 years and is of higher incidence in men. African American men with a history of alcoholism and heavy smoking have a higher incidence of squamous cell esophageal carcinoma. Poor oral hygiene and chronic irritation from tobacco, alcohol, and other agents contribute to the development of this problem. Barrett's esophagus, a condition in which the normal lining of the esophagus is replaced by a type of lining usually found in the intestines (intestinal metaplasia), is associated with an increased risk of developing this cancer (Peters, 2003); the risk of developing adenocarcinoma is 30 to 125 times higher in people who have Barrett's esophagus than in people who do not (National Institute of Diabetes and Digestive and Kidney Disease, 2007).

Dysphagia, weight loss, excessive salivation, thirst, hiccups, anemia, and chronic bleeding are symptoms of the disease. Unfortunately, symptoms often are not recognized until the disease is advanced, contributing to a poor prognosis. Barium swallow, esophagoscopy, and biopsy are performed as diagnostic measures. Treatment options include surgical resection, radiation, chemotherapy, laser therapy, and photodynamic therapy. Benign tumors of the esophagus are rare in older people.

Peptic Ulcer

In addition to stress, diet, and genetic predisposition as causes, particular factors are believed to account for the increased incidence of ulcers in older persons, including longevity; more precise diagnostic evaluation; and the fact that ulcers can be a complication of chronic obstructive pulmonary disease, which is increasingly prevalent. Drugs commonly prescribed for older adults that can increase gastric secretions and reduce the resistance of the mucosa include aspirin, reserpine, tolbutamide, phenylbutazone, colchicine, and adrenal corticosteroids. Other risk factors include smoking,

heavy alcoholic beverage consumption, caffeine, stress, and *Helicobacter pylori* infection.

Peptic ulcers tend to present with more acute symptoms in older adults, such as pain, bleeding, obstruction, and perforation. Diagnostic and therapeutic measures resemble those used for younger adults. Addressing risk factors is important. The nurse should be alert to complications associated with peptic ulcer, which are more likely to occur with older adults, such as constipation or diarrhea caused by antacid therapy and pyloric obstruction resulting in dehydration, peritonitis, hemorrhage, and shock.

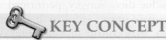

POINT TO PONDER

In what ways do diet, activity, emotions, and other factors affect your appetite, diet, digestion, and bowel elimination? Do you notice any patterns that you could correct, and if so, how?

Cancer of the Stomach

The incidence of gastric cancer increases with age, occurring most frequently in people between 50 and 70 years of age. It is more prevalent among men, poor socioeconomic groups, and African American, Asian, Native American, and Hispanic individuals. Adenocarcinomas account for most gastric malignancies. Anorexia, epigastric pain, weight loss, and anemia are symptoms of gastric cancer; these symptoms may be insidious and easily mistaken for indigestion problems. Bleeding and enlargement of the liver may occur. Symptoms related to pelvic metastasis may also develop. Diagnosis is confirmed by barium swallow and gastroscopy with biopsy. Surgical treatment consisting of a partial or total gastrectomy is preferred. If detected early the prognosis is good but when advanced there is a poor prognosis. A diet low in red meats and high in antioxidants is believed to be helpful in preventing stomach cancer.

KEY CONCEPT

Symptoms of gastric cancer can be insidious and easily mistaken for indigestion.

Diverticular Disease

Multiple pouches of intestinal mucosa in the weakened muscular wall of the large bowel, known as diverticulosis, are common among older persons.

Chronic constipation, obesity, hiatal hernia, and atrophy of the intestinal wall muscles with aging contribute to this problem. The low-fiber, low-residue diets that are common in Western societies are a major reason that diverticulosis is common in this country but rare in many third world countries. Most cases involve the sigmoid colon; many cases are asymptomatic. If symptoms are present, they can include slight bleeding, as well as a change in bowel habits (constipation, diarrhea, or both) and tenderness on palpation of the left lower quadrant. Usually a barium enema identifies the problem. Surgery is not performed unless severe bleeding develops. Medical management is most common and includes an increase in dietary fiber intake, weight reduction, and avoidance of constipation.

Bowel contents can accumulate in the diverticula and decompose, causing inflammation and infection; this is known as diverticulitis. Although fewer than half the patients with diverticulosis develop diverticulitis, most patients who do are old. Older men tend to experience this problem more than any other group.

Overeating, straining during a bowel movement, alcohol, and irritating foods may contribute to diverticulitis in the patient with diverticulosis. Abrupt onset of pain in the left lower quadrant, similar to that of appendicitis but over the sigmoid area, is a symptom of this problem. Nausea, vomiting, constipation, diarrhea, low-grade fever, and blood or mucus in the stool may also occur. These attacks can be severely acute or slowly progressing; although the acute attacks can cause peritonitis, the slower forms can also be serious because of the possibility of lower bowel obstruction resulting from scarring and abscess formation. In addition to the mentioned complications, fistulas to the bladder, vagina, colon, and intestines can develop. During the acute phase, efforts focus on reducing infection, providing nutrition, relieving discomfort, and promoting rest. Usually nothing is ingested by mouth, and intravenous therapy is used. When the acute episode subsides, the patient is taught to consume a low-residue diet. Surgery, performed if medical management is unsuccessful or if serious complications occur, may consist of a resection or temporary colostomy. Continued follow-up should be encouraged.

Colorectal Cancer

Cancer at any site along the large intestine is common with advancing age. The sigmoid colon and rectum tend to be frequent sites for carcinoma; in fact, colorectal cancer is the second most common malignancy in the United States.

Although the pattern of symptoms frequently varies for each person, some common symptoms include:

- bloody stools
- change in bowel pattern
- anorexia
- nausea
- pain over affected region
- anemia

Some older patients ignore bowel symptoms, believing them to be from constipation, poor diet, or hemorrhoids. The patient's description of bowel problems is less reliable than a digital rectal examination, which detects half of all carcinomas of the large bowel and rectum. Fecal occult blood testing is effective for early detection of colonic tumors. The standard diagnostic tests, including barium enema and sigmoidoscopy with biopsy, are used to confirm the diagnosis. Surgical resection with anastomosis or the formation of a colostomy is usually performed. Medical-surgical nursing textbooks can provide information on this surgery, and nurses should consult them for specific guidance on caring for patients with this condition.

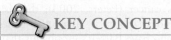 **KEY CONCEPT**

An annual stool occult blood and digital rectal examination are recommended because they can detect many cancers of the large bowel and rectum. In addition, a flexible sigmoidoscopy every 5 years or a colonoscopy every 10 years is advised as an important means to detect colorectal cancer. Risk factors may warrant more frequent screening.

It is important to realize that a colostomy can present many problems for older adults. In addition to having to adjust to many bodily changes with age, a colostomy presents a major adjustment and a threat to a good self-concept. Older adults may feel that a colostomy further separates them from society's view of normal. Socialization may be impaired by the patient's concern over the reactions of others or by fear of embarrassing episodes. Reduced energy reserves, arthritic fingers, slower movement, and poorer eyesight are among the problems that may hamper the ability to care for a colostomy, thus causing dependency on others to assist with this procedure. This need for assistance may be perceived as a significant loss of independence for older persons. Tactful, skilled nursing intervention can promote psychological as well as physical adjustment to a colostomy. Continued follow-up is beneficial to assess the patient's changing ability to engage in this self-care activity, identify problems, and provide ongoing support and reassurance.

Chronic Constipation

Constipation is a common concern for older adults (Nursing Diagnosis Highlight: Constipation). Many factors can contribute to this problem, including:

- inactive lifestyle
- low-fiber and low-fluid intake
- depression
- laxative abuse
- certain medications, such as opiates, sedatives, and aluminum hydroxide gels

- dulled sensations that cause the signal for bowel elimination to be missed
- failure to allow sufficient time for complete emptying of the bowel

A diet high in fiber and fluid and regular activity can promote bowel elimination, and particular foods that patients find effective (e.g., prunes or chocolate pudding) can be incorporated into the regular diet. A mixture of raisins, prunes, dates, and currants can be a nourishing, tasty snack that promotes bowel elimination. (For individuals with chewing impairments, this can be blended with yogurt or applesauce.) Providing a regular time for bowel elimination is often helpful; mornings tend to be the best time for older adults to empty their bowels. Sometimes rocking the trunk from side to side and back and forth while sitting on the toilet will stimulate a bowel movement. Only after these measures have failed should medications be considered.

NURSING DIAGNOSIS HIGHLIGHT

CONSTIPATION

Overview

Constipation is a condition in which there is an infrequent passage of dry, hard stools. Some of the findings consistent with constipation include decreased frequency of bowel movements (as compared with patient's normal pattern); straining to have bowel movement; hard, dry stools; abdominal distension and discomfort; palpable mass and sense of pressure or fullness in rectum; poor appetite; backache, headache; reduced activity level; and request for or use of laxatives or enemas.

Causative or contributing factors

Age-related decrease in peristalsis, inactivity, immobility, hemorrhoidal pain, poor dietary intake of fiber and fluids, dehydration, certain diseases (e.g., hypothyroidism), surgery, dependency on laxatives or enemas, and side effects of medications (e.g., antacids, calcium, anticholinergics, barium, iron, and narcotics)

Goal

The patient establishes a regular pattern of bowel elimination and passes a stool of normal consistency without straining or experiencing discomfort.

Interventions

- Establish and maintain record of frequency and characteristics of bowel movements.
- Ensure patient consumes at least 1,300 mL fluids daily (unless contraindicated).

- Review dietary pattern with patient and educate as needed regarding the inclusion of high-fiber foods in diet; monitor dietary intake.
- Assist patient in developing a program to increase activity level as appropriate.
- Assist patient in developing a regular schedule for toileting; provide toileting assistance as needed; ensure privacy is provided during toileting; if bedpan must be used, be sure patient is in upright position, unless contraindicated, and made comfortable.
- Consider use of herbs with laxative effects, such as aloe, dandelion root, cascara sagrada, senna, and rhubarb.
- Consult with physician regarding use of vitamin C supplements several times daily until stool is soft (not to exceed 5,000 mg/day).
- Administer laxatives, as prescribed; avoid long-term use of laxatives unless patient's condition warrants otherwise.
- Monitor for fecal impaction.
- Assess patient's use of laxatives and enemas; if dependency on laxatives or enemas for bowel elimination exists, educate patient about hazards associated with this dependency and develop a plan to gradually taper usage of laxative or enema (abrupt discontinuation is contraindicated).
- Educate patient as to nonpharmacologic means to stimulate bowel movement.

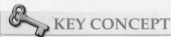

KEY CONCEPT

Measures to promote bowel elimination include scheduling a regular time for this function, incorporating high-fiber foods into the diet, and rocking the trunk from side to side and back and forth while sitting on the toilet.

Older persons may need education concerning bowel elimination. The safe use of laxatives should be emphasized to prevent laxative abuse. The patient should be aware that diarrhea resulting from laxative abuse may cause dehydration, a serious threat to life. Dandelion root, cascara sagrada, senna, and rhubarb are herbs that stimulate bowel movement and can be taken to prevent constipation.

Older adults in a hospital or nursing home may benefit from an elimination chart that reflects the time, amount, and characteristics of bowel movements. This chart can help the nurse prevent constipation and fecal impaction by providing easily accessible data regarding bowel elimination. Even older persons in the community can benefit from the use of an elimination record that they can maintain themselves.

Chronic constipation that does not improve with the usual measures may require medical evaluation, including anal, rectal, and sigmoid examinations, to determine the presence of any underlying cause.

Flatulence/Gas

Flatulence, which is common in older adults, is caused by constipation, irregular bowel movements, certain foods (e.g., the high-fiber foods promoted for increased dietary intake in recent years), and poor neuromuscular control of the anal sphincter. Achieving a regular bowel pattern and avoiding flatus-producing foods may relieve this problem,

as may the administration of specific medications intended for this purpose. Sitting upright after meals is helpful in allowing gas to rise to the fundus of the stomach and be expelled.

Discomfort associated with the inability to expel flatus can occur occasionally. Increased activity can provide relief, as may a knee-chest position, if possible. A flatus bag consisting of a rectal tube with an attached plastic bag that prevents the entrance of air into the rectum can be beneficial.

Intestinal Obstruction

Partial or complete impairment of flow of intestinal contents in the large intestines most often occurs due to cancer of the colon; adhesions and hernias are the primary cause of obstructions in the small intestine. Other causes of blockage include diverticulitis, ulcerative colitis, hypokalemia, vascular problems, and paralytic ileus, a mechanical obstruction that can occur following surgery due to nerves being affected by the extended lack of peristaltic activity.

Symptoms vary depending on the site and cause of the obstruction:

■ Small bowel obstruction causes upper and mid-abdominal pain in rhythmic recurring waves related to the small intestine's attempt to push the contents through the obstruction. Vomiting occurs and may bring some relief.

■ Obstructions occurring past the ileum cause abdominal distension so severe that the raised diaphragm can inhibit respirations. Vomiting is more severe than with small bowel blockages and initially is composed of semi-digested food and later contains bile and is more watery.

■ Obstruction of the colon causes lower abdominal pain, altered bowel habits, distension, and a sensation of the need to defecate. Vomiting usually does not occur until late, when the distension reaches the small intestine.

Basic Metabolic Panel = Electrolyte

CONSIDER THIS CASE

Mr. C is a 75-year-old participant in an adult day care program. In interviewing him, you learn that he had a cerebrovascular accident 2 years ago that left him with some right-sided weakness. His medical record indicates that he also has a history of hiatal hernia, depression, hypertension, and osteoarthritis. He is taking antihypertensive, antidepressant, and nonsteroidal anti-inflammatory drugs.

THINK CRITICALLY

■ What threats to gastrointestinal health exist for Mr. C?
■ What measures could be taken to reduce those threats?

The nurse should review symptoms thoroughly and note bowel sounds. Bowel obstruction can cause high-pitched peristaltic rushes to be heard on auscultation. If the obstruction has persisted for a long time or the bowel has been significantly damaged, bowel sounds decrease and eventually are absent.

Timely intervention is essential to prevent bowel strangulation and serious complications. X-rays and blood evaluation typically are done to determine the cause and extent of the problem. Intestinal intubation is the major treatment and often helps to decompress the bowel and allow the obstruction to be broken. If medical management is unsuccessful or if the cause is due to vascular or mechanical obstructions, surgery is required. In addition to supporting the medical or surgical treatment plan, nurses need to promote the patient's comfort and ensure that fluid and electrolyte balance is restored and maintained.

Fecal Impaction

Prevention of constipation aids in avoiding fecal impaction. Observing the frequency and character of bowel movements may aid in detecting the development of an impaction; a bowel elimination record is essential for older people in a hospital or nursing home for identifying alternations in bowel elimination. Indications of a fecal impaction include:

- distended rectum
- abdominal and rectal discomfort
- oozing of fecal material around the impaction, often mistaken as diarrhea
- palpable, hard fecal mass
- fever

Because policies may vary, nurses should review the permissive procedures of their employing agency to ensure that removal of a fecal impaction is an acceptable nursing action. An enema, usually oil retention, may be prescribed to assist in the softening and elimination process. Manual breaking and removal of feces with a lubricated gloved finger will promote removal of the impaction. Sometimes, injecting 50 mL hydrogen peroxide through a rectal tube will cause breakage of the impaction as the hydrogen peroxide foams. Care should be taken not to traumatize or overexert the patient during these procedures.

Fecal Incontinence

Involuntary defecation, fecal incontinence, refers to the inability to voluntarily control the passage of stool. It is most often associated with fecal impaction in older adults who are institutionalized or physically or cognitively impaired. For this reason, the initial step is to assess for the presence of an impaction. If an impaction is not present, the nurse must assess for other causes. Possible causes of bowel incontinence include decreased contractile strength, impaired automaticity of the puborectal and external anal sphincter (secondary to age-related muscle weakness or injury to the pudendal nerve), loss of cortical control, and reduced reservoir capacity (secondary to surgical resection or the presence of a tumor). Proctosigmoidoscopy, proctography, and anorectal manometry are among the diagnostic tests used to evaluate this disorder. The cause of the incontinence dictates the treatment approach, which could include bowel retraining (Nursing Care Plan 21-2), drugs, surgery, or biofeedback.

Acute Appendicitis

Although acute appendicitis does not occur frequently in older persons, it is important to note that it may present with altered signs and symptoms if it does occur. The severe pain that occurs in younger persons may be absent in older adults, whose pain may be minimal and referred. Fever may be minimal, and leukocytosis may be absent. These differences often cause a delayed diagnosis. Prompt surgery will improve the patient's prognosis. Unfortunately, delayed or missed diagnosis and the inability to improve the general status of the patient before this emergency surgery can lead to greater complications and mortality in older persons with appendicitis.

Cancer of the Pancreas *Greatest cause smoking*

Pancreatic cancer is difficult to detect until it has reached an advanced stage. Anorexia, weakness, weight loss, and wasting are generalized symptoms easily attributed to other causes. Dyspepsia, belching, nausea, vomiting, diarrhea, constipation, and obstructive jaundice may occur as well. Fever may or may not be present. The person may experience epigastric pain radiating to the back. This pain is relieved when the person leans forward and is worsened when a recumbent position is assumed. Surgery is performed to treat this problem. Unfortunately, the disease is generally so advanced by the time diagnosis is made that the prognosis is usually poor.

Biliary Tract Disease *— Pain is big symptom RUQ*

Cholelithiasis, the formation or presence of gallstones in the gallbladder, increases with age and affects women more frequently than men. Pain is the primary symptom. Treatment measures include nonsurgical therapies, such as rotary lithotrite treatment and extracorporeal shock wave lithotripsy,

NURSING CARE PLAN 21-2

THE OLDER ADULT WITH FECAL INCONTINENCE

Nursing Diagnosis: Bowel (Fecal) Incontinence

Goal	Nursing Actions
The patient achieves partial or complete restoration of bowel control.	■ Record and evaluate patient's bowel elimination pattern.
	■ Establish consistent time to toilet based on pattern.
	■ Position patient in best physiologic position for bowel movement: sitting with normal posture.
	■ Have patient lean forward or prop feet on stool to increase intra-abdominal pressure.
	■ Instruct patient to bear down and attempt to defecate.
	■ Record results; ensure patient does not develop fecal impaction.
	■ If necessary, stimulate anorectal reflex with glycerin suppository 30 to 45 minutes before scheduled bowel movement.
	■ Supplement toilet activities with exercise and good fluid (minimally 1,500 mL/day) and fiber intake unless contraindicated.

and the standard surgical procedures. Obstruction, inflammation, and infection are potential outcomes of gallstones and require monitoring.

Cancer of the gallbladder primarily affects older persons, especially women. Fortunately, this disease does not occur frequently. Pain in the right upper quadrant, anorexia, nausea, vomiting, weight loss, jaundice, weakness, and constipation are the usual symptoms. Although surgery may be performed, the prognosis for the patient with cancer of the gallbladder is poor.

SUMMARY

Gastrointestinal symptoms, although common, can indicate serious medical problems in older adults and need to be taken seriously. Diagnosis of these problems can be difficult because of atypical symptomatology, self-medication that masks symptoms, and easy confusion with disorders of other systems. Astute questioning and alertness to subtle symptoms during the assessment can help these conditions to be diagnosed and treated early.

BRINGING RESEARCH TO LIFE

PROFILE OF NURSING HOME RESIDENTS WITH DEMENTIA WHO REQUIRE ASSISTANCE WITH MOUTH CARE

Jablonski, R. A., Kolanowski, A. M., & Litaker, M. (2011). Geriatric Nursing, 32(6), 439–446.

Nursing home residents typically have dependencies that require assistance with activities of daily living (ADL). Mouth care is among the activities for which assistance is needed; however, nursing assistants often are not aware of the need or do not understand the various approaches they can use to assist residents. This study examined the profile of nursing home residents with dementia who needed verbal or physical assistance with oral hygiene. The researchers reviewed demographic data extracted from the medical record and used measures from both direct observation and video recordings. Mouth care was scored according to the type of assistance (verbal or physical) that was required. The study found that participants with higher level of cognitive and ADL function required verbal cueing, whereas those who had lower levels of function and were highly passive required provision of mouth care.

This study highlighted an important although often overlooked aspect of the care of persons with dementia. Nurses need to not only promote oral health in older adults who may lack the cognitive or physical capability to engage in oral hygiene independently but also assess what specific type of assistance is required to assure oral hygiene needs are met. Persons with the capacity to perform their own oral hygiene should have this function preserved and encouraged through verbal cueing and positive reinforcement. Persons unable to perform this function should have it competently provided. Good oral hygiene not only promotes nutritional intake and socialization but also aids in preventing complications such as pneumonia and cardiovascular disease. Thus, this relatively basic care has significant implications.

PRACTICE REALITIES

A local church with a membership of more than 2,000 people has initiated a health ministry program and surveyed their members to assess needs. One of the findings of the survey was that less than 10% of the adults older than 60 years of age had ever had a colonoscopy. All of the respondents had insurance that could cover the cost of the procedure so financial hardship wasn't an obstacle.

The church asks you to assist them in developing a campaign to encourage colorectal screening.

What would you envision the components of this program to be?

What strategies could stimulate interest of the church members?

CRITICAL THINKING EXERCISES

1. What age-related changes affect bowel elimination?

2. Describe the changes in dental care that have occurred since today's older adults were children and the way in which this will affect dental health of future generations of older persons.

3. What preventive measures could you recommend to older adults to promote bowel elimination?

4. What are some actions that a nursing home could take to assess the presence of dysphagia and to monitor their residents for new or worsening of dysphagia symptoms on an ongoing basis?

RESOURCES

American Dental Association
http://www.ada.org

Crohn's & Colitis Foundation of America
http://www.ccfa.org

National Institute of Dental and Craniofacial Research
http://www.nidcr.nih.gov

United Ostomy Associations of America, Inc.
http://www.uoa.org

REFERENCES

National Institute of Diabetes and Digestive and Kidney Disease. (2007). What is the risk of esophageal cancer with Barrett's esophagus? Bethesda, MD: National Digestive Diseases Information Center. NIH Publication No. 02-4546. Available online: http://digestive.niddk.nih.gov/ddiseases/pubs/barretts/index.aspx

Peters, J. H. (2003). Barrett's esophagus: Now what? *Annals of Surgery, 237*(3), 299–300.

RECOMMENDED READINGS

Recommended Readings associated with this chapter can be found on the web site that accompanies the book. Visit **http://thepoint.lww.com/Eliopoulos8e** to access the recommended readings and other additional resources associated with this chapter.

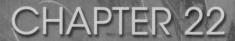

CHAPTER 22

Urinary Elimination

LEARNING OBJECTIVES

After reading this chapter, you should be able to:

1. Describe age-related changes that affect urinary elimination.

2. List measures that promote urinary system health.

3. Outline factors to consider in assessing the urinary system.

4. Describe the incidence, symptoms, and management of selected urinary conditions.

5. Outline a care plan for the patient who is incontinent of urine.

TERMS TO KNOW

Established incontinence: involuntary loss of urine that can have an abrupt or sudden onset and is chronic

Functional incontinence: loss of voluntary control of urine due to disabilities that prevent independent toileting, sedation, inaccessible bathroom, medications that impair cognition, or any other factor interfering with the ability to reach a bathroom

Neurogenic (reflex) incontinence: loss of control of voiding due to inability to sense the urge to void or control urine flow

Nocturia: voiding at least once during the night

(Continued)

Overflow incontinence: involuntary loss of urine due to an excessive accumulation of urine in the bladder

Stress incontinence: involuntary loss of urine when pressure is placed on the pelvic floor (e.g., from laughing, sneezing, or coughing)

Transient incontinence: involuntary loss of urine that is acute in onset and usually reversible

Urgency incontinence: involuntary loss of urine due to irritation or spasms of the bladder wall that cause a sudden elimination of urine

Urinary incontinence: involuntary loss of urine

Urinary problems, although bothersome, frequent, and potentially life-threatening, are disorders not easily discussed by older adults. Some feel embarrassment or believe it is inappropriate to talk about these problems, while other individuals may accept symptoms of urinary disorders as a normal part of aging. These factors often delay early detection and treatment. Untreated, these problems can jeopardize total body health and affect psychosocial well-being. Nurses are in ideal positions to develop close relationships with older patients, which can help patients to more comfortably discuss problems of the urinary tract. By demonstrating sensitivity, acceptance, and understanding of patients' problems, nurses can facilitate prompt, appropriate intervention.

EFFECTS OF AGING ON URINARY ELIMINATION

Age-related changes in the urinary tract may cause various elimination problems. One of the greatest annoyances is urinary frequency, caused by hypertrophy of the bladder muscle and thickening of the bladder, which decreases the ability of the bladder to expand and reduces storage capacity. In addition to frequency during the day, nighttime urinary frequency (nocturia) can be a problem. Often, kidney circulation improves when the person assumes a recumbent position, so voiding may be required a few hours after the individual lies down and at other times during the night. Age-related changes in cortical control of micturition also contribute to nocturia; this problem, along with incontinence (which is not a normal consequence of aging), can be noted in persons with dementia or other conditions affecting the cerebral cortex. Nurses should advise older adults and their caregivers that long-acting diuretics, such as the thiazides, even when administered in the morning, can also cause nocturia. If multiple episodes of nocturia occur, medical evaluation may be warranted to ensure that no urinary tract problem is present.

Inefficient neurologic control of bladder emptying and weaker bladder muscles can promote the retention of large volumes of urine. In women, the most common cause of urinary retention is a fecal impaction; prostatic hypertrophy, present to some degree in most older men, is the primary cause in men. Symptoms of retention include urinary frequency, straining, dribbling, palpable bladder, and the sensation that the bladder has not been emptied. Retention can predispose older individuals to the development of urinary tract infections.

The filtration efficiency of the kidneys decreases with age, affecting the body's ability to eliminate drugs. The nurse should observe the patient for signs of adverse drug reactions resulting from an accumulation of toxic levels of medications. Higher blood urea nitrogen levels may occur due to reduced renal function, causing lethargy, confusion, headache, drowsiness, and other symptoms. Decreased tubular function may cause problems in the concentration of urine; the maximum specific gravity at 80 years of age is 1.024, whereas at younger ages it is 1.032. Reduced ability to concentrate and dilute urine in response to water or sodium excess or depletion occurs . Decreased reabsorption from the filtrate makes a proteinuria of 1.0 usually of no diagnostic significance in older adults. An increase in the renal threshold for glucose is a serious concern, because older individuals can be hyperglycemic without evidence of glycosuria. False-negative results in diabetic urine testing can occur for this reason.

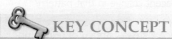

KEY CONCEPT

Changes in the renal threshold for glucose cause older adults to be hyperglycemic without having any evidence of glycosuria.

The inability to control the elimination of urine (i.e., incontinence) is not a normal occurrence with advanced age; however, age-related changes increase the risk of this problem. Incontinence reflects a physical or mental disorder and demands a thorough evaluation. Some stress incontinence may be present, particularly in women who have had multiple pregnancies or in persons who postpone voiding after they sense the urge. More information on incontinence is discussed later in the chapter.

URINARY SYSTEM HEALTH PROMOTION

Basic health practices, which are easily incorporated into the daily schedule, can prevent a variety of urinary tract problems. For instance, a good fluid intake can reduce the amount of bacteria in the bladder. Acidic urine, beneficial in preventing infection, can be enhanced by the intake of vitamin C and foods such as cranberries, prunes, plums, eggs, cheese, fish, and grains. Catheterization significantly increases the risk of infection and should be avoided. Activity can eliminate urinary stasis, and frequent toileting can prevent urinary retention. The nurse can teach older adults specific efforts to enhance voiding and prevent retention, including the following:

- voiding in upright position
- massaging bladder area
- rocking back and forth
- running water
- soaking hands in warm water

The reduced bladder capacity of older adults should be kept in mind when individuals who are unable to ambulate independently are placed in wheelchairs; they will not be able to sit all day without needing to void, and unnecessary incontinence may result if toileting assistance is not provided. Trips and activities should be planned to allow bathroom breaks at frequent intervals.

For older adults experiencing nocturia, nurses can implement measures to promote patients' safety. Because older adults' increased threshold for light perception makes night vision difficult, nocturia could predispose them to accidents when attempting to walk to the bathroom in the dark. Nightlights should be used to improve visibility during trips to the bathroom, and any clutter or environmental hazards that could cause a fall should be removed. Reducing fluids immediately before bedtime may help, although they should not be significantly restricted.

A complete history and examination are essential to pinpoint specific areas that require further investigation; however, obtaining data about urinary function and problems can be difficult. Because older persons may feel embarrassment about discussing these problems, the nurse should set a comfortable tone and display sensitivity during the assessment to facilitate good data collection. Assessment Guide 22-1 describes some of the areas to include in assessing the urinary system; Nursing Diagnosis Table 22-1 outlines some of the nursing diagnoses that could be identified.

ASSESSMENT GUIDE 22-1
URINARY FUNCTION

INTERVIEW

The interview should include a review of function, signs, and symptoms. Ask questions pertaining to the following::

- *Frequency of voiding.* "How often do you need to urinate during the day and during the night? Has there been any recent change in that pattern?"

- *Continence.* "Do you ever lose control of your urine? Do you experience a steady stream of urine dribbling at all times or at certain times? Is urine released when you cough or sneeze? How soon do you need to toilet after getting the urge to void before you lose control?"

- *Retention.* "Do you ever feel that you have not fully emptied your bladder after you have voided? Do you have a sense of fullness in your bladder after voiding?"

- *Pain.* "Does it burn when you void? Do you experience pain in your lower abdomen or anywhere else? Is there any tenderness, discomfort, itching, or pain anywhere along your genital area?"

- *Urine.* "Have you ever seen crystals or particles in your urine? Is your urine ever pink, bloody, or discolored? Is it as clear as tap water or as dark as rusty water? Does your urine ever have a strong odor? If so, what is that odor like?"

- *Medications.* "Do you take any prescription or nonprescription medications? If so, which ones? Do you use any herbal preparations?"

PHYSICAL EXAMINATION

- Inspect, percuss, and palpate the abdomen for bladder fullness, pain, or abnormalities.

- Test women for stress incontinence by doing the following:

  - Have the patient drink at least one full glass of fluid and wait until she senses fullness of the bladder.

  - Instruct the patient to stand. If this is not possible, have her sit as upright as possible.

- Ask the patient to hold a 4 × 4 gauze at her perineum.
- Instruct the patient to cough vigorously.
- The test is negative if no leakage or leakage of only a few drops occurs. If residual urine is a problem, a postvoid residual may be ordered in which the patient is catheterized within 15 minutes of voiding to determine the volume of urine remaining in the bladder.

■ If incontinence is present, refer the patient for a comprehensive evaluation; it can prove useful to maintain a record or have the patient maintain a diary of each occurrence of incontinence and factors associated with these incidents.

EXAMINATION OF URINE SAMPLE

A urinalysis can provide basic information about this system. The specific gravity should range from 1.005 to 1.025, and the pH from 4.6 to 8. Although alkaline urine is most often associated with infections, it can be present if the specimen has been sitting for a few hours. Normally the urine should be free of glucose and protein, but renal changes in the older adult cause proteinuria and glycosuria to be less reliable findings.

Note the color of the urine sample. Examination of the urine's color can yield insight into the presence of health problems. Dark colors can indicate increased urine concentration. Red or rust color usually is associated with the presence of blood. Yellow-brown or green-brown color can be caused by an obstructed bile duct or jaundice. Orange urine results from the presence of bile or the ingestion of phenazopyridine. Very dark brown urine is associated with hematuria or carcinoma.

Also note the urine sample's odor. A faint aromatic odor of the urine is normal. Strong odor can indicate concentrated urine associated with dehydration. Ammonia-like odor can accompany infections.

NURSING DIAGNOSIS

| TABLE 22-1 | Nursing Diagnoses Associated With Aging and Urinary Problems |

Causes or Contributing Factors	Nursing Diagnosis
Ineffective filtration of drugs, wastes from blood due to loss of nephrons and approximately 50% decrease in glomerular filtration rate	Ineffective Health Maintenance
Unreliable urine specimen findings due to decreased resorption of glucose from filtrate and less concentrated urine	Ineffective Health Maintenance
Urgency, frequency, nocturia related to weaker bladder muscles, decreased bladder capacity, slower micturation reflex, and prostate enlargement with age	Impaired Urinary Elimination
Infection, cancer, retention	Acute Pain
Concentrated urine, immobility, more alkaline urine, catheterization	Risk of Infection
Falls on urine puddles	Risk of Injury
Immobility, dementia, weakness	Toileting Self-Care Deficit
Incontinence	Disturbed Body Image
	Impaired Skin Integrity
	Risk of Compromised Human Dignity
Nocturia, retention, dysuria	Disturbed Sleep Pattern
Embarrassment over symptoms, odor, frequency, discomfort	Impaired Social Interaction
Infection, retention, calculi, strictures, incontinence	Impaired Urinary Elimination

SELECTED URINARY CONDITIONS

Urinary Incontinence

A common and bothersome disorder of older adults that requires skillful nursing attention is the involuntary loss of urine, or urinary incontinence. Studies have shown that urinary incontinence is present in 8% to 46% of the community-based older population, at least 50% of the institutionalized older population, as many as 90% of nursing home residents with dementia, and 30% of hospitalized older adults; this problem is twice as prevalent in women as compared with men (Lee, Cigolle, & Blaum, 2009; Ogundele, Silverberg, Sinert, & Guerrero, 2006).

Incontinence can be transient or established. Transient incontinence is acute and reversible and can be caused by infections, delirium, medication reactions, excessive urine production, fecal impaction, mood disorders, or the inability to reach a commode or urinal (e.g., being on bed rest, restrained, and dependent). The onset is abrupt and treatment of the underlying cause can reverse the problem. Established incontinence is chronic and persistent with either an abrupt or gradual onset. The following are various types of established incontinence:

- *Stress incontinence*: caused by weak supporting pelvic muscles. When pressure is placed on the pelvic floor (e.g., from laughing, sneezing, or coughing), urine is involuntarily lost.
- *Urgency incontinence*: caused by urinary tract infection, enlargement of the prostate, diverticulitis, or pelvic or bladder tumors. Irritation or spasms of the bladder wall cause a sudden elimination of urine.
- *Overflow incontinence*: associated with bladder neck obstructions and medications (e.g., adrenergics, anticholinergics, and calcium channel blockers). Bladder muscles fail to contract or periurethral muscles do not relax, leading to an excessive accumulation of urine in the bladder.
- *Neurogenic (reflex) incontinence*: arising from cerebral cortex lesions, multiple sclerosis, and other disturbances along the neural pathway. There is an inability to sense the urge to void or control urine flow.
- *Functional incontinence*: caused by dementia, disabilities that prevent independent toileting, sedation, inaccessible bathroom, medications that impair cognition, or any other factor interfering with the ability to reach a bathroom.
- *Mixed incontinence*: can be due to a combination of these factors.

Nurses should not assume that individuals with incontinence, even long-term incontinence, have necessarily had this problem identified and evaluated. Embarrassment in discussing this disorder or the belief that incontinence is a normal outcome of aging can lead to unreported incontinence. This reinforces the importance of questioning about incontinence during every routine assessment. In addition to referring the patient for a comprehensive medical evaluation, nurses can help identify the cause and determine appropriate treatment measures through the process of nursing assessment. Box 22-1 lists some of the factors to consider in assessing the incontinent individual.

The initial goal for incontinent individuals is to identify the cause of incontinence; thereafter, treatment goals are developed based on the underlying cause. Kegel exercises (Box 22-2), biofeedback, and medications (e.g., estrogen or anticholinergics) may be useful for the improvement of stress incontinence; in some circumstances, surgery may be warranted. Urgency incontinence can be aided by adherence to a toileting schedule, Kegel exercises, biofeedback, and medications (e.g., anticholinergics or adrenergic antagonists). Overflow incontinence may benefit from adherence to a toileting schedule, the use of the Crede method, intermittent catheterization, and medications (e.g., parasympathomimetics). Interventions to assist with functional incontinence could range from improvement of mobility to provision of a bedside commode. Nursing Care Plan 22-1 presents a sample care plan for the older adult with urinary incontinence.

 KEY CONCEPT

Nurses cannot assume that people with long-standing incontinence have received a comprehensive evaluation of this problem. A careful review of the medical history and interview with the patient are important to determine whether diagnostic testing has been done.

Inconsistency on the part of the nursing staff is destructive to the progress of patients and denigrating to their efforts to regain bladder control. Conversely, positive reinforcement and encouragement are most beneficial to the patient during this difficult program. Indwelling catheters should be used only in special circumstances and certainly never for the convenience of staff. Half of patients will develop bacteriuria within the first 24 hours of being catheterized; 35% to 40% of all nosocomial infections are catheter-associated urinary tract

BOX 22-1 **Factors to Assess in the Patient Who is Incontinent of Urine**

- **Medical History:** Note diagnoses that could contribute to incontinence, such as delirium, dementia, cerebrovascular accident, diabetes mellitus, congestive heart failure, urinary tract infection.
- **Medications:** Review all prescription and non-prescription drugs used for those that can affect continence, such as diuretics, antianxiety agents, antipsychotics, antidepressants, sedatives, narcotics, antiparkinsonian agents, antispasmodics, antihistamines, calcium channel blockers, and alpha blockers and alpha-stimulants.
- **Functional Status:** Assess activities of daily living; note impairments; ask about recent changes in function; determine degree of dependency on others for mobility, transfers, toileting.
- **Cognition:** Test cognitive function; review symptoms such as depression, hallucinations; ask about recent changes in mood or intellectual function.
- **Neuromuscular Function in Lower Extremities:** Test patient's ability to keep leg lifted against your efforts to gently push it down; touch various areas along both legs with pin point and smooth side of safety pin to determine patient's ability to detect and differentiate sensations.
- **Urinary Control and Retention:** Test for stress incontinence in women; determine postvoid residual.
- **Bladder Fullness and Pain:** Inspect, percuss, and palpate the bladder for distension, discomfort, and abnormalities.
- **Elimination Pattern:** Record bladder elimination patterns and associated factors for several days; inquire about changes to elimination pattern; note frequency, pattern, amount, and relationship to other factors.
- **Fecal Impaction:** Palpate the rectum for the presence of fecal impaction (unless contraindicated).
- **Symptoms:** Ask about urgency, burning, vaginal itching, pain, pressure in bladder area, fever.
- **Diet:** Assess intake of potential bladder irritants: caffeine, alcohol, citrus fruits/juices, tomatoes, spicy foods, artificial sweeteners.
- **Reactions to Incontinence:** Explore how incontinence has affected activities, lifestyle, self-concept; determine patient's appraisal of problem.

BOX 22-2 **Kegel Exercises**

Kegel exercises are an approach to strengthening the pelvic floor muscles, which can lead to an improvement in control over urine incontinence. Nurses can give the following basic instructions to women.

FIND THE MUSCLES INVOLVED IN THE EXERCISES

You first need to identify the pelvic floor muscles that are involved in the exercises. To do this, stop the flow of urine while voiding and notice how the muscles are tightening in the vaginal area and the pelvic floor is lifting. Another approach is to insert a finger in your vagina and tighten your muscles around your finger. Notice the vagina tightening and the pelvic floor lifting. Stop and start the urinary flow several times until you identify the muscles and understand the muscle movements.

PRACTICE THE EXERCISES

Void prior to starting the exercises. Get in a sitting or standing position and tighten the pelvic floor muscles.

Be sure not to tighten the muscles of the abdomen, buttocks, or thighs but just the pelvic muscles. At first, try to keep the muscles tightened for about 5 seconds, several times in a row. Gradually increase the time the muscles are tightened to 10 seconds with about 10 seconds of muscle relaxation in between flexing.

PERFORM THE EXERCISES

Once you are able to hold the muscles tight for 10 seconds, perform a set of 10 exercises in a row. Repeat these several times throughout the day, every day. Results should be noted in 2 to 3 months. After improvement in incontinence is obtained, it is helpful to continue doing Kegel exercises to maintain the muscle strength. Even if the incontinence is not completely eliminated, its progression can be slowed by doing these exercises.

CONSIDER THIS CASE

Eighty-six-year-old Mr. E lives with his daughter and her family. His bedroom is on the first floor of their two-story home with a bathroom a short distance from his room. The family members pass by Mr. E's bedroom on a regular basis and have noticed a strong urine odor coming from the room. Mr. E has no cognitive impairments, fulfills his activities of daily living independently, and, as has always been his pattern, conducts himself in a proper manner. Mr. E has never mentioned any problem with elimination and, because he launders his own linens and takes care of his own room, the family cannot determine if he is wetting the bed.

THINK CRITICALLY

- What are some of the challenges of this situation?
- What advice could you offer the family in approaching this issue with Mr. E?

NURSING CARE PLAN 22-1

THE OLDER ADULT WITH URINARY INCONTINENCE

Nursing Diagnosis: Impaired Urinary Elimination

Goal	Nursing Actions
The patient achieves partial or complete restoration of bladder control	■ Ensure that a comprehensive evaluation has been conducted to identify cause of incontinence and potential for regained bladder control.
The patient effectively contains expelled urine	■ Identify individual voiding pattern: frequency, sensation of signal to void, time between signal being received and inability to hold urine, amount voided, and symptoms.
	■ If potential for bladder control exists, initiate bladder retraining program.
	■ Monitor intake and output; estimate urine lost on clothing and linens (1 inch diameter is approximately equal to 10 mL of urine).
	■ Ensure that bathroom is easily accessible; provide bedside commode or bedpan if needed.
	■ Offer at least 1,500 mL liquids daily unless contraindicated.
	■ Encourage patient to lean forward while sitting on commode and to press on lower abdomen (Crede method) to promote optimal bladder emptying.
	■ Teach patient methods to stimulate voiding reflex: pouring warm water over perineum, stroking abdomen and inner thigh, drinking water while sitting on commode.
	■ Instruct female patient in Kegel exercises.
	■ Provide urinary sheaths, condom catheters, adult briefs, sanitary pads, or incontinence pants to contain urine.
	■ Avoid indwelling catheter use.
	■ When incontinent episodes occur, discuss cause with patient in a matter-of-fact manner.
	■ Modify environment to accommodate incontinence (e.g., protect mattress and furniture, provide good ventilation, use room deodorizer, keep bathroom well-lighted).

Nursing Diagnosis: Risk of Impaired Skin Integrity related to incontinence

Goal	Nursing Actions
The patient maintains skin integrity.	■ Check patient for wetness every 2 hours; change clothing and linen as necessary.
The patient stays dry and odor free	■ Thoroughly cleanse and dry patient's skin after incontinent episodes.
	■ Assess skin status daily.

Nursing Diagnosis: Risk of Injury related to incontinence

Goal	Nursing Actions
The patient is free from falls related to escaped urine	■ Provide an effective containment device for urine (e.g., adult brief, condom catheter).
	■ Check patient's environment regularly for urine on floor.
	■ Clean urine from floor promptly.

Nursing Diagnosis: Chronic Low Self-Esteem related to incontinence

Goal	Nursing Actions
The patient restores or maintains desired roles and functions	■ Encourage patient to express feelings.
The patient develops or maintains positive view of self	■ Provide realistic explanations as to causes, management, and prognosis of patient's type of incontinence.
	■ Assist patient in dressing In street clothes.
	■ Avoid discussing patient's incontinence in the presence of visitors and other patients.
	■ Ensure that caregivers and family members treat patient with dignity.

infections (Foxman, 2003). In addition, the risk of developing urinary calculi is high when indwelling catheters are present. (Urinary tract infections are discussed in Chapter 30.)

Bladder Cancer

The incidence of bladder cancer increases with age. According to the American Cancer Society (2012), 90% of the cases of bladder cancer are in people over age 55 years and older men have three times the rate of older women. Chronic irritation of the bladder, exposure to dyes, and cigarette smoking—all avoidable factors—are among the risk factors associated with bladder tumors. Some of the symptoms resemble those of a bladder infection, such as frequency, urgency, and dysuria. A painless hematuria is the primary sign and characterizes cancer of the bladder. Standard diagnostic measures for this disease are used with the aged patient, including cystoscopic examination.

Treatment for bladder cancer can include surgery, radiation, immunotherapy, or chemotherapy, depending on the extent and location of the lesion. The nurse should use the nursing measures described in medical-surgical nursing literature. Observation for signs indicating metastasis, such as pelvic or back pain, is part of the nursing care for patients with bladder cancer.

Renal Calculi

Renal calculi occur most frequently in middle-aged adults. In older adults, the formation of stones can result from immobilization, infection, changes in the pH or concentration of urine, chronic diarrhea, dehydration, excessive elimination of uric acid, and hypercalcemia. Pain, hematuria, and symptoms of urinary tract infection are associated with this problem, and gastrointestinal upset may also occur. Standard diagnostic and treatment measures are used for the aged, and the nurse can assist by preventing urinary stasis, providing ample fluids, and facilitating prompt treatment of urinary tract infections.

Glomerulonephritis

Most frequently, chronic glomerulonephritis already exists in older persons who develop an acute condition. The symptoms of this disease may be so subtle and nonspecific that they are initially unnoticed. Clinical manifestations include fever, fatigue, nausea, vomiting, anorexia, abdominal pain, anemia, edema, arthralgias, elevated blood pressure, and an increased sedimentation rate. Oliguria may occur, as can moderate proteinuria and hematuria. Headache, convulsions, paralysis, aphasia, coma, and an altered mental status may be consequences of cerebral edema associated with this disease.

Diagnostic and treatment measures do not differ significantly from those used for the young. Antibiotics, a restricted sodium and protein diet, and close attention to fluid intake and output are basic parts of the treatment plan. If older adults are receiving digitalis, diuretics, or antihypertensive drugs, close observation for cumulative toxic effects resulting from compromised kidney function must

be maintained. The patient should be evaluated periodically after the acute illness is resolved for exacerbations of chronic glomerulonephritis and signs of renal failure.

GENERAL NURSING CONSIDERATIONS FOR URINARY CONDITIONS

Nurses need sensitivity in dealing with patients' urinary problems. In addition to being areas that are considered taboo for discussion for some persons, these disorders may raise fears and anxieties that tales of becoming incontinent in old age perhaps are valid. Realistic explanations and a committed effort to correcting these disorders are vital. All levels of staff need to remember the importance of discretion and dignity in managing these problems. Staff members should not check to see if a patient's pants are wet in front of others, allow someone to sit on a bedside commode in a hallway, bring in a group of students without the patient's permission to observe a catheterization, or scold the patient for having an accident in bed. Every effort should be made to minimize embarrassment and promote a positive self-concept.

BRINGING RESEARCH TO LIFE

URINARY CATHETERS IN THE EMERGENCY DEPARTMENT: VERY ELDERLY WOMEN ARE AT HIGH RISK FOR UNNECESSARY UTILIZATION

Fakih, M. G., Shemes, S. P., Pena, M. E., Dyc, N., Rey, J. E., Szpunar, S. M., & Saravolatz, L. D. (2010). American Journal of Infection Control, 38(9), 683–688.

In this study, the researchers looked at urinary catheterization placement in persons admitted to an emergency department during a 12-week period. Patients who had catheters inserted without an indication were found to be older, with a mean age of 71.3 years. Women were 1.9 times more likely than men to have a catheter inserted, and women aged ≥80 years were 2.9 times more likely than those aged ≤50 years to have a urinary catheter placed without an indication.

The researchers note that urinary tract infections account for more than one third of all hospital-acquired infections and the inappropriate use of urinary catheters contributes to this problem. As more than half of hospital admissions come through the emergency department, this is a significant area of concern.

This study emphasizes the need for gerontological nurses to assure colleagues in all specialty areas not to assume advanced age alone warrants an intervention like urinary catheter insertion and to advocate for older adults by assuring catheters are not inserted without sound justification, using evidence-based criteria. Unnecessary catheterization not only poses risk of infections, to which older adults are highly susceptible, but also has psychosocial implications. This study also demonstrates how essential gerontological nursing knowledge is to nurses in virtually every specialty area; even nurses working in highly acute areas like an emergency department practice gerontological nursing to some degree.

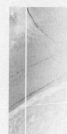

PRACTICE REALITIES

Nurse Adams works part-time in a 25-bed assisted living community. Typically, she works the evening shift but has agreed to relieve a coworker on the day shift for the weekend. On both days, Nurse Adams notices a significant urine odor when she enters the building in the morning. After the residents bathe and dress and their linens are changed, the odor is gone for the remainder of the shift. In reviewing the residents' records, she finds that only two residents wear adult incontinence briefs for occasional urinary incontinence. Based on the strong odor she detected, Nurse Adams suspects there are additional residents with incontinence problems that are more than occasional.

What steps can Nurse Adams take to address her suspicion?

CRITICAL THINKING EXERCISES

1. What factors should be reviewed when assessing urinary incontinence, and what barriers could arise in reviewing them and obtaining accurate answers from older adults?
2. What can be done to reduce each of the major causes of urinary incontinence in older adults?
3. What actions could be taken to promote a positive self-concept of an individual with urinary incontinence?
4. Identify resources in your community to assist patients with incontinence or cancer of the urinary system.

RESOURCES

American Urologic Association
http://www.urologyhealth.org

National Association for Continence
http://www.nafc.org

National Institute of Diabetes and Digestive and Kidney Diseases, National Kidney and Urologic Diseases Information Clearinghouse
http://www.kidney.niddk.nih.gov

Simon Foundation for Continence
http://www.simonfoundation.org

Society of Urologic Nurses and Associates
http://www.suna.org

REFERENCES

American Cancer Society. (2012). *What are the key statistics for bladder cancer? Cancer reference information.* Retrieved June 1, 2012 from http://www.cancer.gov/aboutnci/servingpeople/snapshots/bladder.pdf

Foxman, B. (2003). Epidemiology of urinary tract infections: Incidence, morbidity, and economic costs. *Disease a Month, 49*(2), 53–70.

Lee, P. G., Cigolle, C., & Blaum, C. (2009). The co-occurrence of chronic diseases and geriatric syndromes: The health and retirement study. *Journal of the American Geriatrics Society, 57*(3), 511–516.

Ogundele, O., Silverberg, M. A., Sinert, R., & Guerrero, P. (2006). *Urinary incontinence.* eMedicine. Retrieved August 15, 2007 from http://www.emedicine.com/emerg/topic/91.htm

RECOMMENDED READINGS

Recommended Readings associated with this chapter can be found on the web site that accompanies the book. Visit **http://thepoint.lww.com/Eliopoulos8e** to access the recommended readings and other additional resources associated with this chapter.

Reproductive System Health

LEARNING OBJECTIVES

After reading this chapter, you should be able to:

1. List changes to the male and female reproductive systems that occur with age.

2. Describe measures to promote reproductive system health in older adults.

3. Outline factors to consider in assessing reproductive system health in older adults.

4. Describe the symptoms and management of selected disorders of the reproductive system.

5. Outline care plan measures for the patient who has had prostate surgery.

TERMS TO KNOW

Benign prostatic hyperplasia: nonmalignant enlargement of the prostate gland that commonly occurs with age

Dyspareunia: painful intercourse

Erectile dysfunction: impotence; problems in achieving or sustaining an erection for intercourse

As with urinary problems discussed in the last chapter, reproductive system problems may be difficult topics for older adults to discuss. However, it is important for older adults to consider their reproductive systems when thinking of their overall health. In addition to preventing and detecting serious problems such as cancer and sexually transmitted diseases, understanding health practices related to the reproductive system can promote satisfying sexual activity for older persons, yielding multiple benefits. Gerontological nurses can play an important role in educating older adults about changes that occur with aging and about important health promotion measures to prevent or identify potentially serious reproductive system problems.

EFFECTS OF AGING ON THE REPRODUCTIVE SYSTEM

There are several changes in the female reproductive system that increase the risk of uncomfortable conditions and interfere with satisfying sexual experiences. Hormonal changes cause the vulva to atrophy. There is a flattening of the labia and loss of subcutaneous fat and hair. The vaginal epithelium becomes thin and the vaginal environment is drier and more alkaline; these changes can cause intercourse to be uncomfortable for older women, although orgasms and satisfying sexual experiences are normally possible. The cervix, uterus, fallopian tubes, and ovaries atrophy. The uterus and ovaries also decrease in size; therefore, they may not be palpable during the physical examination. The endometrium continues to respond to hormonal stimulation. The fallopian tubes also undergo shortening and straightening. The breasts sag and are less firm with age due to the replacement of mammary glands by fat tissue after menopause. Some retraction of the nipples may occur as a result of shrinkage and fibrotic changes. Firm linear strands may develop on the breasts from fibrosis and calcification of the terminal ducts.

The genitalia of men undergo changes, as well. There is a reduction in sperm count related to the seminal vesicles having a thinner epithelium, replacement of muscle tissue with connective tissue, and less capacity to retain fluids. Structural changes in the seminiferous tubules include increased fibrosis, thinning of the epithelium, thickening of the basement membrane, and narrowing of the lumen.

There is atrophy of the testes and a reduction in the testicular mass. Fluid ejaculated usually remains the same although it contains lesser amounts of living sperm. Testosterone stays the same or decreases only slightly. More time is required for an erection to be achieved and it is more easily lost than in younger men. Most older men experience an enlargement of the prostate gland as some of the prostate tissue is replaced with a fibrotic tissue. Although most prostatic enlargement is benign, there is an increased risk of malignancy with age.

REPRODUCTIVE SYSTEM HEALTH PROMOTION

An important way that nurses can promote reproductive system health is to stress the value of regular examinations of this system. An annual gynecologic examination, including a Pap smear, is essential for the older woman; she should also be knowledgeable about self-examination of the breasts. Men with prostatic hypertrophy should be examined at least every 6 months to ensure that a malignancy has not developed. Routine prostate-specific antigen (PSA) testing in men with no history of prostate cancer is not recommended. The nurse should also ensure that older men know how to perform testicular self-examination. Finally, a complete history and physical examination are essential to pinpoint specific areas that require further investigation (Assessment Guide 23-1). Nursing Diagnosis Table 23-1 lists diagnoses associated with reproductive system problems that the nurse may identify.

ASSESSMENT GUIDE 23-1
REPRODUCTIVE SYSTEM HEALTH

INTERVIEW

The interview should include a review of function, signs, and symptoms. Ask questions pertaining to the following:

- *Pain.* "Do you experience pain in your lower abdomen or anywhere else? Is there any tenderness, discomfort, itching, or pain anywhere along your genital area? Do you experience pain with intercourse?"

- *Discharge.* "Do you ever have secretions, blood, or other discharge from your genitals?"

- *Sexual dysfunction.* "Can you obtain an erection and hold it through intercourse? What are your ejaculations like? Is your vagina sensitive or overly dry during intercourse? Do you feel extra pressure or that your partner's penis is hitting a blockage during inter-

course? Can you have satisfying orgasms? Has there been any change in your sexual pattern?"

PHYSICAL EXAMINATION

- Inspect the genitalia for lesions, sores, breaks, or masses. Note the bleeding, discharges, odors, and other abnormalities.

- If the female patient has not had a gynecologic examination or mammogram within the past year, refer her accordingly.

- For females, palpate the breasts for masses.

- Review the procedure for self-examination of the breasts with female patients and provide instruction if the patient is unskilled in this technique.

NURSING DIAGNOSIS

TABLE 23-1	Nursing Diagnosis Associated With Reproductive System Problems

Causes or Contributing Factors	Nursing Diagnosis
Sexual dysfunction, pain, embarrassment over symptoms or treatments	Anxiety
Infection, cancer	Acute Pain
More alkaline and fragile vaginal canal, prostatic hypertrophy	Risk for Infection
Infection, pain, altered structures, embarrassment	Sexual Dysfunction
Sexual dysfunction	Disturbed Body Image
Vaginitis	Impaired Skin Integrity
Prostatic enlargement, vaginitis	Impaired Urinary Elimination
	Acute Pain

Chapter 12 discusses nursing considerations in fostering sexual function and expression in older adults.

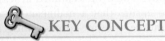

KEY CONCEPT

It is important to ensure that older women know how to perform breast self-examination and that older men know how to perform testicular self-examination.

SELECTED REPRODUCTIVE SYSTEM CONDITIONS

Problems of the Female Reproductive System

Infections and Tumors of the Vulva

Age-related changes to the vulva cause it to be more fragile and more easily susceptible to irritation and infection. Vulvar problems in the aged may reflect serious disease processes such as diabetes, hepatitis, leukemia, and pernicious anemia. Senile vulvitis is the term used to describe vulvar infection associated with hypertrophy or atrophy. Incontinence and poor hygienic practices can also be underlying causes of vulvitis. Pruritus is the primary symptom associated with vulvitis. Patients who are confused and noncommunicative may display restlessness and touch themselves at the genitals; the nurse may discover that patients are suffering from irritation and thickening of the vulvar tissue as a result of scratching. Initially, treatment aims to find and manage any underlying cause. Good nutritional status helps improve the condition, as does special attention to cleanliness. Sitz baths and local applications of saline compresses or steroid creams may be included in the treatment plan. Special attention is required to keep the incontinent patient clean and dry as much as possible.

CONSIDER THIS CASE

Mr. and Mrs. C have been married for 50 years and, with their children all married, they live alone. They shared a healthy sex life, but over the years the frequency of intercourse and sexual play has steadily declined. Recently, Mr. C has heard some of his friends discussing their renewed sexual activity since taking drugs for their erectile dysfunction. These conversations have caused Mr. C to desire sex more frequently; however, his sexual advances have been rejected by his wife who not only shows no interest, but ridicules him for his. Their differences in sexual desires are leading to many arguments between the couple. During her visit for a routine gynecological examination, Mrs. C tells you that her husband "has started to act like a sex maniac and is making a fool of himself by not acting his age."

THINK CRITICALLY

- What are the possible factors causing each of the spouse's reactions?
- How would you respond to Mrs. C?

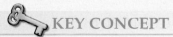

KEY CONCEPT

Age-related changes cause the vulva to be more fragile and more easily susceptible to irritation and infection.

Although pruritus commonly occurs with vulvitis, it may be a symptom of a vulvar tumor. Pain and irritation may also be associated with this problem. Any mass or lesion in this area should receive prompt attention and be biopsied. The clitoris is commonly the site of a vulvar malignancy. Cancer of the vulva, the fourth most common gynecologic malignancy in later life, may be manifested by large, painful, and foul-smelling fungating or ulcerating tumors. The adjacent tissues may also be affected. A radical vulvectomy is usually the treatment of choice and tends to be well tolerated by the older woman. Less commonly used is radiation therapy, which is not tolerated as well as surgery. Counseling regarding self-care practices, body image, and sexual activity should be provided. Early treatment, before metastasis to inguinal lymph nodes, improves prognosis.

Atrophic Vaginitis

The postmenopausal woman experiences a variety of changes that affect the vaginal canal, including reduction in collagen and adipose tissue, shortening and narrowing of the vaginal canal, decreased elasticity, less vaginal lubrication, and a more alkaline vaginal pH as a result of lower estrogen levels. The increased fragility of the fragile vagina in postmenopausal women causes it to be more easily irritated, which heightens the risk of vaginitis. Itching, foul-smelling discharge, and postcoital bleeding are symptoms associated with vaginal infection. Treatment could include topical estrogen creams and estrogen replacement therapy. Nurses should advise the older woman to avoid douches and the use of perfumed soaps and sprays to the genitalia, wear cotton underwear, keep the genital area clean and dry, and use lubricants (e.g., K-Y jelly, vitamin E oil, and aloe vera gel) when engaging in intercourse. (Chapter 30 offers additional discussion of vaginitis.)

Cancer of the Vagina

Cancer of the vagina is rare in older women; it results more frequently from metastasis than from the vaginal area as a primary site. All vaginal ulcers and masses detected in older women should be viewed with suspicion of malignancy and be biopsied. Because chronic irritation can predispose women to vaginal cancer, those who have chronic vaginitis or who wear a pessary should obtain frequent Pap smears. Treatment is similar to that used for younger women and may consist of irradiation, topical chemotherapeutic agents, or surgery, depending on the extent of the carcinoma.

Problems of the Cervix

With age, the cervix becomes smaller, and the endocervical epithelium atrophies. Occasionally, the endocervical glands can seal over, causing the formation of nabothian cysts. As secretions associated with these cysts accumulate, fever and a palpable tender mass may be evident. It is important, therefore, for the older woman to receive regular gynecologic examinations to check the patency of the cervix.

Cancer of the Cervix

The incidence of cervical cancer peaks in the fifth and sixth decades of life and thereafter declines. Although less than 25% of all diagnosed cases of cervical cancer are in older women, over 40% of cervical cancer deaths occur among this group. Despite the fact that most endocervical polyps are benign in older women, they should be viewed with suspicion until biopsy confirms such a diagnosis. Vaginal bleeding and leukorrhea are signs of cervical cancer in aged women. Pain does not usually occur. As the disease progresses, the patient can develop urinary retention or incontinence, fecal incontinence, and uremia. Treatment of cervical cancer can include radium or surgery. The American Cancer Society (2007) suggests annual Pap tests until age 70; for women over 70 years of age who have had at least three normal Pap tests and no abnormal Pap tests in the last 10 years, Pap smears can be done every 2 to 3 years or as recommended by their health care provider.

Cancer of the Endometrium

Although it mainly affects older women at an average age of 55 to 65 years, cancer of the endometrium is not uncommon in the older woman. It is of higher incidence in obese, diabetic, and hypertensive women. Any postmenopausal bleeding should give rise immediately to suspicion of this disease. Dilation and curettage are usually done to confirm the diagnosis because not all cases can be detected by Pap smears alone. Treatment consists of surgery, irradiation, or a combination of both. Early treatment can prevent metastasis to the vagina and cervix. Endometrial polyps can also cause bleeding and should receive serious attention because they could be indicative of early cancer.

Cancer of the Ovaries

Ovarian cancer, which increases in incidence with age, is responsible for only 5% of malignant disease in older women, although it is the leading cause of death from gynecologic malignancies. Early symptoms are nonspecific and can be confused with gastrointestinal discomfort. As this disease progresses, the clinical manifestations include bleeding, ascites, and the presence of multiple masses. Treatment may consist of surgery or irradiation. Benign ovarian tumors commonly occur in older women, and surgery is usually required to differentiate them from malignant ones.

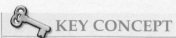

> ### KEY CONCEPT
>
> Although ovarian cancer is less common than endometrial or cervical cancer, it is more deadly when it does occur.

perineum (pelvic floor)

Perineal Herniation :

As a result of the stretching and tearing of muscles during childbirth and of the muscle weakness associated with advanced age, perineal herniation is a common problem among older women. Cystocele, rectocele, and prolapse of the uterus are the types most likely to occur. Associated with this problem are lower back pain, pelvic heaviness, and a pulling sensation. Urinary and fecal incontinence, retention, and constipation may also occur. Sometimes the woman is able to feel pressure or palpate a mass in her vagina. These herniations can make intercourse difficult and uncomfortable. Although rectoceles do not tend to worsen with age, the opposite is true for cystoceles, which will cause increased problems with time. Surgical repair is the treatment of choice and can be successful in relieving these problems.

prolapse of the wall between the rectum and vagina

protrusion of the bladder into the vagina

Dyspareunia : Painful intercourse

Dyspareunia is a common problem among older women that accompanies hormonal changes. Nulliparous women experience this problem more frequently than women who have had children. Because vulvitis, vaginitis, and other gynecologic problems can contribute to dyspareunia, a thorough gynecologic examination is important, and any lesions or infections should be corrected to alleviate the problem. All efforts should be made to help the older woman achieve a satisfactory sexual life. (Chapter 12 presents a more detailed discussion of problems affecting sexual intimacy.)

> ### KEY CONCEPT
>
> Dyspareunia is a common, although not necessarily normal, finding in older women.

Cancer of the Breast

Decreased fat tissue and atrophy in older women's breasts can cause tumors, possibly present for many years, to become more evident. Because breast cancer is the second leading cause of cancer deaths for women, nurses should encourage women to have regular breast examinations. Unfortunately, although the incidence of breast cancer increases with age, the older the woman is, the less likely she is to perform self-examination of breasts or receive yearly mammograms or breast examinations by a health care professional. Diagnostic and treatment measures for women with breast cancer are the same at any age. Annual mammograms are recommended for women starting at age 40, and then at age 75, every 2 to 3 years unless otherwise recommended by a health care provider.

> ### KEY CONCEPT
>
> Although the incidence of breast cancer rises with age, older women are the least likely group to receive mammograms and breast examinations by a professional or to perform self-examinations of their breasts.

Problems of the Male Reproductive System

Erectile Dysfunction

Erectile dysfunction, the inability to achieve and sustain an erection for intercourse, is a problem affecting most men over 70 years of age. Although incidence rates increase with age, erectile dysfunction is not a normal outcome of aging, but rather due to causes such as alcoholism, diabetes, dyslipidemia, hypertension, hypogonadism, multiple sclerosis, renal failure, spinal cord injury, thyroid conditions, and psychological factors. Anticholinergics, antidepressants, antihypertensives, digoxin, sedatives, and tranquilizers are among the medications commonly used among older adults that can cause erectile dysfunction.

A variety of treatments can be used to address erectile dysfunction, including oral erectile agents (e.g., sildenafil citrate [Viagra], vardenafil HCl

[Levitra], and tadalafil [Cialis]), drugs injected into the penis, penile implants, and vacuum pump devices. Some of the erectile drugs can have side effects that may contraindicate their use for some individuals; therefore, careful risk evaluation is essential before these types of drugs are prescribed.

Benign Prostatic Hyperplasia

Most older men have some degree of benign prostatic hyperplasia, which causes approximately one in four of them to have dysuria. Symptoms of this problem progress slowly but continuously, as the enlarging prostate puts pressure on the urethra; they begin with hesitancy, decreased force of urinary stream, frequency, and nocturia as a result of obstruction of the vesical neck and compression of the urethra that causes a compensatory hypertrophy of the detrusor muscle and subsequent outlet obstruction. Dribbling, poor control, overflow incontinence, and bleeding may occur. As the hyperplasia progresses, the bladder wall loses its elasticity and becomes thinner, leading to urinary retention and an increased risk of urinary infection. Unfortunately, some men are reluctant or embarrassed to seek prompt medical attention and may develop kidney damage by the time symptoms are severe enough to motivate them to be evaluated.

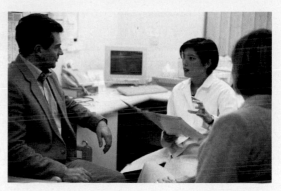

FIGURE 23-1 ■ Men benefit from realistic explanations of the effects of treatments on sexual function.

Treatment can include prostatic massage, the use of urinary antiseptics and, if possible, the avoidance of diuretics, anticholinergics, and antiarrhythmic agents. The most common prostatectomy approach used for older men with prostatism is transurethral surgery. The patient should be reassured that this surgery will not necessarily result in impotence. Realistic explanations are needed, however, so the patient understands that this surgery will not cause a sudden rejuvenation of sexual performance (Fig. 23-1). Nursing Care Plan 23-1 describes care for the older adult recovering from prostate surgery. (Prostatitis is discussed in Chapter 30.)

NURSING CARE PLAN 23-1

THE OLDER ADULT RECOVERING FROM PROSTATE SURGERY

Nursing Diagnosis: Risk for Injury and Infection related to surgery

Goal	Nursing Actions
The patient is free from injury; is free from infection	■ Advise the patient to avoid strenuous activities for 3 to 4 weeks.
	■ Advise the patient to prevent constipation. Recommend dietary adjustments as needed; advise the patient to consult with the physician regarding the use of stool softener if bowel movements are strained or irregular.
	■ Teach the patient to avoid Valsalva maneuver.
	■ Encourage high fluid intake unless contraindicated.
	■ Teach the patient to observe for and promptly report signs of complications, including bright red blood in urine, elevated temperature, severe pain, weakness.

(Continues)

NURSING CARE PLAN 23-1 (Continued)

Nursing Diagnoses: (1) Sexual Dysfunction related to surgery; (2) Deficient Knowledge related to the effect of surgery on sexual function

Goal	Nursing Actions
The patient expresses realistic understanding of the effect of surgery on sexual function; resumes satisfying sexual relationship	■ Consult with the physician regarding sexual restrictions; discuss with the patient. (Typically, sexual intercourse is avoided for about 1 month postoperatively, after which time the patient can usually return to previous sexual function. It is not unusual for complete return of sexual function to take as long as 1 year.)
	■ Assess the patient's understanding of the impact of surgery on sexual function; clarify misinformation as needed.
	■ Listen to the patient's concerns and provide support.
	■ Discuss anticipated return of sexual function with the patient's wife, if acceptable to the patient.
	■ Prepare the patient for possibility of retrograde ejaculation (dry climax), which will make urine appear milky.
	■ Discuss with the couple the potential for anxiety and other psychological factors related to illness and surgery to interfere with sexual function.
	■ Encourage the couple to share other forms of intimacy until intercourse can be resumed.

(handwritten margin note: When semen enters bladder instead of emerging through the penis during orgasm)

Nursing Diagnosis: Risk for Urinary Incontinence: Stress or Urge related to catheter removal

Goal	Nursing Actions
The patient resumes urinary continence	■ Assess bladder control after urinary catheter is removed.
	■ If dribbling of urine occurs, advise the patient that this is common and will subside and instruct the patient in perineal exercises.

Cancer of the Prostate

Prostatic cancer increases in incidence with age. In fact, more than half of men over 70 years of age have histologic evidence of prostate cancer, although less than 3% will die from the disease (National Cancer Institute, 2012). Often, this disease can be asymptomatic; however, most prostatic cancers can be detected by digital rectal examination, which emphasizes the importance of regular physical examinations. Benign hypertrophy should be followed closely because it is thought to be associated with prostatic cancer, the symptoms of which can be similar. Symptoms such as back pain, anemia, weakness, and weight loss can develop as a result of metastasis. A PSA test assists with the diagnosis, which is confirmed through biopsy.

If metastasis has not occurred, treatment may consist of monitoring, irradiation, or a radical prostatectomy; the latter procedure will result in impotency. Estrogens may be used to prevent tumor dissemination. Palliative treatment, used if the cancer has metastasized, includes irradiation, transurethral surgery, orchiectomy, and estrogens. General principles associated with these therapeutic measures are applicable to the aged patient. Many men are able to continue sexual performance after orchiectomy and during estrogen therapy; the physician should be consulted for specific advice concerning the expected outcomes for individual patients.

Tumors of the Penis, Testes, and Scrotum

Cancer of the penis is rare and appears as a painless lesion or wartlike growth on the prepuce or glans. The resemblance of this growth to a chancre can cause a misdiagnosis or reluctance on the part of the patient to seek treatment. A biopsy should be done for any penile lesion. Treatment may consist of irradiation and local excision for small lesions and partial or total penile amputation for extensive lesions.

Testicular tumors are uncommon in older people but are usually malignant when they do occur; testicular enlargement and pain and enlargement of the breasts are suspicious symptoms. Chemotherapy, irradiation, and orchiectomy are among the treatment measures. As part of the assessment, nurses should ascertain the patient's knowledge of testicular self-examination and provide education on this procedure if necessary; the American Cancer Society can provide educational materials to use for this instruction.

Scrotal masses, usually benign, can result from conditions such as hydrocele, spermatocele, varicocele, and hernia. Symptoms and treatment depend on the underlying cause and are the same as for younger men. As with any reproductive system problem, counseling regarding self-care practices, body image, and sexual activity is important.

SUMMARY

The health of the reproductive system has an impact on total body health. Conditions of the reproductive system can be related to undiagnosed disease processes that require attention, such as diabetes and infections. The close relationship and trust that patients often have with nurses can enable patients to more comfortably share concerns and symptoms related to the reproductive system more openly with nurses than with other members of the health care team. Nurses should include a review of the reproductive system in their assessments of patients and assure abnormal findings and symptoms are referred for evaluation and treatment.

BRINGING RESEARCH TO LIFE

SCREENING FOR PROSTATE CANCER: U.S. PREVENTIVE SERVICES TASK FORCE RECOMMENDATIONS STATEMENT

Moyer, V. A.; on behalf of the U. S. Preventive Services Task Force. (2012). Annals of Internal Medicine, 156(10), 812–825; also available on U. S. Preventive Services Task Force website, http://www.uspreventiveservicestaskforce.org/uspstf/uspsprca.htm..

As a result of reviewing data from the U.S. Prostate, Lung, Colorectal, and Ovarian Cancer Screening Trial and the European Randomized Study of Screening for Prostate Cancer, the U.S. Preventive Services Task Force downgraded its assessment of prostate-specific antigen (PSA)–based prostate cancer screening. The U.S. trial did not demonstrate any reduction in prostate cancer deaths as a result of the tests. The European trial found a reduction in prostate cancer deaths of approximately 1 death in 1,000 men screened.

Nearly 90% of the men who were detected to have prostate cancer through PSA testing undergo treatment. Of these, up to 5 in 1,000 die within 1 month of surgery and between 10 and 70 will have serious complications. Overall, the harm resulting from diagnostic and treatment procedures was found to be greater than the benefit.

This new evidence and change in recommendations about PSA testing demonstrate the need for nurses to keep abreast of new research findings and assure their practice is based on current evidence and best practices.

PRACTICE REALITIES

Mr. and Mrs. Noonan, both 66 years old, have enjoyed healthy, satisfying sexual activity throughout their 20 years of marriage. Mrs. Noonan had a mastectomy for breast cancer 4 months ago and confides that, since she was diagnosed, her husband has been more distant. Since the mastectomy, they have not had intercourse and he does not hug her anymore. Mrs. Noonan is interested in resuming sexual activity but her husband makes excuses and appears uninterested.

What could be responsible for Mr. Noonan's reaction? What could be done to help the couple?

CRITICAL THINKING EXERCISES

1. Discuss reasons for older adults not performing breast and testicular self-examinations and measures nurses could take to promote older adults performing these examinations.

2. Outline a program for ensuring regular breast and testicular examinations are done for individuals living in an assisted living community or nursing home.

3. Outline suggestions that could be offered to older women who state that they find sexual intercourse uncomfortable due to the dryness of their vaginal canal.

RESOURCES

Gilda's Club Worldwide
http://www.gildasclub.org

Gynecologic Cancer Foundation
http://www.wcn.org

MaleCare
http://www.malecare.com

National Prostate Cancer Coalition
www.zerocancer.org

Ovarian Cancer National Alliance
http://www.ovariancancer.org

The Wellness Community
http://www.thewellnesscommunity.org

REFERENCES

American Cancer Society. (2007). *American Cancer Society guidelines for early detection of cancer.* Retrieved August 20, 2007 from http://www.cancer.org/Healthy/FindCancer Early/CancerScreeningGuidelines/american-cancer-society-guidelines-for-the-early-detection-of-cancer

National Cancer Institute. (2012). *Cancer Fact Sheet.* Retrieved May 30, 2012 from http://seer.cancer.gov/statfacts/html/prost.html

RECOMMENDED READINGS

Recommended Readings associated with this chapter can be found on the web site that accompanies the book. Visit **http://thepoint.lww.com/Eliopoulos8e** to access the recommended readings and other additional resources associated with this chapter.

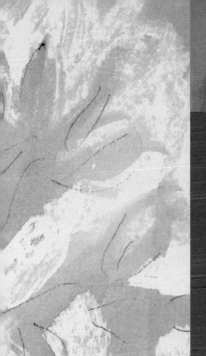

Movement

CHAPTER OUTLINE

LEARNING OBJECTIVES

After reading this chapter, you should be able to:

1. Describe the effects of aging on musculoskeletal function.

2. List the benefits of activity.

3. Describe the adjustments that may need to be made in exercise programs in late life.

4. Discuss the challenges older adults may face in maintaining an active state.

5. List actions that could benefit an older adult who has impaired mobility.

6. Discuss the role of nutrition in musculoskeletal health.

7. Describe factors contributing to, symptoms of, and related nursing care for fractures, osteoarthritis, rheumatoid arthritis, osteoporosis, gout, and podiatric conditions.

8. Discuss pain management measures for musculoskeletal problems.

9. Identify ways to reduce risks of injury associated with musculoskeletal problems.

10. Describe measures to facilitate independence in persons with musculoskeletal problems.

TERMS TO KNOW

Onychomycosis: a fungal infection of the nail or nail bed

Osteoarthritis: degenerative joint disease in which there is progressive deterioration and abrasion of joint cartilage, with the formation of new bone at the joint surfaces

Osteoporosis: bone condition characterized by low bone density and porous bones

Sarcopenia: age-related decrease in muscle mass and/or function resulting from a reduction of protein synthesis and increase in muscle protein degradation

Tinea pedis: athlete's foot; fungal infection of the foot

A variety of physical, psychological, and social benefits are gained through regular activity. Physical activity aids respiratory, circulatory, digestive, excretory, and musculoskeletal functions. Mental acuity and mood are enhanced by the physiological effects of exercise. Physical activity can be a means to engage in social activity; a physically fit state supports older adults in participating in social events. Multiple health problems, such as atherosclerosis, obesity, joint immobility, pneumonia, constipation, pressure ulcers, depression, and insomnia, can be avoided when an active state is maintained. However, maintaining a physically active state is more challenging in late life due to the effects of aging and the symptoms and restrictions imposed by the chronic health conditions that are highly prevalent among older adults. Gerontological nurses can contribute significantly to the health of older adults by guiding them in maintaining and improving their physical condition and by assisting them in effectively managing conditions that could threaten an active physical state.

EFFECTS OF AGING ON MUSCULOSKELETAL FUNCTION

The decline in the number and size of muscle fibers and subsequent reduction in muscle mass decrease the body strength; grip strength endurance declines. Connective tissue changes reduce the flexibility of joints and muscles.

An increasing challenge facing individuals as they age is *sarcopenia*—the age-related reduction of muscle mass and/or function, resulting from a reduction of protein synthesis and an increase in muscle protein degradation. When added to the impaired capacity for muscle regeneration that occurs in late life, this can lead to disability, particularly in patients with diseases or organ impairment. Immobility and lack of exercise, increased levels of proinflammatory cytokines, increased production of oxygen free radicals or impaired detoxification, low anabolic hormone output, malnutrition and reduced neurological drive have been advocated as being responsible for sarcopenia (Di Iorio et al., 2006).

In addition to the effects of aging and disease, activity can be impacted by psychosocial factors. The loss of one's spouse and/or friends can limit the older adult's participation in social and recreational activities, thereby reducing opportunities for physical activity. Retirement is often accompanied by reduced activity as one no longer has to prepare for, travel to, and engage in work; social and recreational activities that could offer opportunities for some exercise may be restricted due to financial limitations or poor health. The relocation from the house in which the older person raised his or her family to a smaller home, apartment, or retirement community reduces housekeeping and maintenance functions that provided some opportunity for movement.

Nursing Diagnosis Table 24-1 describes the effects of aging that challenge the older adult's ability to remain active.

MUSCULOSKELETAL HEALTH PROMOTION

Promotion of Physical Exercise in All Age Groups

Maintaining a physically active state is an increasingly difficult task not only for older adults but also for many younger people. Fewer occupations require hard physical labor, and those that do often use technological innovations to perform the more strenuous tasks. Television viewing, social media, and spectator sports are popular forms of recreation. Automobiles, taxicabs, and buses provide transportation to destinations once

NURSING DIAGNOSIS

TABLE 24-1	Aging and Risks to Maintaining an Active State

Causes or Contributing Factors	Nursing Diagnosis
Decreased cardiac output	Activity Intolerance related to less efficient management of stress
Reduced breathing capacity and efficiency	Activity Intolerance related to shortness of breath
Delayed oxygen diffusion	Ineffective Peripheral Tissue Perfusion related to delayed oxygen diffusion
Decrease in muscle mass, strength, and movements	Activity Intolerance related to muscle weakness and fatigue
Demineralization of bone; deterioration of cartilage, surface of joints	Impaired Physical Mobility related to decreased range of motion
Brittleness of bones	Risk for Injury
Poorer vision and hearing	Social Isolation related to sensory deficit related to sensory deficit
Wrinkling of skin; thinning, loss, and change in hair color	Disturbed Body Image related to age-related changes to appearance
Lower basal metabolic rate	Impaired Physical Mobility related to slower functions
	Risk for Injury and Infection related to decreased bodily functions during resting/sleeping states
Higher prevalence of chronic, disabling disease	Risk for Ineffective Activity Planning related to chronic disease
	Impaired Physical Mobility related to chronic disease
	Chronic Pain related to chronic disease
	Impaired Social Interaction related to chronic disease
Reduced income	Deficient Diversional Activity related to fewer funds available for leisure pursuits
	Chronic Low Self-Esteem related to decreased income
	Social Isolation related to fewer funds available for transportation, entertainment, and leisure pursuits

conveniently reached by walking. Elevators and escalators minimize stair climbing. Modern appliances have considerably eased the physical energy expended in household chores. Youths are spending considerable amounts of time sitting in front of computer screens, texting, and playing video games. Growing numbers of Americans find that it is challenging to find the time for jogging or trips to the gym.

Educating and encouraging persons of all ages to exercise regularly is an important way that gerontological nurses can influence the health of today's and future generations of older people. All exercise programs should address:

- *Cardiovascular endurance.* The ability of the heart, lungs, and blood vessels to deliver oxygen to all body cells is enhanced by aerobic training. Aerobic exercises include walking, jogging, cycling, swimming, rowing, tennis, and aerobic dancing. For cardiac endurance, these exercises must be performed long enough

to require a continuous supply of oxygen, which puts a demand on the cardiopulmonary system to reach at least 55% of its maximum heart rate (Box 24-1). Ideally, the heart rate should fall within the target heart rate range during exercise. Depending on the exercise, these should be done for at least 20 minutes, at least 3 days a week. Adjustments to desirable target heart rate range may need to be made for persons with heart conditions or who are taking certain medications; consultation with a physician is important before initiating an exercise program.

- *Flexibility.* The ability to freely move muscles and joints through their range of motion is another part of physical fitness. Gentle stretching exercises help maintain flexibility of joints and muscles; stretching exercises for about 5 to 10 minutes before and after other exercises can reduce muscle soreness. Major muscle groups should be stretched at least twice weekly.

BOX 24-1 Calculating Maximum and Target Heart Rates

Maximum heart rate = 220 − age
Target heart rate = maximum heart rate × 75%
Target heart rate range = 65% to 80% of maximum
  heart rate

(Commercial heart rate monitors, available at sports supplies stores, can provide feedback on heart rate during exercise without the inconvenience of having to stop to palpate the pulse.)

■ *Strength training.* Strength and endurance are enhanced by exercises that challenge muscles. Key elements of strength training are resistance and progression. Resistance is achieved by lifting weights and the use of weight machines; isometric exercises or the use of one's own body weight through calisthenics, such as push-ups and pull-ups, are also good means of strength training. Progression involves increasing the workload on the muscles, such as by lifting heavier weights. The recommendation for most adults is to exercise a muscle through a set of 8 to 12 repetitions at least twice weekly.

Essential to every health assessment is a review of the quality and quantity of exercise. Nurses should address identified exercise deficits by reviewing desirable exercise goals and strategies. Helping people to develop good exercise habits today promotes a healthier senior population in the future.

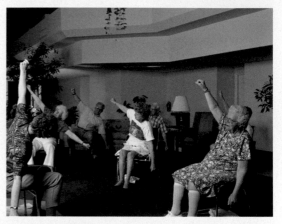

FIGURE 24-1 ■ Planned activities can offer opportunities for socialization as well as exercise.

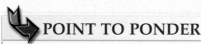

POINT TO PONDER

Do you have regular exercise built into your life? If not, what factors prevent this?

Exercise Programs Tailored for Older Adults

The fitness craze is popular in our society, and older adults are not untouched by this movement. Regular physical activity can delay or prevent some of the age-related losses in cardiovascular function and improve maximal oxygen uptake. It can also lower resting systolic and diastolic blood pressure. Physical activity can increase muscle strength and flexibility and slow the rate of bone loss.

Exercise can improve body tone, circulation, appetite, digestion, elimination, respiration, immunity, sleep, and self-concept. Participation in exercise programs can also provide opportunities for socialization and recreation (Fig. 24-1). Growing numbers of older adults understand the benefits of and are engaging in exercise programs.

Although exercise is highly beneficial to older adults, it can create problems if adjustments are not made for their advanced age. In addition to the effects of aging on musculoskeletal function described previously, age-related changes affect a person's ability to exercise. The reduced stroke volume experienced with age is usually adequate during mild exercise, although it is unable to increase in response to more strenuous exercise as compared with younger hearts. This causes the heart rate to accelerate to supply adequate circulation to the tissues. Not only does an increased resistance to blood flow result in a higher systolic blood pressure during rest but also systolic pressures can rise above 200 mm Hg during exercise. Reduced vital capacity and increased residual capacity limit the air movement, causing the respiratory muscles to work harder and the respiratory rate to increase. The proportionate increase in body fat in older bodies causes heat to dissipate less effectively, making older persons more susceptible to heat stroke if they exercise in hot temperatures. The 10% to 15% decline in total body fluid that is experienced by late life means that older persons can dehydrate more easily from perspiration during exercise. These factors emphasize the importance of assessing older adults before they start an exercise

BOX 24-2 Guidelines for Exercise Programs for Older Adults

- Ensure that a recent physical examination has been done to detect conditions that could affect or be affected by an exercise program (e.g., heart disease and diabetes). If health conditions are present, consult with the physician as to restrictions or modifications to the exercise program.
- Assess the older adult's current activity level, range of motion, muscle strength and tone, and response to physical activity. In collaboration with the patient, develop an exercise program that recognizes interests, capacities, limitations, and realistic potential.
- Emphasize exercises that focus on good speed and rhythm (e.g., low weights and high repetitions). Keep resistance exercises at a low level and avoid isometric exercises.
- Determine the training heart rate and evaluate heart rate during exercise to ensure that the rate stays within a safe range.
- To determine an age-adjusted training heart rate, subtract the person's age from 220 and multiply that answer by 70% (Heyward, 1998). This calculates the maximum rate that will provide vascular

and other benefits without causing deleterious effects. The resting heart rate can serve as the lower level and the training heart rate as the upper level for a safe heart rate range during exercise.
- Monitor pulse during exercise and reduce intensity and length of exercise if heart rate is more than 10 beats above the target heart rate.
- Consult the physician as to the appropriateness of the exercise program for persons who have a resting heart rate exceeding 100 beats per minute.
- Advise the older adult to wear proper-fitting shock-absorbing shoes with traction soles.
- Encourage warm-up exercises (e.g., gentle stretching and flexing) for at least 10 minutes before the person engages in the full exercise program.
- Provide for a period of cooling down after exercises.
- Begin with a conservative exercise program and gradually increase activity. Monitor vital signs and symptoms at various activity levels. Note arrhythmias, significant changes in blood pressure, dyspnea, shortness of breath, fatigue, angina, and intermittent claudication.

program and monitoring their status during physical activity. Box 24-2 describes some of the guidelines that can assist older adults to obtain maximum benefit from exercise programs.

Exercise programs are best followed if they match the individual's interests and needs. Some people dislike playing organized sports but enjoy dancing, so helping them to find church and community groups that regularly sponsor evenings of dancing may do more to promote exercise than describing all the benefits of joining a tennis or bowling team. Likewise, people who may not be able or willing to work out at a gym may be open to lifting weights or jogging on a mini-trampoline in their homes. A range of options should be considered, such as brisk walking, swimming, yoga, and aerobic exercises. In addition, people can take advantage of opportunities to enhance physical activity during daily routines, such as climbing stairs instead of taking an elevator, parking the car farther away from the destination to increase walking, taking the dog on a longer route during regular walks, and doing one's own yard work and housecleaning (Fig. 24-2).

It is advisable to pace exercises throughout the day and avoid fatigue from exercising

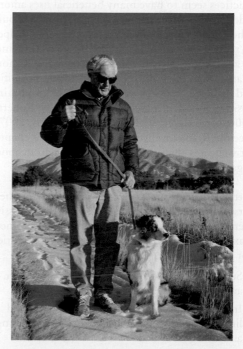

FIGURE 24-2 ■ Walking the dog outdoors can provide an opportunity to incorporate physical activity into the older adult's daily routine.

because of potential muscle pain and cramping. Morning stretching exercises loosen the stiff joints and muscles, which encourages activity, whereas bedtime exercises promote relaxation and encourage sleep. If an older person is not accustomed to a great deal of physical activity, he or she should begin exercises gradually and increase them according to individual progress. Some tachycardia normally may occur during the exercises and continue for as long as several hours thereafter in older adults. Longer periods must be allowed for the older person to perform exercises, and rest periods should follow the activity. Warm water and warm washcloths or towels wrapped around the joints may ease joint motion and facilitate exercising.

The thinner, weaker, and more brittle bones of older people heighten the risk of fractures. Exercises that stress an immobilized joint, strenuous sports, and running and jumping exercises should be avoided to prevent trauma. Older adults with cardiac or respiratory problems should seek advice from their physician about the amount and type of exercise best suited for their unique capacities and limitations.

Increasing numbers of older adults are using exercises that were once limited to the complementary and alternative therapy arena. T'ai chi and yoga are examples of such practices. These practices seem to have many beneficial uses among older adults. After the first major study was published that showed that t'ai chi exercises helped to reduce falls in older adults by 25% (Province et al., 1995), several other studies have demonstrated that in addition to improving flexibility and balance, t'ai chi is beneficial in promoting positive mood in older adults (Adler & Roberts, 2006; Greenspan, Wolf, Kelly, & O'Grady, 2007). (See the Resources listing at the end of this chapter for web sites that provide more information about yoga and t'ai chi.)

Some older individuals may be unable to participate in formal exercise programs. For these persons, it can be beneficial to build less aggressive exercises into their daily activities and promote maximum activity during routine care activities. For example:

■ Suggest that the patient do foot, leg, shoulder, and arm circling while watching television.

■ Instruct the patient to do deep-breathing and limb exercises in the period between awakening and rising from bed.

■ Encourage the patient to wash dishes or light laundry by hand to exercise the fingers with the benefit of warm water.

■ When greeting a patient in the hall, ask the person to raise both arms as high as possible and wave.

■ When giving a medication, ask the patient to bend each extremity several times.

■ During bathing activities, ask the patient to flex and extend all body parts.

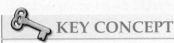

KEY CONCEPT

People who are unable to participate in an aggressive exercise program can stretch and exaggerate movements during routine activities to promote joint mobility and circulation.

Figure 24-3 depicts several exercises that can easily be incorporated into the older adult's daily activities.

At times, older persons may need partial or complete assistance with exercises. The nurse or other caregivers will find it useful to remember the following points:

■ Exercise all body joints through their normal range of motion at least three times daily.

■ Support the joint and distal limb during the exercise.

■ Do not force the joint past the point of resistance.

Chapter 35 reviews the range-of-motion exercises and some of the assistive devices that can help older adults to be active.

The Mind–Body Connection

Cognitive and emotional states can influence the physical activity. Depressed individuals may be poorly motivated to engage in exercise or lack the energy to be physically active. Persons with Alzheimer's disease and other cognitive impairments may lack the memory, judgment, or coordination to safely exercise. However, inactive states lead to the ill effects of immobility (e.g., poor circulation, fatigue, and reduced release of endorphins) that can affect the mind. Promotion of physical activity, therefore, can have positive effects on mood and cognition. Nurses can help patients with mood or cognitive disorders in the development and implementation of an exercise program appropriate for their capabilities and needs. Activities must be planned according to the unique interests of the individual and could include arts, crafts,

Exercises to Do While in Bed

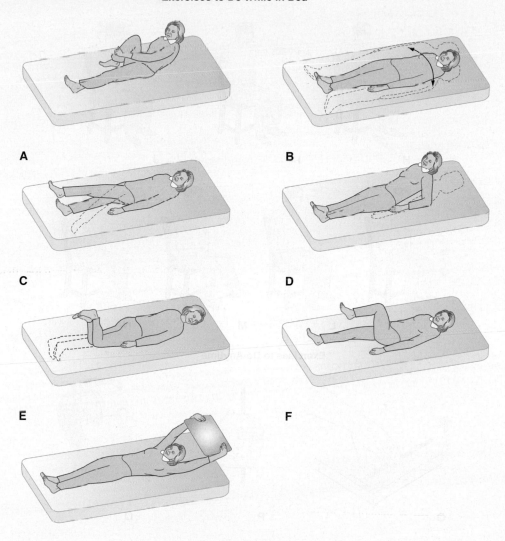

G

FIGURE 24-3 ■ Exercises to do while in bed: **(A)** Flexing the knee with the opposite hand holding the foot for assistance. **(B)** Rolling from side to side. **(C)** Scissorlike crossing of the legs. **(D)** Raising the chest. **(E)** Flexing the knees while lying on the abdomen. **(F)** Bicycling. **(G)** Lifting a pillow over the head with the arms straight. **Exercises to do while sitting: (H)** Circling motion of the shoulder joint with the arm at the side. **(I)** Circling the arms. **(J)** Rotating the head. **(K)** Flexing and extending the neck. **(L)** Pushing up in a chair with the use of the arms. **(M)** Kicking the legs while sitting. **(N)** Rolling the foot on a can.

All exercises can be built into regular activities. **Exercises to do anytime: (O)** Rolling a pencil on a hard surface. **(P)** Flexing the fingers around a pencil. **(Q)** Exaggerating chewing motions. **(R)** Rubbing the back with a towel. **(S)** Tightening the rectoperineal muscles. **(T)** Holding the stomach in to tighten the abdominal muscles.

Exercises to Do While Sitting

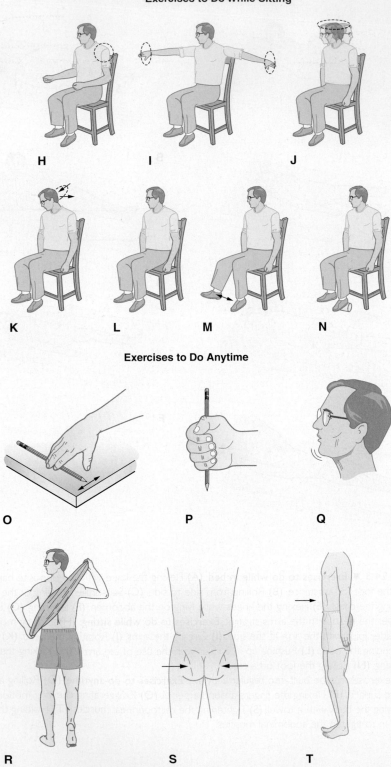

Exercises to Do Anytime

FIGURE 24-3 ■ (Continued)

travel, classes, gardening, auto repair, dancing, listening to music, people watching, and collecting. Pets are frequently a source of interest, activity, and companionship for older adults. Older adulthood can also be a time for the development of new hobbies and interests.

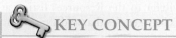

KEY CONCEPT

Mental stimulation is as vital to an individual's physical well-being as physical activity. Likewise, physical activity can improve mood and cognition.

Therapeutic recreation is structured leisure with a specific goal in mind, for example, working with clay to exercise fingers, painting to express feelings, and cooking classes to restore or maintain roles. Specialists in recreation, music, art, or dance therapy can provide valuable assistance in matching activities to the unique needs, interests, and capacities of older persons.

With any activity, adequate time and patience are necessary. Slower passage of impulses through the nervous system, sensory deficits, and the vast storehouse of information being triggered and sorted in response to psychological stimuli are just a few of the factors that interfere with rapid reactions in older people.

Prevention of Inactivity

As listed in Box 24-3, the deconditioning effects of inactivity are significant to older adults and

exaggerate the age-related effects of sarcopenia. For a person of any age, maintaining an active state can be challenging. For older adults, age-related changes in muscle strength and endurance, reduced opportunities for activity, and fatigue, pain, dizziness, dyspnea, and other symptoms associated with health problems prevalent in later life can further reduce activity levels.

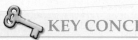

KEY CONCEPT

Inactivity can result in deconditioning, which compounds the effects of sarcopenia.

Because these real obstacles get in the way of being physically active in later life, special efforts are demanded by older adults and those caring for them to compensate for this problem. A crucial measure is to educate the public, especially caregivers, about the importance of physical activity for older adults (e.g., lowering blood pressure, maintaining muscle strength, preventing falls, aiding lymphatic circulation, sharpening mental acuity, elevating mood, and improving digestion and elimination). Sometimes families believe they are assisting their older relatives by "doing for" and allowing them to be sedentary. Often, assisting with household responsibilities not only enhances good functioning of the body's systems but also promotes a sense of worth by providing an opportunity for productivity. Although physical activity may be more uncomfortable or demanding than inactivity,

---

BOX 24-3   Deleterious Effects of Inactivity

- Changes in physiologic function
  - Reduced pulse rate
  - Increased cardiac workload
  - Decreased aerobic capacity
  - Decreased chest expansion and ventilation
  - Reduced muscle strength, tone, and endurance
  - Demineralization of bones, increased ease of fractures
  - Slower gastrointestinal motility
  - Slower metabolism and lymphatic circulation
- Increased risk of complications
  - Postural hypotension
  - Hypostatic pneumonia
  - Pressure ulcers
  - Poor appetite
  - Obesity
  - Constipation
  - Fecal impaction
  - Incontinence
  - Renal stone formation
  - Urinary tract infection
  - Joint stiffness, limited range of motion
- Changes in mood and self-concept
  - Increased feelings of helplessness, depression
  - Perception of self as incapable, frail
- Increased dependency
- Reduced opportunities for socialization

future health problems and disability may be spared by its regular practice.

Creativity in suggesting pastimes that can stimulate movement may be a key to increasing opportunities for activity. For instance, encouraging membership in a senior citizen's club can motivate many types of activities because the individual will have a reason to perform the following tasks, among others:

- get out of bed
- prepare and eat breakfast
- bathe
- dress
- comb hair
- travel to the club
- negotiate a new environment
- interact with others
- participate in activities
- travel home
- undress

Those caring for older people can enhance motivation by demonstrating a sincere interest in their activities, for example, asking how they spent their day, admiring crafts they made, or listening to the details of a trip. Recognizing housekeeping efforts, using their handmade gifts, and commenting on a well-groomed appearance are small but meaningful ways to reinforce the older person's efforts to be active.

Nurses can inform older adults about local resources that can promote activity, such as senior centers, exercise classes, educational and recreational programs at local schools or colleges, volunteer opportunities, and local clubs. In addition, they can promote activity by arranging transportation for older adults to and from activities. For homebound older people, special services offered by libraries, vision associations, Pets on Wheels, social service organizations, faith communities, and other agencies can provide resources and companionship that promote activity. Refer to the Resources listing at the end of chapters for agencies that address specific needs.

An older adult's unique capacities and limitations, as well as interests, will dictate the appropriate activities for that individual. Learning about an older adult's individual interests, preferences, and abilities can assist nurses in identifying activities that will be familiar and enjoyable. Stereotyping older adults by assuming they all enjoy exactly the same activities violates the underlying nursing principle of individualized care and severely limits the opportunities available for older persons. If it is assumed that older persons are normally inactive, disinterested in exercise, and unable to participate in physical activity, and if they are treated as though they are, they most likely will fulfill these expectations. If, however, they are expected to keep active and interested in the world around them, they have a better probability of remaining capable, independent, and physically and mentally functional.

Nursing Diagnosis Highlight: Impaired Physical Mobility describes additional interventions for promoting mobility. Gerontological nurses can make a difference by identifying patients at high risk for developing musculoskeletal problems, implementing interventions to prevent them, and implementing a reconditioning program for persons with chronic deconditioning.

CONSIDER THIS CASE

Since retiring 6 years ago from his job as a delivery man, 74-year-old Mr. E has become progressively more inactive. His wife, who is of the same age and considerably more active, urges him to exercise more, but Mr. E responds that he worked hard all his life and now that he is retired he deserves to "kick back and take it easy." Mr. E's increasingly stiff joints and reduced respiratory capacity cause him to have difficulty walking more than a city block and climbing stairs. He frequently nods off and has few interests other than television. His wife is unhappy because they do not participate in activities together.

THINK CRITICALLY
- What can be done to affect a change in Mr. E's behavior?
- How could you assist both Mr. and Mrs. E?

IMPAIRED PHYSICAL MOBILITY

Overview

Impaired physical mobility is a state in which movement is limited. Some degree of mobility limitation is observed, ranging from the use of special equipment for movement to total dependency on others for movement. Other signs associated with this diagnosis could include decreased muscle strength or control, restricted range of motion, impaired coordination, altered gait, decreased level of consciousness, pain, paralysis, and imposed restrictions on movement.

Causative or contributing factors

Arthritis, malnutrition, neuromuscular disease, sensory deficits, edema, missing limb, cardiovascular disease, pulmonary disease, obesity, side effects of medications, altered mood, and cognition.

Goals

The patient will increase mobility to optimal level. The patient will be free from complications associated with impaired mobility.

Interventions

- Assess muscle strength and tone, active and passive range of motion, and mental status.
- Review history for conditions that can limit mobility or require alteration in the level of mobility. Consult with

the physician as to restrictions on mobility and any necessary modifications for exercises.

- Develop an individualized exercise program, which could include passive or active range-of-motion exercises, structured exercise classes, and walking programs (see Box 24-2).
- Assist patient in maintaining good body alignment and hourly position changes.
- Promote a good nutritional status. Consult with nutritionists as needed.
- If necessary, refer for canes, walkers, wheelchairs, braces, traction devices, and other aids to increase mobility. Provide related health teaching as needed.
- Collaborate with physical therapist, occupational therapist, recreational therapist, and other health team members to develop a program to increase the patient's mobility.
- Encourage family and significant others to assist in efforts to increase the patient's mobility.
- Provide diversional activities based on the patient's interests and level of function.
- Observe for complications associated with immobility and seek prompt correction. Instruct the patient in the recognition of complications.

Nutrition

Finally, although potentially overlooked, good nutrition is an important factor in preventing and managing musculoskeletal problems. A well-balanced diet rich in proteins and minerals will help maintain the structure of the bones and muscles. A minimum of 1,500 mg calcium should be included in the diet daily for older men and women who are not taking estrogen (1,000 mg for women taking estrogen). Table 24-2 details good sources of calcium. If dietary intake of calcium does not meet the daily requirement, supplements should be taken to compensate for the deficient amount (i.e., if a person who should consume 1,500 mg daily only derives an average of 1,000 mg from his or her diet, a 500-mg supplement is appropriate).

In addition to quality of the diet, quantity is also important. Obesity places strain on the joints, which aggravates conditions such as arthritis. Weight reduction frequently will ease musculoskeletal discomforts

TABLE 24-2	Good Sources of Calcium	
Source	**Portion**	**Calcium (mg)**
Plain low-fat yogurt	1 cup	250–400
Sardines	½ cup	375
Fruit juice, calcium fortified	1 glass	300
Skim milk	1 cup	302
Buttermilk	1 cup	300
Instant, enriched cooked farina	1 cup	200
Swiss cheese	1 ounce	272
Ice cream	1 cup	175
Low-fat (2%) cottage cheese	1 cup	155
Cooked turnip greens	½ cup	150
Tofu	½ cup	150
Broccoli	1 cup	136

and reduce limitations and should be promoted as a sound health practice for persons of all ages.

SELECTED MUSCULOSKELETAL CONDITIONS

It is the rare older individual who does not experience some degree of discomfort, disability, or deformity from musculoskeletal disorders. In fact, musculoskeletal diseases are the leading cause of functional impairment in older adults. Because activity and mobility are vital to the total health of older adults, musculoskeletal problems that limit functional capacity can have devastating effects (Nursing Diagnosis Table 24-3). Assessment for musculoskeletal problems should consider not only the presence of these conditions but also the effect they have on the older adult's function (Assessment Guide 24-1). Prevention of these problems and aggressive intervention to minimize their impact if they are present should be integral parts of gerontological nursing care.

Fractures

Trauma, cancer metastasis to the bone, osteoporosis, and other skeletal diseases contribute to fractures in older persons. The neck of the femur is a common site for fractures in older people, especially in older women, and most of these fractures result from falls. Colles' fracture (break at the distal radius) is one of the most frequent upper extremity fractures and often occurs when attempting to stop a fall with an outstretched hand. Older adults are also at risk for compression fractures of the vertebrae, resulting from falls or lifting heavy objects. The more brittle bones of older persons not only fracture more easily but also heal at a slower rate than in younger persons, potentially predisposing older adults to the many complications associated with immobility.

Knowing that the risk of fracture and its multiple complications is high among older adults, the gerontological nurse must aim toward prevention, drawing on the effectiveness of basic common sense measures. Because their coordination and equilibrium are poorer, older people should be advised to avoid risky activities (e.g., climbing on ladders or chairs to reach high places). To prevent dizziness and falls resulting from postural hypotension, older individuals should rise from a kneeling or sitting position slowly. Safe, properly fitting shoes with a low, broad heel can prevent stumbling and loss of balance, and hand rails for climbing stairs or rising from the bath tub provide support and balance. Placing both feet near the edge of a curb or bus before stepping up or down is safer than a poorly balanced stretch of the legs (Fig. 24-4). Older persons should be careful where they are walking to avoid tripping in holes and on damaged sidewalks or slipping on pieces of ice. Older eyes are more sensitive to glare, so sunglasses may be helpful for

NURSING DIAGNOSIS

TABLE 24-3	Nursing Diagnoses Related to Musculoskeletal Problems
Causes or Contributing Factors	**Nursing Diagnosis**
Muscle fatigue, pain, deformity	Activity Intolerance
Pain, fear of injury	Anxiety
Inactivity or immobility from pain or disability	Constipation
Fracture, contracture, spasms, arthritis	Pain (Acute, Chronic)
Change or loss of function or appearance	Fear
Arthritis, contracture, pain, impaired range of motion	Impaired Home Maintenance
Unsteady gait, pain, improper use of heat	Risk for Injury
Spasms, atrophy, pain, deformity	Impaired Physical Mobility
Impaired self-care capacity	Powerlessness
Immobility, pain, deformity	Self-Care Deficit
Change in body structure or function, pain, immobility, increased dependency	Disturbed Body Image
Pain, fatigue, positioning difficulties, altered body image	Sexual Dysfunction
Pain, spasms, cramps	Disturbed Sleep Pattern
Change in body structure or function, altered self-concept, pain	Impaired Social Interaction
Immobility, pain, disfigurement	Social Isolation

ASSESSMENT GUIDE 24-1

MUSCULOSKELETAL FUNCTION

GENERAL OBSERVATION

Assessment of the musculoskeletal system can begin even before the formal examination by noting the patient's actions, such as transfer activities, ambulation, and use of hands. Note observations regarding the following:

- abnormal gait (Table 24-4)
- abnormality of structure
- dysfunction of a limb
- favoring of one side
- tremor
- paralysis
- weakness
- atrophy of a limb
- redness, swelling of a joint
- use of cane, walker, wheelchair

INTERVIEW

Although it may seem tedious, it is best to go from head to toe and question the patient about limited function or discomfort in specific parts of the body. Examples of questions could include the following:

- "Does your jaw ever get stiff or hurt when you chew?"
- "Do you get a stiff neck?"
- "Does your shoulder ever tighten?"
- "Do your ribs ache or feel tender?"
- "Do your hips hurt after you have walked for a while?"
- "Are your joints stiff in the morning?"
- "Do you have back pain or stiffness?"
- "Do you have muscle cramps?"
- "How far are you able to walk?"
- "Are you able to take care of your home, get in and out of a bathtub, and climb stairs?"

Also make specific inquiry into how the patient manages musculoskeletal pain, particularly in reference to the use of analgesics, heat, and topical preparations.

PHYSICAL EXAMINATION

Examine the active and passive range of motion of all joints. Note the degree of movement with and without assistance. Specific areas to review include the following:

- *Shoulder.* The patient should be able to lift both arms straight above the head. With arms straight at the

sides, the patient should be able to lift them laterally above the head (i.e., 180°) with hands supine and 110° with hands prone. The patient should be able to extend the arms 30° behind the body from the sides.
- *Neck.* The patient should be able to turn the head laterally and to flex and extend the head approximately 30° in all directions.
- *Elbow.* The patient should be able to open the arms fully and flex the joint enough to allow the hand to touch the shoulder.
- *Wrist.* The patient should be able to bend the wrist 80° in the palmar direction and 70° in the dorsal direction. With a hand-waving motion, the patient should be able to bend the wrist laterally 10° toward the radial or thumb side and 60° in the direction of the ulnar side. The patient should be able to move the hand to 90° in the prone and supine positions.
- *Finger.* The patient should be able to bend the distal joint of the finger approximately 45° and the proximal joint 90°. Hyperextension of 30° should be possible.
- *Hip.* While lying down, the patient should be able to abduct and adduct the leg 45°. With the patient lying on his back, the leg should be able to be lifted 90° with the knee straight and 125° with the knee bent.
- *Knee.* While lying on the stomach, the patient should be able to flex the knee approximately 100°.
- *Ankle.* The patient should be able to point the toes 10° toward the head and 40° toward the foot of the bed or examining table. There should be a 35° inversion and a 25° eversion.
- *Toe.* The patient should be able to flex and hyperextend the toes approximately 30°. Note the patient's active and passive range of motion, as well as any weakness, tightness, spasm, tremor, or contracture that may be evident.

Some muscle weakness can be anticipated, although the exact degree will vary among individuals. The upper extremity usually shows greater strength on the side of the dominant hand; there should be equal strength in the lower extremities. To test the muscle strength in holding its shortest position, have the patient hold the muscle in its shortest position and apply force to cause the muscle to extend. Normally, a muscle will be able to hold its shortest position under moderate resistance. Palpate all muscles for tenderness, contractures, and masses.

TABLE 24-4	Gait Disturbances	
Gait Pattern		**Associated Disorder**
Ataxic		
Unsteady, uncoordinated, feet raised high while stepping and then dropped flat on floor		Cerebellum disease Intoxication
Foot Slapping		
Wide based, feet raised high while stepping and then slapped down against floor, no staggering or weaving		Lower motor neuron disease Paralysis of pretibial and peroneal muscles
Hemiplegic		
Unilateral foot drop and foot dragging, leg circumducted, arm flexed and held close to side		Unilateral upper motor neuron disease
Parkinsonian		
Trunk leans forward, slight flexion of hip and knees, no arm swing while stepping, short and shuffling steps, starts slowly and then increases in speed		Parkinsonism
Scissors		
Slow, short steps; legs cross while stepping		Spastic paraplegia Dementia Cerebral palsy
Spastic		
Uncoordinated, jerking gait; legs stiff; toes drag		Spastic paraplegia Spinal cord tumor Multiple sclerosis

improving vision outdoors. A nightlight is extremely valuable in preventing falls during night visits to the bathroom. Other fall prevention measures are discussed in Chapter 17.

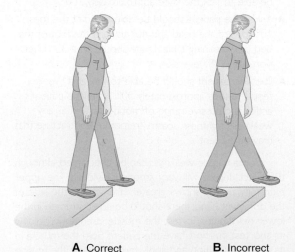

A. Correct   **B.** Incorrect

FIGURE 24-4 ■ **A.** The correct method for stepping to or from a curb is to place both feet near the edge of the curb before stepping up or down. **B.** The incorrect method is to stretch the legs apart before stepping.

Because of the high prevalence and ease of fractures in older adults, fracture should be suspected whenever older adults fall or otherwise subject their bones to trauma. Symptoms include pain, change in the shape or length of a limb, abnormal or restricted motion of a limb, edema, spasm of surrounding tissue, discoloration of tissue, and bone protruding through the tissue. The absence of these symptoms does not rule out the possibility of a fracture. Overt signs and symptoms can be absent; in addition, the position of the fracture can prevent it from being apparent on the initial roentgenogram. As the patient is transported for evaluation, immobility of the injured site and control of bleeding are essential.

KEY CONCEPT

The absence of typical signs of fracture does not guarantee that a bone is not broken; therefore, close nursing observation is essential whenever a bone has been subjected to trauma.

Fractures heal more slowly in older adults, and the risk of complications is greater. Pneumonia, thrombus formation, pressure ulcers, renal calculi, fecal impaction, and contractures are among the complications that special nursing attention can help prevent. Activity within the limits determined by the physician should be promoted, including deep-breathing and coughing exercises, isometric and range-of-motion exercises, and frequent turning and position changes. Fluids should be encouraged, and the characteristics of urine output noted. Good nutrition will facilitate healing, increase resistance to infection, and decrease the likelihood of other complications. Joint exercise and proper positioning can prevent contractures. Correct body alignment can be maintained with the use of foot boards, trochanter rolls, and sandbags. Keeping the skin dry and clean, preventing pressure, stimulating circulation through massage, and frequently turning the patient may reduce the risk of decubiti. Sheepskin, water beds, and alternating pressure mattresses are beneficial, but they are not substitutes for good skin care and frequent position changes.

The patient should be mobilized as early as possible. Because the patient may fear using the fractured limb and avoid doing so, explanations and reassurance are required to help the individual understand that the healed limb is safe to use. Progress in small steps may be easier for the patient to tolerate physically and psychologically; the first attempt at ambulation may be to stand at the bedside, the next to walk to a nearby chair, and the next to walk to the bathroom. Initially, it may be helpful for two people to assist the patient with ambulation, especially because weakness and dizziness are common. The principles of nursing management for specific types of fractures are available in medical–surgical nursing textbooks, and the nurse is advised to explore that literature for more detailed information.

Osteoarthritis

Osteoarthritis is the progressive deterioration and abrasion of joint cartilage, with the formation of new bone at the joint surfaces. This problem occurs increasingly with advanced age and affects most persons over age 55 to some extent. It occurs in women more than men and is the leading cause of physical disability in older adults. Unlike rheumatoid arthritis, osteoarthritis does not cause inflammation, deformity, and crippling—a fact that is reassuring to the affected individual who fears the severe disability often seen in persons with rheumatoid arthritis. For many years, it was believed that the wear and tear of the joints as an individual ages were responsible for the development of osteoarthritis; however, greater insights into the pathophysiology of the condition have afforded

a new understanding. Disequilibrium between destructive (matrix metalloprotease enzymes) and synthetic (tissue inhibitors of matrix metalloprotease) elements lead to a lack of homeostasis necessary to maintain cartilage, causing the joint changes. Excessive use of the joint, trauma, obesity, low vitamin D and C levels, and genetic factors may also predispose an individual to this problem. Patients with acromegaly have a high incidence of osteoarthritis. Usually, osteoarthritis affects several joints rather than a single one. Weight-bearing joints are most affected, the common sites being the knees, hips, vertebrae, and fingers.

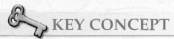

KEY CONCEPT

Osteoarthritis is the leading cause of physical disability in older people.

Systemic symptoms do not accompany osteoarthritis. Crepitation on joint motion may be noted, and the distal joints may develop bony nodules (i.e., Heberden nodes). The patient may notice that the joints are more uncomfortable during damp weather and periods of extended use. Although isometrics and mild exercises are beneficial, excessive exercise will cause more pain and degeneration.

Analgesics may be prescribed to control pain. Acetaminophen is the first drug of choice because of its safety over nonsteroidal anti-inflammatory drugs. Because individual response to analgesics varies, nurses should assess the effectiveness of various analgesics for the patient. Rest, heat or ice, t'ai chi, aquatherapy, ultrasound, and gentle massage help relieve joint aches. Acupuncture has been shown to bring about short-term relief. Splints, braces, and canes provide support and rest to the joints. Some research suggests that oral calcitonin may effectively protect postmenopausal women from the ongoing pain and ultimate disability of joint destruction associated with osteoarthritis and may provide some hope (Sondergaard, Oestergaard, Christiansen, Tankó, & Karsdal, 2007). The nurse should emphasize the importance of maintaining proper body alignment and using good body mechanics when educating the patient. Cold water fish and other foods high in the essential fatty acids have anti-inflammatory effects and should be abundant in the diet. Vitamins A, B, B6, C, and E and zinc, selenium, niacinamide, calcium, and magnesium are among the nutritional supplements that could prove useful in controlling symptoms. The over-the-counter supplements glucosamine and chondroitin have proved helpful for some people. Weight reduction may improve the obese patient's status and should be encouraged. It is beneficial if a homemaker service or other household assistance relieves the patient of strenuous activities that cause the joints to bear weight. Occupational and physical therapists can be consulted for assistive devices to promote independence in self-care activities. Nursing Care Plan 24-1 presents a sample care plan for the patient with osteoarthritis.

NURSING CARE PLAN 24-1

THE OLDER ADULT WITH OSTEOARTHRITIS

Nursing Diagnosis: Chronic Pain related to joint inflammation, stiffness, and fluid accumulation

Goal	Nursing Actions
The patient expresses relief or control of pain, is unrestricted by pain to engage in activities of daily living (ADL), is free from adverse effects of analgesics.	■ Ask patient to self-evaluate pain on a scale of 0 to 10 (0 = no pain, 10 = most severe); monitor daily. ■ Review with patient factors that precipitate, worsen, or relieve pain; incorporate this information into care to prevent and control pain. ■ Apply heat as ordered to relieve discomfort and promote mobility. Encourage the patient to use socks, blankets, and adequate clothing to keep muscles and joints warm. ■ Administer analgesics as ordered or instruct patient in proper self-administration. Monitor effectiveness, tolerance, and side effects. ■ Assist patient in maintaining good body alignment and posture. ■ Assess the impact of pain on ability to fulfill ADL. Consult with physical and occupational therapists regarding exercises and assistive devices that can promote independence. ■ Instruct patient in ways to minimize stress to joints and muscles. ■ Instruct patient in the use of guided imagery, biofeedback, and relaxation techniques; offer massages and other forms of therapeutic touch.

Nursing Diagnosis: Impaired Physical Mobility related to pain and limited joint movement

Goal	Nursing Actions
The patient maintains or achieves functional positions of joints, maintains or achieves optimal joint mobility, is free from flexion contractures.	■ Assess range of joint motion on admission or at first visit and regularly thereafter; note for each joint: swelling, warmth, tenderness, and structural or functional abnormalities. ■ Instruct or assist the patient in maintaining proper body alignment, good posture, correct use of joints. ■ Advise the patient to avoid stressing joints (e.g., by heavy lifting, running, and hammering).

- Schedule analgesic administration and other pain relief measures before activities.
- During exacerbation of pain, provide adequate rest for joints and assist the patient in positioning joints in functional alignment.
- Consult with rehabilitation specialists regarding appropriate exercise to improve muscle strength, tone, and mobility, and possible use of assistive devices and mobility aids (e.g., canes, walkers, customized eating utensils, and dressing aids).
- Encourage or assist the patient to perform range-of-motion exercises at least twice daily.
- Provide warm-up of muscles and joints prior to activities and exercises and a cool-down period afterward.

Nursing Diagnosis: Bathing/Dressing/Feeding/Toileting Self-Care Deficit related to pain or joint immobility

Goal	Nursing Actions
The patient is able to eat, bathe, dress, transfer, ambulate, and toilet independently; uses assistive aids properly and effectively.	<ul><li>Assess the patient's ability to eat, bathe, dress, transfer, ambulate, and toilet independently. Identify deficits in independently meeting ADL and plan measures to compensate for deficits; identify risks and potential deficits and plan measures to prevent the loss of independent function.</li><li>Allow patient maximum independence and participation in care activities.</li><li>Educate the patient as to proper management of condition and measures that can reduce risk of losing independence (e.g., exercise to maintain mobility and use of assistive devices).</li><li>Encourage the patient to express feelings about actual or potential dependency and provide realistic explanations and emotional support.</li></ul>

Nursing Diagnoses: (1) Body Image Disturbance related to joint abnormality, immobility, altered self-care ability; (2) Self-esteem Disturbance related to changes in body appearance and function

Goal	Nursing Actions
The patient expresses acceptance of and realities associated with chronic condition, expresses feelings regarding body changes, develops effective mechanisms to cope with body changes, identifies constructive ways to function with body changes, is free from complications associated with body image and self-esteem disturbances.	<ul><li>Assess impact of altered function and appearance on the patient.</li><li>Encourage the patient to express concerns, fears, and feelings.</li><li>Help the patient to identify effective coping measures (e.g., effective measures used to cope with problems in the past, counseling, and development of new interests).</li><li>Help the patient to identify and focus on capabilities rather than limitations.</li></ul>

If other treatments fail to improve the condition or the person suffers severe functional limitation or pain, arthroplasty may be indicated. Arthroplasty, or joint replacement, can be done to restore joint motion, improve function, and reduce pain. At one time, older people were not considered good candidates for arthroplasty; however, that thinking has changed and increasing numbers of people over the age of 65 are having joint replacements. Hip and knee joint replacements are those most common, although arthroplasty can be performed on any joint. This procedure is not advised for patients with neurotrophic joints or joint sepsis or persons who are obese or have dementias or other conditions that would interfere with their ability to cooperate with rehabilitation therapy. Conditions such as peripheral vascular disease and diabetes mellitus increase the risk of infection and interfere with wound healing. As moderate to severe pain is often present postoperatively, analgesics are administered around the clock. While assuring that pain is controlled adequately to support early rehabilitation efforts, consideration must be given to the high risk of adverse effects from analgesics that also can hamper rehabilitation; it is important to closely observe patients' reactions. Arthroplasty is associated with a high risk of deep venous thrombosis and pulmonary embolism for older patients; warfarin may be used prophylactically. Patients and their caregivers need to be advised of precautions related to anticoagulant therapy. Patients receive specific instructions pertaining to their exercise, weight-bearing, and activity restrictions. Nurses must see that patients and their caregivers understand instructions and adhere to the plan of care to ensure a successful outcome for the surgery.

Rheumatoid Arthritis

Rheumatoid arthritis affects many persons, particularly those aged 20 to 40 years; it is a major cause of arthritic disability in later life as a result. Fortunately, the incidence decreases after 65 years of age; most older patients with this disease developed it earlier in life. Specifically, the deformities and disability associated with this disease primarily begin during early adulthood and peak during middle age; in old age, greater systemic involvement occurs. This disease occurs more frequently in women and in persons with a family history of the problem.

In rheumatoid arthritis, the synovium becomes hypertrophied and edematous with projections of synovial tissue protruding into the joint cavity. The affected joints are extremely painful, stiff, swollen, red, and warm to the touch. Joint pain is present during rest and activity. Subcutaneous nodules over bony prominences and bursae may be present, as may deforming flexion contractures. Systemic symptoms include fatigue, malaise, weakness, weight loss, wasting, fever, and anemia.

Encouraging patients to rest and providing support to the affected limbs are helpful measures. Limb support should be such that pressure ulcers and contractures are prevented. Splints are commonly made for the patient in an effort to prevent deformities. Range-of-motion exercises are vital to maintain musculoskeletal function; the nurse may have to assist the patient with active exercises. Physical and occupational therapists can provide assistive devices to promote independence in self-care activities, and heat, gentle massage, and analgesics can help control pain. Patients with rheumatoid arthritis may be prescribed anti-inflammatory agents (particularly prostaglandins), corticosteroids, antimalarial agents, gold salts, and immunosuppressive drugs. The nurse should be familiar with the many toxic effects of these drugs and detect them early if they occur.

Some patients with rheumatic heart disease are sensitive to the "nightshade" foods: potatoes, peppers, eggplant, tomatoes, and other solanines; eliminating these from the diet could prove beneficial. Herbs that could improve symptoms include turmeric, ginger, skullcap, and ginseng.

Patients with rheumatoid arthritis and their families need considerable education to be able to manage this condition. Patient education should include information about the disease, treatments, administration of medications, identification of side effects, exercise regimens, use of assistive devices, methods to avoid and reduce pain, and an understanding of the need for continued medical supervision. Accepting this chronic disease is not an easy task for either the patient or the family. Finally, the patient may be a prime target for salespeople offering a quick cure or relief for arthritis and should be advised to consult a nurse or physician before investing many dollars on useless fads.

Osteoporosis

Osteoporosis is the most prevalent metabolic disease of the bone; it primarily affects adults in middle to later life, with some groups being at higher risk than others (Box 24-4). Demineralization of the bone occurs, evidenced by a decrease in the mass and density of the skeleton. Any health problem associated with inadequate calcium intake, excessive calcium loss, or poor calcium absorption can cause osteoporosis. Many of the following potential causes are problems commonly found among older persons.

BOX 24-4   Risk Factors for Osteoporosis

- Advanced age (women over 65 years, men over 80 years)
- Ethnicity
  - white women with a northwestern European or British Isles background
  - Asian women
- Calcium deficiency
- Vitamin D deficiency
- Small-framed, thin women
- History of early menopause

- Estrogen deficiency
- History of multiple pregnancies
- Cigarette smoking
- High alcohol consumption
- Prolonged immobility
- Diseases or chronic use of drugs that increase bone loss (e.g., corticosteroids, thyroid hormones, and anticonvulsants)
- Family history of osteoporosis

- *Inactivity or immobility.* A lack of muscle pull on the bone can lead to a loss of minerals, especially calcium and phosphorus. This particularly may be a problem for limbs in a cast.

- *Diseases.* Cushing syndrome, an excessive production of glucocorticosteroids by the adrenal gland, is believed to inhibit the formation of bone matrix. The increased metabolic activity of hyperthyroidism causes more rapid bone turnover and the faster rate of bone resorption to bone formation causes osteoporosis. Excessive diverticulitis can interfere with the absorption of sufficient amounts of calcium. Although the direct relationship is uncertain at this time, diabetes mellitus can contribute to the development of osteoporosis. The percentage of cases of osteoporosis that result secondary to other diseases is relatively small.

- *Reduction in anabolic sex hormones.* Decreased production or loss of estrogens and androgens may be responsible for insufficient bone calcium; therefore, postmenopausal women are at high risk.

- *Diet.* An insufficient amount of calcium, vitamin D, vitamin C, protein, and other nutrients in the diet can cause osteoporosis. Excessive consumption of caffeine or alcohol decreases the body's absorption and retention of calcium.

- *Drugs.* Heparin, furosemide, thyroid supplements, corticosteroids, tetracycline, and magnesium- and aluminum-based antacids can lead to osteoporosis.

Osteoporosis may cause kyphosis and a reduction in height. The person may experience spinal pain, especially in the lumbar region. The bones may tend to fracture more easily. However, patients are often asymptomatic and unaware of the problem until it is detected by radiography. Bone mass density can be measured through several different types of noninvasive techniques, including single-photon absorptiometry, dual-photon absorptiometry, quantitative computed tomography, and dual-energy x-ray absorptiometry, which is the most widely used and recommended method (Anders, Turner, & Wallace, 2007).

Treatment depends on the underlying cause of the disease and may include calcium supplements, vitamin D supplements, progesterone, estrogen, anabolic agents, fluoride, or phosphate. A relatively recent drug that has been shown beneficial in producing modest increases in bone mass is a synthetic form of calcitonin, a hormone produced in the thyroid that is a powerful inhibitor of osteoclastic activity (the cells that continuously reabsorb bone). Bisphosphonates are another beneficial new category of drugs that are primarily antiresorptive (i.e., they prevent or significantly slow the normal osteoclastic activity responsible for the resorption of bone). A diet rich in protein and calcium is encouraged. Braces may be used to provide support and reduce spasms. A bed board is also beneficial and should be recommended.

The nurse must advise the patient to avoid heavy lifting, jumping, and other activities that could result in a fracture. Persons providing care for these patients must remember to be gentle when moving, exercising, or lifting them because fractures can occur easily. Compression fractures of the vertebrae are a potential complication of osteoporosis. Range-of-motion exercises and ambulation are important to maintain function and prevent greater damage.

POINT TO PONDER

To what risk factors for osteoporosis are you subject, and what can you do to reduce them?

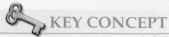

KEY CONCEPT

The bodies of persons with osteoporosis must be handled gently to avoid fractures.

Gout

Gout is a metabolic disorder in which excess uric acid accumulates in the blood. As a result, uric acid crystals are deposited in and around the joints, causing severe pain and tenderness of the joint and warmth, redness, and swelling of the surrounding tissue. During an acute attack, the pain can be quite severe; the person may not be able to bear weight or have a blanket or clothing rest on the affected joint. Attacks can last from weeks to months, with long remissions between attacks possible.

Treatment aims to reduce sodium urate through a low-purine diet (e.g., avoidance of bacon, turkey, veal, liver, kidney, brain, anchovies, sardines, herring, smelt, mackerel, salmon, and legumes) and the administration of drugs. Alcohol should also be avoided because it increases uric acid production and reduces uric acid excretion. Colchicine or phenylbutazone can be used to manage acute attacks; long-term management could include colchicine, allopurinol, probenecid, or indomethacin. Gout attacks can be precipitated by the administration of thiazide diuretics, which raise the uric acid level of the blood. Vitamin E, folic acid, and eicosapentaenoic acid can be useful dietary supplements. Herbs such as yucca and devil's claw reduce symptoms in some persons. Nurses should monitor pain and encourage a good fluid intake to prevent the formation of renal stones.

Podiatric Conditions

By age 65, nearly 90% of all people have some type of foot problem that causes some degree of discomfort or dysfunction. Not surprisingly then, the foot problems of old age have commanded a specialty of their own: podogeriatrics. Lifelong foot problems, changes in gait, diseases that affect the feet (e.g., gout, diabetes, and peripheral vascular disease), and age-related loss of fat padding of the foot contribute to foot conditions.

The older person's own shaving, cutting, and chemical treatment of podiatric conditions can result in serious complications; therefore, patients should be referred to podiatrists for the treatment of foot conditions. Nurses should teach older adults about proper foot care (e.g., keeping feet clean and dry, wearing safe and proper-fitting shoes, exercising feet, and cutting nails straight across and even with the top of the toe) and the importance of seeking professional podiatric care for problems. Nurses can offer foot massages because they can aid in stimulating circulation, reducing edema, and promoting comfort. (Foot massages may be contraindicated in patients with peripheral vascular disease or lesions, so it is important to consult with the physician first.)

Because of the impact of podiatric problems on mobility and independence, these conditions need to be effectively identified and treated. Some of the common conditions are discussed below.

Calluses

Calluses (plantar keratoses) are caused by friction and irritation on the feet that create layers of thickened skin. Reduced fat padding of the foot, dryness of the skin, decreased toe function, and poor fitting shoes contribute to callus formation. They usually appear on the heels and soles and, although not painful, can be unsightly. There is the risk that people will attempt to shave or cut off calluses from their feet and risk injuring their skin. Massaging the feet with lotions and oils can aid in preventing calluses.

Corns

Corns are cone-shaped layers of thick, dry skin that form over a bony prominence. Pressure on the area causes discomfort as the tip of the cone presses into the tissue. Additional pressure increases the size of the corn and, consequently, the pain. U-shaped corn pads and loosely wrapping the toe in lamb's wool are superior to oval or round corn pads, which can restrict circulation. As with calluses, patients should be advised not to attempt to remove corns on their own.

Bunions (Hallux Valgus)

A bunion or bursa is a bony prominence over the first metatarsal head (Fig. 24-5A). There is a medial deviation of the first metatarsal with abduction of the great toe in relation to that metatarsal. Bunions occur more often in women—not surprising considering women's shoe styles that commonly have tight toe fit and the tight hosiery that pull toes together. Some bunions are hereditary in nature. The increased width of the foot caused by the bunion can cause difficulty in finding properly fitting shoes. Shoe repair shops can stretch shoes to accommodate bunions; custom-made shoes are also beneficial. Surgery may be indicated for some cases.

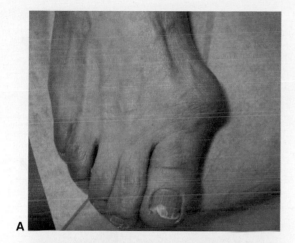

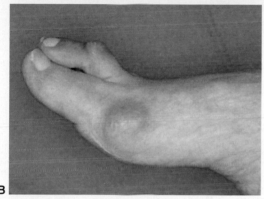

FIGURE 24-5 ■ Foot disorders can cause pain and dysfunction. **A.** Bunion. **B.** Hammer toe.

Hammer Toe (Digiti Flexus)

Hammer toe is a hyperextension at the metatarsophalangeal joint with flexion and often corn formation at the proximal interphalangeal joint. The toe begins to resemble the shape of the hammers inside a piano, thus its name (Fig. 24-5B). Although the joint itself is not painful, pressure to the area results in discomfort. Orthotics can provide symptomatic relief, but surgery is necessary for correction.

Plantar Fasciitis

A common cause of heel pain, often mistaken for a spur, is plantar fasciitis. The plantar fascia is a thick ligamentous band in the bottom of the foot that runs from the ball of the foot to the heel, where it is attached. Poor alignment of the foot that causes pronation or supination of the foot during walking results in stretching and stress of the plantar fascia. Plantar fasciitis is an inflammation of this band at its heel attachment. Pain is the primary symptom and occurs in the center or the inner side of the heel. Pain is worse after a period of rest; most people experience the most pain in the morning. After walking, the pain may subside but tends to increase as pressure is put on the heel from walking or standing. Pain can radiate to the ankle or arch of the foot if nerves become irritated secondary to the swollen plantar fascia.

Symptomatic treatment can include stretch exercising of the foot (pulling up on the ball of the foot), applying ice to the heel for 30-minute periods, and wearing cushions in the heel and shoes with heels elevated about 2 inches. The most effective means of relieving pain and preventing inflammation is to have the foot realigned through the use of custom-made orthotics. Patients need to be advised that they may not note improvement until several months after beginning treatment.

Infections

Housing of the foot in shoes, particularly the ones made from synthetic materials, creates a warm, moist environment that facilitates fungus and bacterial growth. *Onychomycosis* is a fungal infection of the nail or nail bed in which the toenail appears enlarged, thick, brittle, and flaky. As the fungus forms under the nail and displaces it up, the sides of the nail are pushed into the skin and cause pain. Antifungal preparations assist in eliminating the infection, but these infections are stubborn to treat.

Tinea pedis, better known as athlete's foot, is a fungal infection of the foot that can cause burning and itching; the skin surface will peel, crack, and be red, often with vesicle eruptions. The breaks in the skin surface provide easy entry for bacteria.

Ingrown Nails (Onychocryptosis)

Ingrown nails can occur due to tight-fitting shoes or cutting the nail excessively short. As the nail grows, its edge cuts into the tissue, leading to inflammation. Soaks and topical antibiotics may be prescribed; usually, a podiatrist can correct this problem by removing the ingrown portion and cleaning the area.

GENERAL NURSING CONSIDERATIONS FOR MUSCULOSKELETAL CONDITIONS

Managing Pain

Pain often accompanies musculoskeletal problems. Degenerative changes in the tendons and arthritis are often responsible for painful shoulders, elbows, hands, hips, knees, and spines. Cramps, especially during the night, are common in calves, feet, hands, hips, and thighs. Joint strain and damp weather more frequently cause musculoskeletal pain in the old than in the young.

Pain relief is essential in promoting optimal physical, mental, and social function. Unrelieved pain can interfere with older persons' abilities to engage in self-care, manage their households, and maintain social contact. To enrich the quality of life, every effort should be made to minimize or eliminate pain. Often, heat relieves muscle spasms; a warm bath at bedtime and keeping the extremities warm with blankets and clothing can reduce spasms and cramps throughout the night and promote uninterrupted sleep. Because older adults are at high risk for burns, care must be taken to avoid injury if heat applications or soaks are used. Passive stretching of the extremity can be helpful in controlling muscle cramps. Excessive exercise and musculoskeletal stress should be avoided, as well as situations known to cause pain, such as heavy lifting or damp weather. Back rubs using slow, long, rhythmic strokes can promote relaxation and comfort. Pain in the weight-bearing joints can be alleviated by resting those joints, supporting painful joints during transfers, and using a walker or cane (Fig. 24-6). Correct positioning, whereby all body parts are in proper alignment, can help prevent and manage pain. Accidental bumping against the patient's bed or chair and rough handling of the patient during care activities must be prevented. Nurses may also need to emphasize to other caregivers the need for extra gentleness in turning and lifting older patients.

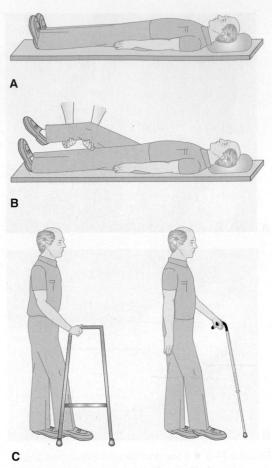

FIGURE 24-6 ■ Methods for reducing musculoskeletal pain. **A.** Good body alignment. **B.** Support of parts of the limb adjacent to the painful joint when moving or lifting. **C.** Use of a walker or cane.

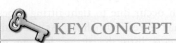

KEY CONCEPT

Unrelieved pain can significantly affect an older person's independence and quality of life.

Diversional activities are useful in preventing the patient's preoccupation with pain. Acupuncture, acupressure, and chiropractic therapy are among the alternative therapies that may help some patients control pain. Guided imagery and therapeutic touch may also prove helpful. The goal is to aid the patient in achieving the maximum level of activity with the least degree of pain.

Preventing Injury

Safety considerations are essential for all older persons because of their high incidence of accidents and musculoskeletal injuries and the prolonged time required for healing. Prevention includes paying attention to the area where one is walking; climbing stairs and curbs slowly; using both feet for support as much as possible; using railings and canes for added balance; wearing properly fitting, safe shoes for good support; and avoiding long trousers, nightgowns, or robes. The importance of the safe use of heat has already been mentioned; it is useful for patients to learn how to measure water temperature and use hot-water bottles and heating pads safely. Patients with peripheral vascular disease must be warned that the local application of heat can cause circulatory demands that their body will be unable to meet; other means of pain relief may be more beneficial to them. Warm baths can reduce muscle spasm and provide pain relief, but they can also cause hypotensive episodes leading to dizziness, fainting, and serious injury.

Carelessly turning patients so that legs hit the bed rail, dropping them into a chair during a transfer, restraining them in an unaligned position, roughly handling a limb, or attempting to use force to straighten a contracture can lead to muscle strain and fractures. Gentle handling will prevent unnecessary musculoskeletal discomfort and injury.

Promoting Independence

Any loss of independence associated with the limitations imposed by musculoskeletal problems has a serious impact on physical, emotional, and social well-being. Therefore, nurses must explore all avenues to help patients minimize limitations and strengthen capacities, thereby promoting the highest possible level of independence. Canes, walkers, and other assistive devices can often provide significant aid in compensating for handicaps and should be used when feasible (Fig. 24-7). Physical and occupational therapists can be valuable resources in determining appropriate assistive devices for use with specific deficits. Chapter 35 discusses the mobility aids in more detail.

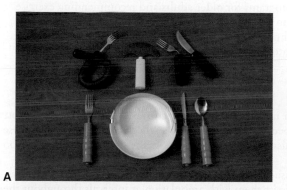

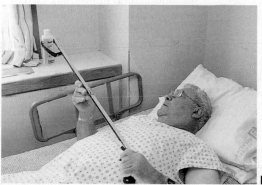

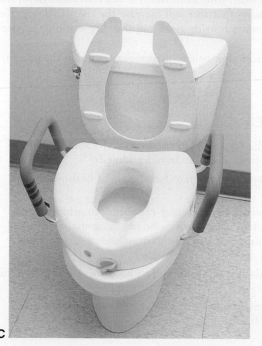

FIGURE 24-7 ■ Self-care devices can help the client with musculoskeletal problems to achieve the maximum independence possible. **A.** Assistive feeding devices help the client to grasp and get food on the utensils. **B.** A reacher is a handy device for the client with mobility restrictions. **C.** A raised toilet seat makes it easier for a person who has trouble lowering him- or herself to the toilet seat to safely use the toilet at home.

BRINGING RESEARCH TO LIFE

EXERGAMING AND OLDER ADULT COGNITION: A CLUSTER RANDOMIZED CLINICAL TRIAL

Anderson-Hanley, C., Arciero, P. J., Brickman, A. M., Nimon, J. P., Okuma, N., Nimon, J. P., Okuma, N., Zimmerman, E. A., et al. (2012). American Journal of Preventive Medicine, 42(2), 109–119.

Exercise is known to yield many physical and cognitive benefits, yet few older adults exercise. The researchers sought to test the hypothesis that stationary cycling with virtual reality tours ("cybercycle") would enhance aspects of cognitive function and clinical status more than traditional exercise. Older adults (102) from eight retirement communities were enrolled in the study and by random selection divided into traditional exercise and cyber-cycle groups. Executive intellectual function, clinical status, and exercise effort and fitness were measured. The older adults who cybercycled achieved better results for the same effort as those who engaged in traditional exercises. The researchers suggested that simultaneous cognitive and physical exercise has significant potential for preventing cognitive decline.

This finding has implications not only for older adults but also for persons of younger ages in that exercises that work out cognitive and physical function could yield better benefit than exercises that focus only on physical activity. Gerontological nurses can use this information in planning exercise programs for older adults and recommending exercise strategies that promote healthy aging in persons of all ages. This study also demonstrates the importance of integrating new technology that may not seem to be directly related to health care (e.g., video games) to gerontological care.

PRACTICE REALITIES

While working on a hospital unit you notice that older patients are allowed to spend most of their time in bed and when out of bed they are pushed in a wheelchair. Nearly all of these patients were ambulatory prior to admission. You observe that many of these patients are too weak to safely ambulate at discharge.

At a team meeting you raise the issue and suggest plans be developed to reduce unnecessary immobility in older patients and assist them with ambulation at intervals throughout the day. Several of the other nurses object, stating that this will increase the risk of falls on the unit. They add that this also will require more nursing time and they are working at barebones staffing.

You want to have harmony with your team but believe their views are not in the patients' best interest.

What are your options?

CRITICAL THINKING EXERCISES

1. What obstacles do older adults face when trying to maintain an active state? What aspects of society at large discourage physical activity in older adults?

2. Outline the contents of an exercise education program for a group of healthy senior citizens.

3. List special problems the following older individuals may experience in achieving adequate exercise: a resident of a long-term care facility who has dementia, a depressed widow who lives alone in the community, and a man who must seek re-employment after retiring.

4. Describe how a nurse's attitude toward older adults can affect his or her participation in activities that promote movement.

5. What situations could an older adult encounter during an acute hospitalization that could increase the risk of sustaining a fracture?

RESOURCES

Arthritis Foundation
http://www.arthritis.org

International Association of Yoga Therapists
http://www.iayt.org

National Arthritis and Musculoskeletal and Skin Diseases Information Clearinghouse
http://www.nih.gov/niams/

National Institute of Arthritis and Musculoskeletal and Skin Diseases (NIAMS)
http://www.niams.nih.gov

National Osteoporosis Foundation
http://www.nof.org

Tai Chi Network
http://www.taichinetwork.org

Tai Chi Tao Center
http://www.taichitaocenter.com

REFERENCES

Adler, P. A., & Roberts, B. L. (2006). The use of Tai Chi to improve health in older adults. *Orthopedic Nursing, 25*(2), 122–126.

Anders, M., Turner, L., & Wallace, L. S. (2007). Use of decision rules for osteoporosis prevention and treatment: Implications for nurse practitioners. *Journal of American Academy of Nurse Practitioners, 19*(6), 299–305.

Di Iorio, A., Abate, M., DiRenzo, D., Russolillo, A., Battaglini, C., Ripari, P., Abate, G., et al. (2006). Sarcopenia: Age-related skeletal muscle changes from determinants to physical disability. *International Journal of Immunopathology and Pharmacology, 19*(4), 703–719.

Greenspan, A. I., Wolf, S. L., Kelly, M. E., & O'Grady, M. (2007). Tai chi and perceived health status in older adults who are transitionally frail: A randomized controlled trial. *Physical Therapy, 87*(5), 525–535.

Heyward, V. H. (1998). *Advanced fitness assessment & exercise prescription.* Champaign, IL: Human Kinetics.

Province, M. A., Hadley, E. C., Hornbrook, M. C., Lipsitz, L. A., Miller, J. P., Mulrow, C. D., Wolf, S. L., et al. (1995). The effects of exercise on falls in elderly patients. *Journal of the American Medical Association, 273*(17), 1341–1347.

Sondergaard, B. C., Oestergaard, S., Christiansen, C., Tankó, L. B., & Karsdal, M. A. (2007). The effect of oral calcitonin on cartilage turnover and surface erosion in an ovariectomized rat model. *Arthritis & Rheumatism, 56*(8), 2674–2678.

RECOMMENDED READINGS

Recommended Readings associated with this chapter can be found on the web site that accompanies the book. Visit **http://thepoint.lww.com/Eliopoulos8e** to access the recommended readings and other additional resources associated with this chapter.

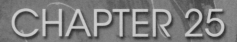

CHAPTER 25

Neurologic Function

LEARNING OBJECTIVES

After reading this chapter, you should be able to:

1. Describe the effects of aging on the nervous system.

2. List risk factors for neurologic problems in older adults.

3. Describe measures to promote neurologic health in older adults.

4. Identify signs and symptoms of neurologic disorders in older adults.

5. Describe the symptoms, unique features, and related nursing care for Parkinson's disease, transient ischemic attacks, and cerebrovascular accidents in older adults.

6. Discuss actions that promote independence in older persons with neurologic problems.

7. Describe measures to reduce the risk of injury in older persons with neurologic problems.

TERMS TO KNOW

Bradykinesia: slow movement

Cerebrovascular accident: stroke; interruption in blood supply to the brain

Hemiparesis: weakness on one side of the body

Hemiplegia: paralysis on one side of the body

(Continued)

The nervous system has a profound influence on our interaction with the world. A healthy system enables us to sense the pleasures around us, protect ourselves from harm, solve problems, derive intellectual stimulation, interact socially, and communicate our needs, thoughts, and desires. Every aspect of our basic activities of daily living depends on a good neurologic status. Dysfunction of this system has a ripple effect on other systems and can profoundly affect health, safety, normalcy, and general well-being.

Parkinson's disease: progressive degeneration of neurons in the basal ganglia resulting in the reduced production of dopamine

Transient ischemic attack (TIA): temporary or intermittent neurological event that can result from any situation that reduces cerebral circulation

EFFECTS OF AGING ON THE NERVOUS SYSTEM

With age, loss of nerve cell mass causes some atrophy of the brain and spinal cord, and brain weight decreases. The number of nerve cells declines, each cell has fewer dendrites, and some demyelinization of the cells occurs. These changes slow nerve conduction. Response and reaction times are slower; reflexes become weaker.

Plaques, tangles, and atrophy occur in the brain to varying degrees; there is not always a relationship between these changes and cognitive function. Free radicals accumulate with age and may have a toxic effect on certain nerve cells. Cerebral blood flow decreases about 20% as fatty deposits gradually accumulate in the blood vessels, and decreases are even greater in persons with small-vessel cerebrovascular disease due to diabetes and hypertension; this contributes to an increased risk of strokes. The brain has a greater ability to compensate after injury than does the spinal cord, but this ability to compensate declines with age.

Intellectual performance tends to be maintained until at least age 80, although a slowing in central processing delays the time required to perform tasks. Verbal skills are well maintained until age 70, after which there is a gradual reduction in vocabulary, a tendency to make semantic errors, and abnormal prosody (rhythm and intonation). Other age-related changes in intellectual function are subtle but can be detected as difficulty learning, especially languages, and forgetfulness in noncritical areas.

The general lack of replacement of neurons affects the sensory organs' function, which becomes less acute with age. The number and sensitivity of sensory receptors, dermatomes, and neurons decrease, resulting in dulling of tactile sensation. There is also some decline in the function of cranial nerves mediating taste and smell. Increased levels of taste, sound, scents, touch, and lighting are required for perception by older persons as compared with younger adults.

It must be remembered that these changes do not affect all individuals similarly. Genetic makeup, diet, lifestyle practices, and other factors influence the health and function of the neurologic system.

NEUROLOGIC HEALTH PROMOTION

Many neurologic disorders occur for reasons beyond one's control, but some can be prevented or minimized. For instance, cigarette smoking, obesity, ineffective stress management, elevated cholesterol, and hypertension are significant risk factors for neurovascular disease. The risk of injury to the head and spinal column is increased with unsafe actions, such as failure to use seatbelts, incompetent driving skills, alcohol and drug abuse, and falls. Infections of the ear or sinuses and sexually transmitted infections can lead to neurologic dysfunction. Most of these factors are within an individual's control to prevent. Nurses can educate persons of all ages in preventive measures that promote neurologic health in late life.

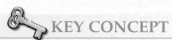

KEY CONCEPT

Maintaining weight and cholesterol levels within their ideal range, avoiding cigarette smoking, effectively managing stress, driving safely, and controlling infections can prevent some neurologic conditions.

The close relationship and regular contact nursing staff have with patients puts them in an ideal position to detect new or subtle symptoms of neurologic diseases that otherwise may be missed (Box 25-1). Recognizing symptoms and taking prompt action to ensure that patients are evaluated in a timely manner can help prevent irreversible or serious dysfunction.

In addition, nursing assessment of neurologic function (Assessment Guide 25-1) can help reveal specific problems that warrant intervention. Nursing Diagnosis Table 25-1 lists nursing diagnoses the nurse may identify through assessment.

POINT TO PONDER

Review your health status and lifestyle for risk factors for neurologic disorders. If risks are present, how can you reduce them?

BOX 25-1 Subtle Indications of Neurologic Problems

- New headaches that occur in the early morning or interrupt sleep
- Change in vision (e.g., sudden decreased acuity, double vision, and blindness in portion of visual field)
- Sudden deafness, ringing in ears
- Mood, personality changes
- Altered cognition or level of consciousness
- Clumsiness, unsteady gait
- Numbness, tingling of extremity
- Unusual sensation or pain over nerve

ASSESSMENT GUIDE 25-1
NEUROLOGIC FUNCTION

GENERAL OBSERVATIONS AND INTERVIEW

Keen observation while interviewing the patient can aid in detecting a variety of neurologic problems:

- On initial inspection of the patient, observe for asymmetry, deformity, weakness, paralysis, tremors, and other abnormalities.
- Explore the presence of symptoms of neurologic disorders, such as pain, tingling sensations, numbness, blackouts, headaches, twitching, seizures, sleep disturbances, dizziness, distortions of reality, weakness, and changes in mental status.
- If clinical abnormalities or symptoms are identified, inquire into their origin, length of time present, and resulting limitations or problems.

SPEECH ASSESSMENT

During something as basic as simple introductions, speech disorders can become evident. If speech problems exist, it is important to differentiate problems with articulation (i.e., dysarthria) and problems with the use of symbols (i.e., dysphagia):

- With dysarthria, the symbols (in this case, words) are used correctly, but speech may be slurred or distorted as a result of poor motor control. Subtle dysarthrias can be disclosed by asking the patient to pronounce the following syllables:

   me, me, me (to test the lips)

   la, la, la (to test the tongue)

   ga, ga, ga (to test the pharynx)

- Dysphasias can be receptive, expressive, or a combination of both:
   - To test for a receptive aphasia, ask the patient to follow a command (e.g., pick up the pencil); the patient's inability to understand what these symbols mean will prevent the command from being followed.
   - The patient with expressive aphasia will be able to understand commands but will not be able to put symbols together into an intelligent speech form. Point to several objects and ask the patient to name them; mild dysphasias (i.e., paraphasia) may be noted if the patient substitutes a close, although inaccurate, word for the right one, such as calling a shoe a boot or a watch a clock.
   - The ability to understand and express oneself through the written word is important to evaluate also. Ask the patient to write a short sentence that you dictate and to read a sentence from a newspaper. Ensure that the patient has the educational and visual abilities to fulfill these demands.

PHYSICAL EXAMINATION

Sensation

Ask the patient to close his or her eyes and to describe the sensations felt. To help document areas where problems are identified, a figure drawing may prove useful.

- Touch various parts of the body (e.g., forehead, cheeks, arms, hands, legs, and feet) lightly with your finger or a cotton wisp and note if the patient is able to feel the sensations. Compare analogous areas on both sides of the body and distal and proximal areas on the same extremity.
- If these primary sensations are intact, test the patient's ability to identify two simultaneous stimuli (e.g., touch the right cheek and the left forearm).
- To test cortical sensation (i.e., stereognosis), have the patient, again with closed eyes, identify various objects placed in each hand (e.g., key, marble, and coin). The inability to sense these objects is known as astereognosis.

Coordination and Cerebellar Function

- Hold up your finger and ask the patient to touch it and then touch his nose; have the patient continue this action as you move your fingers to different areas. Do this point-to-point testing with both arms of the patient, and note uneven, jerking movements and the inability to touch your finger or his nose.
- To test coordination in the lower extremity, have the patient lie down and run the heel of one foot against the shin of the other leg.
- Test the ability to make rapid alternating movements by having the patient rapidly tap his or her index finger on the thigh or a table surface.
- Tandem walking, in which the patient walks heal to toe as though walking a tightrope, also tests coordination; patients with arthritic deformities may not be able to perform this test. Have weak or poorly coordinated patients hold your hand during the tandem walking test.

Reflexes

Nurses can perform some tests of reflexes:

- To test the corneal reflex, gently touch the cornea with a wisp of clean cotton. Tissue and gauze are too rough and can cause corneal abrasions. Normally, the eye should blink.
- Test the Babinski reflex (i.e., plantar response) by stroking the sole of the patient's foot. Normally, the toes should flex; an abnormal response is extension and fanning of the toes.

Additional Tests

Each of the cranial nerves can be tested to identify further problems. Lumbar puncture, cerebral angiography, pneumoencephalography, and computed tomography scans are among other screening devices used to evaluate neurologic problems. A review of mental status is included in the assessment of the nervous system. (For information on mental status examination, refer to Chapter 32.)

NURSING DIAGNOSIS

TABLE 25-1 — Nursing Diagnoses Related to Neurologic Problems

Causes or Contributing Factors	Nursing Diagnosis
Impaired sensory or motor function, fatigue, pain, depression, need for equipment or aids that use energy	Activity Intolerance
Altered self-concept, inability to communicate, dependency	Anxiety
Inability to sense signal, lack of motor control, immobility	Constipation
Poor positioning, pressure on brain, neuritis	Acute Pain
Dysphasia, dysarthria, altered mental status	Impaired Verbal Communication
Altered body structure or function, dependency	Ineffective Coping
Demands, dependency, and role changes due to patient's illness	Interrupted Family Processes
Altered body structure and function, dependency	Disturbed Body Image
Loss of function, lifestyle change	Grieving
Dependency, disability, altered self-concept	Self-Neglect
Disability, dependency, pain, impaired mental status	Impaired Home Maintenance
Immobility, lack of sensation	Risk for Infection
Impaired sensory function, fatigue, altered mental status, improper use of aids, altered mobility or coordination	Risk for Injury
Paralysis, weakness, vertigo, poor coordination	Impaired Physical Mobility
Swallowing disorder, inability to feed self or express desires, depression, altered taste, anorexia	Imbalanced Nutrition: Less Than Body Requirements
Inability to provide adequate oral hygiene	Impaired Oral Mucous Membrane
Dependency, disability, impaired communication, role change	Powerlessness

(Continues)

NURSING DIAGNOSIS (Continued)

| TABLE 25-1 | Nursing Diagnoses Related to Neurologic Problems |

Causes or Contributing Factors	Nursing Diagnosis
Weakness, paralysis, poor coordination, visual disorders	Bathing/Dressing/Feeding/Toileting Self-Care Deficit
Altered body structure or function, dependency, role change	Chronic Low Self-Esteem
Decreased or lost sensory function, cerebral vascular accident, sensory deprivation	Risk for Falls, Risk for Injury
Impaired nerve supply, disability, altered self-image, depression	Ineffective Sexual Patterns
Altered ability to feel pressure or pain, immobility	Impaired Skin Integrity
Altered body structure or function, dysphasia, dysarthria, visual or hearing deficits, depression, altered self-concept	Impaired Social Interaction
Inability to communicate, disability, impaired mobility	Social Isolation
Cerebrovascular accident, depression, anxiety, fear, altered cerebral function	Risk for Acute Confusion, Acute Confusion, Chronic Confusion
Lack of sensory awareness to void or ability to control bladder emptying, inability to communicate needs or toilet self	Impaired Urinary Elimination

SELECTED NEUROLOGIC CONDITIONS

Selected neurologic conditions that nurses may see in older adults are discussed in the following sections. A discussion of Alzheimer's disease, a neurodegenerative condition, is provided in Chapter 33.

Parkinson's Disease

Parkinson's disease affects the ability of the central nervous system to control body movements. It occurs when neurons that produce dopamine in the substantia nigra die or become impaired. Dopamine is necessary for smooth motor movement and has a role in emotions. With the damage of a significant number of these dopamine-producing cells, the symptoms of Parkinson's disease appear.

Parkinson's disease is more common in men and occurs most frequently after the fifth decade of life. The incidence rises with age, although most cases have been diagnosed by the time people reach their seventh decade of life. Although its exact cause is unknown, this disease is thought to be associated with a history of exposure to toxins, encephalitis, and cerebrovascular disease, especially arteriosclerosis. A finding in people with Parkinson's disease compared with individuals who have other causes of tremors is the presence of the Lewy body, an intracellular inclusion body, in the brain. The death of substantia nigra cells within the basal ganglia leads to a significant reduction in dopamine, which is responsible for the symptoms.

A faint tremor in the hands or feet that progresses over a long time may be the first clue to Parkinson's disease (Fig. 25-1). The tremor is reduced when the patient attempts a purposeful movement.

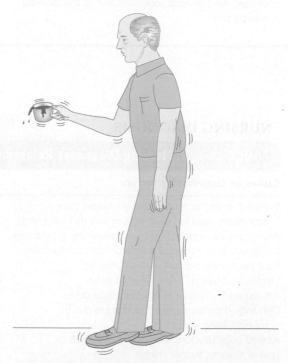

FIGURE 25-1 ■ Tremors and shuffling gait are characteristic of Parkinson's disease.

Muscle rigidity and weakness develop, evidenced by drooling, difficulty in swallowing, slow speech, and a monotone voice. The patient's face assumes a mask-like appearance, and the skin is moist. Bradykinesia (slow movement) and poor balance occur. Appetite frequently increases, and the person may demonstrate emotional instability. A characteristic sign is a shuffling gait while leaning forward at the trunk.

The rate of movement increases as the patient walks, and the patient may not be able to voluntarily stop walking. As the disease progresses, the patient may become entirely unable to ambulate. Secondary symptoms include depression, sleep disturbances, dementia, forced eyelid closure, drooling, dysphagia, constipation, shortness of breath, urinary hesitancy, urgency, and reduced interest in sex.

A variety of measures are used to control the tremors and maintain the highest possible level of independence. Anticholinergics may be prescribed to decrease the patient's symptoms. Nurses need to be aware that anticholinergics can exacerbate glaucoma, warranting close monitoring of the condition when it is present. Also, anticholinergics can cause temporary anuria. Close monitoring during drug therapy is important. While they are taking levodopa, patients should avoid foods that are high in vitamin B6, such as avocados, lentils, and lima beans, because they will counteract the drug; dietary restrictions are not necessary if the patient is taking carbidopa–levodopa (Sinemet). Technology to control symptoms, such as pulse generators that send electrical impulses that block tremor-causing brain signals, drug infusion systems, and gene therapy, may benefit some people who have Parkinson's disease (Aebischer & Pralog, 2003; Senatus et al., 2004); the neurologist should be consulted regarding the potential usefulness to the patient.

Active and passive range-of-motion exercises maintain and improve joint mobility; warm baths and massage may facilitate these exercises and relieve muscle spasms caused by rigidity. Contractures are a particular risk of older persons with Parkinson's disease. Physical and occupational therapists should be actively involved in the exercise program to help the patient find devices that increase self-care ability. Surgical intervention is rare for older patients because they do not tend to respond well.

Tension and frustration will aggravate the patient's symptoms; therefore, it is important for the nurse to offer psychological support and minimize emotional upsets. Teaching helps patients and their families gain realistic insight into the disease. The nurse should emphasize that the disease progresses slowly and that therapy can minimize the disability. Although intellectual functioning may be impaired as the disease progresses, the person with Parkinson's disease cannot be assumed to be cognitively impaired; it is important that others do not underestimate the mental abilities of the patient due to the speech problems and helpless appearance, as this can be extremely frustrating and degrading to the patient, who may react by becoming depressed or irritable. Continuing support by the nurse can help the family maximize the patient's mental capacity and understand personality changes that may occur. Communication and mental stimulation should be encouraged on a level that the patient always enjoyed.

As the disease progresses, the patient requires increased assistance. Skillful nursing assessment is essential to ensure that the demands for assistance are met while the maximum level of patient independence is preserved. The nurse should also assess family caregivers for stress and fatigue.

Transient Ischemic Attacks

Transient ischemic attacks (TIAs) are temporary or intermittent neurological events that can result from any situation that reduces cerebral circulation. Hyperextension and flexion of the head, such as when an individual falls asleep in a chair, can impair cerebral blood flow. Reduced blood pressure resulting from anemia and certain drugs (e.g., diuretics and antihypertensives) and cigarette smoking, due to its vasoconstrictive effect, will also decrease cerebral circulation, as will sudden standing from a prone position. Hemiparesis, hemianesthesia, aphasia, unilateral loss of vision, diplopia, vertigo, nausea, vomiting, and dysphagia are among the manifestations of a TIA, depending on the location of the ischemic area. These signs can last from minutes to hours, and complete recovery is usual within a day. Treatment may consist of correction of the underlying cause, anticoagulant therapy, or vascular reconstruction. A significant concern regarding TIAs is that they increase the patient's risk of sustaining a cerebrovascular accident (CVA).

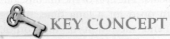

KEY CONCEPT

Good alignment and support of the head and neck can prevent hyperextension and flexion of the head that can lead to impaired cerebral blood flow.

Cerebrovascular Accidents

CVAs are the third leading cause of death and a major cause of disability in older adults. Older persons with hypertension, severe arteriosclerosis, diabetes, gout, anemia, hypothyroidism, silent myocardial infarction, TIAs, and dehydration and those who smoke are among the high-risk candidates for a CVA. The major types of CVA are ischemic, usually resulting from a thrombus or embolus, and hemorrhagic, which can occur from a ruptured cerebral blood vessel. Most CVAs in older individuals are ischemic, caused by partial or complete cerebral thrombosis. Light-headedness, dizziness, headache, drop attack (feeling of being strongly and suddenly pulled to the ground), and memory and behavioral changes are some of the warning signs of a CVA. A drop attack is a fall caused by a complete muscular flaccidity in the legs but with no alteration in consciousness. Patients describing or demonstrating these symptoms should be referred for prompt medical evaluation. Because nurses are in a key position to first learn of these signs, they can be instrumental in helping the patient avoid disability or death from a stroke. CVAs can occur without warning, however, and show highly variable signs and symptoms, depending on the area of the brain affected. Major signs tend to include hemiplegia, aphasia, and hemianopsia.

Although older adults have a higher mortality rate from CVAs than the young, those who do survive have a good chance of recovery. Good nursing care can improve the patient's chance of survival and minimize the limitations that impair a full recovery. In the acute phase, nursing efforts have the following aims:

- Maintain a patent airway.
- Provide adequate nutrition and hydration.
- Monitor neurologic and vital signs.
- Prevent complications associated with immobility.

In addition, unconscious patients need good skin care and frequent turning because they are more susceptible to pressure ulcer formation. If an indwelling catheter is not being used, it is important for the nurse to examine the patient for indications of an overdistended bladder and promptly remedy the situation if it occurs. The eyes of the unconscious patient may remain open for a long time, risking drying, irritation, and ulceration of the cornea. Corneal damage can be prevented by eye irrigations with a sterile saline solution followed by the use of sterile mineral oil eye drops. Eye pads may be used to help keep the eyelids closed; these are changed daily and frequently checked to make sure the lids are actually closed. Regular mouth care and range-of-motion exercises are also standard measures.

POINT TO PONDER

How would your life and the lives of your family members be affected if you suffered a stroke?

When the patient regains consciousness and stabilizes, more active nursing efforts can focus on rehabilitation. It may be extremely difficult for patients to understand and participate in their rehabilitation because of speech, behavior, and memory problems. Although these problems vary depending on the

side of the brain affected, some general observations can be noted. Attention span is reduced, and long, complicated directions may be confusing. Memory for old events may be intact, whereas recent events or explanations are forgotten, a characteristic demonstrated by many older persons without a history of CVA. Patients may have difficulty transferring information from one situation to another. For example, they may be able to remember the steps in lifting from the bed to the wheelchair but be unable to apply the same principles in moving from the wheelchair to an armchair. Confusion, restlessness, and irritability may arise from sensory deprivation. Emotional lability may also be a problem. To minimize the limitations imposed by these problems, the nurse may find the following actions helpful:

- Talk to the patient during routine activities.
- Briefly explain the basics of what has occurred, the procedures being performed, and the activities to expect.
- Speak distinctly but do not shout.
- Devise an easy means of communication, such as a picture chart to which one can point.
- Minimize environmental noise, traffic, and clutter.
- Aim for consistency of those providing care and of care activities.
- Use objects familiar to patients (e.g., their own clothing and clock).
- Keep a calendar or sign in the room showing the day and date.
- Supply sensory stimulation through conversation, radio, television, wall decorations, and objects for patients to handle.
- Provide frequent positive feedback; even a minor task may be a major achievement for the patient.
- Expect and accept errors and failures.

General medical–surgical textbooks provide more detailed guidance in the care of patients who have suffered a stroke. Local chapters of the American Heart Association also provide much useful material for the nurse, the patient, and the family on the topic of stroke. Nursing Care Plan 25-1 outlines care plan considerations for the patient who is recovering from a stroke.

Nurses should also promote activities that reduce patients' risk of stroke. Managing hypertension is important in decreasing fatal and nonfatal strokes in older adults. Likewise, smoking cessation is helpful. Older persons who stop smoking could improve cerebral perfusion levels, which is an important measure in preventing strokes.

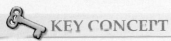

KEY CONCEPT

Controlling hypertension is important in reducing stroke risk in older adults.

GENERAL NURSING CONSIDERATIONS FOR NEUROLOGIC CONDITIONS

Promoting Independence

Older patients with neurologic conditions face limitations imposed by both the disease and the aging process. Skillful and creative nursing assistance can help patients achieve maximum levels of independence. Some assistive devices—such as rails in the hallways, grab bars in bathrooms, and numerous other household modifications—can extend the time that patients can live independently in the community. Periodic home visits by a nurse, regular contact with a family member or friend, and a daily call from a local telephone reassurance program can help the patient feel confident and protected, which promotes independence. Although these individuals may perform tasks awkwardly and slowly, family members need to understand that allowing independent function is physically and psychologically more beneficial than doing tasks for them. Continuing patience, reassurance, and encouragement are essential to maximize patients' capacities for independence.

Personality changes often accompany neurologic problems. Patients may become depressed as they realize their limitations and become frustrated by their need to be dependent on others. They may grieve loss of former roles and identities. Their reactions may be displaced and evidenced by irritability toward others, often their loved ones or immediate caregivers. Family members and caregivers may need help in understanding the reasons for this behavior and in learning effective ways of dealing with it. Getting offended or angry at such patients may only anger or frustrate them further. Understanding, patience, and tolerance are needed.

KEY CONCEPT

Caregivers should be prepared for the personality changes that often occur in individuals who have neurologic disorders; caregivers may benefit from nursing support also.

NURSING CARE PLAN 25-1

THE OLDER ADULT WITH A CEREBROVASCULAR ACCIDENT: CONVALESCENCE PERIOD

Nursing Diagnosis: (1) Self-Care Deficits related to sensory or motor impairment, visual deficits, fatigue, aphasia; (2) Activity Intolerance related to depression, poor motivation, prolonged immobility, fatigue

Goal	Nursing Actions
The patient progressively increases independence in activities of daily living (ADL).	■ Assess patient's independence–dependence in each of the ADL. ■ Assess cognition and emotional status; repeat monthly or whenever there is a change in physical or mental status. ■ Consult with the physical therapist (PT) and develop plans for exercises, transfer techniques, and mobility aids. ■ Consult with the occupational therapist and develop plans for measures to improve independence in ADL and adaptive or assistive equipment. ■ Ensure that the patient properly uses mobility aids and adaptive or assistive equipment. ■ Encourage the patient to use existing capabilities and recognize efforts to be independent. ■ Offer assistance with ADL as needed; ensure that caregivers provide adequate time for tasks to be performed by the patient when possible.

(Continues)

NURSING CARE PLAN 25-1 (Continued)

- Monitor nutritional status, intake, and output.
- Review patient's progress regularly with multidisciplinary team, patient, and family.

Nursing Diagnosis: Impaired Physical Mobility related to altered sensory and motor function

Goal	Nursing Actions
The patient is free from complications related to immobility; progressively increases independent mobility.	<ul><li>Determine the active and passive range of motion of every joint; reassess at least monthly.</li><li>Guide patient through range-of-motion exercises at least three times each day; provide assistance as needed.</li><li>Use isometric, resistance, muscle-setting exercises if possible.</li><li>Ensure that the patient is properly positioned and maintained in proper alignment.</li><li>Establish the amount of time patient can remain in one position before showing indications of pressure. To do this, check the patient's skin after he or she has been in the same position for half an hour; if no redness is noted, increase the amount of time the patient remains in position by half hour increments up to 2 hours. Develop a repositioning schedule based on the amount of time the patient has been assessed to be able to remain in a position without redness of tissues.</li><li>Instruct the patient to cough and deep breathe at least every 2 hours.</li><li>Encourage adequate fluid intake and a high-fiber intake, unless contraindicated.</li><li>Use massage, lotion, or protective padding as needed to protect skin integrity.</li><li>Assist the patient with proper use of mobility aids.</li><li>Consult with PT regarding ways to increase mobility.</li><li>Monitor progress and give feedback to patient.</li></ul>

Nursing Diagnoses: (1) Ineffective Role Performance related to loss of body function, physical changes, role changes; (2) Interrupted Family Process related to changes in function, dependency on family for caregiving, ineffective coping

Goal	Nursing Actions
The patient expresses acceptance of altered lifestyle and functions; develops or maintains satisfying interactions with family.	<ul><li>Interview patient and family to identify patient's previous interests, roles, and functions; assess patient's ability or readiness to resume activities.</li><li>Identify and implement measures to enable patient to engage in previous interests, roles, and functions with modifications.</li><li>Acknowledge patient's frustrations with altered capabilities; encourage expression of feelings.</li><li>Encourage the patient to participate in family and social functions in community; assist patient and family in identifying measures and aids to facilitate activities.</li><li>Monitor patient's mood; intervene if problems are noted.</li><li>Confer with family regarding their feelings and needs; plan accordingly.</li></ul>

Mr. J, aged 68 years, experienced a cerebrovascular accident 1 week ago that left him with right-sided weakness, aphasia, and incontinence. His wife is eager to have him discharged from the hospital and to care for him at home. You have heard her state to Mr. J that he "needn't worry about a thing because she'll do everything that needs to be done and all he has to do is stay in bed and take it easy."

TI IINK CRITICALLY

- Based on the information provided, what problems Mr. and Mrs. J face?
- What goals for the care plan will help them address their needs?

Preventing Injury

Protecting older adults with a neurologic disorder from hazards is particularly important. Uncoordinated movements, weakness, and dizziness are among the problems that cause these patients to be at high risk for accidents. Whether in a health facility setting or the patient's own home in the community, the nurse should scrutinize the environment for potential sources of mishaps, such as loose carpeting, poorly lit stairwells, clutter, and ill-functioning appliances, as well as the lack of fire warning systems, fire escapes, tub rails, nonslip tub surfaces, or other safeguards. Safety considerations also include the prevention of contractures, pressure ulcers, and other risks to health and well-being. Allowing preventable complications to hamper progress and compound disability is an injustice to the patient.

BRINGING RESEARCH TO LIFE

TOTAL ANTIOXIDANT CAPACITY OF DIET AND RISK OF STROKE: A POPULATION-BASED PROSPECTIVE COHORT OF WOMEN

Rautiainen, S., Larrson, S., Virtamo, J. & Wolk, A. (2012). Stroke, 43(2):335–340.

The purpose of this study was to determine if total antioxidant capacity (a measurement of the ability of foods to reduce free radicals) has a role in reducing inflammation and oxidative stress, which could decrease stroke risk. Nearly 37,000 women completed questionnaires related to their diet. Information was also collected pertaining to their body mass index, smoking status, activity level, alcohol use, medical conditions, presence of cardiovascular disease, and history of stroke (as ascertained from hospital discharge records).

Women who consumed high amounts of fruits and vegetables, took vitamins, were better educated, and did not smoke had a lower risk of stroke. The researchers noted a significant inverse relationship between total antioxidant capacity and stroke, supporting the belief that a high-oxidant diet offers protection against stroke.

A diet rich in antioxidants has many health benefits and should be encouraged in persons of all ages to facilitate a healthy aging process and health in late life. In addition, the diets of older adults should be reviewed for intake of fruits and vegetables and teaching provided as needed as to strategies to increase antioxidant intake.

PRACTICE REALITIES

Sixty-three-year-old Ms. Trotta works in the billing department of the hospital where you are employed. One of her coworkers with whom you are friends shares that he is concerned that "something is going on with Ms. Trotta." He describes her as having developed a blank expression and monotone speech. When she picks up papers her hands shake considerably and she does not walk with the same bounce that she once did. He is uncomfortable discussing his observations with Ms. Trotta but is concerned for her health. He asks for your help.

Over the next few weeks you sit at the same lunch table as your friend and Ms. Trotta. You notice the symptoms your friend described and suspect there could be a neurologic problem. What would be an appropriate way to address your friend's concerns and help Ms. Trotta?

CRITICAL THINKING EXERCISES

1. Outline the content of a health education program to instruct older adults on practices that could reduce their risks of neurologic problems.
2. What factors will worsen the symptoms of the patient with Parkinson's disease? What suggestions could you give caregivers to promote maximum function of this patient?
3. What resources exist in your community to assist patients with Parkinson's disease, stroke, or other neurologic disorders?

RESOURCES

American Heart Association Stroke Connection
http://www.strokeassociation.org

American Parkinson Disease Association
http://www.apdaparkinson.org

Epilepsy Foundation of America
http://www.efa.org

Michael J. Fox Foundation for Parkinson's Research
http://www.michaeljfox.org

National Institute of Neurological Disorders and Stroke
http://www.ninds.nih.gov

National Multiple Sclerosis Society
http://www.nmss.org

National Parkinson Foundation
http://www.parkinson.org

National Stroke Association
http://www.stroke.org

Paralyzed Veterans of America
http://www.pva.org

Parkinson Alliance
http://www.parkinsonalliance.org

Parkinson's Action Network (PAN)
http://www.parkinsonsaction.org

Parkinson's Disease Foundation (PDF)
http://www.pdf.org

Parkinson's Institute
http://www.thepi.org

Parkinson's Resource Organization
http://www.parkinsonsresource.org

WE MOVE (Worldwide Education & Awareness for Movement Disorders)
http://www.wemove.org

REFERENCES

Aebischer, P., & Pralog, W. (2003). Gene therapy approaches for Parkinson's disease. *Journal of Neurochemistry, 85* (6 Suppl 2), 8.

Senatus, P. B., McClelland, S. 3rd, Ferris, A. D., Ford, B., Winfield, L. M., Pullman, S. L., Goodman, R. R., et al. (2004). Implantation of bilateral deep brain stimulators in patients with Parkinson disease and preexisting cardiac pacemakers. Report of two cases. *Journal of Neurology, 101*(6), 1073–1077.

RECOMMENDED READINGS

Recommended Readings associated with this chapter can be found on the web site that accompanies the book. Visit http://thepoint.lww.com/Eliopoulos8e to access the recommended readings and other additional resources associated with this chapter.

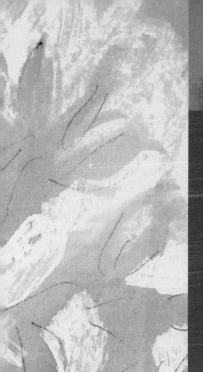

Sensation

LEARNING OBJECTIVES

After reading this chapter, you should be able to:

1 Explain the importance of sensory function and the impact of sensory deficits on older adults.

2 Describe the effects of aging on sensory function.

3 List measures to promote healthy sensory function in older adults.

4 Identify signs of and nursing interventions for older adults with cataracts, glaucoma, macular degeneration, detached retina, corneal ulcers, and hearing impairment.

TERMS TO KNOW

Cataract: clouding of crystalline lens of eye

Glaucoma: eye disease involving increased intraocular pressure

Macular degeneration: loss of central vision due to the development of drusen deposits in the retinal pigmented epithelium

Presbycusis: age-related high-frequency sensorineural hearing loss

Presbyopia: age-related decrease in eye's ability to change the shape of lens to focus on near objects

Good sensory function is an extremely valuable asset that is often taken for granted. For instance, people are better able to protect themselves from harm when they can see, hear, smell, touch, and communicate. The reduced ability to protect oneself from hazards because of sensory deficits can result in serious falls from unseen obstacles, missed alarms and warnings, ingestion of hazardous substances from not recognizing bad tastes, an inability to detect the odor of smoke or gas, and burns and skin breakdown because of decreased cutaneous sensation of excessive temperature and pressure.

Intact senses also facilitate accurate perception of the environment. When sensory function is impaired, perception of the environment is distorted (e.g., people might suspect they are being talked about if they are unable to hear the conversation of those around them). Impaired sensory function affects everyday experiences. For example, poor eyesight can hamper reading the newspaper and recognizing a familiar face on the street. Food tastes bland without properly functioning taste buds. The pleasant experience of smelling freshly cut flowers is lost when olfactory functioning is poor.

Finally, sensory function is essential to communication. Social interaction, the sharing of experiences, and the exchange of feelings are more complete when all the senses can participate. Through communication, people share joys and burdens, derive feelings of normalcy, validate perceptions, and maintain a link with reality.

POINT TO PONDER

How would being blind or deaf affect your daily life? What reactions do you think you would experience?

A variety of intrinsic and extrinsic factors, including alterations during the aging process, excessive use and abuse of certain medications, and the disease processes that affect all age groups, contribute to the sensory problems of older adults. Sensory deficits compound other problems that threaten the health, well-being, and independence of older persons—their increased vulnerability to accidents, their social isolation and declining physical function, and many other limitations regarding self-care activities. Gerontological nurses must be aware of the factors that influence sensory function in older adults and help to ensure that sensory problems are properly evaluated and corrected when possible.

EFFECTS OF AGING ON SENSORY FUNCTION

One of the most significant areas of changes that occur with age is that affecting vision. The reduced elasticity and stiffening of the muscle fibers of the lens of the eye that begins in the fourth decade

of life interferes with the ability to adequately focus and is the factor responsible for most older people requiring some form of corrective lenses; this condition is known as *presbyopia*. Visual acuity progressively declines due to reduced pupil size, opacification of the lens and vitreous, and loss of photoreceptor cells in the retina. The light perception threshold decreases causing difficulty with vision at night and in dimly lit areas. Dark and light adaptation takes longer. Sensitivity to glare increases due to cataract formation. Visual changes cause depth perception to become distorted, making the ability to judge the height of walking surfaces more challenging. Visual fields become smaller reducing peripheral vision. The eyes produce fewer tears and are drier.

Approximately half of all individuals who are identified as legally blind each year are 65 years of age or older. Visual limitations can make communication problematic because facial expressions and gestures, which are as important as the words themselves, may be missed or misinterpreted. Lip reading to compensate for hearing deficits may be difficult, and written correspondence may be limited because independent reading and writing become almost impossible tasks. Remaining aware of current events through newspapers and socialization through playing cards and other games may be hampered.

Hearing changes are also common and may negatively impact communication. Presbycusis (age-related sensorineural hearing loss) reduces the ability to hear s, sh, f, ph, and w sounds and may cause speech to be inaudible or distorted, as can impacted cerumen, which is a common problem in older adults. Older people may be self-conscious of this limitation and avoid situations in which they must interact. In turn, others may avoid them because of this difficulty. Telephone conversations can be affected by this problem, limiting social contact even further for the individual who may be socially isolated for other reasons. Approximately 10% of the older population has some difficulty hearing telephone conversations. Assessing the underlying cause of a hearing problem through professional evaluation, including an audiometric examination, is the first step in the management or correction of the problem.

POINT TO PONDER

Cellular phones have widespread use. In what ways do you believe these have both facilitated and impaired communication?

In addition to the changes affecting vision and hearing, other sensations are also reduced with age. The number of functioning taste buds may be significantly decreased, especially those responsible for sweet and salty flavors. Pressure is not sensed as easily in late life. Age-related effects on tactile sensation may also be noted by the difficulty some older persons have in discriminating between temperatures. Some loss of olfactory function may be noted as well; this can also affect the ability to taste.

SENSORY HEALTH PROMOTION

Promoting Vision

Despite age-related changes, most older persons have sufficient visual capacity to meet normal self-care demands with the assistance of corrective lenses. Serious visual problems can develop, however, and should be recognized early to prevent significant visual damage. Routine and thorough eye examinations, including tonometry, by an ophthalmologist are important in detecting and treating eye problems early in older individuals. The nurse should stress the importance of an annual eye examination, to detect vision changes and needs not only for alterations in corrective lenses but also for early discovery of problems, such as cataracts, glaucoma, and other disease processes. The nurse must also evaluate the older adult's financial ability to afford an eye examination and glasses because health insurance seldom covers this important service; community resources or the negotiation of special payment plans may help older adults to acquire the necessary aid. Medicare may cover eye examinations for people who have or are at risk for certain conditions.

In addition to annual eye examinations, prompt evaluation is required for any symptom that could indicate a visual problem, including burning or pain in the eye, blurred or double vision, redness of the conjunctiva, spots, headaches, and any other change in vision. The nurse should review the diet to ensure an adequate intake of nutrients that promote good vision (Box 26-1). A variety of disorders can threaten the older individual's vision. For instance, arteriosclerosis and diabetes can cause damage to the retina, and nutritional deficiencies and hypertension can result in visual impairment. Refer to the sections of this book that describe these diseases to understand the pathophysiology involved.

Promoting Hearing

Gerontological nurses have a responsibility to help aging persons protect and preserve their hearing as well. Some hearing deficits in old age can be avoided by good care of the ears throughout the life. Such care should include prompt and complete treatment of ear infections, prevention of trauma to the ear (e.g., from a severe blow or a foreign object in the ear), and regular audiometric examinations.

The nurse should examine an older adult's ears frequently for cerumen accumulation. Cerumen removal can be aided by gentle irrigation of the external auditory canal with warm water or a hydrogen peroxide and water solution; commercial preparations are also available. A forceful stream of solution should not be used during this procedure because it can cause perforation of the eardrum. It is wise for older persons to have assistance when irrigating ears because dizziness often occurs during the procedure. Even allowing water to run in the ears during showers or shampoos can aid in loosening cerumen. Avoid the use of cotton-tipped applicators for cerumen removal, because they can push the cerumen back into the ear canal and cause an impaction. Hairpins or similar devices should never be used.

| **BOX 26-1** | **Nutrients Beneficial to Vision** |

Zinc: Promotes normal visual capacity and adaptation to dark; supplementation can reduce visual loss in macular degeneration; deficiency can facilitate cataract development.

Selenium: May aid in preventing cataracts; supplementation with vitamin E can reduce visual loss in macular degeneration.

Vitamin C: Promotes normal vision; supplementation may improve vision in persons with cataracts.

Vitamin A: Maintains healthy rods and cones in retina.

Vitamin E: May aid in preventing cataracts; supplementation in large doses can prevent macular degeneration.

Riboflavin: Aids in preventing cataracts.

Ginkgo biloba: May prevent degenerative changes in eye.

Flavonoid: Improves night vision and adaptation to dark; promotes visual acuity; improves capillary integrity to reduce hemorrhage risk in diabetic retinopathy.

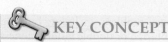

KEY CONCEPT

Ear irrigations can help to remove cerumen accumulations; however, care must be taken to protect the older person from the potential dizziness associated with this procedure.

In addition, it is beneficial for nurses to provide health education about the effects of environmental noise on hearing and general health. Protection from exposure to loud noises, such as those associated with factory and construction work, vehicles, loud music or drums, and explosions is important throughout the life; earplugs or other sound-reducing devices should be used when exposure is unavoidable. Nurses can take an active role in advocating legislation to control noise pollution and the enforcement of that legislation.

Assessing Problems

Because it is the rare older individual who does not suffer from some sensory deficit, it behooves the nurse working with older adults to be skilled in assessing sensory function (Assessment Guide 26-1); to ensure that sensory problems are properly evaluated; and to implement associated assistive techniques to promote maximum sensory functioning. Nursing Diagnosis Table 26-1 lists some of the nursing diagnoses associated with sensory deficits.

ASSESSMENT GUIDE 26-1

SENSORY FUNCTION

GENERAL OBSERVATIONS

During interactions with the patient, note the signs of hearing deficits such as missed communication, requests to have words repeated, reliance on lip reading, and cocking of the head to one side in an effort to hear better. Identify eye problems by noticing if the patient uses eyeglasses, demonstrates difficulty seeing (e.g., bumping into objects and unable to see small print), or possesses eye abnormalities such as drooping eyelids, discolored sclera, excess tearing, discharge, and unusual movements of the eyes. Foul odors (e.g., associated with incontinence or vaginitis) that do not seem to bother the patient could reflect diminished olfactory function; cigarette burns on finger or unrecognized pressure ulcers may indicate that the patient has reduced ability to sense pressure and pain.

INTERVIEW

- Ask the patient about the date and type of the last ophthalmic and audiometric examinations (e.g., Where was the examination done? Was an ophthalmologist or optometrist seen? Did the eye examination include tonometry? Was a full audiometric evaluation or basic hearing screening done?).

- If eyeglasses or hearing aids are used, ask questions about where, when, and how these appliances were obtained (e.g., reading glasses purchased from the local pharmacy versus prescription glasses; hearing aid obtained via television advertisement).

- Ask questions such as the following to disclose the presence of sensory problems:
  - "Has there been any change in your vision? Please describe."
  - "Are your glasses as useful to you as they were when you first obtained them?"
  - "Do you experience pain, burning, or itching in the eyes?"
  - "Do you ever see spots floating across your eyes? How often does this happen and how large and numerous are the spots?"
  - "Do you ever see flashes of light or halos?"
  - "Are your eyes ever unusually dry or watery?"
  - "Do you have difficulty with vision at night, in dimly lit areas, or in bright areas?"
  - "Does anyone in your family have glaucoma or other eye problems?"
  - "Have you noticed any change in your ability to hear? Please describe."
  - "Are certain sounds more difficult for you to hear than others?"
  - "Do you ever experience pain, itching, ringing, or a sense of fullness in your ears?"
  - "Do your ears accumulate a lot of wax? How do you manage this?"
  - "Is there ever drainage from your ears?"

- "Is your sense of smell as keen as it was in earlier years? Describe any differences."
- "Do you have any problems or have you noticed changes in your ability to feel pain, pressure, or different temperatures?"

PHYSICAL EXAMINATION

Eyes

- Inspect the eyes for unusual structure, drooping eyelids, discoloration, and abnormal movement. Loss of elasticity around the eyes, indicated by bags, is a common finding. Black-skinned persons may normally have a slight yellow discoloration of the sclera. Note any lesions on the eyelids.

- Palpation of the eyeballs with the eyelids closed can reveal hard-feeling eyes with extremely elevated intraocular pressure and spongy-feeling eyes with fluid volume deficits.

- Perform a gross evaluation of visual acuity by having the patient read a Snellen chart or various sized lettering on a newspaper. If the patient is unable to see letters on the chart or newspaper, estimate the extent of the visual limitation by determining if the patient is able to see fingers held up before him or can merely make out figures.

- To perform a gross test of the visual field, have the patient focus straight ahead. While facing the patient, bring your finger into the field of view. Note when the patient indicates seeing your finger compared with when you are able to see it. If the patient has restrictions in seeing all portions of the visual field, review the exact nature of this problem. A blind spot in the visual field (i.e., scotoma) can occur with macular degeneration, a narrowing of the peripheral field may be associated with

glaucoma, and blindness in the same half of both eyes (i.e., homonymous hemianopia) can be present in persons who have experienced a cerebrovascular accident.

- Test extraocular movements by having the patient follow your finger as you move it to various points, horizontally and vertically. Irregular, jerking eye movements can result from disturbances in cranial nerves III, IV, or VI.

Ears

- Inspection of the ears usually shows cerumen accumulation, increased hair growth, and atrophy of the tympanic membrane, which causes it to appear white or gray.

- Cerumen impactions should be noted and removed.

- A small, crusted, ulcerated lesion on the pinna can be a sign of basal or squamous cell carcinoma.

- Perform a gross evaluation of hearing by determining the patient's ability to hear a watch ticking. Check both ears.

- Weber and Rinne tests can be performed to assess sounds at different frequencies. These tests involve placing a vibrating tuning fork next to the ear or against the skull, this will stimulate the inner ear to vibrate. The Rinne tuning fork test helps evaluate a patient's hearing ability by air conduction compared with that of bone conduction. The Weber tuning fork test helps determine a patient's hearing ability by bone conduction only, and this test is useful when hearing loss is asymmetrical.

- In addition to presbycusis and conductive hearing losses, ear or upper respiratory infections, ototoxic drugs, and diabetes can be responsible for diminishing hearing.

NURSING DIAGNOSIS

TABLE 26-1	Nursing Diagnoses Associated with Sensory Deficits

Causes or Contributing Factors	Nursing Diagnosis
Sensory deprivation or overload, impaired communication	Activity Intolerance
Impaired communication, altered self-concept, reduced ability to protect self	Anxiety
Acute glaucoma, corneal ulcer, detached retina	Acute Pain
Hearing deficit	Impaired Verbal Communication
Impaired vision or hearing	Deficient Diversional Activity
Visual deficits, inability to protect self	Impaired Home Maintenance
Reduced tactile sensations	Risk for Infection
Inability to see, hear, smell, or feel hazards	Risk for Injury

(Continue)

NURSING DIAGNOSIS (Continued)

TABLE 26-1	Nursing Diagnoses Associated with Sensory Deficits

Causes or Contributing Factors	Nursing Diagnosis
Inability to protect self, care for self, communicate	Powerlessness
Dependency, impaired interactions, altered self-concept	Disturbed Body Image
Impairment of any of the sensory organs	Disturbed Sensory Perception
Reduced tactile sensations	Impaired Skin Integrity
Misperception of environment	Disturbed Sleep Pattern
Visual or hearing deficits	Impaired Social Interaction
Visual or hearing deficits, frustration of patient or others in attempting to communicate	Social Isolation
Misperceptions or sensory deprivation due to altered sensory function	Risk for Acute Confusion
	Anxiety

SELECTED SENSORY CONDITIONS AND RELATED NURSING INTERVENTIONS

Visual Deficits

Cataracts

A cataract is a clouding of the lens or its capsule that causes the lens to lose its transparency. Cataracts are common in older people because everyone develops some degree of lens opacity with age. In fact, cataracts are the leading cause of low vision in older adults. Exposure to ultraviolet B increases the risk of developing cataracts, emphasizing the importance of wearing proper sunglasses to protect the eyes. Diabetes, cigarette smoking, high alcohol consumption, and eye injury are also contributing factors. Most older adults do have some degree of lens opacity with or without the presence of other eye disorders.

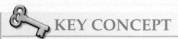 KEY CONCEPT

Everyone develops some degree of lens opacity with age, although it is more severe in persons who have had significant exposure to sunlight.

Symptoms No discomfort or pain is associated with cataracts. At first, visual acuity is not affected, but as opacification continues, vision is distorted, night vision is decreased, and objects appear blurred. People may have trouble seeing street signs while driving and feel that there is a film over the eye. Eventually, lens opacity and vision loss are complete. Glare from sunlight and bright lights is extremely bothersome to the affected person; this is due to the cloudy lens causing light to scatter

more than it would in a clear lens. Nuclear sclerosis develops, causing the lens of the eye to become yellow or yellow-brown; eventually the color of the pupil changes from black to a cloudy white. Some individuals may report an improvement in the ability to see small print and objects ("second sight"), which is due to changes in the lens that increase nearsightedness.

Treatment and Cataract Surgery Although surgery to remove the lens is the only cure for a cataract, cataracts affect people differently. Therefore, the need for surgery must be assessed based on an individual's unique situation. Patients with a single cataract may not necessarily undergo surgery if vision in the other eye is good, and these individuals should concentrate on strengthening their existing visual capacity, reducing their limitations, and using the safety measures applicable to any visually impaired person (Box 26-2). Sunglasses, sheer curtains over windows, furniture placed away from bright light, and several soft lights instead of a single bright light source minimize annoyance from glare. It is beneficial to place items within the visual field of the unaffected eye, a consideration when preparing a food tray and arranging furniture and frequently used objects. Regular evaluations of the patient by an ophthalmologist are essential to detect changes or a new problem in the unaffected eye.

For most patients, surgery improves vision. Cataract surgery is an outpatient procedure and older people usually withstand it well. Gerontological nurses are in a position to reassure older patients and their families that age is no deterrent to cataract surgery. Patients typically can resume nonstrenuous activities within a day. The simple surgical procedure and several weeks of rehabilitation can result

BOX 26-2 **Measures to Compensate for Visual Deficits in Older Adults**

- Face the person when speaking.
- Use several soft indirect lights instead of a single glaring one.
- Avoid glare from windows by using sheer curtains or stained windows.
- Use large print reading material.
- Place frequently used items within the visual field.

- Avoid the use of low-tone colors and attempt to use bright ones.
- Use contrasting colors on doorways and stairs and for changes in levels.
- Identify personal belongings and differentiate the room and wheelchair with a unique design rather than by letters or numbers.

in years of improved vision and, consequently, a life of higher quality. Two types of surgical procedures are used for removing the lens. Intracapsular extraction is the surgical procedure of choice for the older patient with cataracts and consists of removing the lens and the capsule. Extracapsular extraction is a simple surgical procedure in which the lens is removed and the posterior capsule is left in place. A common problem with extracapsular extraction is that a secondary membrane may form, requiring an additional procedure for discission of the membrane.

The most common method of replacing the surgically removed lens is the insertion of an intraocular lens at the time of cataract surgery. For older patients, this method has been more successful than adjusting to a contact lens or special cataract glasses. The intraocular lens tends to distort vision less than cataract glasses do and does not require the care of a contact lens. Some patients do develop complications with a lens implant, such as eye infection, loss of vitreous humor, and slipping of the implant.

Glaucoma

Glaucoma is a degenerative eye disease in which the optic nerve is damaged from an above-normal intraocular pressure (IOP). It ranks after cataracts as a major eye problem in older persons and is the second leading cause of blindness in this population, accounting for 10% of all blindness in the United States. Glaucoma tends to occur in people over age 40 and increases in prevalence with age. African-American individuals tend to develop glaucoma at earlier ages than whites and have a significantly higher incidence; women are affected more than men in all groups. Although the exact cause is unknown, glaucoma can be associated with increased size of the lens, iritis, allergy, endocrine imbalance, emotional instability, and a family history of this disorder. Drugs with anticholinergic properties can exacerbate glaucoma due to their

effects of dilating the pupil. An increase in IOP occurs rapidly in acute glaucoma and gradually in chronic glaucoma.

Acute Glaucoma With acute glaucoma, also called closed-angle or narrow-angle glaucoma, the patient experiences severe eye pain, headache, nausea, and vomiting. In addition to the rapid increased tension within the eyeball, edema of the ciliary body and dilation of the pupil occur. Vision becomes blurred, and blindness will result if this problem is not corrected within a day, emphasizing that this is a medical emergency demanding prompt attention. The ophthalmologist will examine the eye with an ophthalmoscope and conduct a visual field test (perimetry). Diagnosis is confirmed by placing a tonometer on the anesthetized cornea to measure IOP (Fig. 26-1). The normal pressure is within 20 mm Hg. A reading between 20 and 25 mm Hg is considered potential glaucoma. Another diagnostic test (i.e., gonioscopy) uses a contact lens and a binocular microscope to allow direct examination of the anterior chamber and differentiate closed-angle from open-angle glaucoma. In the past, if IOP did not decline within 24 hours, surgical intervention would be necessary. However, medications are now effective in treating the acute attack (e.g., carbonic anhydrase inhibitors, which reduce the formation of aqueous solution; mannitol, urea, and glycerin, which reduce fluid because of their ability to increase osmotic tension in the circulating blood). An iridectomy may be performed after the acute attack to prevent future episodes of acute glaucoma.

Chronic Glaucoma Chronic, or open-angle, glaucoma is more common than acute glaucoma. It often occurs so gradually that affected individuals are unaware that they have a visual problem. Peripheral vision becomes slowly but increasingly impaired so that people may not realize for a long time why they bump or knock over items

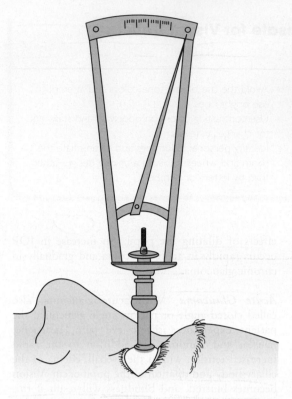

FIGURE 26-1 ■ Measuring intraocular pressure by the use of a tonometer.

at their side. They may need to change eyeglasses frequently. As the impairment progresses, central vision is affected. People may complain of a tired feeling in their eyes, headaches, misty vision, or seeing halos around lights—symptoms that tend to be more pronounced in the morning. The cornea may have a cloudy appearance, and the iris may be fixed and dilated. Although this condition usually involves one eye, both eyes can become affected if treatment is not sought. The same procedures as mentioned with acute glaucoma are used to diagnose this problem. Treatment, aimed toward reducing the IOP, may consist of a combination of a miotic and a carbonic anhydrase inhibitor or of surgery to establish a channel to filter the aqueous fluid (e.g., iridectomy, iridencleisis, cyclodialysis, and corneoscleral trephining).

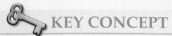

KEY CONCEPT

Open-angle glaucoma, the most common form of the disease, can be asymptomatic until an advanced stage; therefore, glaucoma screening is important.

Care and Prevention of Complications Vision lost due to glaucoma cannot be restored. However, additional damage can be prevented by avoiding any situation or activity that increases IOP. Physical straining and emotional stress should be prevented. Miotics may be instilled into the eye; acetazolamide may be used. Mydriatics, stimulants, and agents that elevate the blood pressure must not be administered. It may benefit patients to carry a card or wear a bracelet indicating their problem to prevent administration of these medications in situations in which they may be unconscious or otherwise unable to communicate. Abuse and overuse of the eyes must also be prevented. Periodic evaluation by an ophthalmologist is an essential part of the continued care of the patient with glaucoma.

Patient compliance with treatment for glaucoma can be challenging. The silent nature of this condition, difficulties with instilling eyedrops, and the cost of medications contribute to a lack of adherence to the plan of care. Nurses need to teach patients about the disease and its care and counsel them about the importance of compliance. The care plan for these patients needs to include ongoing reinforcement of self-care measures for disease management. Nursing Care Plan 26-1 presents a sample care plan for the patient with open-angle glaucoma.

NURSING CARE PLAN 26-1

THE OLDER ADULT WITH OPEN-ANGLE GLAUCOMA

Nursing Diagnosis: Deficient Knowledge related to management of disease

Goals	Nursing Actions
The patient expresses knowledge of facts about glaucoma and related care; administers eye drops correctly.	■ Assess patient's knowledge about disease in relation to what it is, the care required, symptoms to note and report, and precautions.

- Clarify misunderstandings and provide instruction as necessary.
- Ensure that the patient understands the importance of regular administration of eye drops.
- Evaluate patient's ability to manipulate dropper and instill drops (particularly in cases of arthritic hands). Instruct as necessary. If the patient is unable to independently use dropper and instill drops, determine the ability of family member to assist and provide instruction to family member.
- Instruct the patient to discuss any asthma condition with the physician as pilocarpine hydrochloride should be used with caution in persons with asthma.
- Reinforce importance of patient sharing complete medical history with every health care provider with whom he or she has contact.
- Prepare the patient for side effects from pilocarpine hydrochloride, such as blurring of vision for 1 to 2 hours after administration; review related safety considerations.
- Teach the patient to avoid situations that can increase intraocular pressure, such as aggressive coughing, sneezing, and straining during defecation.
- Advise the patient to avoid self-medication for treatment of colds because cold remedies can contain mydriatic agents that can increase intraocular pressure.
- Discuss the chronic nature of glaucoma and the need for lifetime administration of medications and attention to precautions and recognition of symptoms that should be reported. Reinforce that although lost vision cannot be restored, additional loss usually can be avoided with control of the disease.

Nursing Diagnosis: Risk for Injury related to impaired vision and risks associated with glaucoma

Goals	Nursing Actions
The patient is free from injury related to impaired vision; uses preventive measures to avoid complications associated with glaucoma.	- Explain the impact of reduced peripheral vision and related safety precautions, such as placing frequently used objects in visual field, keeping clutter off floor, turning head to fully see objects to the side, avoiding driving. - Instruct the patient to avoid situations that could damage vision by increasing intraocular pressure, such as aggressive coughing, sneezing, straining to have a bowel movement, strenuous exercise, and emotional stress. - Encourage the patient to keep bathroom and hallways well lit because vision may be impaired at night or in dimly lit areas as a result of pilocarpine hydrochloride use. - Advise the patient to avoid activities for several hours following administration of eye drops to accommodate blurred vision that could occur during this time. - Assist the patient in obtaining medical identification bracelet to assure others are informed of his or her condition in the event he or she is unable to communicate.

(Continues)

NURSING CARE PLAN 26-1 (Continued)

Nursing Diagnoses: Anxiety and Fear related to loss of vision

Goal	Nursing Actions
The patient lives a satisfying lifestyle with effective management of disease; is free from anxiety and fear.	■ Encourage the patient to express feelings regarding loss of vision and impact on function. Listen and offer support. ■ Clarify misconceptions; offer realistic explanations. ■ Determine activities that are important to patient and those that are at risk of being threatened by condition. Develop strategies to preserve and promote these activities. ■ Assist the patient in locating resources that can promote function, independence, and enjoyment. Contact local offices of agencies for the visually impaired for assistance.

Nursing Diagnosis: Constipation

Goal	Nursing Actions
The patient eliminates feces without straining at least every 2 to 3 days.	■ Assess bowel elimination pattern; if no problem exists, reinforce current practices; if constipation is a problem, initiate measures to promote regular bowel elimination, such as increasing fiber in diet, establishing regular time for bowel elimination, and using stool softener to avoid increases in intraocular pressure that can occur when straining with a bowel movement.

Macular Degeneration

Macular degeneration, the most common cause of blindness in people over age 65, involves damage or breakdown of the macula, which results in a loss of central vision. The most common form is involutional macular degeneration, which is associated with the aging process, although macular degeneration can also result from injury, infection, or exudative macular degeneration. Figure 26-2 compares vision loss experienced with cataracts, glaucoma, and macular degeneration.

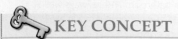

KEY CONCEPT

A loss of central vision accompanies macular degeneration.

Routine ophthalmic examinations can identify macular degeneration and promote treatment that can prevent additional vision loss. Laser therapy has been used for the treatment of some forms of macular degeneration, but the involutional type does not respond well to this procedure.

Magnifying glasses, high-intensity reading lamps, and other aids can prove helpful to patients with this condition.

Detached Retina

Older persons may experience detachment of the retina, a forward displacement of the retina from its normal position against the choroid. The symptoms, which can be gradual or sudden, include the perception of spots moving across the eye, blurred vision, flashes of light, and the feeling that a coating is developing over the eye. Blank areas of vision progress to complete loss of vision. The severity of the symptoms depends on the degree of retinal detachment. There does not tend to be pain.

Prompt treatment is required to prevent continued damage and eventual blindness. Initial measures most likely to be prescribed, bed rest and the use of bilateral eye patches, can be frightening to the older patient, who may react with confusion and unusual behavior. The nurse should help the patient feel as secure as possible; frequent checks and communication, easy access to a call light or other means of assistance, and

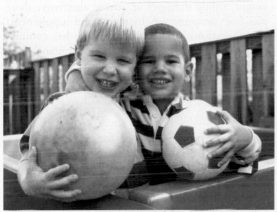
Normal vision

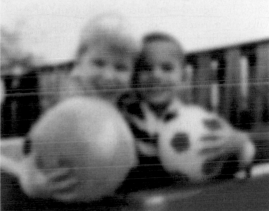
Cataracts

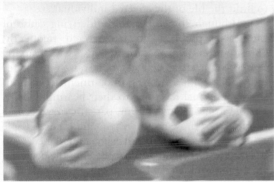
Macular degeneration

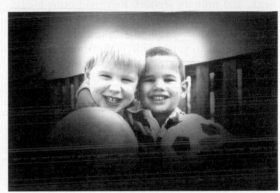
Glaucoma

FIGURE 26-2 ■ Examples of normal vision, vision with cataracts, vision with age-related macular degeneration, and vision with glaucoma. (Images courtesy of the National Eye Institute, National Institutes of Health.)

full, honest explanations will help provide a sense of well-being. After time has been allowed for the maximum amount of "reattachment" of the retina to occur, surgery may be planned. Several surgical techniques are used in the treatment of detached retinas. Electrodiathermy and cryosurgery cause the retina to adhere to its original attachment; scleral buckling and photocoagulation decrease the size of the vitreous space. Eye patches remain on the patient for several days after surgery. Specific routines vary according to the type of surgery performed. The patient needs frequent verbal stimuli to minimize anxiety and enhance psychological comfort. Physical and emotional stress must be avoided. Approximately 2 weeks after surgery, the success of the operation can be evaluated. A minority of patients must undergo a second procedure. It is important for the patient to understand that periodic examination is important, especially because some patients later suffer a detached retina in the other eye.

Corneal Ulcer

Inflammation of the cornea, accompanied by a loss of substance, causes the development of a corneal ulcer, a problem more common in older adults than in younger aged individuals. Febrile states, irritation, dietary deficiencies, lowered resistance, and cerebrovascular accident tend to predispose the individual to this problem. Corneal ulcers, which are extremely difficult to treat in older persons, may scar or perforate, leading to destruction of the cornea and blindness. The affected eye may appear bloodshot and show increased lacrimation. Pain and photophobia are also present.

Nurses should advise patients to seek prompt assistance for any irritation, suspected infection, or other difficulty with the cornea as soon as it is identified. Early care is often effective in preventing the development of a corneal ulcer and preserving visual capacity. Cycloplegics, sedatives, antibiotics, and heat may be prescribed to treat a corneal ulcer. Sunglasses will ease the discomfort associated with photophobia. It is important that the underlying cause be treated—an infection, abrasion, or presence of a foreign body. Corneal transplants are occasionally done for more advanced corneal ulcers.

Hearing Deficits

A significant number of older people, including a majority of those residing in nursing homes, have some degree of hearing loss, resulting from a variety of factors in addition to aging. Exposure to noise from loud music, jets, traffic, heavy machinery, and guns cause cell injury and loss. The higher incidence of hearing loss in men may be associated with their more frequent employment in occupations that subject them to loud noises (e.g., truck driving, construction work, heavy factory work, and military service). Recurrent otitis media and trauma can damage hearing. Certain drugs may be ototoxic, including aspirin, bumetanide, ethacrynic acid, furosemide, indomethacin, erythromycin, streptomycin, neomycin, karomycin, and Rauwolfia derivatives; the delayed excretion of these drugs in many older persons may promote this effect. Diabetes, tumors of the nasopharynx, hypothyroidism, syphilis, other disease processes, and psychogenic factors can also contribute to hearing impairment.

Particular problems affect the ears of the older person (Fig. 26-3). Vascular problems, viral infections, and presbycusis are often causes of inner ear damage. In otosclerosis, an osseous growth causes fixation of the footplate of the stapes in the oval window of the cochlea. This may be a middle ear problem; it is more common among women and can progress to complete deafness. Tinnitus, a ringing or other sound in the ear, can be associated with age-related hearing loss, ear injury, medications, or cardiovascular disease. If correcting the underlying problem does not eliminate the tinnitus, medications may be prescribed (e.g., tricyclic antidepressants,

gabapentin, and acamprosate); patients may be taught coping strategies or offered alternative therapies (e.g., acupuncture, hypnosis, and supplements) also. Infections of the middle ear are less common in older individuals; they usually accompany more serious disorders, such as tumors and diabetes. The external ear can be affected by dermatoses, furunculosis, cerumen impaction, cysts, and neoplasms.

Patient Care

The first action in caring for someone with a hearing deficit should be to encourage audiometric examination. Hearing impairment should not be assumed to be a normal consequence of aging and ignored. It would be most sad and negligent if the cause of the hearing problem was easily correctable (e.g., removal of cerumen or a cyst) but was allowed to limit the life of the affected individual.

Although sometimes the underlying cause of the hearing problem can be corrected, frequently, older persons must learn to live with varying degrees of hearing deficits. It is not unusual for individuals with a hearing impairment to demonstrate emotional reactions to their hearing deficits. Unable to hear conversation, patients may become suspicious of those around them and accuse people of talking about them. Anger, impatience, and frustration can result from repeatedly unsuccessful attempts to understand conversation. Patients may feel confused or react inappropriately on receiving distorted verbal communications. Limited ability to hear danger and protect themselves may make them feel insecure. Being self-conscious of their limitation may make them avoid social contact to escape embarrassment and frustration. Social isolation can be a serious threat; people sometimes avoid an older person with a hearing deficit because of the difficulty in communication. Physical, emotional, and social health can be seriously affected by this deficit. Helping older adults live with hearing deficits is a

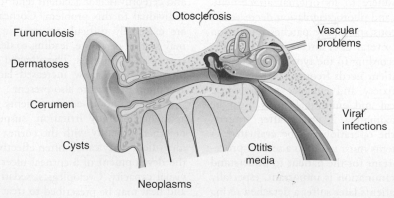

FIGURE 26-3 ■ Problems affecting the ears of older adults.

challenge but an important responsibility in gerontological care.

A neighbor should be alerted to the individual's hearing problem so that he or she can be protected in an emergency. In an institutional setting,
such patients should be located near the nurse's
station. People with hearing loss should be advised
to request explanations and instructions in writing
so that they receive the full content.

Hearing Aids

Hearing aids can benefit persons with some hearing
disorders, but they may not solve all hearing
problems. The otologist can determine if the specific hearing problem can be improved by using
a hearing aid and can recommend the particular
aid best suited to the patient's needs (Fig. 26-4). A
variety of styles of hearing aids are available, including in the ear, behind the ear, over the ear, and in the
ear canal. A hearing aid should never be purchased
without being specifically prescribed. Sometimes
older persons will attempt to improve hearing by
purchasing an aid through a private party or a mail-
order catalog, which often results in disappointment and a waste of money from an already limited
budget. The nurse is in a key position to educate the
older individual on the importance of consulting an
otologist before purchasing a hearing aid.

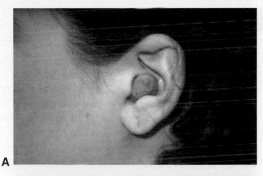

A

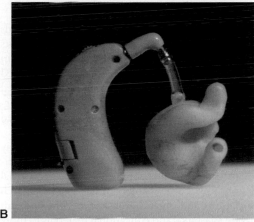

B

FIGURE 26-4 ■ Types of hearing aids. **A.** In-the-ear
model. **B.** Behind-the-ear model.

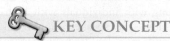

KEY CONCEPT

Nurses should advise patients to avoid purchasing a hearing aid without a complete audiometric
examination.

Patients must understand that, even with a
hearing aid, their problems will not be solved.
Although hearing will improve, it will not return
to normal. Speech may sound distorted through

the aid because when speech is amplified, so are all
environmental noises, which can be most uncomfortable and disturbing to the individual. Sounds
may be particularly annoying in areas where rever-
beration can easily occur (e.g., a church or large
hall). Some persons never make the adjustment
to a hearing aid and choose not to wear the appliance rather than to tolerate these disturbances and
distortions. New hearing aid users need support
during the adjustment phase and should be advised

CONSIDER THIS CASE

You meet Mr. and Mrs. R as you are providing influenza vaccines at a local senior center. When Mr. R does not
respond to your questions, his wife, in an impatient manner, tells you that her husband is not responding because
"he can't hear you and is too stubborn to get a hearing aid." Mr. R, sensing his wife's annoyance with him and
hearing a little of what she is saying comments, "I can hear; she just talks too low sometimes."

THINK CRITICALLY

- Although the time you can spend with the couple during this encounter is limited, you do want to help.
  What actions can you take? What referrals could you make?
- What quick facts about the importance of hearing screening and safety issues related to the inability to hear
  could you share?

BOX 26-3 | **Hearing Aid Care**

- Turn the aid off or remove the battery when the aid is not being worn. Store it in a safe, padded container.
- Clean the aid at least weekly. Wipe the aid off and use a toothpick, pipe cleaner, or pick that may have come with the aid to clean the channel. Do not use alcohol to clean the aid as this can cause

drying and cracking. Avoid having hairspray, gels, or other chemicals come in contact with the aid.
- Protect the aid from exposure to extreme heat (e.g., hair dryers), cold weather, or moisture.
- When changing the battery, turn off the aid first.
- Keep several new batteries available. Typically, a battery will last about 80 hours.

---

to wear the aid for progressively longer periods each day until comfort is gained and to avoid its use in noisy environments, such as airports, train stations, and stadiums. The aid must be checked regularly to ensure that the earpiece is not blocked with cerumen and that the battery is working. Some suggestions for hearing aid care are offered in Box 26-3.

When used appropriately, hearing aids may correct hearing problems and allow older individuals to maintain communication and social relationships. Local chapters of hearing and speech associations and organizations serving the deaf can provide assistance and educational materials to those affected by and interested in hearing problems.

GENERAL NURSING CONSIDERATIONS FOR SENSORY DEFICITS

To compensate for the multiple sensory deficits older persons may experience, special attention must be paid to stimulation of all the senses during routine daily activities. The diet can be planned to include a variety of flavors and colors. Perfumes, fresh flowers, and scented candles, safely used, can provide interesting fragrances. In an institutional setting, having a pot of fresh coffee brewing in the patients' area can provide a pleasant and familiar aroma during the early morning hours; likewise, a tabletop oven can allow for cookie baking and other cooking activities in the patients' area, providing a variety of stimuli. Different textures can be used in upholstery and clothing fabrics. Clocks that chime, music boxes, and wind chimes can vary environmental sounds. The design of facilities for older people should take into consideration the use of different shapes and colors. Intellectual stimulation, through conversation, music, and books, for instance, is also vital.

To compensate for visual limitations, one should face the individual and exaggerate gestures and facial expressions when speaking. To compensate for poor peripheral vision, which is common in

older people, one should approach these individuals from the front rather than the side where their vision is limited and ensure that seating allows for full sight of persons or objects with which they are interacting. Ample lighting is important and should be provided by several soft indirect lights rather than a single, bright, glaring source. Using large print games and playing cards and telephone dials with enlarged numbers that glow in the dark can promote interaction. Books and magazines with large print and recordings of current events and popular literature can provide a source of recreation and a means of keeping informed.

To compensate for a hearing problem that is not corrected by a hearing aid, efforts should be made to minimize the limitations caused by the deficit. When talking with individuals with high-frequency hearing loss, the speaker should talk slowly, distinctly, and in a low-frequency voice. Raising the voice or shouting will only raise the sounds to a higher frequency and compound the deficit. Methods for promoting more accurate and complete communication include talking into the less impaired ear, facing the individual when talking, using visual speech (e.g., sign language, gestures, and facial expressions), allowing the person to lip read, using a stethoscope to amplify sounds (speaking into the diaphragm while the earpieces are in the patient's ears), and using flash cards, work lists, and similar aids and devices. Cupping the hands over the less deficient ear and talking directly into the ear may also be helpful.

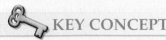

KEY CONCEPT

Shouting raises the frequency of the voice, potentially reducing what the older ear can hear.

Finally, touch is not only a means of sensory stimulation but also an expression of warmth and caring. Too frequently, the nurse may touch the patient only during specified procedures. It is easy for patients to begin to feel that others perceive them only in terms of tasks rather than as total human beings. How often are patients referred to as "a complete bath," "a dressing change," or "a feed?" How often are these labels nonverbally communicated when the nurse's only encounters with the patient are for the sake of these activities? Holding a hand, rubbing a cheek, and patting a shoulder, basic as they may seem, can convey a message to patients that they are still valued as unique human beings. Acceptance of the patient's efforts to touch is also important. The universal language of touch can often communicate a friendship, warmth, and caring that overcomes the most severe sensory deficit.

BRINING RESEARCH TO LIFE

VISUAL ACUITY'S ASSOCIATION WITH LEVELS OF LEISURE TIME PHYSICAL ACTIVITY IN COMMUNITY-DWELLING OLDER ADULTS

Swanson, M. W., Bodner, E., Sawyer, P., & Allman, R. M. (2012). Journal of Aging and Physical Activity, 20(1), 1–14.

As common as reduced vision is among older adults, little is understood about the effect of visual deficits on physical activity. This study examined the association of visual acuity level, self-reported vision, and ocular disease conditions with leisure time physical activity and calculated caloric expenditure in 911 community-based individuals aged 65 years and older who were part of the University of Alabama at Birmingham Study of Aging. A review of vision-related variables to weekly kilocalorie expenditure was calculated from the 17-item Leisure Time Physical Activity Questionnaire. Findings revealed that reduced visual acuity was associated with lower levels of physical activity.

This study demonstrates the impact of vision on multiple aspects of a person's function. Although not blind, older adults with reduced vision may have restricted physical activity and limitations in their ability to participate in activities and benefit from physical therapy. Muscle wasting and weakness associated with low physical activity could have a vision impairment as a root cause. Older adults should be instructed in ways to promote eye health and the necessity for regular visual screening and advised of the impact of good vision on their ability to be physically active. This study also reinforces the importance of comprehensive assessment of older adults.

PRACTICE REALITIES

Mrs. Wynn has recently been admitted to an assisted living community. At 82 years of age, she is able to function and independently perform most activities of daily living; however, she has experienced some minor injuries as a result of bumping into furniture in her room. Once, she tripped when walking from her dark bedroom to the brightly lighted bathroom during the night. Mrs. Wynn is frustrated and claims she never had this problem in her home.

What can be done to assist Mrs. Wynn?

CRITICAL THINKING EXERCISES

1. What can be done to prevent vision and hearing losses with aging?
2. Why are older adults unaware of the signs of glaucoma?
3. Outline a teaching plan for a patient with newly diagnosed glaucoma.
4. Outline modifications to the average home that could benefit a person with impaired vision.
5. List assistive devices to promote the independent function of persons with impaired vision or hearing.
6. Locate resources in your community to assist persons with visual and hearing impairments.

RESOURCES

Alexander Graham Bell Association for the Deaf
http://www.agbell.org

American Council of the Blind
http://www.acb.org

American Humane Association Hearing Dog Program
http://www.americanhumane.org

American Speech-Language-Hearing Association
http://www.asha.org

Blinded Veterans Association
http://www.bva.org

Guide Dogs for the Blind
http://www.guidedogs.com

Guiding Eyes for the Blind
http://www.guiding-eyes.org

Leader Dogs for the Blind
http://www.leaderdog.org

Lighthouse National Center for Vision and Aging
http://www.lighthouse.org

National Association for the Deaf
http://www.nad.org

National Association for the Visually Handicapped
http://www.navh.org

National Braille Association
http://www.nationalbraille.org

National Federation of the Blind
http://www.nfb.org/

National Library Service for the Blind and Physically Handicapped
http://www.lcweb.loc.gov/nls

Recordings for the Blind and Dyslexic
http://www.rfbd.org

RECOMMENDED READINGS

Recommended Readings associated with this chapter can be found on the web site that accompanies the book. Visit **http://thepoint.lww.com/Eliopoulos8e** to access the recommended readings and other additional resources associated with this chapter.

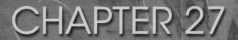

CHAPTER 27

Endocrine Function

CHAPTER OUTLINE

LEARNING OBJECTIVES

After reading this chapter, you should be able to:

1. Summarize the effects of aging on endocrine function.

2. Describe unique manifestations of diabetes in older adults.

3. Outline a teaching plan for the older person with diabetes.

4. List symptoms of hypothyroidism and hyperthyroidism in older adults.

TERMS TO KNOW

Dupuytren contracture: fixed flexion of the hands due to a thickening of the fibrous tissue under the skin of the palm and fingers; a risk for persons with diabetes mellitus

Goiter: nonmalignant swelling of the thyroid gland

Metabolic syndrome: group of conditions (high triglycerides, low high-density lipoprotein, elevated fasting blood sugar, elevated blood pressure, and central obesity) occurring together that increase the risk of diabetes, stroke, and coronary artery disease

The endocrine system enables the body to grow and develop, reproduce, metabolize energy, maintain homeostasis, and respond to stress and injury. This complex system consists of glands that synthesize and secrete hormones—substances that are transported from glands through the blood to targeted tissues where they exert specific effects either directly or indirectly by interacting with specific cell receptors. There are two major classes of hormones: steroids and thyronines, which are lipid soluble, and polypeptides and catecholamines, which are water soluble. With aging, the endocrine system experiences changes that can be diverse and interrelated in that some changes are compensatory responses for others. Knowledge of these changes and their effects is beneficial in interpreting symptoms and advising older adults regarding practices to promote optimal health.

EFFECTS OF AGING ON ENDOCRINE FUNCTION

With age, the thyroid gland progressively atrophies and thyroid gland activity decreases, resulting in a lower basal metabolic rate, reduced radioactive iodine uptake, and less secretion and release of thyrotropin. Thyroid activity can be further reduced by diminished adrenal function. Despite these changes, thyroid function remains adequate to meet daily needs. Adrenocorticotropic hormone secretion decreases with age, which in turn reduces the secretory activity of the adrenal gland which reduces the secretion of estrogen, progesterone, androgen, 17-ketosteroids, and glucocorticoids. The volume of the pituitary gland decreases with age; somatotropic growth hormone blood levels may be reduced. Insulin secretion is also affected by age; there is insufficient release of insulin by the β cells in the pancreas and reduced tissue sensitivity to the circulating insulin. Many older adults have reduced ability to metabolize glucose, particularly when a sudden high concentration of glucose is consumed.

Endocrine health promotion includes giving attention to these effects of aging and any symptoms of endocrine dysfunction in older adults in order to facilitate intervention and treatment.

SELECTED ENDOCRINE CONDITIONS AND RELATED NURSING CONSIDERATIONS

Diabetes Mellitus

A blend of various knowledge and skills is required when caring for older adults who have diabetes. Type 2 diabetes, the seventh leading cause of death among older adults, affects 20% of the older population and has a particularly high prevalence among African Americans and people who are 65 to 74 years of age. Consequently, nurses must be adequately informed of how the detection and management of diabetes in older adults differs from that in other age groups.

Glucose intolerance is a common occurrence among older adults; several explanations are offered

for this. At one time it was thought that a physiologic deterioration of glucose tolerance occurred with increasing age; however, increased amounts of fat tissue present in older persons who are obese and inactive are now considered significant to the development of this condition. This may be a factor in the high incidence of diabetes throughout the general population. Also, diagnostic techniques have been improved, enabling more persons with the condition to be detected. Regardless of the reason, it is agreed that different standards must be applied in evaluating glucose tolerance in older adults.

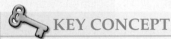

KEY CONCEPT

Obesity and inactivity contribute to the high prevalence of diabetes mellitus.

Diagnosis

Early diagnosis of diabetes in older persons is often difficult. The classic symptoms of diabetes may be absent, leaving nonspecific symptoms as the only clues. For this reason, screening with the use of fasting blood sugar is recommended every 3 years for persons over 45 years of age. Some indications of diabetes in older adults include orthostatic hypotension, periodontal disease, stroke, gastric hypotony, impotence, neuropathy, confusion, glaucoma, Dupuytren contracture, and infection. Laboratory tests, as well as symptoms, may be misleading. Because the renal threshold for glucose increases with age, older individuals can be hyperglycemic without evidence of glycosuria, thus limiting the validity of urine testing for glucose.

Among all the diagnostic measures, the glucose tolerance test is the most effective. To avoid a false-positive diagnosis, more than one test should be performed. The American Diabetes Association recommends that a minimum of 150 g of carbohydrates be ingested daily for several days before the test; older, malnourished individuals may be prescribed 300 g. Recent periods of inactivity, stressful illness, and inadequate dietary intake should be communicated to the physician because these situations can contribute to glucose intolerance. In such circumstances, more accurate results can be obtained if the test is postponed for 1 month after the episode. Nicotinic acid, ethacrynic acid, estrogen, furosemide, and diuretics can decrease glucose tolerance and should not be administered before testing. Monoamine oxidase inhibitors, propranolol, and high dosages of salicylates may lower blood sugar levels and also interfere with testing. Standard nursing measures are applied during glucose tolerance testing of older adults. If unusual symptoms such as confusion develop during the test, it is important to tell the physician.

The diagnosis of diabetes is usually established if one of three criteria exists:

1. Symptoms of diabetes and a random blood glucose concentration > 200 mg/dL (11.1 mmol/L).
2. Fasting blood glucose concentration ≥ 126 mg/dL (7.0 mmol/L).
3. Blood glucose concentrations 2 hours after an oral glucose intake ≥ 200 mg/dL (11.1 mmol/L) during an oral glucose tolerance test. The test should be performed as described by the World Health Organization, using a glucose load containing the equivalent of 75-g anhydrous glucose dissolved in water.

These results are usually confirmed by repeat testing on a different day.

Management of the Illness

As drug therapy to control hyperglycemia is used with most older persons with diabetes, careful attention to patient education, compliance with the prescribed plan, and monitoring are essential.

Patient Education   Once the diagnosis has been confirmed, the nurse should establish a teaching plan (Box 27-1). Diabetes is known as a serious and chronic problem to most lay individuals, and being diagnosed with this disease can be frightening. Fear and anxiety can interfere with the learning process for older people with newly diagnosed diabetes, who may have witnessed the crippling or fatal effects of diabetes in others and anticipate such occurrences in themselves. Having lived through a period in which diabetes was not successfully managed and was often severely disabling or fatal, the older individual may not be aware of the advances in diabetes management.

BOX 27-1   Content for Diabetic Patient Education

GENERAL OVERVIEW

Definition and description of diabetes mellitus
Basic anatomy and physiology
Basic metabolism of nutrients
Impact of advanced age on glucose metabolism, presentation of symptoms, complications

NUTRITION

Food groups, food exchange system
Dietary requirements
Consistent pattern of food intake
Menu plans
Understanding food labels
Flexibility of diet

ACTIVITY AND EXERCISE

Coordination and goal setting with the health care provider
Planning exercise in relation to glucose levels
Precautions
Monitoring glucose, vital signs
Recognizing complications
Importance of good fluid intake

MEDICATIONS

Actions
Dosage

Proper administration
Precautions
Adverse effects
Interactions

MONITORING

Purpose, goals
Types
Procedure

RECOGNIZING HYPOGLYCEMIA AND HYPERGLYCEMIA

Description and definition of hypoglycemia and hyperglycemia
Prevention

RECOGNITION OF SYMPTOMS

Actions to take for each
Signs that warrant contacting the health care provider

PREVENTION OF COMPLICATIONS

Foot care
Eye examinations
Adjustments for diabetes care during illnesses
Recognition of complications (e.g., infections and neuropathies)

look up

Gliclazide + Metformin

Older people may be depressed or angry that this disease threatens to reduce the quality of the remainder of their lives; they may question the value of exchanging an unrestricted lifestyle for a potentially longer but restricted one. Concerns may arise about how a special diet and medications will be afforded on an already limited budget. Social isolation may develop from fear of becoming ill in public or facing restrictions that make them different from their peers. They may question their ability to manage their diabetes independently and worry that institutionalization will be necessary. Such concerns must be recognized and dealt with by the nurse to reduce the risk of other limitations and promote the individual's self-care capacities (Nursing Diagnosis Table 27-1). Reassurance, support, and information can reduce barriers to learning about and managing diabetes. The information in Box 27-2, helpful in any patient education situation, offers guidance in teaching the older diabetic patient.

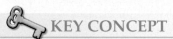

KEY CONCEPT

As diabetes impacts and is impacted by many facets of a person's life, patient education must be comprehensive and individualized.

Drug Therapy A variety of medications may be used to control hyperglycemia. Sulfonylurea drugs, such as glibenclamide, stimulate insulin secretion by blocking adenosine triphosphate–sensitive potassium channels on pancreatic β cells. However, the use of glibenclamide in older persons carries a risk of severe hypoglycemia, and this is believed to be related to delayed clearance of the active metabolites of this drug. Also, research suggests that glibenclamide is associated with significantly higher annual mortality when combined with metformin than other insulin-secreting medications (Monami et al., 2007). Due to these risks, glipizide and gliclazide, which have shorter half-lives and few or no active metabolites, are preferred sulfonylurea agents in older persons with diabetes. The latest generation sulfonylurea, glimepiride, appears to be more selective than the earlier agents and carries a lower risk for causing vasoconstriction of small vessels. Besides exhibiting less hypoglycemia compared with glibenclamide, this drug appears to be more specific for islet cell potassium channels and is less likely to produce coronary artery vasoconstriction. Sulfonylurea tablets should be taken a half-hour before meals. It is recommended that the drug be started at a low dose, about half of the usual adult dosage, and gradually increased if required.

NURSING DIAGNOSIS

TABLE 27-1 **Nursing Diagnoses Related to Diabetes Mellitus**

Causes or Contributing Factors	Nursing Diagnosis
Fear of disease's impact	Anxiety
High risk for loss of body part or function	Fear
Hyperglycemia	Risk for Infection
Decreased sensations, confusion, or dizziness from hypoglycemia	Risk for Injury
Diagnostic tests, care demands, denial	Deficient Knowledge
Lack of knowledge, self-care limitation	Noncompliance
Insufficient calories to meet energy, insulin demands	Imbalanced Nutrition: Less than Body Requirements
Caloric intake in excess of energy, insulin coverage	Imbalanced Nutrition: More than Body Requirements
Inability to meet therapeutic demands, feeling that disease is controlling life	Powerlessness
Peripheral neuropathies, retinopathy	Disturbed Sensory Perception
Peripheral neuropathy, vaginitis	Sexual Dysfunction
Susceptibility to fungal infections, pruritus from hyperglycemia	Impaired Skin Integrity
Urinary frequency	Disturbed Sleep Pattern
Altered neurovascular function secondary to neuropathies	Risk for Ineffective Peripheral Tissue Perfusion

| BOX 27-2 | **General Guidelines for Patient Education** |

ASSESS READINESS TO LEARN

Discomfort, anxiety, and depression may block learning and the retention of knowledge. Relieving these symptoms, and allowing time for patients to develop to the point where they desire and can cope with information, may be necessary.

ASSESS LEARNING CAPACITIES AND LIMITATIONS

Consider the patient's educational level, language problems, literacy, present knowledge, willingness to learn, cultural background, previous experience with the illness, memory, vision, hearing, speech, and mental status.

OUTLINE CONTENT OF PRESENTATION

Your outline should not only be specific and clear but also consider learning priorities. Nurses sometimes feel obligated to teach every detail about an illness, condensing a multitude of new facts and procedures into a short time frame. Most people need time to receive, absorb, sort, and translate new information into behavioral changes; older adults are no different. Altered cerebral function or slower responses may further interfere with learning in the aged. Patients and their families should have a role in setting teaching priorities; the most vital information should be given first, followed by other relevant material. Visiting nurses and other resources should be used after hospital discharge to continue the teaching plan if the proposed outline is not completed during the hospitalization.

ALTER THE TEACHING PLAN IN VIEW OF CAPACITIES AND LIMITATIONS

The nurse may feel that an explanation of the physiologic effects of diabetes is significant for new diabetics. However, the older person who tends to be confused or has a poor memory may not have long-range benefit from this type of information. It may be better to use that time to reinforce diet information or to make sure the most significant information required for self-care is retained.

PREPARE THE PATIENT FOR THE TEACHING–LEARNING SESSION

Patients should understand that education is an integral part of care. Whenever possible, arrange a specific time in advance to avoid conflict with other activities and to allow the family to be present if desired.

PROVIDE ENVIRONMENT CONDUCIVE TO LEARNING

An area that is quiet, clean, relaxing, and free from odors and interference will help create a good atmosphere for learning. Distraction should be minimal, especially in view of the aged people's reduced capacity to manage multiple stimuli.

USE THE MOST EFFECTIVE INDIVIDUALIZED EDUCATIONAL MATERIAL

It is important to recognize the limitations of standard teaching aids and the importance of individualized methods. An aid that was successful for one person may not be effective for another. The variety of sophisticated audiovisual aids that are commercially prepared and available in many agencies as resources for nurses are impressive, but they may not necessarily be effective for the given patient. The quality of an audio recording may be excellent, but it is of little benefit to the older person with a hearing problem. A slide presentation, even slowly paced, may present facts more rapidly than can be absorbed by an older person with delayed response time. The print on a commercial pamphlet may appear minute to older eyes. The language used in many commercial materials may not be one to which the person is accustomed. Original handmade aids suited for the individual's unique needs may have a value equal to or greater than commercially prepared ones. Selectivity in methodology is essential.

USE SEVERAL APPROACHES TO THE SAME BODY OF KNOWLEDGE

The greater the number of different exposures to new material, the higher the probability that the material will be learned. Combine verbal explanation with charts, diagrams, pamphlets, demonstrations, discussions with other patients, and audiovisual resources.

LEAVE MATERIAL WITH THE PATIENT FOR LATER REVIEW

Often, it is helpful to summarize the teaching session in writing, using language familiar to the patient. This provides concrete material that the patient can review independently later and share with the family.

REINFORCE KEY POINTS

Reinforcement should be regular and consistent, with all staff members supporting the teaching plan. For example, if the objective of the nurse caring for the patient has been to increase competency in self-injection of insulin, then the person substituting on the nurse's day off should comply with the established objectives rather than administering the insulin for the individual. Informal reinforcement of information during other daily activities should also be planned.

OBTAIN FEEDBACK

Evaluate whether the patient and family have received and understood accurately the information communicated. This can be done by observing return demonstrations, asking questions, and listening to discussions among patients.

REEVALUATE PERIODICALLY

To ascertain retention and effectiveness of the teaching sessions, informally reevaluate at a later time. Remember that retention of information may be especially difficult for the older individual.

DOCUMENT

Describe specifically what was taught, when, who was involved, what methodology was used, the patient's reaction and understanding, and future plans for remaining learning needs. This assists the staff caring for patients during their hospitalization and serves as a guide for those providing continued care after discharge.

In overweight and obese people with diabetes who have no abnormality in renal, cardiac, or respiratory functions, biguanides (e.g., metformin) can be used if diet alone is not sufficient or as an add-on therapy with sulfonylureas. When used alone, they do not produce hypoglycemia. Metformin should not be used when there is renal insufficiency, hepatic disease, alcoholism, severe congestive cardiac failure, severe peripheral vascular disease, and severe chronic obstructive pulmonary disease. Metformin should be administered immediately after meals to avoid gastrointestinal disturbances; starting with a smaller dose can reduce this side effect.

Acarbose, an α-glucosidase inhibitor, reduces postprandial hyperglycemia with lesser effect on fasting glucose levels and is safe for older adults. Gastrointestinal disturbance, particularly flatulence, is the major side effect of acarbose, which can be minimized by starting with a smaller dose and gradually increasing the dosage if required. Repaglinide is a short-acting insulinotropic antidiabetic agent that has similar effectiveness and safety in older and younger adults. It acts principally by augmenting endogenous insulin secretion from the pancreas in response to a meal. This drug can be taken with meals.

Rosiglitazone and pioglitazone are thiazolidinediones that can be used alone or in combination with sulfonylureas, metformin, or insulin for the management of type 2 diabetes mellitus. They act principally by increasing insulin sensitivity in target tissues, as well as decreasing hepatic gluconeogenesis; they do this without stimulating insulin release from pancreatic β cells, thereby reducing the risk of hypoglycemia. The reduced risk of hypoglycemia makes them well suited for use in older adults. Cardiac function must be assessed in all patients before starting these drugs as they can precipitate cardiac failure in patients with cardiac dysfunction. Caution is needed in patients with liver disease; liver enzymes should be monitored closely for all patients using these drugs.

Some individuals require only oral hypoglycemic agents to control their diabetes. Those on insulin therapy who have lost weight or have not been ketoacidotic may have their insulin substituted by oral hypoglycemic agents. Still others will need periodic changes in their insulin dosages to meet changing demands. These factors, combined with other management difficulties in the older diabetic person, necessitate frequent reevaluation of the patient's status. The continuation of health supervision is an essential part of diabetic management.

Patient Self-Care and Monitoring If an older person with diabetes must self-inject insulin, one factor that must be considered is the patient's ability to handle a syringe and vial of insulin. Several repeat demonstrations of this skill should be performed during the hospitalization, especially on days when arthritis discomfort is present. Also, because most older persons have some degree of visual impairment, the nurse must evaluate their ability to read the calibrations on an insulin syringe. Some of the new insulin pens that are available can assist older adults in delivering the correct amount of insulin easily.

The older individual can be hyperglycemic without being glycosuric. Higher blood glucose levels are common in older adults, and minimal or mild glycosuria is usually not treated with insulin. Although nurses are not responsible for prescribing insulin coverage, they need to be aware that the insulin requirements of older patients are individualized. Responses to various insulin levels should be carefully observed and communicated to the physician.

Many diabetic patients must perform blood glucose level testing using a finger-prick method. Patients must be instructed in this technique and must demonstrate competence in performing it. The finger-prick technique will most likely be replaced in the near future by an infrared device that determines the blood glucose level by measuring how light is absorbed by the body. The patient sticks a finger into a small meter that shines an infrared light through the skin. The infrared method should make glucose testing more convenient and pain free for diabetic persons.

The hemoglobin A1c test (also called HbA1c, glycated hemoglobin test, or glycohemoglobin) measures the amount of glycosylated hemoglobin in the blood and is used to monitor the effectiveness of disease control. Glycosylated hemoglobin is a molecule in red blood cells that attaches to glucose. Hemoglobin A1c provides an average of the patient's blood glucose control over a 6- to 12-week period; the normal range is between 4% and 6%. For persons with diabetes, the goal is HbA1c below 7%. This test is usually performed quarterly.

Triglyceride monitoring is also important. People with diabetes are at risk for metabolic syndrome, characterized by the combination of high triglycerides, low high-density lipoprotein, and central obesity. The risk of premature death from cardiovascular disease is increased in persons with these factors. The American Diabetes Association recommends that people with diabetes maintain their triglyceride levels below 150 mg/dL.

Exercise and Nutrition Regular exercise is important for older diabetic patients and provides multiple health benefits, including improved glucose tolerance, increased muscle strength, decreased body fat, improved maximal oxygen consumption, and improved lipid profile (Fig. 27-1). Physical activity can improve the patient's response to insulin during the period in which the exercise regimen is done, if the exercise is sufficient to lower the resting heart rate. In the diabetic individual, however, a vigorous exercise program or changes in an exercise program must be reviewed with the physician to prevent adverse consequences. For example, moderate to vigorous exercise increases

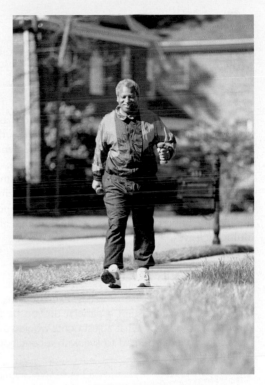

FIGURE 27-1 ■ Regular exercise provides multiple health benefits for older diabetic patients.

the absorption of insulin and heightens the use of glucose by the exercising muscles, potentially leading to hypoglycemia.

Attempts should be made to maintain a consistent daily food intake because an insulin dosage is prescribed to cover a specific amount of food. This may be difficult if the older person has a minimal food intake during the week when alone but an increased intake when visiting with family on weekends or if the patient skimps on meals when financial resources are low. Older people may also be limited in their ability to purchase and prepare adequate meals because of financial, energy, or social limitations. This can interfere with management of the illness. Meals on wheels, food stamps, the assistance of a neighbor, and other appropriate resources should be used to assist the individual. Psychosocial factors can influence consistent food intake as much as physical factors. The nurse and physician must carefully assess, plan, and manage insulin needs in view of the individual's unique problems and lifestyle. Older adults in a hospital or nursing home setting require special attention to ensure that food intake is regular and adequate.

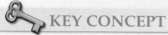

KEY CONCEPT

Psychosocial factors can alter food intake from day to day and affect insulin requirements.

A diet high in complex carbohydrates and fibers controls the release of glucose into the bloodstream and can reduce insulin requirements. Nutritional supplements can reduce the risk of complications; such supplements include vitamin B_6, folic acid, riboflavin (B_2), magnesium, zinc, and chromium. Herbs with hypoglycemic properties include bilberry, fenugreek, garlic, ginseng, and mulberry leaves.

POINT TO PONDER

Consider your schedule of eating, exercise, sleep, and rest. How consistent a pattern do you have from day to day, and what adjustments would you need to make if you had to live with a condition such as diabetes?

Complications

Older people are subject to a long list of complications from diabetes and have a greater risk of developing these complications than younger adults. Hypoglycemia seems to be a greater threat to older patients than ketoacidosis, and this is especially problematic because of the possible presentation of a different set of symptoms. Classic symptoms such as tachycardia, restlessness, perspiration, and anxiety may be totally absent in the older individual with hypoglycemia. Instead, any of the following may be the first indication of the problem: behavior disorders, convulsions, somnolence, confusion, disorientation, poor sleep patterns, nocturnal headache, slurred speech, and unconsciousness. Uncorrected hypoglycemia can cause tachycardia, arrhythmias, myocardial infarctions, cerebrovascular accident, and death.

KEY CONCEPT

Rather than the classic symptoms of hypoglycemia that one would anticipate in younger adults, older individuals instead may experience confusion, abnormal behavior, altered sleep patterns, nocturnal headache, and slurred speech.

Peripheral vascular disease is a common complication in the older individual who has diabetes and is influenced by the poorer circulation and atherosclerosis often associated with increased age. Symptoms may range from numbness and weak pulses to infection and gangrene. The nurse should identify and promptly communicate to the physician the symptoms of peripheral vascular disease. Educating the patient in proper foot care and in the early detection of foot problems can help reduce the risk of this problem; referral to a podiatrist also can prove beneficial. (See Chapter 20 for a discussion of foot care.)

Another significant vascular problem of older patients with diabetes is retinopathy with consequent blindness. Individuals who are hypertensive or who have had diabetes for a long time have a greater risk of developing this complication. Hemorrhage, pigment disturbances, edema, and visual disorders are manifested with this problem.

Many older patients taking sulfonylureas experience hypoglycemia. There are many age-related factors that increase the risk of hypoglycemia, including the age-related changes in hepatic and renal functions that alter drug metabolism and excretion. Aging is also associated with impairments in the autonomic nervous system and reductions in adrenergic receptor function, suggesting decreased response to hypoglycemia in older adults. This can be dangerous as older people may not display warning symptoms such as tremors, sweating, and palpitation; before it is recognized, their hypoglycemia can progress to convulsions or coma.

Drug interactions can be a major source of complications for older diabetic patients. Older adults are frequent users of drugs that are known to increase the risk of hypoglycemia, including β-blockers, salicylates, warfarin, sulfonamides, tricyclic anti-depressants, and alcohol. Nurses should review all medications the patient is taking to identify those drugs that may interact with antidiabetic medications. Nurses also must consider asking about the use of herbal remedies that could affect blood glucose levels.

A variety of additional complications can affect older individuals who are living with diabetes. Cognitive impairment can be a complication. Older persons may develop neuropathies, demonstrated through tingling sensations progressing to stinging or stabbing pain; carpal tunnel syndrome; paresthesias; nocturnal diarrhea; tachycardia; and postural hypotension. They have twice the mortality rate from coronary artery disease and cerebral arteriosclerosis and a higher incidence of urinary tract infections. They also have a higher risk of problems developing in virtually every body system. Early detection of complications is essential and can be facilitated by nursing intervention and patient education. Competent management of the older patient with diabetes is a vital activity that requires considerable skill and poses a great challenge and responsibility to the practice of nursing. The recognition of differences in symptomatology, diagnosis, management, and complications is crucial. Box 27-3 lists some potential care plan goals. Resources of benefit to patients with diabetes are listed at the end of this chapter.

Hypothyroidism

Thyroxine (T4) and triiodothyronine (T3) are essential hormones produced by the thyroid gland. Aging affects the thyroid gland in several ways, including moderate atrophy, fibrosis, increasing colloid nodules, and some lymphocytic infiltration. Although production of T4 declines with age, this is believed to be a compensatory process related to decreased tissue use of the hormone; serum levels of thyroid hormones do not significantly change.

A subnormal concentration of thyroid hormone in the tissues is known as hypothyroidism. This condition increases in prevalence with age and is more common in women than men. Hypothyroidism can be either primary, resulting from a disease process that destroys the thyroid gland, or secondary, caused by insufficient pituitary secretion of thyroid-stimulating hormone (TSH). Primary hypothyroidism is characterized by low free T4 or free T4 index with an elevated TSH level; secondary hypothyroidism displays low free T4 or free T4 index and low TSH. A subclinical hypothyroidism can exist in which the person is asymptomatic but has an elevated TSH level and normal T4. If symptoms are present but TSH, T3, and T4 levels are normal, checking the thyrotropin-releasing hormone (TRH) level may benefit the patient; the TRH level is more sensitive than the other thyroid levels and could help reveal subnormal thyroid function.

Symptoms

Symptoms of hypothyroidism can be easily missed or attributed to other conditions and include:

- fatigue, weakness, and lethargy
- depression and disinterest in activities
- anorexia
- weight gain and puffy face
- impaired hearing
- periorbital or peripheral edema
- constipation
- cold intolerance
- myalgia, paresthesia, and ataxia
- dry skin and coarse hair

Treatment

Treatment includes replacement of thyroid hormone using a synthetic T4 (e.g., Synthroid and thyroxine). Initially, a low dose is recommended to avoid exacerbation of asymptomatic coronary artery disease that could occur from rapid replacement. Desiccated thyroid preparations are avoided. Regular monitoring provides feedback for the need for dosage adjustments.

 KEY CONCEPT

Initially, thyroid replacement is prescribed at a low dose and gradually increased under close supervision to prevent cardiac complications.

BOX 27-3 **Care Plan Goals for the Patient With Diabetes**

To verbalize understanding of diabetes and its management
To demonstrate proper technique for administration of antidiabetic medication
To demonstrate correct method of blood glucose testing
To be free from signs of hypoglycemia and hyperglycemia
To describe signs and symptoms of hypoglycemia and insulin shock
To adapt management of diabetes to lifestyle
To maintain weight at appropriate level or to lose specified amount
To engage in a regular exercise program
To be free from injury
To be free from infection
To be free from impairments in skin integrity
To be free from complications associated with diabetes

Nursing measures should support the treatment plan and assist patients with the management of symptoms (e.g., prevention of constipation and provision of extra clothing to compensate for cold intolerance). It is important that patients understand that thyroid replacement will most likely be a lifelong requirement.

Hyperthyroidism

At the other extreme from hypothyroidism is a condition known as hyperthyroidism. In this disorder, the thyroid gland secretes excess amounts of thyroid hormones. Hyperthyroidism is less prevalent than hypothyroidism in older adults; it affects women more than men. A potential cause of hyperthyroidism in older patients that should be considered is iodine-induced hyperthyroidism, often related to the use of amiodarone, a cardiac drug containing iodine that deposits in tissue and delivers iodine to the circulation over very long periods of time. Amiodarone may also interfere with thyroid hormone transport into cells and with pathways of intracellular thyroid hormone metabolism (Reed & Wheeler, 2005).

Diagnostic testing can be challenging because blood tests do not always reflect hyperthyroidism. This is particularly true in malnourished older people, whose T3 levels are reduced due to their nutritional status; thus, the excess secretion will cause the T3 to fall within a normal range. Diagnosis relies on evaluation of T4 and free T4, TSH, and increased uptake of radionuclide thyroid scans.

Symptoms

Classic symptoms of hyperthyroidism include diaphoresis, tachycardia, palpitations, hypertension, tremor, diarrhea, stare, lid lag, insomnia, nervousness, confusion, heat intolerance, increased hunger, proximal muscle weakness, and hyperreflexia. However, as with hypothyroidism, hyperthyroidism can present with atypical symptoms in older adults. For example, increased perspiration may not occur, and for the person with a history of chronic constipation, diarrhea may be displayed by now having regular bowel movements.

Treatment

Treatment of hyperthyroidism depends on the cause. In Graves' disease, an autoimmune disorder that leads to the production of an antibody to the TSH receptor that stimulates thyroid growth and overproduction of thyroid hormone, or when there is a single autonomous nodule, treatment typically includes antithyroid medications or radioactive iodine. If toxic multinodular goiter is the underlying cause, surgery may be preferred due to the delayed and incomplete response to medications. Hypothyroidism can develop as a complication in persons who have had surgery or radioactive iodine therapy.

Patients with a history of thyroid disease need special monitoring when experiencing an acute illness, surgery, or trauma because this can precipitate extreme thyrotoxicosis (thyroid storm). Hospitalization may be required to return their thyroid level to a normal range.

BRINGING RESEARCH TO LIFE

TELEVISION VIEWING AND RISK OF TYPE 2 DIABETES, CARDIOVASCULAR DISEASE, AND ALL-CAUSE MORTALITY: A META-ANALYSIS

Grontved, A. & Hu, F. B. (2011). *Journal of the American Medical Association,* 305(23), 2248–2255.

Throughout the world, television (TV) viewing is the most common daily activity, apart from working and sleeping. In the United States, people watch an average of 5 hours of TV daily. TV viewing is associated with reduced physical activity, unhealthy eating patterns, and exposure to advertisements that could promote unhealthy behaviors. Physical inactivity and unhealthy eating patterns are risk factors of various diseases, including type 2 diabetes. The researchers in this study intended to quantify the relationship between TV viewing and the risk of these health outcomes.

A meta-analysis of studies published from 1970 to 2011 was conducted to examine the relationship between TV viewing and health outcomes. Among the findings was a direct relationship between TV viewing and the risk of developing type 2 diabetes, along with higher rates of cardiovascular disease and obesity. The risk of developing diabetes increased by 20% for every additional 2 hours of TV viewing.

TV viewing habits need to be considered when gerontological nurses assess older adults and educate about healthy practices. As long-established patterns, insufficient financial resources, and limited opportunities for other recreation are factors influencing TV viewing, nurses could assist older adults in engaging in healthy practices by helping them to locate free or low-cost recreation that is easily accessible. It is also beneficial to educate persons of all ages of the impact of TV viewing on health and encourage them to engage in healthier recreation.

The amount of time that baby boomers and younger generations spend in front of a computer or phone screen could produce the same risks as extended times of TV viewing. These aging individuals need to be reminded that these behaviors could increase their risk of diabetes, obesity, and cardiovascular disease; they need to balance these behaviors with sufficient physical activity to minimize their risks.

PRACTICE REALITIES

Eighty-three-year old Mr. Vincent has been diagnosed with diabetes mellitus. At 5′ 7″ and 290 lb, his excess weight is contributing to his problem. He and his wife, who is also obese, have been counseled and educated on the need to reduce weight and to follow good dietary practices.

At his first follow-up visit Mr. Vincent is found to have gained 4 lb. When questioned, he admits to not following his dietary plan and instead eating the heavy pastas, fried foods, and cakes that his wife continues to prepare. "She's a great cook and I love the dishes she makes," he said.

Mrs. Vincent who accompanies him on the visit adds, "He's been so worried about his diabetes and these little treats help to calm him. After all, at our age good eating is one of the few pleasures we have."

The record indicates that Mr. Vincent has been advised that he has circulatory and visual problems that are most likely related to his diabetes, so he has been informed of the risks associated with noncompliance.

How do you balance Mr. Vincent's lifelong eating habits and desires against the risks he is subjecting himself to? What actions could you take?

CRITICAL THINKING EXERCISES

1. Discuss reasons for different norms to be used to interpret the outcomes of glucose tolerance tests in older adults.

2. Describe the challenges to physical and psychosocial well-being faced by the older diabetic patient.

3. In what ways do age-related changes affect the presentation of symptoms and risks associated with diabetes and thyroid disease?

4. Outline a teaching plan for the person with hyperlipidemia that includes natural and alternative/complementary therapies.

RESOURCES

American Diabetes Association
http://www.diabetes.org

American Heart Association
http://www.americanheart.org

National Diabetes Education Program
http://www.ndep.nih.gov

National Diabetes Information Clearinghouse
http://www.diabetes.niddk.nih.gov

REFERENCES

Monami, M., Luzzi, C., Lamana, C., Chiaserrini, V., Adante, F., Desideri, C. M., Mannucci, E., et al. (2007). Three-year mortality in diabetic patients treated with different combinations of insulin secretagogues and metformin. *Diabetes/Metabolism Research Review, 22*(6), 477–482.

Reed, J. R., & Wheeler, S. F. (2005). Hyperthyroidism: Diagnosis and treatment. *American Family Physician*, August 15, 2005. Retrieved May 12, 2008 from http://www.aafp.org/afp/2005/0815/p623.html

RECOMMENDED READINGS

Recommended Readings associated with this chapter can be found on the web site that accompanies the book. Visit **http://thepoint.lww.com/Eliopoulos8e** to access the recommended readings and other additional resources associated with this chapter.

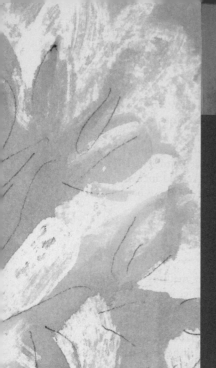

CHAPTER 28

Integumentary Function

LEARNING OBJECTIVES

After reading this chapter, you should be able to:

1. Summarize the effects of aging on the skin.
2. List practices that promote good skin health in older adults.
3. Describe signs of and nursing care for pruritus, keratosis, seborrheic keratosis, skin cancer, stasis dermatitis, and pressure ulcer in older adults.
4. Discuss measures that help older patients cope with skin problems and feel normal.
5. Identify alternative therapies that promote good skin health in older adults.

TERMS TO KNOW

Epidermis: outer layer of skin

Keratosis: small, light-colored benign lesions on epidermis

Melanocytes: epidermal cells that give skin its color

Mongolian spots: irregular, dark areas (resembling bruises) that may be found on the buttocks, lower back, and to a lesser extent on the arms, abdomen, and thighs; more prevalent in persons of African, Asian, or Native American backgrounds

Photoaging (solar elastosis): skin changes resulting from exposure to ultraviolet rays

Pressure ulcer: localized injury to skin and/or underlying tissue resulting from pressure or pressure combined with shear or friction

Pruritus: itching

Turgor: elasticity

Perhaps, the most obvious effects of growing old are the changes involving the integumentary system. In addition to the effects of aging, past health practices largely influence the status of the integument in old age; its status in old age, in turn, influences older persons' general health. In other words, problems involving other body systems can result from an unhealthy integumentary system. Because gerontological nurses often have more direct contact with older adults than the other health care professionals, they play an important role in promoting healthy skin and identifying signs of problems.

EFFECTS OF AGING ON THE INTEGUMENT

Lines and wrinkles, thicker nails, and graying hair are constant reminders of the aging process. These result from common aging changes to the integumentary system that include flattening of the dermal–epidermal junction, reduced thickness and vascularity of the dermis, decreased rate of epidermal turnover, degeneration of elastic fibers, increased coarseness of collagen, reduction in melanocytes (pigment cells that gives hair its color), atrophy of hair bulbs, and decline in rate of hair and nail growth. The increased fragility of the skin poses challenges to older adults and their caregivers in that there are heightened risks for skin tears, bruising, ulcer formation, and skin infections. In addition, the effects of this system's aging on appearance are highly visible signs of the aging process, potentially affecting body image, self-concept, reactions from others, socialization, and other psychosocial factors.

INTEGUMENTARY HEALTH PROMOTION

Some general measures can help prevent and manage dermatologic problems in older persons. It is important to avoid drying agents, rough clothing, highly starched linens, and other items irritating to the skin. Good skin nutrition and hydration can be promoted by activity, bath oils, lotions, and massages. Although skin cleanliness is important, excessive bathing may be hazardous to the skin; daily partial sponge baths and complete baths every third or fourth day are sufficient for the average older person. Early attention to and treatment of pruritus and skin lesions are advisable for preventing irritation, infection, and other problems.

Exposure to ultraviolet rays damages the skin, causing a condition known as *solar elastosis*, or *photoaging*. Loss of elasticity and wrinkling of the skin characterize this sun-induced premature aging of the skin. Fair-skinned individuals who easily burn when in the sun are at particularly high risk for this condition. The skin changes associated with exposure to ultraviolet radiation may not be apparent for years; therefore, sunbathing practices in youth affect the skin condition in late life. Sun-screening lotions are beneficial in protecting the skin; the sun protection factor (SPF) required will depend on the ease with which the skin burns and could range from an SPF of 15 or more in highly sensitive persons to an SPF of 4 to 6 in people who seldom burn and tan dark brown easily. Nurses can remind patients that skin damage can occur on overcast days because ultraviolet rays can penetrate clouds.

With the increased prevalence of skin cancer in late life, educating older adults in skin inspection for abnormalities is a beneficial action. Nurses should encourage older adults to examine their entire bodies with special attention to moles that could indicate possible carcinomas. To help them remember signs to bring to their health providers' attention, nurses can instruct older adults in the A, B, C, and Ds for detecting unhealthy moles:

A—Asymmetry: If a mole is not round or symmetrical, or one half of the mole is not similar to the other half, it could be a sign of melanoma.

B—Border Irregularity: Cancerous moles have irregular borders that may be uneven, ragged, notched, or blurred.

C—Color: The typical color of a mole is consistently brown throughout. A mole that has changed color over time or is varied in a shade of brown, tan, and black may be cancerous. If melanoma has progressed, the mole may become red, blue, or white.

D—Diameter: Cancerous moles can be more than 6 mm in diameter (about ¼ inch or the size of a pencil eraser).

Other mole variations that may indicate melanoma include elevation in height from the skin surface both horizontally or vertically; a change in feeling, such as itchiness, tenderness, or pain; and the tendency to bleed if scratched. Knowing these signs can enable older individuals in being proactive in their health care and obtaining evaluations and treatment while problems are in an early stage.

Although less serious than the possibility of skin cancer, integument issues affecting the appearance are another area for health promotion. All individuals should be encouraged to look their best and make the most of their appearance. However, efforts to avoid the normal outcomes of the aging process can be fruitless and frustrating. Money that could be applied to more basic needs is sometimes invested in attempts to defy reality. The nurse should emphasize to persons young and old that no cream, lotion, or miracle drug will remove wrinkles and lines or return youthful skin. While clarifying misconceptions regarding rejuvenating products, the nurse can encourage the use of cosmetics to protect the

CONSIDER THIS CASE

Seventy-year-old Mrs. J is a well-dressed, attractive woman who appears younger than her actual age. She mentions to you that she was widowed earlier this year and has begun to date. "I tend to be attracted to younger men, and many of them like being with a mature woman," she comments. "I had a facelift when I was 55 and looked great, so I'm thinking about having another one so that I can look young again."

THINK CRITICALLY

- How would you respond to Mrs. J?
- What advice could you give her?

skin and maintain an attractive appearance; many benefits may be derived from this practice.

Because increasing numbers of aging individuals are seeking cosmetic surgery, gerontological nurses will find it beneficial to be informed of the various types of surgical interventions. Nurses can also help patients locate competent cosmetic surgeons. Patients need to be aware that not all surgeons are skilled in cosmetic surgery, and some unfortunate complications have resulted from unskilled physicians performing cosmetic surgery or injecting patients with collagen or silicone. Nurses should also explore patients' reasons for seeking cosmetic surgery to ensure that it is a rational decision rather than a symptom of an underlying problem, such as depression or a neurotic disorder; counseling and therapy may be a more pressing need than surgical intervention in some circumstances. Perhaps as society achieves a greater acceptance and understanding of the aging process, the masking of the effects of aging with cosmetics

and surgery will be replaced by an appreciation of the natural beauty of age.

POINT TO PONDER

How much of your self-concept is based on your physical appearance? How do you anticipate reacting to the physical manifestations of aging?

Direct contact with patients allows nursing staff to detect skin problems that may not be apparent to other health care professionals. It is important for nurses to regularly assess patients' skin status (Assessment Guide 28-1) and identify nursing diagnoses (Nursing Diagnosis Table 28-1) and problems in need of referral for medical attention. Because serious complications, such as new pressure ulcers, can result from undetected skin problems, astute attention to skin status is crucial.

NURSING DIAGNOSIS

TABLE 28-1	Nursing Diagnoses Related to Dermatologic Problems

Causes or Contributing Factors	Nursing Diagnosis
Altered body appearance	Anxiety
Pruritus, infection, ulcer	Acute Pain
Ulcer, fragile skin	Risk for Infection
More fragile skin	Risk for Injury
Age-related changes to skin, hair, and nails; pain	Disturbed Body Image
Altered self-concept due to age-related changes, more fragile vaginal epithelium	Sexual Dysfunction
Fragile skin, immobility	Impaired Skin Integrity
Altered self-concept due to age-related changes to integument	Impaired Social Interaction
Pressure sites, ulcers	Risk for Ineffective Peripheral Tissue Perfusion

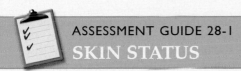

ASSESSMENT GUIDE 28-1
SKIN STATUS

GENERAL OBSERVATIONS

Much of the status of the integumentary system is evident to the naked eye. A quick observation can assist in evaluating skin color, moisture, and cleanliness; the presence of lesions; hair condition and grooming; and the condition of the nails. Signs such as pallor or flushing can provide clues to health problems.

INTERVIEW

Ask the patient about itching, burning sensations on the skin surface, hair loss, increased fragility of nails, and other symptoms associated with integumentary system problems. Also use this opportunity to review bathing and shampooing practices.

PHYSICAL EXAMINATION

- *Skin surface.* Examine the entire skin surface from head to toe, including behind the ears, within skin folds, under the breasts, and between the toes. Bathing and massages are good opportunities to inspect the skin in the course of patient care. Note moles, skin tears, bruises, discoloration, and any other unusual finding. Be aware that areas of pressure may be difficult to detect in dark-skinned persons.

- *Lesions.* Describe any lesions as specifically as possible in regard to their color (e.g., purple, black, and hypopigmented), configuration (e.g., linear, separate, confluent, and annular), size (e.g., measurement of depth and diameter), drainage, and type. Terms used to describe the types of lesions include the following:

  Macule: a small nonpalpable spot or discoloration

  Papule: a discoloration <1/2 cm in diameter with palpable elevation

  Plaque: a group of papules

  Nodule: a lesion 1/2 to 1 cm in diameter with palpable elevation; the skin may or may not be discolored

  Tumor: a lesion >1 cm with palpable elevation; the skin may or may not be discolored

  Wheal: a red or white palpable elevation that may occur in variable sizes

  Vesicle: a lesion <1/2 cm in diameter that contains fluid and has a palpable elevation

  Bulla: a lesion >1/2 cm in diameter that contains fluid and has a palpable elevation

  Pustule: a lesion containing purulent fluid; of variable size and palpable elevation

  Fissure: a groove in the skin

  Ulcer: an open depression in the skin that may occur in variable sizes.

- *Mongolian spots.* Consider that many persons of African, Asian, or Native American backgrounds have Mongolian spots. These are irregular, dark areas (resembling bruises) that may be found on the buttocks, lower back, and to a lesser extent on the arms, abdomen, and thighs.

- *Skin turgor.* Test skin turgor by gently pinching various areas of the skin. Skin turgor tends to be poor in most older adults; however, the areas over the sternum and forehead do experience less of an age-related reduction in turgor and are good areas for turgor assessment.

- *Pressure tolerance.* Assess pressure tolerance by inspecting a pressure point after the patient has been in the same position for half an hour; if redness is present, the patient must be on a turning schedule of every half an hour. If redness is not present, allow the patient to remain in the same position for 1 hour and inspect; if redness is not apparent increase increments by half an hour up to 2 hours.

- *Temperature.* Obtain a gross assessment of skin temperature by using the back of the hands and touching various areas. Note coldness or temperature inequalities between the extremities.

SELECTED INTEGUMENTARY CONDITIONS

Pruritus

The most common dermatologic problem among older adults is pruritus. Although atrophic changes alone may be responsible for this problem, pruritus can be precipitated by any circumstance that dries the person's skin, such as excessive bathing and dry heat. Diabetes, arteriosclerosis, hyperthyroidism, uremia, liver disease, cancer, pernicious anemia, and certain psychiatric problems can also contribute to pruritus. If not corrected, the itching may cause traumatizing scratching, leading to breakage and infection of the skin. Prompt recognition of this problem and implementation of corrective measures are, therefore, essential. If possible, the underlying cause should be corrected. Careful assessment is required to assure conditions, such as scabies, that demand special precautions are not present. Bath oils, moisturizing lotions, and massage are beneficial in treating and preventing pruritus. Vitamin supplements and a high-quality, vitamin-rich diet may be recommended. Topical application of zinc oxide is effective in controlling itching in some individuals. Antihistamines and topical steroids may also be prescribed for relief.

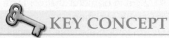

KEY CONCEPT

Excessive bathing and dry heat dry the skin and can promote pruritus.

Keratosis

Keratoses, also referred to as actinic or solar keratoses, are small, light-colored lesions, usually gray or brown, on exposed areas of the skin. Keratin may be accumulated in these lesions, causing the formation of a cutaneous horn with a slightly reddened and swollen base. Freezing agents and acids can be used to destroy the keratotic lesions, but electrodesiccation or surgical excision ensures a more thorough removal. Close nursing observation for changes in keratotic lesions is vital because these lesions are precancerous.

Seborrheic Keratosis

Seborrheic keratoses are dark, wartlike projections on the skin (Fig. 28-1). Older adults commonly have these lesions on various parts of their bodies. The lesions may be as small as a pinhead or as large as a quarter. They tend to increase in size and number with age. In the sebaceous areas of the trunk, face, and neck and in persons with oily skin, these lesions appear dark and oily; in less

sebaceous areas, they are dry in appearance and of a light color. Normally, seborrheic keratoses will not have swelling or redness around their base. Sometimes abrasive activity with a gauze pad containing oil will remove small seborrheic keratoses. Larger, raised lesions can be removed by freezing agents or by a curettage and cauterization procedure. Although these lesions are benign, medical evaluation is important to differentiate them from precancerous lesions. In addition, the cosmetic benefit of removal should not be overlooked for the older patient.

Skin Cancer

There are three major skin cancers that are common in late life: basal cell carcinoma, squamous cell carcinoma, and melanoma. Basal cell carcinoma, the most common form of skin cancer, grows slowly and rarely metastasizes. Risk factors for its development include advanced age, and exposure to the sun, ultraviolent radiation, and therapeutic radiation. It commonly occurs on the face, although it can erupt anywhere on the body. The growths tend to be small, dome-shaped elevations covered by small blood vessels that often resemble benign, flesh-colored moles with a "pearly" surface (Fig. 28-2 A). The surface sometimes is dark,

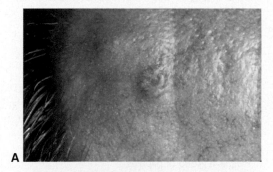

A

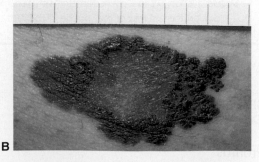

B

FIGURE 28-2 ■ Common types of skin cancer. (**A**) Basal cell carcinoma. (**B**) Melanoma. (From Rosenthal, T. C., Williams, M. E., & Naughton, B. J. [2007]. *Office care geriatrics*. Philadelphia, PA: Lippincott Williams & Wilkins.)

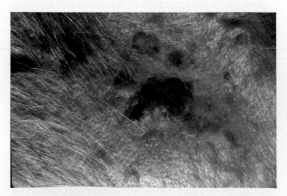

FIGURE 28-1 ■ Seborrheic keratosis. (From Rosenthal, T. C., Williams, M. E., & Naughton, B. J. [2007] *Office care geriatrics*. Philadelphia, PA: Lippincott Williams & Wilkins.)

rather than shiny, if the growth contains melanin pigments.

As the name implies, squamous cell carcinoma arises in the squamous cells that are on the surface of the skin, the lining of the hollow organs of the body, and the passages of the respiratory and digestive tracts. Sun exposure is the most prevalent factor contributing to the development of this cancer, although some less common factors (e.g., exposure to hydrocarbons, arsenic, and radiation) can facilitate its growth. Squamous cell carcinoma can develop in scar tissue and is also associated with suppression of the immune system. These cancers typically appear as firm, skin-colored or red nodules. Squamous cell carcinoma usually stays in the epidermis but can metastasize; the lower lip is a common site of metastasis.

Melanoma tends to metastasize, or spread, more easily than the other forms of skin cancer, making it more deadly if not caught early. The incidence of melanomas has been rising in the United States, probably due to sun exposure. Fair-skinned individuals are at higher risk for melanomas than the general population, and the incidence increases with age.

Melanomas can be classified as follows:

- *Lentigo maligna melanoma.* This black, brown, white, or red pigmented flat lesion occurs predominately on sun-exposed areas of the body. With time it enlarges and becomes progressively irregularly pigmented. The mean age at diagnosis is 67.
- *Superficial spreading melanoma.* Most melanomas are of this type. The lesion appears as variable pigmented plaque with an irregular border. It can occur on any area of the body. Its incidence peaks in middle age and continues to be high through the eighth decade.
- *Nodular melanoma.* This melanoma can be found on any body surface and presents as a darkly pigmented papule that increases in size over time.

Suspicious lesions should be evaluated and biopsied (Fig. 28-2B). Usually, melanomas are excised with removal of some of the surrounding tissue and subcutaneous fat. Some physicians recommend removal of all palpably enlarged lymph nodes. The prognosis depends on the depth of the melanoma rather than the type.

Nurses should teach older adults to inspect themselves for melanomas, identify moles that demonstrate changes in pigmentation or size, and seek evaluation of suspicious lesions. Early detection improves the prognosis.

Vascular Lesions

Age-related changes can weaken the walls of the veins and reduce the veins' ability to respond to increased venous pressure. Obesity and hereditary factors compound this problem. Weakened vessel walls cause varicose veins. The poor venous return and congestion that result lead to edema of the lower extremities, which leads to poor tissue nutrition. As the poorly nourished legs accumulate debris, inadequately carried away with the venous return, the legs gain a pigmented, cracked, and exudative appearance. Stasis dermatitis, an inflammatory condition associated with chronic venous insufficiency, can result. Subsequent scratching, irritation, or other trauma (which can result from tight elastic-band stockings) that occurs with stasis dermatitis can then easily lead to the formation of leg ulcers. These ulcers, known as *stasis ulcers,* often appear on the medial aspect of the tibia above the malleolus and, prior to skin breakdown, present as a dark discoloration of the skin.

Stasis ulcers need special attention to facilitate healing. Infection must be controlled and necrotic tissue removed before healing will occur. Good nutrition is an important component of the therapy, and a diet high in vitamins and protein is recommended. Once healing has occurred, concern should be given to avoiding situations that promote stasis dermatitis. The patient may need instruction regarding a diet for weight reduction or the planning of high-quality meals. Venous return can be enhanced by elevating the legs several times a day and by preventing interferences to circulation, such as standing for long periods, sitting with legs crossed, and wearing garters. Elastic support stockings may be prescribed and, although effective, can be a challenge for some older adults to apply. The nurse needs to assess the older adult's ability to properly put on these stockings and provide instruction as needed. Some patients may require ligation and stripping of the veins to prevent further episodes of stasis dermatitis.

Pressure Ulcers

Tissue anoxia and ischemia resulting from pressure can cause the necrosis, sloughing, and ulceration of tissue. This is commonly known as a pressure ulcer, or decubitus ulcer. Box 28-1 describes the recommended system for describing the stages of ulcers. This staging system is used in the Minimum Data Set tool for assessing nursing home residents.

BOX 28-1 | Stages of Pressure Ulcers

STAGE I

A persistent area of skin redness (without a break in the skin) that does not disappear when pressure is relieved.

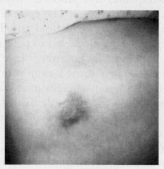

STAGE II

A partial thickness loss of skin layers involving the epidermis that presents clinically as an abrasion, blister, or shallow crater.

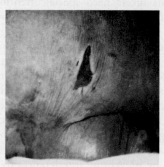

STAGE III

A full thickness of skin is lost extending through the epidermis and exposing the subcutaneous tissues; presents as a deep crater with or without undermining adjacent tissue.

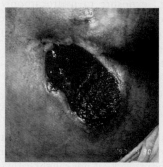

STAGE IV

A full thickness of skin and subcutaneous tissue is lost, exposing muscle, bone, or both; presents as a deep crater that may include necrotic tissue, exudate, sinus tract formation, and infection.

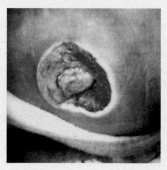

Any part of the body can develop a pressure ulcer, but the most common sites are the sacrum, greater trochanter, and ischial tuberosities (Fig. 28-3). Older adults are at high risk for pressure ulcers because they:

- have skin that is fragile and damages easily
- are often in a poor nutritional state
- have reduced sensation of pressure and pain
- are more frequently affected by immobile and edematous conditions, which contribute to skin breakdown.

In addition to developing more easily in older persons, pressure ulcers require a longer period to

heal than in younger people. Therefore, the most important nursing measure is to prevent their formation; to do this, it is essential to avoid unrelieved pressure. Encouraging activity or turning the patient who cannot move independently is necessary. The patient's individual pressure tolerance (see Assessment Guide 28-1) determines the frequency of turning; a turning schedule of every 2 hours may not be sufficient for every patient, and pressure ulcers can develop under that turning schedule. Shearing forces that cause two layers of tissue to move across each other should be prevented by not elevating the head of the bed more than 30°, not allowing patients to slide in bed, and lifting instead of pulling patients when moving

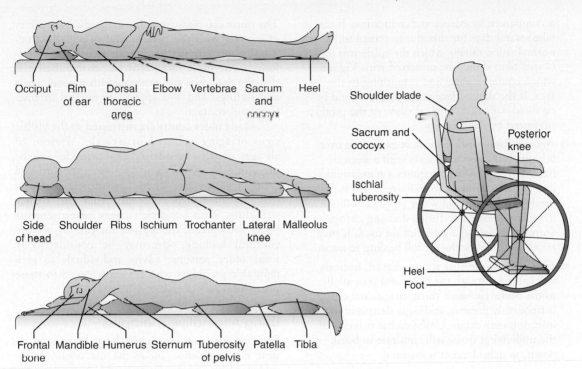

FIGURE 28-3 ■ Common locations for pressure sores when supine and sitting. (From Miller, C. [2009] *Nursing for wellness in older adults.* [5th ed.] Philadelphia, PA: Lippincott Williams & Wilkins.)

them. Use of pillows, floatation pads, alternating pressure mattresses, and water beds can disperse pressure from bony prominences. However, it must be emphasized that these devices do not eliminate the need for frequent position changes. When sitting in a chair, patients should be urged to move and should be assisted with shifting their weight at certain intervals. Lamb's wool and heel protectors are useful in preventing irritation to bony prominences. The nurse should make sure that sheets are kept wrinkle free and check the bed frequently for foreign objects, such as syringes and utensils, which the patient may be lying on unknowingly.

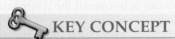

KEY CONCEPT

Some older patients may develop signs of pressure ulcers, even with a turning schedule of every 2 hours, and require more frequent repositioning.

A high-protein, vitamin-rich diet to maintain and improve tissue health is also essential to avoid formation of pressure ulcers. Good skin care is another essential ingredient in prevention. Skin should be kept clean and dry; blotting the patient

dry will avoid irritation from rubbing the skin with a towel. Bath oils and lotions, used prophylactically, help keep the skin soft and intact. Massage of bony prominences and range-of-motion exercises promote circulation and help keep the tissues well nourished. The person who is incontinent should be thoroughly cleansed with soap and water and dried after each episode to avoid skin breakdown from irritating excreta.

Once evidence of an ulcer is noted, aggressive intervention is necessary to avoid the multiple risks associated with this impairment of skin integrity. Treatment measures depend on the state of the pressure ulcer as identified by the following signs:

■ *Hyperemia.* Redness of the skin appears quickly and can disappear quickly if pressure is removed. There is no break in the skin and the underlying tissues remain soft. Relieving the pressure by the use of a square of adhesive foam is useful; it is advisable to protect the skin with a product such as DuoDerm (Squibb) or Tegasorb (3M) before applying the adhesive.

■ *Ischemia.* Redness of the skin develops from up to 6 hours of unrelieved pressure and is often accompanied by edema and induration. It can take several days for this area to return to its normal color, during which the epidermis may blister. Skin should be protected with Vigilon, which contains water and is soothing to the area. If the skin surface is broken, it should be cleansed daily with normal saline or the product suggested by your agency.

- *Necrosis.* Unremitting pressure extending over 6 hours can cause ulceration with a necrotic base. This type of sore requires a transparent dressing that protects from bacteria but is permeable to oxygen and water vapor. Thorough irrigation is essential during dressing changes. Sometimes topical antibiotics are used. It may take weeks to months for full healing to occur.

- *Ulceration.* If pressure is not relieved, necrosis will extend through the fascia and potentially to the bone. Eschar, a thick, coagulated crust, is frequently present, and bone destruction and infection may occur. Unless eschar is removed, the underlying tissue will continue to break down, so debridement is essential.

Because the risk of pressure ulcer formation is high among older patients, it is wise for gerontological nurses to assess patients' risk of pressure ulcers upon admission or first contact. Several tools that have been used for several decades can assist in objective assessment of pressure ulcer risk, such as the Braden Scale (Bergstrom, Allman, & Carlson, 1994) and the Norton scale (Norton, McLaren, & Exton-Smith, 1962). The Pressure Sore Status Tool (PSST) (Bates-Jensen, 1996) is an instrument that offers a means for assessing and monitoring existing pressure ulcers using 13 indexes (e.g., size, exudate, necrotic tissue, edema, and granulation). Depending on the patient population served and types of clinical setting, agencies and facilities may develop their own tools to assess risk and monitor pressure ulcers.

GENERAL NURSING CONSIDERATIONS FOR INTEGUMENTARY CONDITIONS

Promoting Normalcy

Psychological support can be especially important to the patient with a dermatologic problem. Unlike respiratory, cardiac, and other disorders, dermatologic problems are often visibly unpleasant to the patient and others. Visitors and staff may unnecessarily avoid touching and being with the patient in reaction to his or her skin problems.

The nurse can reassure visitors regarding the safety of contact with the patient and provide instruction for any special precautions that must be followed. The most important fact to emphasize is that the patient is still normal, with normal needs and feelings, and will appreciate normal interactions and contact.

Many older adults are distressed at the visible signs of aging reflected in wrinkles. Persons of all ages need to be advised that wrinkles can be prevented by avoiding excess sun exposure and using a sunscreen. There are topical products (e.g., α- or β-hydroxy acids) that can reduce wrinkling. With cosmetic surgery advertisements being widespread, this option for gaining a more youthful looking skin may be considered by some older persons; advise individuals to seek reputable providers who are experienced in these procedures.

Using Alternative Therapies

For centuries, various herbs have been used to treat skin problems. Today the use continues, as evidenced by creams, lotions, and shampoos containing aloe, chamomile, and other plant products. Aloe vera has emollient properties when used externally, and many people find it useful for treating minor cuts and burns. The external application of chamomile extract is used for skin inflammation. Witch hazel has long been used for its astringent effects and is applied externally for the treatment of bruises and swelling.

Essential oils are also increasingly used for the prevention and treatment of skin problems, including thyme oil as an antiseptic, thyme linalol and rosewood oil for topical acne, rosemary oil for cell regeneration, and the oils of basil, cinnamon, garlic, lavender, lemon, sage, savory, and thyme for insect bites or stings. Topical application of peppermint oil can have an anti-inflammatory effect and speed the healing of wounds and mild burns.

Some homeopathic and naturopathic remedies are being used to treat skin eruptions, as is acupuncture. Biofeedback, guided imagery, and relaxation exercises can help control the symptoms of some dermatologic disorders.

There is a belief that nutritional supplements can also be beneficial for skin disorders; those most commonly recommended are zinc, magnesium, essential fatty acids, and vitamins A, B complex, B_6, and E. Nurses should urge patients to discuss the use of alternative therapies with their physicians.

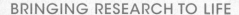

BRINGING RESEARCH TO LIFE

PREDICTIVE VALIDITY OF THE BRADEN SCALE FOR PRESSURE ULCER RISK IN ELDERLY RESIDENTS OF LONG-TERM CARE FACILITIES

de Souza, D. M. S. T., de Gouveia Santos, V. I., C., In, H. K., Oguri, M. Y. S. (2010). Geriatric Nursing, 31(2), 95–104.

In the late 1980s, the Braden Scale was developed as a tool to identify pressure ulcer risk. It is composed of six subscales: sensory perception, activity, mobility, moisture, nutrition, and friction and shear. The sum of the ratings could yield a score ranging from 6 to 23, with the lower scores indicating a higher risk.

Although the Braden Scale has been tested and shown to have predictive validity, few studies have been done on its ability to predict pressure ulcer risk in older residents of long-term care facilities. This study explored the predictive value of the Braden Scale among this population. A group of older long-term care residents at high risk was compared with the total group. Each resident underwent complete skin examination and Braden Scale rating every 2 days for 3 months.

Strong evidence has supported the validity and reliability of the Braden Scale, and the findings of this study were consistent with previous studies. Although previous studies identified cutoff scores of 19 as predictive for pressure ulcers, this study found lower cutoff scores in the older long-term care residents who were at risk for pressure ulcers.

Nurses should assure that tools used to predict risk have been tested and can be used with confidence. The Braden Scale is a tool that can be trusted, based on this and previous studies. This study also reminds us that assessment tools need to be tested in special populations (e.g., long-term care facility and intensive care unit) to assure their universal validity and reliability.

PRACTICE REALITIES

You are working in an intensive care unit and notice that although the nursing staff is highly skilled in monitoring patients and providing complex treatments, they are less attentive to changing patients' positions and checking skin status. It is not uncommon for older patients to develop pressure ulcers during their stay in the unit. You mention this to one of the nurses who responds, "That is the least of their problems. Our concern is keeping them alive."

Although you appreciate the complexities of the care offered, you still believe that patients should not be allowed to develop pressure ulcers while on the unit.

What can you do to address this issue while maintaining harmony with coworkers?

CRITICAL THINKING EXERCISES

1. Discuss the psychosocial implications of pressure ulcers and malignant melanoma.
2. Describe the method for determining an individualized turning schedule.
3. Develop a protocol for the prevention of pressure ulcers.

RESOURCES

Agency for Healthcare Research and Quality

Pressure Ulcers in Hospitals: A Toolkit for Improving Quality of Care
http://www.ahrq.gov/research/ltc/pressureulcertoolkit/

American Academy of Facial and Reconstructive Plastic Surgery
http://www.aafprs.org/patient/procedures/proctypes.html
American Cancer Society
http://www.cancer.org
Braden Scale for Predicting Pressure Ulcer Risk
http://www.in.gov/isdh/files/Braden_Scale.pdf

National Arthritis and Musculoskeletal and Skin Diseases Information Clearinghouse
http://www.nih.gov/niams

National Pressure Ulcer Advisory Panel
http://npuap.org

Skin Cancer Foundation
http://www.skincancer.org

Wound, Ostomy, and Continence Nursing Society
http://www.wocn.org

REFERENCES

Bates-Jensen, B. M. (1996). *Why and how to assess pressure ulcers.* Presented at the Ninth Annual Symposium on Advanced Wound Care, Atlanta, April 20, 1996.

Bergstrom, M., Allman, R. M., & Carlson, E. D. (1994). *Treatment of pressure ulcers.* Clinical Practice Guideline No. 15, AHCPR Pub No 95-0652. Rockville, MD: U.S. Department of Health and Human Services, Public Health Service, Agency for Health Care Policy and Research.

Norton, D., McLaren, R., & Exton-Smith, A. N. (1962). *An investigation of geriatric nursing problems in the hospital.* London: National Corporation for the Care of Old People.

RECOMMENDED READINGS

Recommended Readings associated with this chapter can be found on the web site that accompanies the book. Visit **http://thepoint.lww.com/Eliopoulos8e** to access the recommended readings and other additional resources associated with this chapter.

CHAPTER 29

Immune Function

CHAPTER OUTLINE

Effects of Aging on Immune Function

Immunologic Health Promotion
    Diet
    Exercise
    Immunization
    Stress Management
    Mind–Body Connection
    Careful Use of Antibiotics

Our bodies are exposed to many bacteria over the course of the average day, yet we do not develop infectious diseases from each exposure. Our ability to protect ourselves is the result of the effectiveness of the immune system. However, *immune senescence*, an age-related decline in the immune system's function, increases the body's susceptibility to infections and diminishes the strength of the immune response. In addition, the high prevalence of chronic conditions in late life enables infectious agents to invade easily, and the high rate of hospitalization and institutionalization increases the exposure to pathogens. The result is that older adults experience infectious diseases that are usually more severe than those of younger adults. Strengthening the older adult's immune system and protecting against factors that promote infection are essential to gerontological nursing care.

LEARNING OBJECTIVES

After reading this chapter, you should be able to:

1. List major changes in immunologic function as the result of aging.

2. Discuss natural approaches to promoting immunologic health.

3. Describe the risks associated with overuse and misuse of antibiotics.

TERMS TO KNOW

Antibody: protein produced in the immune system that attacks antigens

Antigen: foreign substance that invades the body

Autoimmune: immune system attacks the host's body

Immunosenescence: age-related dysfunction in immune response

Inflammatory response: body's reaction to infection, usually producing redness, warmth, and swelling of affected tissue

Macrophage: immune cell that engulfs foreign substances and dead tissue through phagocytosis

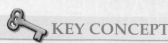

KEY CONCEPT

An age-related decline in the immune system's function, known as *immune senescence*, increases susceptibility to infections.

EFFECTS OF AGING ON IMMUNE FUNCTION

Simply put, the immune system works in the following manner:

1. An antigen (invading bacteria) enters the body.
2. A macrophage attacks the antigen and retains some of the antigen's protein on its surface.
3. The macrophage carries the protein markers to lymphoid tissue where T lymphocytes interpret them as foreign.
4. Stimulated by this activity, antibodies are produced by a white blood cell called a B cell and attack the antigens.

This process is called the antigen–antibody reaction. Once the body has been exposed to an antigen, it stores information about the antigen in its memory system to use in the future for protection of the body. (This is the principle on which vaccination works.) When functioning optimally, the immune system offers resistance to infection that maintains health.

There are changes within the immune system and some differences in the way in which it responds in late life. The thymus gland progressively declines in size with age, although the number of T and B cells in circulation does not significantly decrease; however, there is an increased number of immature T cells in the thymus and blood. T-cell function declines, resulting in a reduced response to foreign antigens because of decreases in cell-mediated immunity and humoral immunity. Cell-mediated immunity is deficient. The inability of many older adults to raise a delayed cutaneous hypersensitivity

response (e.g., with a tuberculin test) is related to this. The total concentration of immunoglobulins (Ig) in the blood is not significantly altered with age, although there are changes in the serum distribution of IgA and IgG, which increase, and IgM and IgD, which decrease. A reduced antibody response to pneumococcus, influenza, and tetanus vaccines is noted (although these are recommended for older people). The skin loses macrophages (Langerhans cells), and when this is combined with reduced thickness and circulation to the skin, local defenses against infections are weakened.

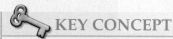

KEY CONCEPT

The inability of many older adults to raise a delayed cutaneous hypersensitivity response can alter the results of skin tests.

IMMUNOLOGIC HEALTH PROMOTION

To compensate for older adults' compromised immune function and high prevalence of health conditions that increases the risk of infections, health practices that stimulate immunity are essential nursing interventions in gerontological care. Some interventions that could prove useful are discussed in the following sections and outlined in the Nursing Diagnosis Highlight: Risk for Infection.

Diet

In addition to maintaining a good nutritional state, older people can include foods in their diet that positively affect immunity; some of these include milk, yogurt, nonfat cottage cheese, eggs, fresh fruits and vegetables, nuts, garlic, onion, sprouts, pure honey, and unsulfured molasses. A daily multivitamin and mineral supplement is also helpful; specific nutrients that have immune-boosting effects are listed in Box 29-1. Intake of refined carbohydrates, saturated and polyunsaturated fats, caffeine, and alcohol should be limited.

BOX 29-1   Nutrients With Immune-Boosting Effects

Protein
Vitamins A, E, B_1, B_2, B_6, B_{12}, C
Folic acid
Pantothenic acid
Iron

Magnesium
Manganese
Selenium
Zinc

Fasting, the abstinence of solid foods for 1 to 2 days, is becoming increasingly popular as a means to promote health and healing. The effects of fasting on the immune system include (Muller, 2001; Steinman, Conlin, Maki, & Foster, 2003):

- increased macrophage activity, Ig levels, and neutrophil antibacterial activity
- improvement of cell-mediated immunity, ability of monocytes to kill bacteria, and natural killer cell activity
- reductions in free radicals and antioxidant damage

For most persons, a day or two without food is safe; however, an assessment of health status is essential before beginning a fast because fasting can alter some health conditions and medication needs. Also, maintaining good fluid intake during a fast is essential.

POINT TO PONDER

In what types of practices do you engage that boost your immune system and offer you protection from infection? What can you do to improve on this?

Exercise

Any type of regular physical activity can enhance immune function. Exercises such as yoga and t'ai chi are low impact and have a positive effect on immunity. There are exercises that can benefit persons with various levels of physical function, and nurses can assist patients in developing a regular exercise program that is tailored to their unique needs (see Chapter 24 for more information on physical activity and exercise).

Immunization

General immunizations that are recommended for older persons, unless contraindicated, include:

- pneumococcal polysaccharide vaccine: once in a lifetime unless the primary vaccination occurred 5 years or more before age 65
- influenza vaccine: annually
- zoster vaccine: once in a lifetime regardless of history of zoster
- tetanus and diphtheria toxoids: every 10 years

If there is significant risk of exposure and immunity does not exist as a result of having the disease or being vaccinated, older adults should be immunized against:

- measles, mumps, and rubella: once
- varicella: once

NURSING DIAGNOSIS HIGHLIGHT

RISK FOR INFECTION

Overview
Risk for infection implies that an individual has a potential to develop an infection resulting from factors such as age, residence, lifestyle, and health conditions.

Causative or contributing factors
Age-related decline in immune system's function, high prevalence of chronic conditions, high rate of hospitalization and institutionalization, and age-related changes to body systems (e.g., enlarged prostate, weaker bladder muscles, increased residual capacity of lungs, and increased fragility of skin).

Goal
The patient will be free from infection.

Interventions
- Promote good general health.
- Ensure patient is current for all immunizations.

- Encourage dietary intake of foods that have positive effect on immunity, such as nonfat dairy products, fresh fish, fruits, vegetables, garlic, grains, pure honey, unsulfured molasses.
- Assist patient in maintaining skin integrity.
- Instruct in stress management techniques.
- Encourage and assist with regular exercise.
- Counsel patient against overuse of antibiotics. Consider use of immune-boosting herbs, such as *Echinacea*, garlic, ginseng, and goldenseal.
- Instruct patient in infection control measures and early recognition of infection.
- Ensure all caregivers adhere to strict infection prevention and control measures.

Special circumstances demand immunization against hepatitis:

- hepatitis A: for individuals who are IV drug users, engage in homosexual sexual activity, or who reside or travel in areas with high rates of infection
- hepatitis B: for persons who are IV drug users, engage in homosexual sexual activity, receive hemodialysis, or have received blood transfusions

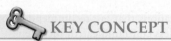

KEY CONCEPT

Vaccinations for older adults should include pneumococcal vaccination once in a lifetime, influenza vaccination annually, and tetanus and diphtheria vaccinations every 10 years. Other vaccines may be administered under special conditions.

Stress Management

The thymus, spleen, and lymph nodes are involved in the stress response; therefore, stress can affect the function of the immune system. Some stress-related diseases, including arthritis, depression, hypertension, and diabetes mellitus, cause a rise in serum cortisol, a powerful immunosuppressant. Elevated cortisol levels can lead to a breakdown in lymphoid tissue, inhibition of the production of natural killer cells, increases in T-suppressor cells, and reductions in the levels of T-helper cells and virus-fighting interferon. Some stress reduction measures that nurses can encourage older adults to use include progressive relaxation, meditation, prayer, yoga, imagery, exercise, diversional activity, and replacement of caffeine and "junk" foods with juices and nutritious snacks (Fig. 29-1).

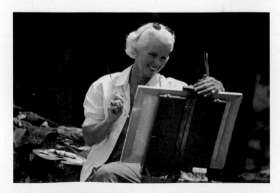

FIGURE 29-1 ■ Managing stress and developing an optimistic attitude can promote good immunologic health.

Mind–Body Connection

It is recognized that a person's psychological state can affect physical health; in fact, the specialty of psychoneuroimmunology has emerged in recognition that thoughts and emotions affect the immune system. Studies have identified traits consistent with strong immune systems to include the following (Cohen, 2002; Cohen & Miller, 2001):

- assertiveness
- faith in God or a higher power
- ability to trust and offer unconditional love
- willingness to be open and confide in others
- purposeful activity
- control over one's life
- acceptance of stress as a challenge rather than a threat
- altruism
- development and exercise of multiple facets of personality

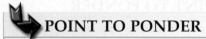

POINT TO PONDER

Do your psychological traits positively support your immunity?

Nursing interventions that assist older adults with the developmental tasks of aging (see Chapter 2) and maintaining satisfying relationships with others are useful in promoting an immune-enhancing psychological state.

In addition to releasing endorphins and increasing the body's oxygenation and heart rate, laughter and humor can stimulate immunologic function. Nurses can use therapeutic humor by sharing jokes, providing comedy videos or audiotaped comedy programs, and finding laughter and levity among the occurrences in the average day.

Careful Use of Antibiotics

A significant number of antibiotics are prescribed to older adults annually, and serious consequences have resulted from their overuse and misuse. Some strains of bacteria are resistant to penicillin and ampicillin, and many are resistant to all antibiotics except highly potent and toxic form. Furthermore, antibiotics can produce side effects and adverse reactions that can cause serious consequences (Table 29-1). A trend has been noted in long-term care facilities in which multiple antibiotic-resistant

TABLE 29-1	Adverse Effects of Antibiotics
Antibiotic	**Adverse Effect**
Cephalosporin, penicillin, fluoroquinolones, macrolides, erythromycin	Nausea, gastrointestinal upset
Vancomycin, cotrimoxazole	Kidney toxicity
Isoniazid, penicillin, cephalosporin, erythromycin, cotrimoxazole	Liver toxicity
Penicillin-like antibiotics	Neutropenia
Nalidixic acid, metronidazole	Convulsions
Aminoglycosides	Hearing impairments
Tetracyclines	Photophobia
Penicillin	Muscle inflammation

Klebsiella and *Escherichia coli* are being observed, attributable to the use of broad-spectrum oral antibiotics and poor infection control techniques (El Solh, Pietrantoni, Bhat, Bhora, & Berbary, 2004; Wick, 2006).

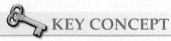

KEY CONCEPT

Overuse and misuse of antibiotics have resulted in many strains of bacteria becoming resistant to antibiotics.

Nurses play a significant role in promoting safety in antibiotic use. Some suggestions include:

- assist patients in health promotion efforts to increase their resistance to infections
- adhere to strict infection control practices
- use alternatives to antibiotics whenever possible (Box 29-2)
- educate consumers about the realities and risks of antibiotics
- advise patients not to save and use antibiotics for future illnesses

BOX 29-2	Alternatives to Antibiotics

Some herbs have gained popularity for their effectiveness in preventing and treating infections:

- *Echinacea,* long used by Native Americans, has been shown to increase the number and activity of white blood cells, promote phagocytosis, and stimulate the reproduction of T-helper cells and cytokines (Libster, 2002). Because *Echinacea* can activate autoimmune aggressions and other

overreactive immune responses, it is contraindicated in persons with AIDS, multiple sclerosis, or tuberculosis.
- *Garlic* is known for its antibiotic, antifungal, and antiviral properties.
- *Siberian ginseng* is a general tonic that can boost the immune system.

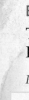

BRINGING RESEARCH TO LIFE

THE ROLE OF NUTRITION IN ENHANCING IMMUNITY IN AGING

Pae, M., Meydani, S.N., & Wu, D. (2012). Aging and Disease, 3(1), 91–129.

A variety of nutritional interventions have been promoted as having value in reversing impaired immune function and strengthening resistance to infection in older adults; however, controversy exists regarding the various nutritional supplements' effectiveness and

(Continues)

safety. This chapter surveys the research that has been done in the area of nutrition and immunity in aging. Some of the findings include:

- Vitamin E intake above the recommended daily allowance can enhance T-cell function in older humans and contribute toward reduced incidence of upper respiratory infections.

- Zinc deficiency can impair immune function and increase the risk of infection.

- Increased intake of fish oils can be beneficial to inflammatory and autoimmune disorders but may have an immunosuppressive effect on T-cell–mediated function that can reduce resistance to infection.

- Caloric restriction has been shown to delay the decline of the immune system in animals, but its effectiveness in humans has not been verified.

Although there is some evidence that nutritional interventions could improve immune function as people age, additional research is needed that can establish specific benefit, optimal dose/amount, and characteristics of the population who could benefit and for whom the intervention would be contraindicated.

With the popularity of nutritional supplements, it is important that nurses advise individuals to weigh claims carefully. People need to understand that just because they read an article with claims about the value of a supplement that does not mean it is supported by evidence. Even if a claim is made that "studies have proven" the value, caution is needed as the studies may not have been sound ones or used a good sample size. It is useful for nurses to keep abreast of research that could support the role of diet, nutritional supplements, and other factors that could positively impact the aging immune system.

PRACTICE REALITIES

One of the leading corporations in the state has identified that it has a considerable number of employees between the ages of 55 and 70 years. Noticing a trend for its employees retiring at older ages, the corporation is concerned for their health and wants to develop a series of health promotion programs. It has conducted a needs assessment and identified stress as a major problem.

You are the nurse in the health office of the corporation and have been given the responsibility of developing a stress management program for the employees. The leadership of the corporation has committed to supporting programs offered during work hours and making some environmental modifications. You are to give them a plan for the program within the next month.

Create a plan for a stress management program for the employees.

CRITICAL THINKING EXERCISES

1. What major points would you discuss if you were presenting a health education class at a senior citizen center on the topic of "Boosting Your Immunity"?

2. What are the differences between your generation and that of your grandparents in regard to lifestyle and environmental factors that could influence immunity to infection and disease?

3. What factors have contributed to the overuse of antibiotics? How were these factors related to society's attitude and priorities?

4. How did conventional medical care in the United States contribute to antibiotic overuse? What can be done to change this?

RESOURCES

National Center for Preparedness, Detection, and Control of Infectious Diseases
http://www.cdc.gov/ncpdcid/

Norman Cousins Center for Psychoneuroimmunology
http://www.cousinspni.org

REFERENCES

Cohen, S. (2002). Psychosocial stress, social networks, and susceptibility to infection. In H. G. Koenig & H. J. Cohen (Eds.), *The link between religion and health: Psychoneuroimmunology and the faith factor*. New York, NY: Oxford University Press.

Cohen, S., & Miller, G. E. (2001). Stress, immunity, and susceptibility to upper respiratory infections. In R. Ader, D. Felten, & N. Cohen (Eds.), *Psychoneuroimmunology* (3rd ed.). New York, NY: Academic Press.

El Solh, A. A., Pietrantoni, C., Bhat, A., Bhora, M., & Berbary, E. (2004). Indicators of potentially drug-resistant bacteria in severe nursing home-acquired pneumonia. *Clinical Infectious Diseases, 39*(4), 474–480.

Libster, M. (2002). *Delmar's integrative herb guide for nurses* (pp. 263–272). Florence, KY: Delmar/Thompson Learning.

Muller, H. (2001). Fasting followed by vegetarian diet in patients with rheumatoid arthritis: A systematic review. *Scandinavian Journal of Rheumatology, 30*(1), 1–10.

Steinman, L., Conlin, P., Maki, R., & Foster, A. (2003). The intricate interplay among body weight, stress, and the immune response to friend or foe? *Journal of Clinical Investigation, 111,* 183–185.

Wick, J.Y. (2006). Infection control and the long-term care facility. *Consultant Pharmacist, 21*(6), 467–480.

RECOMMENDED READINGS

Recommended Readings associated with this chapter can be found on the web site that accompanies the book. Visit **http://thepoint.lww.com/Eliopoulos8e** to access the recommended readings and other additional resources associated with this chapter.

Multisystemic Disorders

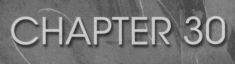

CHAPTER 30

Infections

CHAPTER OUTLINE

Unique Manifestations of Infection In Older Adults

Common Infections
Urinary Tract Infection
Prostatitis
Pneumonia
Influenza
Tuberculosis
Vaginitis
Herpes Zoster
Scabies
HIV and AIDS
Clostridium difficile Infection
Antibiotic-Resistant Microorganisms

As described in Chapter 29, age-related changes in the immune system and the high prevalence of diseases in the older population heighten the risk of infections. Infections tend to have more profound effects in older adults, causing them significant consequences. Since the mid-1980s, the rates of hospitalization for septicemia among older adults have more than doubled, with the primary sources being urinary tract infections (UTIs), cystitis, pneumonia, pressure ulcer, cellulitis, and renal infections (DeFrances & Paul, 2006). Older adults have a high rate of iatrogenic infections associated with their increased exposure to health care settings (i.e., hospitalizations and nursing home residence). Understanding the predisposing factors and related interventions to prevent the development of infections is basic to gerontological nursing practice.

LEARNING OBJECTIVES

After reading this chapter, you should be able to:

1. Describe unique aspects of infection in older adults.
2. Describe features of common infections in older adults and related nursing interventions.

TERMS TO KNOW

Antibiotic resistance: when a bacteria has built up resistance to an antibiotic

Postherpetic neuralgia: pain that persists along a dermatome after vesicular lesions from herpes zoster have resolved

Shingles: herpes zoster, caused by varicella virus that typically has been latent after initial exposure to it from chickenpox

406

UNIQUE MANIFESTATIONS OF INFECTION IN OLDER ADULTS

The challenges presented by the increased risk and incidence of infections in older adults are compounded by the fact that infections often do not present in the typical manner that is seen in adults of younger ages (Box 30-1). Fever, the primary clinical sign of an infection, can be undetected in older persons because their lower baseline temperatures can cause them to be febrile at temperatures of 99°F; consequently, caregivers accustomed to the fevers of 101°F in other age groups may miss the presentation of fever in older individuals. Often, older adults manifest infections through lethargy, weakness, and anorexia; these symptoms may be attributed to advanced age or other health conditions rather than an infection. Changes in mental status, incontinence, and increased incidence of falls may be related to the presence of infections in older adults, but could be erroneously attributed to other causes. The failure to interpret the atypical symptoms can result in delayed diagnosis of infections.

COMMON INFECTIONS

Urinary Tract Infection

Infections of the urinary tract are the most common infection of the aged, affecting as many as 1 in 10 older adults annually (Graves et al., 2007). Furthermore, UTIs increase in prevalence with age. Although UTIs occur more frequently in women than in men at younger ages, the gap between the sexes narrows in late life, which is attributable to reduced sexual intercourse in women and a higher incidence of bladder outlet obstruction secondary to benign prostatic hyperplasia in men. Organisms primarily responsible for UTIs are *Escherichia coli* in women and *Proteus* species in men. The presence of any foreign body in the urinary tract or anything that slows or obstructs the flow of urine (e.g., immobilization, urethral strictures, neoplasms, or a clogged indwelling catheter) predisposes the individual to these infections. UTIs can result from poor hygienic practices, improper cleansing after bowel elimination, a predisposition created by low fluid intake and excessive fluid loss, and hormonal changes, which reduce the body's resistance. Persons in a debilitated state or who have neurogenic bladders, arteriosclerosis, or diabetes also have a high risk of developing UTIs. Of major consideration are catheter-associated UTIs, which are the single most common health care–associated infections.

 KEY CONCEPT

Urinary tract infections can result from poor hygienic practices, prostate problems, catheterization, dehydration, diabetes, arteriosclerosis, neurogenic bladders, and general debilitated states.

The gerontological nurse should be alert to the signs and symptoms of UTIs. Early indicators include burning, urgency, and fever. Some older adults develop incontinence and delirium with UTIs. Awareness of the patient's normal body

---

BOX 30-1   **Possible Signs of Infection in Older Adults**

- Delirium
- Fever
- Chills
- Hypotension
- Increased pulse
- Increased respiration
- Flank pain
- Hematuria, pyuria
- Dysuria, burning
- Urinary frequency
- Incontinence
- Cough
- Chest discomfort
- Purulent sputum
- Rhinorrhea

- Nasal congestion
- Headache
- Malaise
- Anorexia
- Weight loss
- Vomiting
- Diarrhea
- Mucus or blood in stool
- Purulent drainage
- Pain or swelling over joint
- >10,000 white blood cells in blood
- >100,000 bacteria/mL in urine
- Decreased arterial blood gases
- Positive blood, sputum, cerebrospinal fluid, or wound culture

temperature helps the nurse recognize the presence of fever, for instance, 99°F (37°C) in a patient whose normal temperature is 96.8°F (35°C). Some urologists believe that many UTIs in older adults seem asymptomatic due to lack of awareness of elevations in normal temperature from the baseline norm. The nurse can significantly facilitate diagnosis by informing the physician of temperature increases from the patient's normal level. Bacteriuria greater than 105 CFU/mL confirms the diagnosis of UTI. As a UTI progresses, retention, incontinence, and hematuria may occur.

Treatment aims to establish adequate urinary drainage and control the infection through antibiotic therapy. The nurse should carefully note the patient's fluid intake and output. Forcing fluids is advisable, provided that the patient's cardiac status does not contraindicate this action. Observation for new symptoms, bladder distention, skin irritation, and other unusual signs should continue as the patient recovers.

Severe UTIs leading to septicemia occur more frequently among older persons than among the young, as do recurrent UTIs. Urosepsis (septicemia secondary to UTI) is a common complication of persons with indwelling catheters, so selective use of catheters is important.

Asymptomatic bacteriuria is a common finding in older adults and is usually not treated, although it is important to assess underlying factors that could contribute to this condition.

Cranberry juice has long been promoted as a means to reduce UTIs; research now supports this belief. A study conducted at the Harvard Medical School demonstrated a reduction in the frequency of bacteria and white blood cells in the urine of women who regularly consumed cranberry juice (Jepson & Craig, 2007). The gerontological nurse may want to promote the daily inclusion of cranberry juice in the diet of older adults. (It may be best to use forms such as capsules that have no sugar added to avoid the high sugar content of some commercial brands; these capsules and other freeze-dried forms of cranberry juice are available at most health food stores.)

An important measure to assist in the prevention of UTIs is to avoid the use of urinary catheters. Nurses should question the rationale for orders for indwelling catheters and consider other options. The convenience of staff (e.g., reducing the need to change soiled linens or to toilet a person) is not justification for inserting an indwelling catheter and exposing the individual to the risk of UTI. Early removal of the catheter should be encouraged as this has been found to reduce the risk of UTI.

Prostatitis

Prostatitis is the most common UTI among older men. Although nonbacterial prostatitis is responsible for some cases, most infections are bacterial in origin. Acute bacterial prostatitis is characterized by the systemic symptoms of fever, chills, and malaise, whereas these symptoms are uncommon with chronic bacterial prostatitis. Both types will present urinary symptoms of frequency, nocturia, dysuria, and varying degrees of bladder obstruction secondary to an edematous, enlarged prostate, as well as lower back and perineal pain. A simple urinalysis usually can identify the pathogen responsible for acute bacterial prostatitis; with the chronic form, a special process may be used to collect a clean-catch urine sample, with prostatic secretions obtained by massaging the prostate during the procedure. Acute prostatitis usually responds well to antibiotic therapy; chronic prostatitis responds less well to antibiotics and is more difficult to treat.

Pneumonia

Pneumonia, especially bronchopneumonia, is common in older adults and is one of the leading causes of death in this age group (Table 30-1). Several factors contribute to its high incidence:

- poor chest expansion and more shallow breathing due to age-related changes to the respiratory system
- high prevalence of respiratory diseases that promote mucus formation and bronchial obstruction
- lowered resistance to infection

TABLE 30-1 **Deaths From Pneumonia in the Older Population**

Age Group	Death Rate/100,000 Population
45–54 years	4.5
55–64 years	10.7
65–74 years	34.0
75–84 years	137.0
85+ years	571.2

Source: U.S. Department of Health and Human Services. Centers for Disease Control and Prevention (2012). *Trends in Influenza and Pneumonia among Older Persons in the United States. Table 1.* http://www.cdc.gov/nchs/data/ahcd/agingtrends/08influenza.pdf

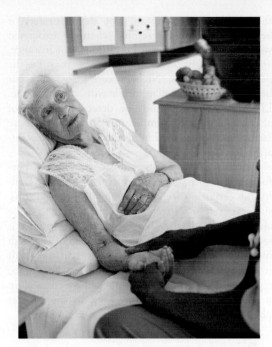

FIGURE 30-1 ■ Immobile states increase the risk of pneumonia in older adults.

■ reduced sensitivity of pharyngeal reflexes that promotes aspiration of foreign material

■ high incidence of conditions that cause reduced mobility and debilitation (Fig. 30-1)

■ greater likelihood for older adults to be hospitalized or institutionalized and develop nosocomial pneumonia than younger persons

Pneumococcal pneumonia caused by *Streptococcus pneumoniae* is the most common type of pneumonia in older adults. Other pneumonias are caused by gram-negative bacilli (*Klebsiella pneumoniae*), *Legionella pneumophila*, anaerobic bacteria, and influenza (*Haemophilus influenzae*).

The signs and symptoms of pneumonia may be altered in older persons, and serious pneumonia may exist without symptoms being evident. Pleuritic pain, for instance, may not be as severe as that described by younger patients. Differences in body temperature may cause minimal or no fever. Symptoms may include a slight cough, fatigue, and rapid respiration. Confusion, restlessness, and behavioral changes may occur as a result of cerebral hypoxia. Nursing care for the older patient with pneumonia is similar to that used for the younger patient. Close observation for subtle changes is especially important. The aged patient can also develop the complication of paralytic ileus, which can be prevented by mobility.

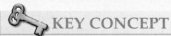

KEY CONCEPT

Productive cough, fever, and chest pain may be atypical in older adults because of age-related changes and cause a delayed diagnosis of pneumonia.

Although their effectiveness continues to be debated, pneumococcal vaccines are recommended for persons over 65 years of age. The vaccine should not be administered during a febrile illness. Concurrent administration with influenza and some other vaccines is acceptable, provided that different injection sites are used. Common side effects are local redness, fever, myalgia, and malaise. Some individuals may experience arthritic flare-ups and, more rarely, paresthesias and other neuropathies. The Centers for Disease Control and Prevention (CDC) recommends a pneumococcal vaccination and a one-time booster after 5 years if the person was under 65 years of age when the initial vaccination was administered. Nurses should be sure to document the administration of the vaccine, along with the name of the manufacturer, lot number, and expiration date. The CDC also advises that if there is doubt whether the vaccine has already been given, it is best to administer the vaccine rather than risk pneumonia. The revaccination of older adults with pneumococcal vaccines has been shown to cause local site reactions lasting several days but no life-threatening effects (High, 2007; Jackson et al., 2003).

Influenza

Most deaths from influenza occur in the older population, emphasizing the seriousness of this infection to older adults. Of the two subtypes of influenza, influenza A is the most frequent cause of serious illness and death in older adults; influenza B is less severe, although it can produce serious problems for older adults. Age-related changes, including an impaired immune response to the virus, cause older persons to be highly susceptible to influenza. Typically, influenza causes fever (although not as high as in younger adults), myalgia, sore throat, and nonproductive cough. Once it attacks, influenza destroys ciliated epithelial cells of the respiratory tract and depresses mucociliary clearance. Secondary bacterial infections and other complications increase the risk of older adults dying as a result of influenza. Patients with chronic respiratory, cardiac, or metabolic disease are at particularly high risk for developing secondary bacterial pneumonia. Nonpulmonary complications can include myositis, pericarditis, Guillain-Barré syndrome, encephalitis, and a temporary loss of smell or taste.

The serious consequences of influenza for older adults necessitate preventive measures. Because influenza is acquired through inhalation of infected droplets, reducing contact with persons with known or suspected influenza is important. Prevention also can be achieved by annual influenza vaccination, which is recommended for persons over age 65 years. Although older persons have lower antibody titers after vaccination than younger adults, vaccination can prevent severe complications associated with influenza, even if it does not prevent the disease itself. Approximately 2 weeks are needed for an antibody response to the vaccine; therefore, administration of the vaccine in October is recommended. Because the flu season can last through February, vaccinations for older adults can be administered after October. Daily vitamin and mineral supplements with enhanced antioxidants have been shown to increase antibody titers in older people after influenza vaccines have been administered (Wouters-Wesseling et al., 2002), suggesting that the relatively safe practice of administering supplements be considered in gerontological care. Immunity gradually declines in the months following vaccination, so annual revaccination is needed. The vaccine is contraindicated in persons with febrile conditions and egg allergy and those with a history of Guillain-Barré syndrome. The blood level of carbamazepine, phenobarbital, phenytoin, theophylline, and warfarin can rise within 1 to 4 weeks after vaccination; therefore, patients using these drugs need to be closely monitored for toxic reactions. It is advisable for persons who work with older adults to be immunized.

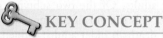 **KEY CONCEPT**

Although older adults have lower antibody titers than younger persons after vaccination, influenza vaccines can prevent severe complications associated with the disease, even if they do not prevent the disease itself.

Tuberculosis

The incidence of tuberculosis has been decreasing. A reactivation of an earlier asymptomatic or improperly treated infection is more common than new infection in older adults, and older adults in institutional settings are at higher risk for contracting this infection than community-based older persons. Diagnosis may be delayed, either because

the classic symptoms are not demonstrated or because symptoms resemble changes associated with many other geriatric conditions. For instance, anorexia, weight loss, and weakness may be the primary symptoms. Night sweats may not occur because of reduced diaphoresis with advanced age. Likewise, fever may not be detected because of alterations in body temperature in late life. These factors emphasize the importance of periodic evaluation for this disease.

Screening for tuberculosis should be performed for all patients entering a hospital or facility for geriatric care, and groups of older persons, such as senior citizen organizations, should be checked periodically. A two-step Mantoux test is recommended for older adults because of the high incidence of false-negative results (i.e., if the result is negative after the first test, the test should be repeated in 1 week, which could cause a conversion if the infection is present, owing to the booster phenomenon associated with a waned response).

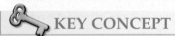 **KEY CONCEPT**

Because of the risk of false-negative results, a two-step Mantoux test is recommended for tuberculosis screening in older adults.

Treatment for tuberculosis follows the same principles as for any age group, basically consisting of rest, good nutrition, and medications. Some of the side effects of medications commonly prescribed for tuberculosis have special implications for older persons. Streptomycin can cause damage to the peripheral and central nervous systems, demonstrated through hearing limitations and disequilibrium, which create safety risks. *Para*-aminosalicylic acid can cause irritation to the gastrointestinal tract, anorexia, nausea, vomiting, and diarrhea, which can predispose older adults to the risk of malnutrition. Changes in gastric secretions can cause these tablets to pass through the gastrointestinal system without being dissolved, thereby preventing a therapeutic benefit; stools should be examined for undissolved tablets. Isoniazid, although not as toxic as the other drugs mentioned, can have toxic effects on the peripheral and central nervous systems. The nurse must assess the patient regularly for the presence of adverse reactions to such medications.

A diagnosis of tuberculosis can be extremely difficult for some older persons to accept. Having lived through an era when people with tuberculosis were sent to sanitariums for long periods of time, older adults may be unaware of new approaches to treatment and fear institutionalization. Believing they could infect family and friends, they may avoid contact with others, promoting social isolation. Other people may fear contracting the disease and be reluctant to maintain social contact. Educating patients, their families, and friends is essential to clarify these misconceptions and promote a normal lifestyle.

Nurses must teach patients their responsibilities in managing this disease. Medication is essential for the treatment of tuberculosis, and because the older person may have a problem remembering to take it, nurses should devise a system for helping the patient remember how to administer the medication. For example, medications and denture cream container could be placed in the same box so that during daily denture care the patient would remember to take the medications. The patient, a family member, or a visiting nurse could fill seven envelopes with medications, labeling them for each day of the week, and devise a chart for recording when medication is taken. A family member or friend could call the patient daily to ask whether medication was taken. With prompt and proper therapy, the older person can recover from tuberculosis with minimal residual effects.

Vaginitis

With advancing age, the vaginal epithelium thins, which is accompanied by a loss of tissue elasticity. Secretions become alkaline and of lesser quantity. The flora changes, affecting the natural protection that the vagina normally provides. These changes predispose the older woman to the common infection, senile vaginitis. Soreness, pruritus, burning, and a reddened vagina are symptoms, and the accompanying vaginal discharge is clear, brown, or white. As it progresses, vaginitis can cause bleeding and adhesions.

Local estrogens in suppository or cream form are usually effective in treating senile vaginitis. Nurses should ensure that patients understand the proper use of these topical medications and do not attempt to administer them orally. Boric acid, zinc, lysine, or gentian violet douches may also be prescribed. Some herbal medicine practitioners recommend a douche of antiseptic herbs, such as St. John's wort, goldenseal, *Echinacea*, garlic, self-heal, and calendula. If the patient is to administer a douche at home, it is important to emphasize the need to measure the solution's temperature. Altered receptors for hot and cold temperatures and reduced pain sensation predispose the patient to burns from solutions excessively hot for fragile vaginal tissue. Good hygienic practices help treat and prevent vaginitis.

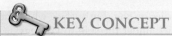

KEY CONCEPT

Older women should be advised to measure the temperature of douche solutions because altered receptors for temperatures and reduced pain sensations predispose them to burns.

Women can be advised to use a variety of natural approaches to the treatment of vaginitis. Vaginal infections have responded well to vitamins A, B complex, C, E, and β-carotene. An increased intake of acidophilus yogurt and garlic can help fight fungal infections, as can the avoidance of fermented foods and refined sugars.

Herpes Zoster

Herpes zoster, or shingles, is an acute viral infection usually caused in older adults by a reactivation of the latent varicella virus (the same virus that causes chickenpox) in the dorsal root ganglia. The weakening of immunity associated with aging is believed to contribute to the increased incidence of this problem with age; radiation, chemotherapy, stress, or other factors that disturb immune mechanisms also can cause shingles.

The disease begins with pain and itching of the skin, followed in several days by the formation of vesicles. The eruption follows the path of a sensory nerve and can occur anywhere on the body, although the thoracic and abdominal areas are the most common sites. Treatment is symptomatic, consisting of analgesics, corticosteroids, and topical preparations to dry the lesions. Older adults are more likely than other age groups to experience postherpetic neuralgia. If herpes zoster is recurrent or if dissemination is widespread, the patient should be evaluated for the possibility of an underlying lymphoma or other immune deficiency. It is recommended that all people over age 60 be vaccinated against shingles.

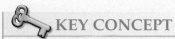

KEY CONCEPT

Older adults are more likely than younger persons to experience postherpetic neuralgia.

Scabies

Scabies is a highly contagious, pruritic skin eruption caused by a mite, the *Sarcoptes scabiei*. On contact, the female itch mite burrows under the skin and lays eggs. In 8 to 17 days, the larvae mature and travel to the skin surface to mate. After mating, the male dies on the skin surface while the female burrows back under the skin to lay eggs.

Intense pruritus, caused by an allergic reaction to the mites and their waste products, is characteristic of scabies. Pruritus worsens at night. On inspection, the skin appears excoriated. The rash is typically present in the interdigital webs, hands, wrists, elbows, abdominal folds, around the nipples, and on the genitalia, although older adults can also have a rash on the face, scalp, back, buttocks, and knees. Close examination of the rash can detect the burrow (a linear ridge with a vesicle on one end) where the mite is located. Without careful examination, the rash can be incorrectly attributed to other dermatologic conditions, such as eczema; therefore, astute assessment is essential.

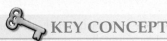

KEY CONCEPT

On inspection of the scabies rash, a burrow can be detected where the mite is located.

Diagnosis is made by scraping the lesions with a scalpel and having the material examined under a microscope for evidence of mites, eggs, or their wastes. A burrow ink test or application of mineral oil on the lesions can be done to enhance visualization of the burrows. Even with a negative finding on the scrapings, the patient may be treated if symptoms are consistent with scabies.

The case study in Box 30-2 describes the treatment and nursing care of patients with scabies.

HIV and AIDS

Although human immunodeficiency virus (HIV) and acquired immunodeficiency syndrome (AIDS) are thought of as younger persons' diseases, a little more than 10% of all cases occur in people over age 65—a number that has been consistent since the beginning of the AIDS epidemic (Centers for Disease Control and Prevention, 2007). Unfortunately, HIV and AIDS can be misdiagnosed due to the low index of suspicion in this age group. Health care professionals may

---

BOX 30-2 **Control of a Scabies Outbreak in a Long-Term Care Facility**

For the past 2 weeks, a growing number of residents of Great Oaks Nursing Home have been complaining of severe itching and presenting with a skin rash. The skin rash showed no consistent pattern among residents: some experienced a rash on the hands, wrists, and between the fingers, and others had a rash on the back and buttocks. Nursing staff initially applied moisturizing lotions, but residents obtained no relief. Observation revealed that itching worsened when residents were in bed, giving rise to the suspicion that perhaps the laundry was using an irritating detergent to wash linens; however, a review of the laundry's practice demonstrated no change in their procedures or chemicals used. When some nursing staff began to develop similar symptoms, it was suspected that the rash was contagious rather than a contact dermatitis. Close inspection of the rashes revealed thin, wavy, brown lines, characteristic of scabies. The diagnosis was confirmed through microscopic examination of scraped lesions.

Residents and staff with evidence of the infection were prescribed Lindane to kill the scabies and oral antihistamines and mild topical corticosteroid agents to control pruritus (a rash and pruritus could persist for as long as 1 month after treatment is initiated). Other staff and visitors who had had close contact

with infected residents were also encouraged to be treated. In addition, the following measures were taken to control the infection from spreading:

- Wearing of gowns and gloves for staff and visitors who have close contact with infected persons for the initial 24-hour period after treatment has begun
- Meticulous handwashing
- Laundry isolation during the entire period of treatment. Laundering of all linens and previously worn clothing in hot water or dry-cleaned. Sealing items that cannot be laundered (e.g., shoes and coats) in plastic bags and not used for 2 weeks
- Disinfection of surfaces of mattresses; turning of mattresses on the side that was not in contact with residents
- Disinfection of furniture surfaces (mites are able to live up to 3 days on a surface off the body)
- Notification of the health department (although it is usually not required to report isolated cases, the health department may want to investigate and provide consultation for outbreaks of this scope)
- Education of residents, visitors, and staff about cause and nature of infection, treatment, precautions, and prognosis
- Ongoing monitoring by the facility's infection control nurse

---

BOX 30-3   Symptoms That Can Develop Years After HIV Has Invaded the Body

Persistent fever	Herpes zoster
Drenching night sweats	Lymph node swelling
Headaches	Meningitis
Fatigue	Palsies
Chronic diarrhea	Pain
Thrush	Dementia
Persistent vaginitis	

---

not consider that older adults could be practicing unprotected sex (although without pregnancy to worry about, the probability of this is high) or be homosexual. Also, this infection can be overlooked due to the similarity of symptoms to common conditions in older adults. For example, cognitive impairment may be attributed to Alzheimer's disease rather than HIV-related dementia. In addition, as a result of advances in treatments, people are surviving into late life with these diseases so nurses will encounter more older adults with HIV.

Risk factors for HIV are the same for older people as for younger adults and include vaginal or anal sex without using a condom; sharing needles or syringes; receiving transfusions, blood products, or organ transplants between 1978 and 1985; and getting tattoos or body piercings with a contaminated needle. More than half of the cases in women are the result of having intercourse with an infected man; the changes in the vaginal canal after menopause heighten the risk of vaginal trauma and tissue tears during intercourse and, consequently, transmittal of the infection.

Initial symptoms appear within the first few weeks of being infected with the virus and resemble those of the flu, such as low-grade fever, headache, sore throat, fatigue, nausea, and a rash. These symptoms can last for several months, and then the infected person can be asymptomatic for several years. Blood will test positive for the HIV antibody about 2 months after the infection is contracted. Years after HIV has invaded the body, symptoms may appear again (Box 30-3). Infection with HIV needs to be considered when these symptoms are present. AIDS is diagnosed when people who are HIV positive develop decreased CD4+ lymphocyte count, an opportunistic infection (e.g., pneumonia or septicemia), an opportunistic cancer (e.g., Kaposi's sarcoma or invasive cervical cancer),

wasting syndrome (loss of at least 10% of body weight), or dementia.

The high risk of infection of older adults is compounded when they have HIV/AIDS. Infection prevention measures need to be strictly adhered to, and signs of infection need to be identified early. Promotion of good nutrition can offer protection from infection and improve general health status. As these patients may become easily fatigued, mealtime assistance can spare their energy and facilitate good intake.

Emotional support is a crucial part of the care of any person with HIV/AIDS, and this may be even more significant for older adults, particularly if their infection is associated with unprotected sex. Many people still feel uncomfortable with the notion of older adults being sexually active or engaging in homosexual relationships; therefore, older adults may have difficulty admitting their infection to close friends and family. In addition, the infected older adult may be rejected or treated with disdain by family and friends. A nonjudgmental attitude, listening ear, and emotional support are crucial components of the care of these patients.

POINT TO PONDER

What values and attitudes do you hold that influence your feelings about people who have contracted HIV/AIDS in extramarital or homosexual relationships? How could this influence your care of these patients?

Clostridium difficile Infection

Clostridium difficile has become the most common cause of nosocomial infectious diarrhea in nursing home settings. The consequences of *C. difficile* in causing a wide range of clinical illnesses, as well as severe and life-threatening disease, have led to it being renamed *C. difficile*–associated disease (Bartlett & Makris, 2007).

Age-related changes and the compromised health status of many older adults contribute to the high risk of *C. difficile* infections; other risk factors include overuse of antibiotics, immunosuppressant therapy, gastrointubation, and gastric feeding tubes. A significant number of hospitalized older adults develop this infection. Oral–fecal transmission of *C. difficile*, from the hands of caregivers or contaminated surfaces, causes the spread of this infection.

Diarrhea and abdominal cramps are common symptoms associated with *C. difficile* infections. Other symptoms can include delirium, low-grade fever, nausea, anorexia, and general malaise. Diagnosis is confirmed through laboratory tests of stool, including antigen detection assays and toxin testing.

The first line of treatment for mild cases of *C. difficile* is metronidazole. Vancomycin is recommended for serious cases or when patients do not respond to metronidazole within a few days of treatment. For some patients with recurrent *C. difficile*–associated disease, probiotics or biotherapy with *Saccharomyces boulardii* or *Lactobacillus* GG can be effective. Correction of fluid and electrolyte imbalances is crucial.

Because this infection can spread from infected fecal matter being transported by contaminated objects or hands, the use of gloves, strict handwashing techniques, cleaning of environmental surfaces (usually with a bleach solution), and use of enteric or contact precautions are crucial. Monitoring hydration status is important due to the risk of dehydration secondary to diarrhea.

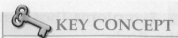

KEY CONCEPT

The spores of pathogens like *C. difficile* can persist on the surfaces of furniture and equipment for months and contaminate the hands of caregivers; strict adherence to handwashing procedures is crucial to protect both patients and caregivers from developing infections.

Antibiotic-Resistant Microorganisms

Methicillin-Resistant Staphylococcus aureus

A serious situation has evolved in recent years with the inability to control certain infections due to the resistance of pathogens to antibiotics. *Staphylococcus aureus*, a bacterium commonly found on the skin of healthy people, can enter the body and cause infections. The infections can range from minor (e.g., boils or pimples) to quite serious (e.g., pneumonia or septicemia). Until the introduction of penicillin, the fatality rate for bacteremia caused by *S. aureus* was 90%, but the use of the antibiotic significantly improved survival. However, within a short period, a strain of *S. aureus* grew that was resistant to penicillin. Methicillin was introduced in the 1960s as an effective new means of treating these infections, but in the 1980s, the pathogen grew resistant to this antibiotic, and health care settings began to see epidemics of methicillin-resistant *S. aureus* (MRSA) infections.

MRSA infection typically develops in hospitalized or institutionalized people who are old, are debilitated, or have an open wound or catheter that allows the bacteria to enter the body. It spreads through nasopharyngeal secretions and hands. For a time, vancomycin was effective against MRSA, but resistance to this antibiotic led to the need for new drugs. Linezolid (Zyvox) and the combination of

CONSIDER THIS CASE

You are having a clinical experience in a nursing home and observe several of the nursing caregivers not washing their hands between the care of different residents or after emptying bedpans. You know this violates basic infection prevention principles but want to be tactful, as the staff does not look positively at having students present. You nicely ask one of the caregivers, "How often am I supposed to wash my hands?" in the hopes that this may drop a hint to improve their handwashing practices. "Wash them before you eat and before you leave," the caregiver responds. "If you do it more, you'll just make your hands raw."

THINK CRITICALLY

■ How can you help to correct this practice?

quinupristin with dalfopristin (Synercid) have since offered treatment options.

Vancomycin-Resistant *Enterococcus* (VRE)

In the 1990s, strains of vancomycin-resistant *Enterococcus* (VRE) began to appear, which have now become significant sources of nosocomial infection. VRE infections tend to be resistant to most of the drugs previously used to treat such infections; furthermore, it is believed that genes present in VRE can be transferred to other gram-positive microorganisms, such as *S. aureus*. Persons who are severely ill, who are debilitated, or who are immunosuppressed or who have had major surgical procedures, an indwelling urinary or central venous catheter or antibiotic therapy are at risk for VRE infection. At present, Zyvox and Synercid are the only drugs effective against VRE. Like so many other infections, VRE is easily transmitted through the hands of health care workers and contaminated devices and surfaces.

It is important to promote immunologic health as part of infection prevention and control. Chapter 29 provides specific measures that can prove beneficial.

POINT TO PONDER

What self-care practices do you follow to strengthen your defenses against infection? In what ways could you improve this?

BRINGING RESEARCH TO LIFE

EMPIRIC ANTIBIOTIC THERAPY AND RESISTANCE PATTERNS IN LONG-TERM CARE–ACQUIRED URINARY TRACT INFECTIONS

Parish, A. (2012). Geriatric Nursing, 33(1), 68–69.

This study retrospectively examined data on long-term care residents over the age of 65 who were prescribed an antibiotic for a facility-acquired urinary tract infection (UTI). Ciprofloxacin was selected as the antibiotic of choice by prescribing health care providers 76% of the time. Of the persons for whom ciprofloxacin was prescribed, the predominant pathogen causing the UTI was susceptible to ciprofloxacin only 45% of the time. Approximately 43 days of incorrect therapy were used, and the patients grew a variety of resistant pathogens.

Particularly in long-term care settings (e.g., nursing homes and assisted living communities), the absence of laboratory services onsite can delay the time between the collection of a urine culture and the reporting of results. Nurses need to be aware of this and be proactive in demonstrating antibiotic stewardship, including contacting the laboratory for specimen results, communicating findings to prescribing providers promptly, and assuring patients are receiving antibiotics that are effective for their specific infection.

PRACTICE REALITIES

Seventy-year-old Ms. Marks is a new patient in the community medical practice. You are conducting the intake assessment and, when asking about her history of infections, Ms. Marks confides that she has had repeated urinary tract infections and vaginitis. You question her as to how these have been managed in the past and what her health care providers have said about them. She shares that the physicians have prescribed antibiotics and that was all. She then adds, "I've been embarrassed to discuss this with the doctors as they probably would have some choice thoughts about me, but I wonder if it could be related to my having sex. There is a man who I occasionally see and it seems I get an infection right after we have sex."

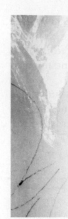

You advise her that she can openly discuss this with her physician but she says she can't, particularly as he is a young man.

How can you help Ms. Marks?

CRITICAL THINKING EXERCISES

1. What would you include in a health education session to teach older adults about prevention, recognition, and care of influenza and pneumonia?

2. What are some of the reasons for HIV/AIDS not being identified in older adults?

3. Describe potential implications for your community if the residents of a local senior citizen housing complex developed an acute respiratory infection that was resistant to all currently available antibiotics. What actions could be taken to protect the community?

REFERENCES

Bartlett, J. G., & Makris, A. T. (2007). *Clostridium difficile*-associated disease in the long-term care setting: Strategies for identification, management, and infection control. *Caring for the Ages, supplement,* Elsevier Society News Group.

Centers for Disease Control and Prevention. (2007). Epidemiology of HIV/AIDS—United States, 1981–2005. *Morbidity and Mortality Weekly Report, 55*(21), 589–592.

DeFrances, M. J., & Paul, C. J. (2006). 2005 National hospital discharge survey. *Advance Data, 12*(385), 1–19.

Graves, N., Tong, E., Mortaon, A. P., Holton, K., Curtis, M., Lairson D, & Whitby M. (2007). Factors associated with health care-acquired urinary tract infection. *American Journal of Infection Control, 35*(6), 387–392.

High, K. (2007). Immunizations in older adults. *Clinical Geriatric Medicine, 23*(3), 669–685.

Jackson, L. A., Neuzil, K. M., Yu, O., Benson, P., Barlow, W. E., Adams, A. L., Thompson, W. W., et al. (2003). Effectiveness of pneumococcal polysaccharide vaccine in older adults. *New England Journal of Medicine, 348*(18), 1747–1755.

Jepson, R. G., & Craig, J. C. (2007). A systematic review of the evidence for cranberries and blueberries in UTI prevention. *Molecular Nutrition and Food Research, 51*(6), 738–745.

Wouters-Wesseling, W., Rozendaal, M., Snijder, M., et al. (2002). Effect of a complete nutritional supplement on antibody response to influenza vaccine in older people. *Journals of Gerontology Series A: Biological Sciences and Medical Sciences, 57*(9), M563.

RECOMMENDED READINGS

Recommended Readings associated with this chapter can be found on the web site that accompanies the book. Visit **http://thepoint.lww.com/Eliopoulos8e** to access the recommended readings and other additional resources associated with this chapter.

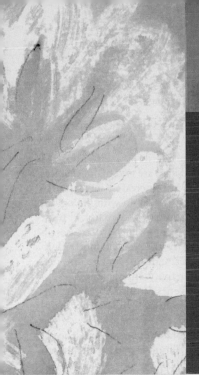

CHAPTER 31

Cancer

CHAPTER OUTLINE

LEARNING OBJECTIVES

After reading this chapter, you should be able to:

1. Discuss the prevalence and risks of cancer in the older population.
2. Describe reasons for cancer being more complex in older adults.
3. List factors that increase the risk of cancer.
4. Outline preventive measures that can reduce the risk of cancer in older adults.
5. Describe increased risks for older adults receiving conventional cancer treatment.
6. Discuss reasons for patients' choice to use complementary and alternative medicine (CAM).
7. List issues to evaluate in the selection of CAM for patients with cancer.
8. Discuss nursing considerations in caring for older patients with cancer.

TERMS TO KNOW

BRCA: breast cancer gene; blood tests can be done to identify mutations in either one of two breast cancer susceptible genes (*BRAC1* and *BRAC2*)

CAM: complementary and alternative medicine therapies; those therapies that fall outside of mainstream Western medical practices; includes alternative medical systems, mind–body interventions, manipulative and body-based methods, biologically based therapies, and energy therapies

SPF: sun protection factor; rating used for sunscreens to indicate the protection they offer from sun

Caring for older adults with cancer is a nearly inescapable aspect of gerontological nursing. Cancer is a disease of older people, being the second leading cause of death in persons aged 65 years and older (National Center for Health Statistics, 2012). Most new cases are diagnosed in older adults, with a mean age of cancer diagnosis of 66 years, and the probability of developing this disease dramatically increases with advancing age. The National Cancer Institute acknowledges that age is the single most important risk factor for cancer. Cancer rates increase from childhood on, with the most dramatic increases being in late life. The rates peak at age 80 to 84 years for males and at age 85 and above for females; the rates for white and black females do not increase as rapidly as those for their male counterparts. The rates for white females are similar to those for black females until age 70 years and older, when they are slightly higher. Even if there were no increase in cancer rates, the prevalence of cancer in older adults will rise in the future as the older population continues to grow.

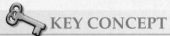

KEY CONCEPT

More than half of the persons diagnosed with cancer are over age 65 years.

Gerontological nurses have a significant role to play in the prevention, diagnosis, and treatment of cancer. Encouraging healthy lifestyle habits in persons of all ages can help reduce the risk factors for developing cancer. Educating patients about cancer screening and facilitating their efforts to obtain tests can enable cancers to be detected in early stages, thereby increasing survival rates. Creative, holistic, and skillful nursing interventions that offer support—physical, emotional, and spiritual—to individuals diagnosed with cancer and their significant others promote the best possible quality of life in the presence of the disease.

AGING AND CANCER

Unique Challenges for Older Persons With Cancer

Cancer in any age group presents many clinical challenges; however, in older adults, the complexities are even greater. Despite having the highest rate of most cancers, older adults have the lowest rate of receiving early detection tests; thus, their disease may be in an advanced stage when diagnosed (Bradley, Given, Dahman, Luo, & Virnig, 2007; Walker & Covinsky, 2001). In addition, it is the rare older adult who does not have another health condition (e.g., heart disease, diabetes mellitus, arthritis, or chronic obstructive pulmonary disease) present when diagnosed with cancer. The presence of multiple health conditions elevates the risk of complications, disability, and death for older patients diagnosed with cancer. Further, concern regarding how the older patient's already compromised organs will tolerate chemotherapy and other cancer therapies could impact treatment decisions. Survival rates for older adults are lower than in

younger persons for most types of cancer, even if they are diagnosed at the same stage.

Explanations for Increased Incidence in Old Age

As mentioned, cancer primarily is a disease of old age, but why is that so? There are two major theories that attempt to explain the increased incidence of cancer with age. The first has to do with biological, age-related changes that impair the ability to resist diseases. This theory is supported by decreases in the mitochondrial activity of the cell that reduce its ability to resist cancer. Changes in the immune system (reduced T-cell activity, interleukin-2 levels, and mitogen responsiveness) impair the body's ability to recognize cancerous cells and destroy them.

Prolonged exposure to carcinogens over the years is another explanation for the rising incidence of cancer with age. This is demonstrated by the growth of melanomas on the skin of persons who have had chronic exposure to damaging ultraviolet rays and the development of lung cancer in industrial workers who regularly breathed toxic substances.

Although the extent of responsibility that either age-related changes or exposure has in the development of cancer cannot be clearly stated at this time, it is evident that aging adults face an increased risk of developing cancer; therefore, the reduction of risk factors is beneficial.

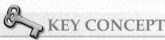

KEY CONCEPT

The increased incidence of cancer with age could result from age-related changes that reduce the ability to resist the disease or prolonged exposure to carcinogens.

RISK FACTORS, PREVENTION, AND SCREENING

The risk factors for cancers offer insights into some of the preventive measures that could prove useful in avoiding these diseases. Many cancers can be prevented by healthy lifestyle practices that minimize risks. Box 31-1 connects risk factors with some preventive measures that nurses can incorporate into health education and counseling.

Women have special risks. Because most breast and ovarian cancers occur in women over age 50 years, increased age is a factor (Turchetti, Cortesi, Federico, Romagnoli, & Silingardi, 2002). In addition, women who had their first menstrual period before the age of 12 years or experienced menopause after age 55 years have a slightly increased risk of breast cancer, as do women who had their first child

BOX 31-1   Cancer Risk Factors and Actions to Reduce Risk

Avoid the use of and exposure to tobacco products.

Cigarette smoking is the leading cause of lung cancer death in both men and women. Smoking is also responsible for one third of all cancer deaths and for most cancers of the larynx, oral cavity, and esophagus. It is highly associated with the development of, and deaths from, bladder, kidney, pancreatic, and cervical cancers (National Cancer Institute, 2012).

Limit exposure to the sun. Use sunscreens (rated between 15 and 30 SPF [sun protection factor]) and avoid sunbathing.

Repeated exposure to ultraviolet rays from the sun, sunlamps, and tanning beds can increase the risk of skin cancer, particularly in persons with fair skin.

Eat a diet rich in fiber, fruits, and vegetables; limit intake of red meats, fats, fried foods, and pickled, smoked, or cured foods.

Researchers have discovered that people who ate diets high in animal fat had higher rates of stomach and colorectal cancer than those who ate low–animal fat diets (Doyle, 2007; Palli et al., 2000). Additional studies have shown that an increased risk of developing pancreatic and breast cancer is associated with high intakes of well-done, fried, or barbecued meats. Microwaving meats at least 2 minutes before cooking can reduce the risk (Thomas, 2003).

Maintain weight within an ideal range; exercise and be physically active.

Obesity increases the rates of cancer of the prostate, pancreas, uterus, colon, and ovary and breast cancer in older women. Exercise could decrease the risk of breast cancer.

Protect against exposure to known carcinogens.

The contamination of drinking water from nitrate, a chemical used in fertilizers, has been associated with an increased risk of non-Hodgkin's lymphoma (Ward, Cerhan, Colt, & Hartge, 2006). The risk is directly correlated to the level of nitrates consumed and is particularly high in rural areas. Vegetables high in nitrate content do not carry the same risk.

Before the 1950s, x-rays were used to treat acne, ringworm of the scalp, and enlarged thymus, tonsils, and adenoids. This exposure to radiation increases the risk of thyroid cancer. Exposure to asbestos, nickel, cadmium, uranium, radon, vinyl chloride, benzene, and other substances also can increase the risk of cancer.

Radon can enter homes through cracks in the foundation. In areas without adequate ventilation, radon gas can accumulate to levels that substantially increase the risk of lung cancer (Boffetta, 2006; Duckworth, Frank-Stromborg, Oleckno, Duffy, & Burns, 2002).

Limit alcohol consumption.

Heavy alcohol consumption increases the risk of cancer of the mouth, throat, esophagus, larynx, and liver.

Discuss chemoprevention with your physician if family history increases the risk of cancer.

Inherited alterations in the genes called BRCA1 and BRCA2 (short for breast cancer 1 and breast cancer 2) are involved in many cases of hereditary breast and ovarian cancer. The risk that BRCA1 or BRCA2 is associated with these cancers is highest in women with a family history of multiple cases of breast cancer, with at least one family member having two primary cancers at different sites, or who are of Eastern European (Ashkenazi) Jewish background (American Cancer Society, 2007; Brekelmans et al., 2001).

---

after age 30 years. Women who have a first-degree relative (mother, sister, or daughter) or other close relative with breast and/or ovarian cancer may be at increased risk for developing these cancers. Women whose mothers took diethylstilbestrol during pregnancy have an increased risk of vaginal cancer (Li, Hursting, Davis, McLachlan, & Barrett, 2003). In addition, women with relatives who have had colon cancer are at increased risk for developing ovarian cancer. Excess estrogen is suspected to contribute to breast cancer because of its natural role in stimulating breast cell growth. Long-term hormonal replacement therapy may increase a woman's risk of breast and ovarian cancer, although research is inconclusive at this time.

Gerontological nurses need discretion to sort through risk factors, so that while promoting positive health habits, they do not alarm patients with unsupported claims. For instance, some people think that because stress and other "toxic" emotions can depress immune function, they also can contribute to cancer. Evidence currently does not conclusively support this relationship. Another example is the fear many people have that artificial sweeteners cause cancer, but this link has not been proven (Samuels, 2007). Nor has the National Cancer Institute proved any link between coffee and cancer, another common belief. Further, there is no clear evidence that food additives are risk factors for cancer.

There has also been considerable debate regarding the role of fluoridated water in the development of cancer. However, numerous studies have not shown that fluoride increases the risk of cancer, and the National Cancer Institute (2012) supports this position.

In addition to preventive measures, nurses should educate older adults about cancer screening, an important measure to improve outcomes in patients who develop cancer. Early detection can improve prognosis of cancer and should be encouraged for persons of all ages. Medicare provides reimbursement for screening tests for breast, cervical, colorectal, and prostate cancers. Some of the recommended tests are outlined in Box 31-2.

TREATMENT

Conventional Treatment

The plan of treatment depends on the specific cancer; however, most conventional forms of treatment include surgery, radiation, chemotherapy, and biologic therapy. Although the same basic care measures apply to older patients undergoing these treatments as to adults of any age, there are some unique risks. Persons over age 70 years have a higher risk of mortality and complications from all surgeries, and this risk is heightened with emergency or unplanned surgeries, as can occur with an unexpected detection of a mass. Advanced age can affect the pharmacokinetics and

pharmacodynamics of cytotoxic drugs and increase the risk of complications (e.g., cardiotoxicity, neurotoxicity, and myelodepression). Doses need to be adjusted carefully to account for altered glomerular filtration rates and other differences. Fortunately, there is no significant difference between the older persons and adults of other ages in the ability to tolerate radiation therapy.

POINT TO PONDER

What would be your primary concerns if you faced treatment for cancer?

Complementary and Alternative Medicine

Complementary and alternative medicine (CAM) therapies are used by nearly half of all Americans and by more than 80% of people with cancer (Hlubocky, Ratain, Web, & Daughtery, 2007). These therapies include special diets, psychotherapy, spiritual practices, vitamin supplements, and herbal remedies.

CAM therapies often are attractive to patients with cancer because of the healing philosophies and approaches used. CAM practitioners tend to have a holistic orientation. They are not only concerned with treating the disease but also likely to be equally, if not more, concerned with caring for the whole person. CAM practitioners offer:

- *Relationship-centered care:* They invest the time in learning about the unique characteristics of patients and enter a unique journey with each patient.
- *Support:* Learning to live with cancer is challenging and demanding. Even if the malignant cells are eliminated, emotional and spiritual pain may be present. CAM practitioners provide unconditional acceptance and understanding of patients "where they are."
- *Healing partnerships:* CAM practitioners honor patients' rights to control their care and their lives, seeing their role as empowering, facilitating, and supporting patients in the healing process.
- *Comfort:* Many CAM therapies are high touch (i.e., "hands-on" therapies such as massage, Therapeutic Touch, Healing Touch) and relieve stress and discomfort. Practitioners provide psychological comfort as they take the time to listen, to reassure, and to be emotionally available.
- *Hope:* Particularly when conventional medicine has exhausted its treatments, CAM practitioners provide options that can offer

---

BOX 31-2 Recommended Cancer Screening for Older Adults

- Annual checkup that examines oral cavity, thyroid, breasts, ovaries, testicles, and skin
- Annual mammogram
- Annual fecal occult blood test
- Flexible sigmoidoscopy every 5 years or colonoscopy every 10 years
- Double contrast barium enema every 5 years
- Pap test every 2 to 3 years if there have been three consecutive normal tests; the American Cancer Society suggests that women 70 years of age or older who have had three consecutive normal Pap tests and no abnormal Pap tests in the last 10 years may choose to discontinue cervical screening
- Annual endometrial biopsy for women at high risk for hereditary nonpolyposis colon cancer

hope and encouragement through knowing that something is being attempted. Patients can heal—that is, feel a sense of wholeness and live the best possible quality of life—despite having an incurable disease.

POINT TO PONDER

Why might you seek complementary and alternative therapies if you or a loved one were diagnosed with cancer?

Although CAM can contribute to a patient's care, it is unwise for patients to use these therapies without carefully weighing risks and benefits. The labels *natural* or *holistic* do not ensure that the therapy is safe or the best option for the patient for his or her given circumstances. Box 31-3 offers some questions that nurses can use in assisting patients in evaluating CAM. Nurses can provide a useful service to patients in helping them to research claims made by promoters of therapies and products to treat cancer. The National Cancer Institute and National Center for Complementary and Alternative Medicine (see Resource listings) can offer assistance in evaluating CAM claims.

Knowledge about CAM is rapidly growing, and today's hypotheses could be proved or disproved tomorrow. Nurses are challenged to stay current of this expanding field so that they can integrate CAM into their practice safely and effectively.

KEY CONCEPT

Ask about the use of CAM during every assessment and encourage patients to inform their physicians of all therapies and products being used.

NURSING CONSIDERATIONS FOR OLDER ADULTS WITH CANCER

Providing Patient Education

Gerontological nurses have a commitment to promoting healthy aging. One means of demonstrating this is to increase awareness of measures that can prevent cancer (see Box 31-1). Opportunities for educating individuals can range from teaching formal group classes to discussing options for change when risk factors are identified during individual assessments. This education need not be limited to older adults. Cancer prevention to younger people can promote a healthier senior population in the future.

Nurses play an important role in ensuring that patients understand the warning signs of cancer.

The American Cancer Society's (2012) use of the word CAUTION, in which each letter represents the first letter of a warning sign, provides a useful way to remember them:

- **C**hange in bowel or bladder habits
- **A** sore that does not heal
- **U**nusual bleeding or drainage
- **T**hickening or lump in the breast or elsewhere
- **I**ndigestion or swallowing difficulty
- **O**bvious change in a wart or mole
- **N**agging persistent cough or hoarseness

In addition, nurses assess patients' knowledge of self-examination for cancer (e.g., breast examination, testicular examination, and skin inspection) and provide instruction as needed. For the patient who

BOX 31-3 Questions to Ask When Evaluating a Complementary and Alternative Therapy

- What is the purpose or expected outcome of the therapy?
- Is the therapy compatible with other treatments being used?
- Will serious delays in seeking or using conventional treatment result from using complementary and alternative medicine?
- Is special training, licensure, or certification required by practitioners of the therapy, and if so, is the practitioner being considered to provide the therapy qualified?
- What risks are associated with the therapy? Do the risks outweigh the benefits?
- What are the expected side effects?
- What is the cost?
- How many treatments will be needed; how long will the product need to be used?
- Is the therapy covered by any health insurance?
- What research exists supporting the therapy? How large have the studies been, what were their quality, and who has conducted them?
- Is the therapist willing to offer the names of other patients who have used his or her service?
- Are there any "red flags" (e.g., secretive nature of treatment, unwillingness to disclose ingredients of product, necessity to travel to a foreign country to obtain treatment, requirement that all other treatments be discontinued)?

is unable to perform self-examinations, the nurse develops a plan for caregivers to perform these examinations for the patient on a regular schedule. It is important to inquire about dates of last cancer screening tests and refer for testing as needed.

Promoting Optimum Care

When the diagnosis of cancer is made, the nurse can help the patient to obtain the best possible care. Some oncology centers may specialize in a particular cancer and be able to offer more options to patients than other facilities. Also, as appropriate, the nurse assists patients in contacting the National Cancer Institute to learn about clinical trials that may be beneficial.

Older adults receiving radiation and chemotherapy require the same basic care and face the same general risks as adults of any age who undergo these treatments; oncology nursing literature should be consulted for guidance. However, the challenges with older adults may be increased because of common age-related factors that contribute to increased risks of malnutrition, dehydration, constipation, immobility, impaired skin integrity, and infection. Close monitoring and taking actions to prevent complications (e.g., reporting changes in vital signs or increased fatigue) are essential.

A significant fear associated with cancer is pain. Patients need to be assured that pain can be managed. The nurse should regularly assess for pain and assist in developing a plan to prevent and manage pain. (See Chapter 16 for discussion of comfort measures.)

Further information about specific types of cancers appears in other chapters, e.g., cancer of the colon (Chapter 21); prostate (Chapter 23); lung (Chapter 19); stomach (Chapter 21); testes (Chapter 23); and pancreas (Chapter 21).

Providing Support to Patients and Families

The diagnosis of cancer can be considerably overwhelming and stressful to many patients. Older adults may recall the grim experiences of people with cancer they have known throughout their lives—people who were diagnosed years ago when treatment options were considerably more limited than today—and fear that their outlook will be similar. They may fear that they will experience pain, deformity, and lost independence. The cost of treatment could present significant burdens to patients and their families. Plans and pursuits may have to be forfeited as treatment of the disease takes center stage. Patients will need strong support during this time. It is important to consult with the physician to learn about the patient's diagnosis, treatment plan, and prognosis. The nurse assesses the patient's understanding, clarifies misconceptions, and offers explanations where needed. Providing ample opportunity for the patient to express feelings is important.

Family and significant others may share the patient's concerns and have additional concerns of their own. For example, a wife may worry that the cost of her husband's treatment or his death will place her in a financially vulnerable position. Or a daughter may grieve that her parent may not survive to see her marry. They, too, need support. (Local chapters of the American Cancer Society can provide information on support groups for people with cancer and their loved ones.)

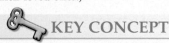

KEY CONCEPT

Remember that the diagnosis of cancer touches lives beyond the patient's.

CONSIDER THIS CASE

Sixty-two year-old Carrie S has been diagnosed with breast cancer and after having a lumpectomy has begun chemotherapy. She has been optimistic and eager to progress with her treatment. During one of her treatments she is accompanied by her 55-year-old sister. The sister appears quite anxious. She shares that her mother had breast cancer at age 65 years and lived until age 82 years, when she died of lung cancer. "Now," she says, "Carrie has the disease, and I know I'm next in line." She tells you that she is "thinking of having bilateral mastectomies to avoid the fate of my mother and sister."

THINK CRITICALLY

- How would you react to the sister's concerns?
- How could her sister's feelings potentially affect Carrie S?
- What support can you offer Ms. S?

Patients may experience a variety of reactions as they cope with their disease, including depression, grief, guilt, anger, bargaining, and acceptance. Similar to the grief experienced with the dying process, they may float in and out of various stages at different times. Sensitivity to the patient's emotional and spiritual status during each encounter is essential. The nurse must remember that family members may experience these same fluctuations in emotions.

Physical, emotional, and spiritual support are required by patients with terminal cancer as they cope with potentially many challenges (Box 31-4). The needs of these patients and their families can change and demand regular reassessment and adjustment to the plan of care. Chapter 39 offers guidelines for end-of-life care that are applicable to patients with terminal cancer.

BOX 31-4 Possible Nursing Diagnoses of Patients With Terminal Cancer

EXCHANGING
Imbalanced Nutrition: Less Than Body Requirements
Risk of Infection
Constipation
Impaired Urinary Elimination
Deficient Fluid Volume
Impaired Gas Exchange
Ineffective Airway Clearance
Ineffective Breathing Pattern
Risk of Injury
Risk of Aspiration
Impaired Tissue Integrity

COMMUNICATING
Impaired Verbal Communication

RELATING
Impaired Social Interaction
Social Isolation
Ineffective Role Performance
Caregiver Role Strain

VALUING
Spiritual Distress

CHOOSING
Ineffective Coping
Ineffective Denial
Decisional Conflict

MOVING
Impaired Physical Mobility
Activity Intolerance
Fatigue
Disturbed Sleep Pattern
Feeding/Bathing/Dressing/Grooming/Toileting Self-Care Deficit
Impaired Swallowing

PERCEIVING
Disturbed Body Image
Hopelessness
Powerlessness

KNOWING
Deficient Knowledge
Acute Confusion

FEELING
Acute Pain
Chronic Pain
Nausea
Anticipatory Grieving
Anxiety
Fear
Risk of Suicide

BRINGING RESEARCH TO LIFE

COLORECTAL CANCER SCREENING AMONG ETHNICALLY DIVERSE, LOW-INCOME PATIENTS: A RANDOMIZED CONTROLLED TRIAL

Lasser, K. E., Murillo, J., Lisboa, S., Casimir, N., Valley-Shah, L., Emmons, K. M., Ayanian, J. Z., et al. (2011). Archives of Internal Medicine, 171(10), 906–912.

Recognizing that one in three adults between the ages of 50 and 75 years does not undergo colorectal cancer screening, this study sought to determine if a strategy using laypeople as health system "navigators" could encourage higher participation in cancer screening. Patients were randomly assigned to a group targeted to receive assistance in navigating the health care system or a control group who received nothing beyond the standard care. Those in the intervention group received a letter and brochure about colorectal screening from their provider, followed by a telephone call from a navigator who was fluent in the patient's primary language. In addition to encouraging colorectal screening, the navigators helped patients in solving insurance problems and scheduling appointments. The navigators were supervised by a nurse.

In the course of 1 year, patients in the group who received the intervention had higher rates of cancer screening and cancer detection.

This study reminds us that the most sophisticated diagnostic tests in the world mean little if people do not access them due to lack of knowledge, language barriers, low motivation, or challenges in navigating the health care system. Laypeople who are peers to patients may be effective in changing perceptions and practices. In addition, nurses can show leadership by advocating and implementing such programs.

PRACTICE REALITIES

Sixty-two year-old Ms. Strand has been diagnosed with breast cancer. She has visited the oncology department where you work and the oncologist has recommended chemotherapy, radiation, and a lumpectomy. A very attractive single woman, Ms. Strand expressed concern about the effects of the treatments on her appearance. When she misses her next appointment and fails to contact the office, you call her to reschedule her appointment. She tells you she isn't going to have the recommended therapies as she has found an alternative practitioner who claims he can cure her of her cancer with a special diet, supplements, and positive thinking exercises. "I can treat my cancer, improve my general health, and I won't have to get cut, burned, or go bald," she says with excitement.

What could you do in this situation?

CRITICAL THINKING EXERCISES

1. Develop an outline of the content for a health education program for a senior citizen group on "Cancer Prevention, Risks, and Diagnosis."
2. Describe current lifestyle factors that may affect the risk of cancer in future generations of older persons.
3. Develop a plan of care for an older adult diagnosed with lung cancer that integrates conventional and CAM therapies.
4. What actions could nurses take in their communities to reduce cancer risks?

RESOURCES

American Cancer Society
http://www.cancer.org

National Breast Cancer Foundation
http://www.nationalbreastcancer.org

National Cancer Institute
http://www.cancer.gov
1-800-4-CANCER (1-800-422-6237)
TTY (for deaf and hard of hearing callers): 1-800-332-8615

National Center for Complementary and Alternative Medicine
http://www.nccam.nih.gov
1-888-644-6226 (toll free)

National Comprehensive Cancer Network
http://www.nccn.org

REFERENCES

American Cancer Society. (2006). *Cancer facts and figures 2002.* Atlanta, GA: American Cancer Society.

American Cancer Society. (2012). *Detailed guide: Breast cancer. What are the risk factors for breast cancer?* Retrieved October 10, 2012 from http://www.cancer.org/Cancer/BreastCancer/DetailedGuide/breast-cancer-risk-factors

Boffetta, P. (2006). Human cancer from environmental pollutants. The epidemiological evidence. *Mutation Research, 608*(2), 157–162.

Bradley, C. J., Given, C. W., Dahman, B., Luo, Z., & Virnig, B. A. (2007). Diagnosis of advanced cancer among elderly Medicare and Medicaid patients. *Medical Care, 45*(5), 410–419.

Brekelmans, C. T. M., Seynaeve, C., Bartels, C. C. M., Tilanus-Linthorst, M. M., Meijers-Heijboer, E. J., Crepin, C. M., Klijn, J. G., et al.; Rotterdam Committee for Medical and Genetic Counseling. (2001). Effectiveness of breast cancer surveillance in BRCA1/2 gene mutation carriers and women with high familial risk. *Journal of Clinical Oncology, 19*(4), 924–930.

Doyle, V. C. (2007). Nutrition and colorectal cancer risk: A literature review. *Gastroenterology Nursing, 30*(3), 178–182.

Duckworth, L. T., Frank-Stromborg, M., Oleckno, W. A., Duffy, P., & Burns, K. (2002). Relationship of perception of radon as a health risk and willingness to engage in radon testing and mitigation. *Oncology Nursing Forum, 29*(7), 1099–1107.

Hlubocky, F. J., Ratain, M. J., Web, M., & Daughtery, C. K. (2007). Complementary and alternative medicine among advanced cancer patients enrolled on phase I trials: A study of prognosis, quality of life, and preferences for decision making. *Journal of Clinical Oncology, 25*(5), 548–554.

Li, S., Hursting, S. D., Davis, B. J., McLachlan, J. A., & Barrett, J. C. (2003). Environmental exposure, DNA methylation, and gene regulation: Lessons from diethylstilbestrol-induced cancers [review]. *Annals of the New York Academy of Science, 983*, 161–169

National Cancer Institute. (2012). *Fluoridated water.* National Cancer Institute's Cancer Facts website. Retrieved October 10, 2012 from http://www.cancer.gov/cancertopics/factsheet/Risk/fluoridated-water/print

National Cancer Institute (2012). Harms of smoking and health benefits of quitting. Accessed October 10, 2012, http://www.cancer.gov/cancertopics/factsheet/Tobacco/cessation

National Center for Health Statistics. (2012). *Leading causes of death.* Retrieved June 22, 2012 from http://www.cdc.gov/nchs/fastats/lcod.htm

Palli, D., Russo, A., Sajeva, C., Salvini, S., Amorosi, A., & Decarli, A. (2000). Dietary and familial determinants of 10-year survival among patients with gastric carcinoma. *Cancer, 89*, 1205–1213.

Samuels, A. (2007). Aspartame consumption and incidence of hematopoietic and brain cancers. *Cancer Epidemiology, Biomarkers, and Prevention, 16*(7), 527–528.

Thomas, C. (2003). *Common sense about food and cancer.* Cancerpage.com. Retrieved May 27, 2003 from http://www.cancerpage.com/news/article.asp?id=2169

Turchetti, D., Cortesi, L., Federico, M., Romagnoli, R., & Silingardi, V. (2002). Hereditary risk of breast cancer: Not only BRCA. *Journal of Experimental Clinical Cancer Research, 21*(3 Suppl.), 17–21.

Walker, L., & Covinsky, K. E. (2001). Cancer screening in elderly patients: A framework for individualized decision making. *Journal of the American Medical Association, 285*, 2750–2765.

Ward, M. H., Cerhan, J. R., Colt, J. S., & Hartge, P. (2006). Risk of non-Hodgkin lymphoma and nitrate and nitrite from drinking water and diet. *Epidemiology, 17*(4), 375–382.

RECOMMENDED READINGS

Recommended Readings associated with this chapter can be found on the web site that accompanies the book. Visit **http://thepoint.lww.com/Eliopoulos8e** to access the recommended readings and other additional resources associated with this chapter.

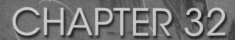

CHAPTER 32

Mental Health Disorders

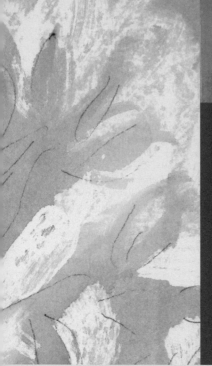

CHAPTER OUTLINE

LEARNING OBJECTIVES

After reading this chapter, you should be able to:

1. Describe the realities of mental health and illness in older adulthood.

2. List measures that promote mental health for older adults.

3. Describe the symptoms and care of the older person with depression.

4. Identify indications of suicidal thoughts in older adults.

5. Describe interventions to reduce anxiety in older adults.

6. Discuss the scope and signs of alcohol abuse in the older population.

7. List reasons for hypochondriasis in older adults.

8. Identify factors to consider in monitoring psychotropic medications in older adults.

9. Describe factors that promote a positive self-concept in older adults.

10. Identify nursing actions to manage disruptive behavior associated with mental health conditions in older adults.

Mental health indicates a capacity to cope effectively with and manage life's stresses in an effort to achieve a state of emotional homeostasis. Older people have an advantage over other age groups in that they probably have had more experience with coping, problem solving, and managing crises by virtue of the years they have lived. Most older persons have few delusions regarding what they are or what they are going to be.

TERMS TO KNOW

Emotional homeostasis: balance of emotions

Hypochondriasis: excessive concern or fear that one has a serious disease

Pseudodementia: false appearance of dementia that occurs when persons demonstrate cognitive deficits secondary to being depressed

They know where they have been, what they have accomplished, and who they really are. Immigrating to a new country, watching loved ones die from epidemics, fighting in world wars, and surviving the Great Depression may be among the numerous stresses that today's older adults have faced and overcome. Such experiences have provided them with unique strength that should not be underestimated.

However, acknowledging this strength does not imply that psychiatric illness is not a problem among the older population. More people than ever are surviving to old age, and many bring to their later years the mental health problems they have possessed throughout their lifetimes. In addition, the many losses and challenges of late life may exceed the physical, emotional, and social resources of some persons and promote mental illness. By promoting mental health, detecting problems early, and minimizing the impact of existing psychiatric problems, nurses can help older people achieve optimal satisfaction and function.

 POINT TO PONDER

What does mental health mean to you?

AGING AND MENTAL HEALTH

Many myths prevail regarding mental health and older people. For instance, many people still believe that loss of mental functioning, "senility," or mental incompetence is a natural part of old age. Descriptions of older adults being childlike, rigid, or cantankerous propagate stereotypes about personality in later life. Frequently, these misconceptions are so widely accepted that when an older person demonstrates pathological signs, it is considered normal and no attempt is made to intervene. Nurses can play a significant role in ensuring that the myths and realities of mental health in old age are understood.

Cognitive function in later life is highly individualized, based on personal resources, health status, and the unique experiences of the individual's life. The incidence of mental illness is higher among the old than among the young. A significant number of older adults in the community and in nursing homes have symptoms of serious mental health problems. Nearly 10% of the older population has a problem with alcoholism, and the rate of completed suicide among older persons continues to be the highest of any age group in the United States, with nearly one fourth of all suicides committed by persons aged 65 years and older (Loebel, 2005). Depression increases in prevalence and intensity with age (Centers for Disease Control and Prevention, 2005). Multiple losses, altered sensory function, and alterations, discomforts, and demands associated with illnesses that older adults frequently encounter set the stage for a variety of mental health problems.

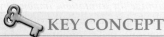 KEY CONCEPT

Cognitive function among older adults is highly individualized based on their health status, experiences, and personal resources.

PROMOTING MENTAL HEALTH IN OLDER ADULTS

Mental health in old age implies a satisfaction and interest in life. This can be displayed in a variety of ways, ranging from silent reflection to zealous activity. The quiet individual who stays at home does not necessarily have less mental capacity or mental health than the person who is actively involved in every possible community program. There is no single profile for mental health; thus, attempts to assess an older individual's mental status based on any given stereotype must be avoided.

Good mental health practices throughout an individual's lifetime promote good mental health in later life. To preserve mental health, people need to maintain the activities and interests that they find satisfying. They need opportunities to sense their value as a member of society and to have their self-worth reinforced. Security through the provision of adequate income, safe housing, the means to meet basic human needs, and support and assistance through stressful situations will promote mental health. Connection with others is also an aspect of mental health. Finally, a basic ingredient in the preservation and promotion of mental health that cannot be overstated is the importance of optimum physical health.

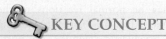 KEY CONCEPT

Good mental health practices throughout the life span promote good mental health in old age.

Nurses must recognize that there are times in everyone's life when disturbances occur and alter the capacity to manage stress. The same principles guiding the care of physical health problems can be applied to the care of persons with mental health problems. The following are actions related to those principles that can be used in care:

- *Strengthen the individual's capacity to manage the condition:* fostering improvement of physical health, good nutrition, increased knowledge, meaningful activity, stress management, income supplements, and socialization.
- *Eliminate or minimize the limitations imposed by the condition:* providing consistency in care, not fostering hallucinations, reality orientation, correction of physical problems, and modifying the environment to compensate for deficits.
- *Act for or do for the individual only when absolutely necessary:* selecting an adequate diet, assisting with bathing, administering medications, managing finances, and coordinating activities for the patient.

Mental health conditions must be seen in the perspective of the patient's total world. Older adults confront many problems that challenge their emotional homeostasis, such as the following:

- *Illness:* coping, related self-care demands, pain, altered function or body image
- *Death:* friends, family, significant support person
- *Retirement:* loss of status, role, income, sense of purpose
- *Increased vulnerability:* crime, illness, disability, abuse
- *Social isolation:* lack of transportation, funds, health, friends
- *Sensory deficits:* decrease in or loss of function of hearing, vision, taste, smell, and touch
- *Greater awareness of own mortality:* increased number of deaths among peers
- *Increased risk of institutionalization, dependency:* loss of self-care capabilities to varying degrees

With these factors in mind, some of the symptoms displayed may be normal reactions to the circumstances at hand (Fig. 32-1). Before labeling the patient with a psychiatric diagnosis, the nurse should explore such factors in the patient's behavior and address the cause of the problem rather than its effects alone.

Astute assessment can help distinguish normal reactions to life events from mental health conditions (Assessment Guide 32-1). Nursing Diagnosis Table 32-1 outlines potential diagnoses that assessment may reveal.

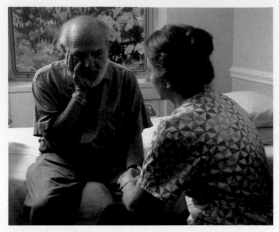

FIGURE 32-1 ■ Astute assessment of behavior and cognitive function aids in differentiating symptoms of psychiatric illness from normal reactions to life events.

SELECTED MENTAL HEALTH CONDITIONS

Depression

Depression is the most frequent problem that psychiatrists treat in older adults, and although major depression declines with age, minor depression increases in incidence with age. Various estimates have placed the prevalence of depression at 15% to 25% in community-based older persons and as many as 25% in older adults who are residents of long-term care facilities; another 20% to 30% of nursing home residents display symptoms of depression although they are not diagnosed with clinical depression (Centers for Disease Control and Prevention, 2005).

Although depressive episodes may have been a lifelong problem for some individuals, it is not uncommon for depression to be a new problem in old age. In fact, most depressions diagnosed in older adults have an initial onset in later life (Fiske, Wetherell, & Gatz, 2009). This is not surprising when one considers the adjustments and losses older persons face, such as the independence of one's children; the reality of retirement; significant changes or losses of roles; reduced income restricting the pursuit of satisfying leisure activities and limiting the ability to meet basic needs; decreasing efficiency of the body; a changing self-image; the death of family members and friends, reinforcing the reality of one's own shrinking life span; and overt and covert messages from society that one's worth is inversely proportional to one's age. In addition, drugs can cause or aggravate depression (Box 32-1).

ASSESSMENT GUIDE 32-1

MENTAL HEALTH

Every comprehensive assessment includes an evaluation of mental status. Because patients may be anxious, embarrassed, or insulted by having their mental status reviewed, explain the importance of and the reasons for the examination. Approach the evaluation in a matter-of-fact manner, not in an apologetic or intimidating one, with reassurance that this evaluation is part of every patient's assessment. Making the patient comfortable and establishing rapport before the assessment can reduce some of the barriers to an effective examination.

GENERAL OBSERVATIONS

Assessment of mental status actually begins the moment the nurse meets the patient. Upon initial observation, pay attention to the following indicators of mental health:

- *Grooming and dress:* Is clothing appropriate for the season, clean and presentable, appropriately worn? Is the patient clean? Is the hair clean and combed? Are makeup and accessories excessive or bizarre?

- *Posture:* Does the patient appear stooped and fearful? Is body alignment normal?

- *Movement:* Are tongue rolling, twitching, tremors, and hand wringing present? Are movements hyperactive or hypoactive?

- *Facial expression:* Is it masklike or overly dramatic? Are there indications of pain, fear, or anger?

- *Level of consciousness:* Does the patient drift into sleep and need to be aroused (i.e., lethargic)? Does the patient offer only incomplete or slow responses and need repeated arousal (i.e., stuporous)? Are painful stimuli the only thing the patient responds to (i.e., semiconscious)? Is there no response, even to painful stimuli (i.e., unconscious)? While observing the patient, general conversation can aid in evaluating mental status.

Note the tone of voice, rate of speech, ability to articulate, use of unusual words or combinations of words, and appropriateness of speech. Also evaluate mood during this time.

INTERVIEW

Effective questioning can reveal much about the patient's mental health. Ask direct questions to unveil specific problems, such as the following:

- "How do you feel about yourself? Would you say others would say you are a good or bad person?"

- "Do you have many friends? How do you get along with people?"

- "Do you feel that anyone is trying to harm you? Who? Why?"

- "Are you moody? Do you quickly go from laughing to crying or from being happy to sad?"

- "Do you have trouble falling asleep or staying asleep? How much sleep do you get? Do you use any drug or alcohol to become sleepy?"

- "How is your appetite? How does your appetite and eating pattern change when you are sad or worried?"

- "Do you ever have feelings of being nervous, such as palpitations, hyperventilating, and restlessness?"

- "Are there any particular problems in your life or anything you are concerned about now?"

- "Do you see or hear things that other people do not? Have you ever heard voices? If so, how do you feel about them?"

- "Does life bring you pleasure? Do you look forward to each day?"

- "Have you ever thought about suicide? If so, what were those ideas like? How would you do it?"

- "Do you feel you are losing any of your mental abilities? If so, describe how."

- "Have you ever been hospitalized or had treatment for mental problems? Has any member of your family?"

Listen carefully to the answers and how they are given. It is important to pick up nonverbal clues.

COGNITIVE TESTING

A variety of reliable, validated tools can be used in assessing mental function, such as the Short Portable Mental Status Questionnaire (Pfeiffer, 1975), the Philadelphia Geriatric Center Mental Status Questionnaire (Fishback, 1977), Mini-Mental Status (Folstein, Folstein, & McHugh, 1975), Symptoms Check List 90 (Derogatis, Lipma, Rickels, Uhlenbath, & Covi, 1974), General Health Questionnaire (Goldberg, 1972), OARS (Duke University, 1978), and, specifically for depression, the Zung Self-Rating Depression Scale (Zung, 1965). Most mental status evaluation tools test orientation, memory and retention, the ability to follow commands, judgment, and basic calculation and reasoning.

Even without the use of a tool, the nurse can assess basic cognitive function in the following ways:

- *Orientation:* Ask the patient his or her name, where he or she is, the date, time, and season.

- *Memory and retention:* At the beginning of the assessment, ask the patient to remember three objects (e.g., watch, telephone, and boat). First, ask the patient to recall the items immediately after being told; then, after asking several other questions, ask for recall of the three items again; near the end of the assessment, ask what the three items were one last time.

(Continues)

ASSESSMENT GUIDE 32-1 (Continued)

- *Three-stage command:* Ask the patient to perform three simple tasks (e.g., "Pick up the pencil, touch it to your head, and hand it to me.").
- *Judgment:* Present a situation that requires basic problem solving and reasoning (e.g., "What is meant by the statement. 'A bird in the hand is worth two in the bush'?").
- *Calculation:* Ask the patient to count backward from 100 by increments of 5; if this is difficult, ask the patient to count backward from 20 by increments of 2. Simple arithmetic problems may also be asked, if they are within the realm of the patient's educational experience.

Whenever cognitive function is tested, consider the unique experiences, educational level, and cultural background of the patient, as well as the role of sensory deficits, health problems, and the stress associated with being examined.

Persons with Alzheimer's disease or other cognitive deficits may become overwhelmed by the assessment and react with anger, tears, or withdrawal. This is referred to as a *catastrophic reaction.* The assessment may need to be discontinued temporarily and the patient reassured and comforted.

PHYSICAL EXAMINATION

Physical health problems are often at the root of many cognitive disturbances; as such, it is essential that a complete physical examination supplements the mental status evaluation. A complete review of medications being used is crucial. In addition, a variety of laboratory tests may be conducted, including the following:

- complete blood count
- serum electrolytes
- serologic test for syphilis
- blood urea nitrogen
- blood glucose
- bilirubin
- blood vitamin level
- sedimentation rate
- urinalysis

Depending on the problem suspected, cerebrospinal fluid may be tested and a variety of diagnostic procedures performed, including electroencephalography, computed tomography, magnetic resonance imaging, and positron emission tomography scan. The mental status evaluation often presents only a snapshot of the individual. Cerebral blood flow, body temperature, blood glucose, fluid and electrolyte balance, and the stress to which the patient is subjected can change from one day to the next and cause different levels of mental function to occur. Repeated assessments may be necessary to obtain an accurate evaluation of the patient's mental status.

Signs and Symptoms

Depression is a complex syndrome and is demonstrated in a variety of ways in older persons. The most common manifestations of this problem are the vegetative symptoms, which include insomnia, fatigue, anorexia, weight loss, constipation, and decreased interest in sex. Depressed persons may express self-deprecation, guilt, apathy, remorse, hopelessness, helplessness, and feelings of being a burden. They may have problems with their personal relationships and social interactions and lose interest in people. Changes in sleep and psychomotor activity patterns can be evident. Hygienic practices may be neglected. Physical complaints of headache, indigestion, and other problems often surface. Altered cognition may be present, caused by malnutrition or other effects of the depression. The symptoms of depression can mimic those of dementia; thus, careful assessment is crucial to avoid misdiagnosis. However, a decline in intellect and personality is usually indicative of dementia (see Chapter 33), not depression. Depression can occur in the early stage of dementia as the patient becomes aware of declining intellectual abilities.

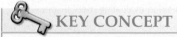

KEY CONCEPT

Some older adults who are depressed demonstrate cognitive deficits secondary to the effects of depression. This pseudodementia can delay or prevent the underlying depression from being recognized and treated.

The prevalence and risk of depression in older adults reinforces the importance of assessing for this problem during routine health visits. Short assessment tools such as the Geriatric Depression Scale, Short Form, can assist in this process (Box 32-2).

Older Native Americans, African Americans, and Asian Americans have been found to have lower

TABLE 32-1 Nursing Diagnoses Related to Mental Health Problems

Causes or Contributing Factors	Nursing Diagnosis
Depression, lack of motivation, sensory overload, fatigue, medications	Activity Intolerance
Threat to self-concept, losses	Anxiety
Psychomotor slowing, medications, inactivity, lack of recognition of need to defecate	Constipation
Anxiety, medications, stress	Diarrhea
Hyperactivity, sensory overload, suicidal attempt	Pain (Acute or Chronic)
Impaired cerebral function, anxiety, suspiciousness	Impaired Verbal Communication
Stress, altered body function, low self-esteem, dependency, sensory overload, loss of significant other	Ineffective Coping
Patient dependency; history of poor family relationships	Disabled Family Coping
Physical, mental, or social limitations	Deficient Diversional Activity
New or misperceived environment, losses	Fear
Loss of body part, function, role, significant other	Grieving
Cognitive impairment, lack of motivation, misperceptions	Ineffective Health Maintenance
Cognitive impairment, misperceptions, lack of motivation	Impaired Home Maintenance
Medications, inactivity, inability to protect self	Risk for Infection
Cognitive impairment, fatigue, medications, suicidal attempt	Risk for Injury
Medications, fatigue	Impaired Physical Mobility
Cognitive impairment, lack of motivation or capacity, suicidal desires	Noncompliance
Depression, anxiety, stress, paranoia, cognitive impairment, suicidal attempt	Impaired Nutrition: Less Than Body Requirements
Depression, anxiety, cognitive impairment, inactivity, suicidal attempt	Impaired Nutrition: More Than Body Requirements
Paranoia, depression, disability, stress	Powerlessness
Cognitive impairment, lack of motivation, knowledge, skill	Self-Care Deficit (Bathing, Dressing, Feeding, Toileting)
Altered body image or function, losses, ageism	Disturbed Body Image
Depression, anxiety, paranoia, guilt, stress, altered self-concept, medications	Sexual Dysfunction
Cognitive impairment (inability to protect self), malnutrition	Impaired Skin Integrity
Anxiety, paranoia, depression, confusion, medications	Disturbed Sleep Pattern
Altered body part or function, cognitive impairment, anxiety, depression, misperceptions, paranoia, hypochondriasis	Impaired Social Interaction
Anxiety, depression, paranoia, cognitive impairment	Social Isolation
Cognitive impairment, fear, depression, anxiety, stress, isolation	Disturbed Thought Processes
Cognitive impairment, anxiety, depression, medications	Impaired Urinary Elimination
Cognitive impairment, paranoia, stress, misperceptions, fear, suicidal attempt	Risk for Other Directed Violence

rates of diagnosed depression, believed to be associated with missed identification or misdiagnosis (Harvath and McKenzie, 2012). This may be less attributed to provider bias than poor reporting of symptoms, language barriers, individuals' beliefs that admitting to depression is shameful or reflects weakness, distrust, or other factors. Missed diagnosis can delay the treatment that could be beneficial in promoting self-care and quality of life; therefore,

nurses and other providers need to be alert to atypical presentation of symptoms (e.g., physical complaints, decline in physical health status due to inattention to health practices, reports of fatigue, feelings of helplessness, unusual risk taking, and self-imposed isolation) and explore the potential for depression being the root cause.

The relationship of life events to the depression is essential to explore during the assessment;

Antihypertensives and cardiac drugs: β-blockers, digoxin, procainamide, guanethidine, clonidine, reserpine, methyldopa, spironolactone

Hormones: corticotropin, corticosteroids, estrogens

Central nervous system depressants, antianxiety agents, psychotropics: alcohol, haloperidol, flurazepam, barbiturates, benzodiazepines

Others: cimetidine, L-dopa, ranitidine, asparaginase, tamoxifen

the approach for a person depressed from the effects of a drug obviously will differ from that for a person who has just become widowed. The underlying problem should be addressed. Although depressions do tend to last longer in older adults, prompt treatment can hasten recovery. Treatment should not be withheld for depression associated with a serious or terminal illness; alleviating the depression may help the individual cope more effectively and be in a better position to manage other health problems.

Treatment

Psychotherapy and antidepressants (Box 32-3) can alleviate many depressions to varying degrees. Electroconvulsive therapy has been shown to be effective in patients who have serious depressions that have been unresponsive to other therapies. Some herbs have been promoted to have antidepressant effects. These include St. John's wort, which has been shown to be effective for mild depressions; it can cause photosensitivity and should not be used with an antidepressant medication (National Health Information, 2003; Pilkington, Rampes, & Richardson, 2006). Acupressure, acupuncture, guided imagery, and light therapy, in conjunction with psychotherapy, can prove helpful. Good basic health practices, including proper nutrition and regular exercise, can also have a positive effect on mood. Box 32-4 describes other helpful nursing measures.

Suicide Risk

Suicide is a real and serious risk among depressed persons. The suicide rate increases with age, is greater than any other age group, and is highest among older white men. All suicide threats from older adults should be taken seriously. In addition to recognizing obvious suicide attempts, nurses must learn to recognize those that are more subtle but equally destructive.

Choose the best answer for how you have felt over the past week:

1. Are you basically satisfied with your life? YES/**NO**
2. Have you dropped many of your activities and interests? **YES**/NO
3. Do you feel that your life is empty? **YES**/NO
4. Do you often get bored? **YES**/NO
5. Are you in good spirits most of the time? YES/**NO**
6. Are you afraid that something bad is going to happen to you? **YES**/NO
7. Do you feel happy most of the time? YES/**NO**
8. Do you often feel helpless? **YES**/NO
9. Do you prefer to stay at home, rather than going out and doing new things? **YES**/NO
10. Do you feel you have more problems with memory than most? **YES**/NO
11. Do you think it is wonderful to be alive now? YES/**NO**
12. Do you feel pretty worthless the way you are now? **YES**/NO
13. Do you feel full of energy? YES/**NO**
14. Do you feel that your situation is hopeless? **YES**/NO
15. Do you think that most people are better off than you are? **YES**/NO

Answers in **bold** indicate depression. Score 1 point for each bolded answer.
  A score > 5 points is suggestive of depression.
  A score > 10 points is almost always indicative of depression.
  A score > 5 points should warrant a follow-up comprehensive assessment.

From Yesavage, J. A., Brink, T. L., Rose, T. L., Lum, O., Huang, V., Adey, M. B., & Leirer, V. O. (1983). Development and validation of a geriatric depression screening scale: A preliminary report. *Journal of Psychiatric Research, 17*, 37–49. Retrieved from http://www.stanford.edu/%7Eyesavage/GDS.html.

BOX 32-3 Antidepressants

SELECTIVE SEROTONIN REUPTAKE INHIBITORS

Escitalopram (Lexapro)
Fluvoxamine (Luvox)
Fluoxetine (Prozac)
Paroxetine (Paxil)
Sertraline (Zoloft)

CYCLIC COMPOUNDS

Amoxapine (Asendin)
Desipramine HCl (Norpramin, Pertofrane)
Doxepin HCl (Adapin, Sinequan)
Imipramine pamoate (Trofanil)
Nortriptyline HCl (Aventyl, Pamelor)

MONOAMINE OXIDASE INHIBITORS

Phenelzine (Nardil)
Tranylcypromine (Parnate)

NURSING GUIDELINES

- Dosages for older adults should begin at about one half that recommended for the general adult population.
- Sedation commonly occurs during the initial few days of treatment; take precautions to reduce the risk of falls.

- At least 1 month of therapy is needed before therapeutic effects will be noted; advise and support the patient during this period.
- Bedtime administration is preferable with antide pressants that produce a sedative effect.
- Prepare patients for side effects, including dry mouth, diaphoresis, urinary retention, indigestion, constipation, hypotension, blurred vision, drowsiness, increased appetite, weight gain, photosensitivity, and fluctuating blood glucose levels. Assist patient in preventing complications secondary to side effects.
- Be alert to anticholinergic symptoms, particularly when cyclic compounds are used.
- Ensure that older adults and their caregivers understand dosage, intended effects, and adverse reactions to the drugs. Instruct about drug–drug and drug–food interactions, e.g., antidepressants can increase the effects of anticoagulants, atropine-like drugs, antihistamines, sedatives, tranquilizers, narcotics, and levodopa; antidepressants can decrease the effects of clonidine, phenytoin, and some antihypertensives; alcohol and thiazide diuretics can increase the effects of antidepressants.

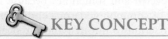 KEY CONCEPT

All suicide threats from older persons should be taken seriously.

Medication misuse, either in the form of overdoses or omission of dosages, may be a suicidal gesture. Self-starvation is another sign and can occur even in an institutional setting if staff members are not attentive to monitoring intake and nutritional

BOX 32-4 Nursing Considerations in Caring for Depressed Patients

- *Help the patient develop a positive self-concept.* It must be emphasized that, although the situation may be bad, the person is not. Opportunities for success, regardless of how minor, should be provided, and new goals should be formed.
- *Encourage the expression of feelings.* Anger, guilt, frustration, and other feelings should be vented. Nurses should afford time to listen and guide patients through these feelings. In addition to verbalization, feelings can be expressed through writing.
- *Avoid minimizing feelings.* Statements such as "Don't worry, things will get better" or "Don't talk that

way; you have a lot to be thankful for" offer little benefit to depressed persons.
- *Ensure that physical needs are met.* Good nutrition, activity, sleep, and regular bowel movements are among the factors that enhance a healthy physical state, which in turn strengthen the patient's capacities to work through depression. Physical care problems must be aggressively addressed.
- *Offer hope.* While being realistic regarding the individual situation, nurses can, by words and deeds, convey their belief that the future will have meaning and that the patient's life is of value.

status. Engaging in activities that oppose a therapeutic need or threaten a medical problem (e.g., ignoring dietary restrictions or refusing a particular therapy) may indicate a desire to die. Walking through a dangerous area, driving while intoxicated, and subjecting oneself to other risks can also be signals of suicidal desires. Suicidal risk can further be assessed by asking the patient about recent losses, lifestyle changes, new or worsening health problems, new symptoms of depression, changes in or a limited support system, and a family history of suicide.

Suicidal older persons need close observation, careful protection, and prompt therapy. Treatment of the underlying depression should be supported. The environment should be made safe by removing items that could be used for self-harm. Nurses need to convey a willingness to listen to and discuss thoughts and feelings about suicide. Being able to reach out for help by expressing their suicidal thoughts to nursing staff may prevent patients from taking actions to end their lives.

Anxiety

Adjustments to physical, emotional, and socioeconomic limitations in old age and the new problems that frequently are encountered due to aging add to the variety of causes for anxiety. Anxiety reactions, not uncommon in older persons, can be manifested in various ways, including somatic complaints, rigidity in thinking and behavior, insomnia, fatigue, hostility, restlessness, chain smoking, pacing, fantasizing, confusion, and increased dependency. An increase in blood pressure, pulse, respirations, psychomotor activity, and frequency of voiding may occur. Appetite may increase or decrease. Anxious individuals often handle their clothing, jewelry, or utensils excessively, become intensively involved with a minor task (e.g., folding a piece of linen), and have difficulty concentrating on the activity at hand.

Treatment of anxiety depends on its cause. Nurses should probe into the patient's history for recent changes or new stresses (e.g., new or worsening of diagnosis, rent increase, increased neighborhood crime, and divorce of child). The consumption of caffeine, alcohol, nicotine, and over-the-counter drugs should be reviewed for possible causes. In addition to drugs, interventions such as biofeedback, guided imagery, and relaxation therapy can prove helpful. Anxious persons need their lives to be simplified and stable, with few unpredictable occurrences. Environmental stimuli must be controlled. Nurses should plan interventions specific to the underlying cause. Basic nursing

interventions that could prove beneficial include the following:

- allow adequate time for conversations, procedures, and other activities
- encourage and respect the patient's decisions over matters affecting his or her life
- prepare the individual for all anticipated activities
- provide thorough, honest, and basic explanations
- control the number and variety of persons with whom the patient must interact
- adhere to routines
- keep and use familiar objects
- prevent overstimulation of the senses by reducing noise, using soft lights, and maintaining a stable room temperature

POINT TO PONDER

What types of situations cause you to become depressed or anxious? What implications does this have for your senior years?

Alcohol Abuse

As the number of people reaching late life increases, so does the number of people with a history of alcohol and illegal drug use. Abuse of, dependency on, or addiction to alcohol among older adults is often a problem that goes unnoticed, sometimes because it is unexpected and sometimes because it mimics symptoms of common geriatric conditions. Alcohol abuse can seriously threaten the physical, emotional, and social health of older persons. Older adults who drink alcohol and who take medications increase their risk of adverse drug consequences. They also increase their risk of falls, reduced cognitive function, abuse, and self-neglect. It is important that gerontological nurses recognize this problem and help patients seek appropriate treatment.

Most older adults who are alcoholics are chronic alcohol abusers who have used it heavily throughout their lives. A significant number of chronic abusers die before reaching old age, contributing to a decreased incidence of alcoholism with age. The other type of older alcoholics is the one who begins abusing alcohol in late life because of situational factors (e.g., retirement, widowhood, or poor health status).

Health care professionals may possess the same stereotype of alcoholics as some people in the general public, believing alcoholics to be sloppy, "skid row" types of people. Consequently, even professionals may fail to detect alcohol abuse in the retired professional who drinks at the country club daily or the frail widow who begins sipping brandy at midmorning. Nurses must keep an open mind and recognize that alcoholics come in many forms.

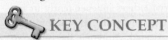

KEY CONCEPT

Alcoholics come in many forms and often do not fit the stereotypical profile.

Alcohol abuse can be manifested in a variety of ways, some of which may be subtle or easy to confuse with other disorders (Box 32-5). Symptoms can develop secondary to complications from alcoholism, such as cirrhosis, hepatitis, and chronic infections (related to suppressed immune system). These signs should be noted during an assessment and trigger questions regarding the patient's drinking pattern. The Short Michigan Alcohol Screening Test-Geriatric Version (Blow et al., 1992) and Alcohol Use Disorders Identification Test (AUDIT) (Babor, Higgins-Biddle, Saunders, & Monteiro, 2001) are screening tools that have proven effective at identifying alcohol abuse in older adults. Box 32-6 describes the criteria for a definitive diagnosis of alcoholism.

Ongoing supervision of the older alcoholics health status can help identify and, in some cases, correct complications early. Chronic alcoholism can cause magnesium deficiencies, gastritis, pancreatitis, and polyneuropathy. Cardiac disorders

---

BOX 32-5 Possible Indications of Alcohol Abuse

Drinking alcohol to calm nerves or improve mood
Gulping or rapidly consuming alcoholic beverages
Memory blackouts
Malnutrition
Confusion
Social isolation and withdrawal
Disrupted relationships
Arrests for minor offenses
Anxiety
Irritability
Depression
Mood swings
Lack of motivation or energy
Injuries, falls
Insomnia
Gastrointestinal distress
Clumsiness

BOX 32-6 Criteria for Diagnosing Alcoholism

- Drinks a fifth of whiskey a day or its equivalent in wine or beer (for a 180-lb person)
- Alcoholic blackouts
- Blood alcohol level greater than 150 mg/100 mL
- Withdrawal syndrome: hallucinations, convulsions, gross tremors, delirium tremens
- Continued drinking despite medical advice or problems caused by drinking

---

can result from alcoholism and can be displayed by hypertension, irregular heartbeat, and heart failure due to cardiomyopathy. Cognition can be impaired by a loss of brain cells and enlargement of the ventricles.

In caring for the patient who has an alcohol problem, the long-term goal is sobriety; this can be achieved only if the patient acknowledges the problem and takes responsibility for doing something about it. Family involvement can be significant to the success of the treatment plan because outcomes can be negatively affected by loved ones denying or enabling the drinking problem.

Alcoholism treatment programs designed specifically for older adults are rare, and it is likely that traditional program staff are unfamiliar with the unique characteristics and needs of the older alcoholics. Gerontological nurses must ensure that the needs of the older alcoholics are competently addressed. For example, benzodiazepines, commonly used for detoxification, can cause toxicity in older people at the same dosage levels that are prescribed for younger adults. Dosage adjustments are necessary, as is close monitoring for complications.

Alcoholics Anonymous (see the Resources at the end of the chapter) is a free program for recovery, available in most communities, which provides counseling and opportunities for alcohol-free socialization for the older alcoholics. Supplying patients with locations, meeting times, and encouragement to attend meetings can be significant to helping them get on the treatment path.

Paranoia

Paranoid states frequently occur in older persons, which is not surprising considering the following:

- sensory losses, so common in later life, easily cause the environment to be misperceived
- illness, disability, living alone, and a limited budget promote insecurity

---

CONSIDER THIS CASE

Seventy-nine-year-old Mrs. B has recently moved into an in-law apartment in the home of her son and daughter-in-law. She shares meals and social time with her son and daughter-in-law, but otherwise, lives independently in her apartment. During the day, Mrs. B entertains friends who share alcoholic beverages with her. By the time her son and daughter-in-law come home from work in the evening, Mrs. B is intoxicated. Although she is able to walk and engage in most normal activities, her speech is slurred and her gait unsteady. There have been occasions when she forgot something was on the stove, setting off the fire alarm, and left doors open and unlocked when she left the house.

THINK CRITICALLY

■ What risks does Mrs. B impose for herself and her family?
■ What approaches can the family use to address the problem with Mrs. B?
■ What resources may be of help?

■ ageism within society sends a message of the undesirability of the old

■ older people are frequent victims of crime and unscrupulous practices

Conditions affecting physical health can contribute to paranoia. Endocrine disorders, such as hyperparathyroidism, can cause paranoia as a symptom (Chiba et al., 2007). Paranoia can also be an adverse response to some drugs. This reinforces the importance of a good physical evaluation and history when psychiatric symptoms present.

The initial consideration in working with paranoid older individuals is to explore mechanisms that could reduce insecurity and misperception. Corrective lenses, hearing aids, supplemental income, new housing, and a stable environment are potential interventions. Psychotherapy and medications can be used when improvement is not achieved through other interventions. Nurses should ensure that these patients do not become withdrawn from the rest of the world because of self-imposed isolation.

Not to be overlooked is the impact of the paranoid state on general health and well-being. Nutritional status can be threatened if the patient refuses to eat, believing his or her food to be poisoned; sleep deprivation can result if there is suspicion that a stranger is in the house; and health problems may not be diagnosed if the person believes the doctor is an enemy. Honest, basic explanations and approaches to dealing with paranoid misperceptions are beneficial; at no time should delusions be supported.

Hypochondriasis

Hypochondriasis may be a problem of some older individuals. Although it is commonly associated with depression, for some older adults it may be

an attention-getting mechanism. Often, health professionals reinforce this behavior by reacting to physical complaints promptly but not reinforcing periods of good function and health. Staff members may not respond to a request to sit down and talk with a patient, but they give undivided attention when that same person expresses physical discomfort. Some older people find hypochondriasis as an effective means of controlling a spouse or children. Older people may use it as a means of socialization; if they do not have travels, professions, or interests they can share with others, they can count on their peers having similar ailments, which can serve as the common ground for conversation.

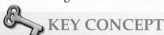 **KEY CONCEPT**

Health care professionals may promote hypochondriac behavior by investing more time and interest reviewing the complaints of the older person than in discussing interests and normal life activities.

Regardless of how unfounded they seem, complaints must be evaluated for their validity before assuming that they are part of hypochondriasis. Even the complaints of a known hypochondriac deserve evaluation, particularly if a new set of complaints emerges. It is beneficial to help these people find alternatives to their obsession with their bodily functions. Spending time in non–illness-related conversation can demonstrate that one can receive attention without resorting to physical complaints. Family members need to understand the dynamics of this problem so that they can reinforce positive behaviors and not be manipulated. Telling these patients that nothing is wrong is of little help; the underlying reason for this reaction must be addressed.

NURSING CONSIDERATIONS FOR MENTAL HEALTH CONDITIONS

Monitoring Medications

Medications used to treat psychiatric disorders can bring significant improvement to patients, but they can also have profound adverse effects on older adults. Some of the adverse effects of these medications can lead to anorexia, constipation, falls, incontinence, anemia, lethargy, sleep disturbances, and confusion. The lowest possible dosage should be used, and any reactions should be observed closely. A checklist for problem identification, as shown in Table 32-2, may be useful to track the impact of medications on behavior and function. Of course, drugs complement and do not substitute for other forms of treatment.

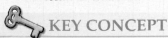
KEY CONCEPT

Drugs should be viewed as an adjunct to rather than as a substitute for other forms of treatment.

Promoting a Positive Self-Concept

The importance of promoting a positive self-concept in all older adults cannot be overemphasized. All people need to feel that their lives have had meaning and that there is hope. A sense of meaninglessness and hopelessness threatens mental health and minimizes the pleasures that the last segment of life can bring. Nurses should take a sincere interest in the lives and accomplishments of their older patients. It must be remembered that the disabled or frail person who now presents to the nurse may once have demonstrated the courage to venture from a native country to America, risked his life to save fellow soldiers in a war, scrubbed floors at night to support a family during the Great Depression, or developed a successful business from scratch. Struggles and accomplishments exist in every life and can be recognized to help promote self-esteem. Activities such as life-review discussions, taping oral histories, and compiling a scrapbook of life events not only help older adults feel a sense of worth about the lives they have lived but also provide a sense of history and legacy for younger generations (see Chapter 4). In addition to the past, the present and future should hold meaning for older adults, and this can be promoted by helping patients participate in relevant activities, engage in meaningful social interactions, have opportunities to do for others, exercise the maximum amount of control possible over their lives, maintain religious and cultural practices, and be respected as individuals.

Managing Behavioral Problems

Behavioral problems are actions that are annoying, disruptive, harmful, or generally deviate from the norm and that tend to be recurrent in nature, such as physical or verbal abuse, resistance to care, repetitive actions, wandering, restlessness, suspiciousness, and inappropriate sexual behavior and undressing. These problems can occur in persons with altered cognitive status who are incapable of thinking rationally and making good judgments. Any type of illness that lowers the patient's ability to cope with changes and stress can also contribute to these problems. Medications, environmental factors, a loss of independence, and insufficient activity can cause problematic behaviors as well.

Assessing the cause of the behavior is the first step in assisting the patient who displays behavioral problems. Factors associated with the behavior should be closely observed and documented and include the following information:

- time of onset
- where it occurred
- environmental conditions
- persons present
- activities that preceded
- pattern of behavior
- signs and symptoms present
- outcome
- measures that helped or worsened the behavior

It is beneficial to correct the underlying cause of the problem whenever possible. Likewise, factors that precipitate the behavioral problem should be avoided (e.g., if it is identified that the patient becomes agitated when seated in a busy hallway, try to avoid seating the patient in this area). Staff or caregivers can prevent behavioral problems by identifying signs and symptoms that precipitate the behaviors and intervening in a timely manner. Environmental considerations that can decrease behavioral problems include maintaining a room temperature between 70°F (21°C) and 75°F (24°C), avoiding wall coverings and linens that have busy patterns, limiting traffic flow, controlling noise, preventing dramatic transitions from daylight to nighttime darkness, and installing safety devices for monitoring, such as alarms on doors and video cameras. Table 32-3 reviews some of the major behavioral problems, their causes, and related nursing interventions.

A full discussion of delirium and dementia is provided in Chapter 33.

TABLE 32-2 Checklist for Documenting Drugs and Behavior

Date	A.M.												P.M.												
	12	1	2	3	4	5	6	7	8	9	10	11	12	1	2	3	4	5	6	7	8	9	10	11
Medications:																									
Disoriented regarding:																									
Self																									
Others																									
Place																									
Day																									
Time																									
Forgetful of:																									
Today's events																									
Past events																									
Inappropriate:																									
Speech																									
Behavior																									
Hallucinations																									
Wandering																									
ADL deficits:																									
Feeding																									
Bathing																									
Dressing																									
Toileting																									
Mobility																									
Incontinence, urinary																									
Pulse																									
Blood pressure																									
Bowel movement																									
Sleeping/napping																									
Other symptoms:																									

Food Intake	100%	75%	50%	25%	0%	Comments
Breakfast						
Lunch						
Dinner						
Snacks						

Use back to describe specific problems or changes

ADL, activities of daily living.

TABLE 32-3	Understanding and Managing Common Behavioral Problems	
Behavior	**Possible Causes**	**Nursing Actions**
Violent/physically abusive (e.g., hitting, kicking, and biting others)	Dementia Paranoia Misinterpretation of actions of others Anger Feeling powerless Anxiety Fatigue	Avoid putting person in situations that trigger behaviors Recognize warning signs (e.g., cursing and pacing) Get help to protect self and others Address in calm, quiet manner Distract Move person to area away from others
Verbally abusive (e.g., insulting, accusing, and threatening)	Dementia Feeling powerless Anger	Avoid arguing, reasoning, and reacting to comments Distract with activities Reinforce positive behaviors Allow maximum decision making and participation
Resisting care	Dementia Misinterpretation of actions, objects, and environment Depression	Prepare for activities Break activities into single, simple steps Use alternatives if possible (e.g., sponge bath instead of tub bath) Monitor hygiene, nutritional status, intake and output, elimination
Undressing inappropriately	Dementia Soiled clothing Irritation from clothing Feeling too warm	Ensure clothing is clean, dry; replace as necessary Examine clothing for irritation, poor fit Inspect skin for irritation Redress Use clothing that is difficult to unfasten Offer positive reinforcement when person remains dressed
Repetitive actions	Dementia Agitation Anxiety Boredom	Ignore Distract with other activities Replace with a more acceptable repetitive activity (e.g., folding laundry and stacking papers)
Wandering	Dementia Boredom Restlessness Anxiety	Schedule times for supervised walking Provide activities Safeguard environment (e.g., alarm doors, install door locks that require punching in code to open, and ensure window screens cannot be removed) Ensure person is wearing some form of identification Familiarize person with environment; orient
Night wandering, restlessness	Dementia Excess daytime sleeping Misinterpretation of environment Sundowner syndrome Medications (e.g., sedatives, hypnotics, diuretics, and laxatives)	Provide daytime activities Provide late day exercise Toilet before bed time Keep night light on in bedroom and bathroom Reassure and orient when person awakens Safeguard environment
Inappropriate sexual behavior	Dementia, leading to poor judgment, loss of inhibition Misinterpretation of actions and messages from others	Relocate person to private area Distract with other activities Set limits and remind of acceptable behaviors Review medications for those that can cause reduced inhibitions (e.g., antianxiety agents) or that increase libido (e.g., L-dopa) Provide acceptable means of touch, human contact

(Continues)

TABLE 32-3	Understanding and Managing Common Behavioral Problems (continued)

Behavior	Possible Causes	Nursing Actions
Suspiciousness	Paranoid state	Assess cause
	Dementia	Do not react to behavior; depersonalize
	Suspicious personality	Protect from harm
	Medications (e.g., anticholinergics, L-dopa, and tolbutamide)	Provide explanations; prepare for activities, changes
		Afford maximum decision making
		Do not try to explain to person that suspicions are unfounded or wrong; this will not be helpful

BRINGING RESEARCH TO LIFE

EFFICACY OF COGNITIVE BEHAVIORAL THERAPY FOR ANXIETY DISORDERS IN OLDER PEOPLE: A META-ANALYSIS AND META-REGRESSION OF RANDOMIZED CONTROLLED TRIALS

Gould, R. L., Coulson, M. C., & Howard, R. J. (2012). Journal of the American Geriatrics Society, 60(2), 218–229.

A systematic critical review of randomized controlled trials were conducted to examine the effects of cognitive behavioral therapy (CBT) for anxiety disorders in older people. CBT typically consists of one-to-one talk therapy between the individual and a therapist to explore the cause of the anxiety and ways to manage it. At 6- but not 3- or 12-month follow-up, older persons receiving CBT had a significant reduction in symptoms as compared with those in the control group but not to the extent of effectiveness in non-elderly adults receiving CBT. The study concluded that although found to have some benefit, effectiveness of CBT for anxiety disorders in older people is suggestive of lower efficacy in older persons than working-age people.

The conclusion could be drawn that CBT is not useful in older adults, but this may not be appropriate. It may be that older adults need more time to show benefit from CBT than persons of younger ages. In addition, individual variation in response can exist. Cultural background, physical and mental health status, and experience with psychotherapy can differ among the diverse older population, thereby affecting the outcome of CBT. Individual assessment for factors that could influence the ability to benefit from CBT and monitoring for effectiveness is necessary.

PRACTICE REALITIES

Mr. Connor has come to the emergency department with chest pain. The evaluation finds no evidence of cardiovascular disease and you are preparing him for discharge. You comment, "I bet it is a relief to hear that you didn't have a heart attack." "I'm not so sure," he responds. "Sometimes I think a heart attack would be a great way to put an end to my troubles."

Concerned, you ask him what he means and he shares that at 66 years of age he finds himself still having to work and has little interest or energy left for anything else. "My kids are grown and barely have time to call me, my wife is unhappy that I don't feel like doing anything, and my employer hints that he could easily replace me with a less expensive younger person. At this age I thought I'd be retired, travelling, golfing, and enjoying life. I never expected it to be so hard. Makes you wonder what the point of it all is." With that, he prepares to sign his discharge papers and leave.

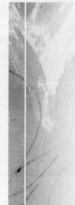

You see a need and want to help Mr. Connor but are pressured with the demands of a very busy day in the emergency department. What can you do?

CRITICAL THINKING EXERCISES

1. Discuss factors associated with aging in America that contribute to mental illness in late life.

2. Why is alcoholism sometimes missed in older adults?

3. Describe questions and observations that could be used in an interview to uncover mental health problems.

4. Describe reasons other than a paranoid disorder for an older adult being suspicious.

5. As the baby boomers enter old age, what type of mental health conditions could be more prevalent than with previous generations of older adults?

RESOURCES

Al-Anon Family Group Headquarters (local chapters available)
http://www.al-anon-alateen.org

Alcoholics Anonymous (local chapters available)
http://www.alcoholics-anonymous.org

Anxiety Disorders Association of America
http://www.adaa.org

Mental Health America
http://www.nmha.org

National Clearinghouse for Alcohol and Drug Information
http://www.ncadi.samhsa.gov/

National Depressive and Manic-Depressive Association
http://www.ndmda.org

National Institute of Alcohol Abuse and Alcoholism
http://www.niaaa.nih.gov

REFERENCES

Babor, T. F., Higgins-Biddle, J. C., Saunders, J. B., & Monteiro, M. G. (2001). *AUDIT: The alcohol use disorders identification test. Guidelines for use in primary care* (2nd ed.). Geneva, Switzerland: World Health Organization.

Blow, F. C., Brower, K. J., Schulenberg, J. E., Demo-Danaberg, L. M., Young, J. P., & Beresford, T. P. (1992). The Michigan Alcoholism Screening Test-Geriatric Version: A new elderly-specific screening instrument. *Alcoholism: Clinical and Experimental Research, 16*(2), 372.

Centers for Disease Control and Prevention, National Center for Injury Prevention and Control. (2005). *Web-based injury statistics query and reporting system (WISQARS)* [online]. Retrieved September 1, 2007 from http://www.cdc.gov/ncipc/wisqars.

Chiba, Y., Satoh, K., Ueda, S., Kanazawa, N., Tamura, Y., & Horiuchi, T. (2007). Marked improvement of psychiatric symptoms after parathyroidectomy in elderly primary hyperparathyroidism. *Endocrine Journal, 54*(3), 379–383.

Derogatis, R. S., Lipma, K., Rickels, E. H., Uhlenbath, E. H., & Covi, L. (1974). The Hopkins symptom checklist: A measure of primary symptom dimensions. *Pharmacopsychiatry, 7,* 79.

Duke University Center for the Study of Aging. (1978). *Multidimensional functional assessment: The OARS methodology.* Durham, NC: Duke University.

Fishback, D. B. (1977). Mental status questionnaire for organic brain syndrome, with a new visual counting test. *Journal of the American Geriatric Society, 25,* 167.

Fiske, A., Wetherell, J. L., & Gatz, M. (2009). Depression in older adults. *Annual Review of Clinical Psychology, 5,* 363–389.

Folstein, M. F., Folstein, S., & McHugh, P. R. (1975). Mini-mental state: A practical method for grading the cognitive state of patients for the clinician. *Journal of Psychiatry Research, 12,* 189.

Goldberg, D. (1972). *The detection of psychiatric illness by questionnaire.* London: Oxford University Press.

Harvath, T.A., & McKenzie, G. (2012). Depression in older adults. In Boltz, M., Capezuti, E., Fulmer, T., & Zwicker, D. (Eds.), *Evidence-based geriatric nursing protocols for best practice* (pp. 141–142). New York, NY: Springer Publishing Company.

Lochel, J. P. (2005). Practical geriatrics: Completed suicides in late life. *Psychiatric Services, 56*(3), 260–262.

National Health Information. (2003). St. John's wort in depression: A new meta-analysis. *Alternative Medicine Research Report, 2*(1), 1–5.

Pfeiffer, E. (1975). A short portable mental status questionnaire for the assessment of organic brain deficit in elderly patients. *Journal of the American Geriatric Society, 23*(10), 433.

Pilkington, K., Rampes, H., & Richardson, J. (2006). Complementary medicine for depression. *Expert Review of Neurotherapeutics, 6*(11), 1741–1751.

Zung, W. W. K. (1965). A self-rating depression scale. *Archives of General Psychiatry, 12,* 63.

RECOMMENDED READINGS

Recommended Readings associated with this chapter can be found on the web site that accompanies the book. Visit **http://thepoint.lww.com/Eliopoulos8e** to access the recommended readings and other additional resources associated with this chapter.

Delirium and Dementia

LEARNING OBJECTIVES

After reading this chapter, you should be able to:

1. Differentiate delirium from dementia.
2. Identify factors that cause delirium in older adults.
3. Describe the progression of symptoms of dementia.
4. List causes of dementia in older adults.
5. Outline nursing considerations for the older adult with dementia.

TERMS TO KNOW

Delirium: acute confusion, usually reversible

Dementia: irreversible, progressive impairment in cognitive function

Mild cognitive impairment: transitional stage between normal cognitive aging and dementia in which the person has short-term memory impairment and challenges with complex cognitive functions

Sundowner syndrome: nocturnal confusion

Although arthritis, heart disease, and other physical diseases are not welcomed by older adults, these conditions tend to be dreaded less than the loss of normal cognition. Impaired cognition threatens the ability to communicate, function independently, make decisions, and comprehend events. With advancing age, there is increased risk of delirium, the reversible reduction in cognition caused by acute conditions, and

TABLE 33-1	Delirium vs. Dementia	
	Delirium	**Dementia**
Cause	Disruption in brain function due to medication side effect, circulatory disturbance, dehydration, low or high blood pressure, low or high thyroid activity, low or high blood glucose, surgery, stress, etc.	Damage to brain tissue due to Alzheimer's or other degenerative diseases, circulatory problems, lack of oxygen, infection, trauma, hydrocephalus, tumor, alcoholism, etc.
Onset	Rapid; change noted within day or days	Slow; months to years before symptoms are evident
Mental Status	Short-term memory impaired more than long-term, disoriented, confused, distorted thinking, incoherent speech, may be suspicious of others, see or hear things that are not there (illusions, hallucinations), exaggeration of personality features	Poor short- and long-term memory, disoriented, confused, difficulty finding proper word to use, impaired judgment, problems with arithmetic and problem-solving, personality changes
Level of Consciousness (Alertness)	Changed, can be highly agitated or very dull	Normal
Behavior	Can be hyperactive, less active than normal, or fluctuate between both extremes	Inappropriate, may be unsteady on feet, have difficulty with coordinated movements
Recovery	Disease can be reversed and normal mental status restored if cause is treated promptly	Progression of disease may be slowed but disease cannot be reversed; usually continues to worsen

dementia, the irreversible impairment in cognition caused by disease or injury to the brain. Although both conditions cause cognitive impairment, there are significant differences (Table 33-1). Assisting with the prevention, diagnosis, and treatment of these cognitive impairments is an important responsibility of the gerontological nurse.

DELIRIUM

A variety of conditions can impair cerebral circulation and cause disturbances in cognitive function

(Box 33-1). Sometimes the history, physical examination, or laboratory tests will indicate the presence of an organic factor that has caused the disturbance; however, without such evidence, the diagnosis of delirium can be established by the symptoms and lack of any nonorganic mental disorder that could cause them.

The onset of symptoms with delirium tends to be rapid and can include disturbed intellectual function; disorientation of time and place but usually not of identity; altered attention span; worsened memory; labile mood; meaningless chatter;

BOX 33-1	Potential Causes of Impaired Cognition
Fluid and electrolyte imbalances	Pain
Medications	Malnutrition
Congestive heart failure	Dehydration
Hyperglycemia and hypoglycemia	Anemias
Hyperthermia and hypothermia	Infection
Hypercalcemia and hypocalcemia	Hypotension
Hypothyroidism	Trauma
Decreased cardiac function	Malignancy
Decreased respiratory function	Alcoholism
Decreased renal function	Hypoxia
CNS disturbances	Toxic substances
Emotional stress	

Source: CNS, central nervous system.

poor judgment; and altered level of consciousness, including hypervigilance, mild drowsiness, and semicomatose status. Significant perceptual changes can occur, such as hallucinations (usually visual) and illusions (e.g., misinterpreting caregivers as police guards). Disturbances in sleep–wake cycles can occur; in fact, restlessness and sleep disturbances may be early clues. The patient may be suspicious, have personality changes, and experience illusions more often than delusions. Physical signs, such as shortness of breath, fatigue, and slower psychomotor activities, may accompany behavioral changes.

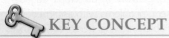

KEY CONCEPT

Delirium alters the level of consciousness, whereas dementia does not.

Nurses can play a significant role by detecting signs of confusion promptly. A good history and assessment of mental status on initial contact can provide the baseline data with which changes can be compared (see Assessment Guide 32-1). Any change in behavior or cognitive pattern warrants an evaluation. There is the risk that delirium may not be recognized if persons unfamiliar with the patient assume that poor cognition is normal for him or her. Likewise, persons with dementia can develop delirium as a response to an acute condition but be undiagnosed because changes are not understood or identified.

Delirium is reversible in most circumstances, and prompt care, treating this condition as a medical emergency, can prevent permanent damage. Treatment depends on the cause (e.g., stabilizing blood glucose, correcting dehydration, and discontinuing a medication). Treating the symptoms rather than the cause or accepting the symptoms as normal and failing to obtain treatment can result not only in worsened mental status but also in the continuation of a physical condition that could be life threatening.

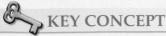

KEY CONCEPT

As older adults often have multiple health conditions, it is important to remember that several coexisting factors can be responsible for a delirium.

During the initial acute stage, establishing medical stability and minimizing stimulation are primary goals. Consistency in care is important; thus, the patient benefits from interaction with only a limited number of people. Providing frequent orientation and explanations fosters function and reduces anxiety and stress. Controlling environmental temperature, noise, and traffic flow is important. Placing this patient in a quiet area away from the mainstream activity is beneficial. Bright lights should be avoided, but ample lighting is needed to enable the patient to adequately visualize the environment. The nurse should ensure that the patient does not harm himself or herself or others and that physical care needs are met. Regardless of the level of intellectual function or consciousness, it is important to speak to the patient and offer explanations of activities or procedures being done. Families may need considerable support and realistic explanations to alleviate their anxieties (e.g., "No, he does not have Alzheimer's disease. His confusion occurred because the level of glucose, or sugar, in his blood dropped too low. He'll be better as soon as the level is brought back to normal.").

DEMENTIA

Dementia is an irreversible, progressive impairment in cognitive function affecting memory, orientation, judgment, reasoning, attention, language, and problem solving. It is caused by damage or injury to the brain. An estimated 5% older adults suffer some form of dementia.

Alzheimer's Disease

Alzheimer's disease is the most common form of dementia; in fact, the likelihood of developing Alzheimer's disease doubles every 5 years after the age of 65 resulting in more than 60% of all cases of dementia (Alzheimer's Association, 2007). Scientists project a dramatic increase in prevalence unless new ways to prevent and treat the disease are discovered (National Institute on Aging, 2006).

Alzheimer's disease is characterized by two changes in the brain. The first is the presence of neuritic plaques, which contain deposits of β-amyloid protein (excess amounts of this are found in persons with Alzheimer's disease and Down syndrome). β-Amyloid protein is a fragment of amyloid precursor protein that helps the neurons grow and repair. The β-amyloid fragments clump together into plaques that impair the function of nerve cells in the brain. It is unclear at this point if the plaques are a cause or by-product of the disease.

The second characteristic brain change is neurofibrillary tangles in the cortex. Microtubules, structures within healthy neurons, are normally stabilized by a special protein called tau. In Alzheimer's disease, tau is changed and begins to pair with other threads of tau that become tangled. This causes the microtubules to disintegrate and collapse the neuron's transport system.

These brain changes lead to a loss or degeneration of neurons and synapses, especially within the neocortex and hippocampus. Interestingly, the cause-and-effect relationship between these brain changes and Alzheimer's disease is unclear at present.

There are also changes in neurotransmitter systems associated with Alzheimer's disease, including reductions in serotonin receptors, serotonin uptake into platelets, production of acetylcholine in the areas of the brain in which plaque and tangles are found, acetylcholinesterase (which breaks down acetylcholine), and choline acetyltransferase. (Cholinesterase inhibitors and nicotinic, muscarinic, and cholinergic agonists are among the neurotransmitter-affecting drugs used in the treatment of Alzheimer's to compensate for the neurotransmitter changes.)

Recent studies have confirmed that there are pathological changes in the brain years before symptoms of Alzheimer's disease appear. The transitional stage between normal cognitive aging and dementia in which the person has short-term memory impairment and challenges with complex cognitive functions is referred to a *mild cognitive impairment*. Persons with mild cognitive impairment have a higher risk of developing Alzheimer's disease; research is currently exploring the reason for some persons with this condition progressing on to developing the disease while others do not.

Possible Causes

Although environmental factors play a role, genetic factors do increase the risk of Alzheimer's disease. Studies have revealed several generations of Alzheimer's disease patients occurring in the same family. Chromosomal abnormalities have been identified. A strong argument for the genetic formulation of the disease stems from its connection with Down syndrome. An extra chromosome 21 exists in persons with Down syndrome; not only do people with Down syndrome begin to develop symptoms of dementia after age 35 but also the prevalence of Alzheimer's disease is higher in families with Down syndrome, and vice versa (Dykens, 2007). An altered chromosome 21 in people with Alzheimer's disease causes production of an abnormal amyloid precursor protein. Chromosomes 14 and 1 have also been found to have mutations within families who have a high prevalence of Alzheimer's disease; these mutations cause abnormal proteins to be produced. If only one of these mutated genes is inherited from a parent with Alzheimer's disease, a person has a

50/50 chance of developing the disease (Robakis, 2007).

POINT TO PONDER

Would you want to know if you had a genetic predisposition toward Alzheimer's disease? What difference could this make in your life?

There is some investigation into the role of free radicals in the development of Alzheimer's disease. Free radicals are molecules that can build up in neurons, resulting in damage (called oxidative damage). The damage blocks substances from flowing in and out of the cell, leading to brain damage. Some studies suggest that a diet rich in antioxidants may offer protection (Ancelin, Christen, & Ritchie, 2007).

Higher than normal levels of aluminum and mercury have been found in the brain cells of Alzheimer's disease patients, causing some speculation regarding the role of environmental toxins in the disease. However, the results are inconclusive as to their role in the development of Alzheimer's disease. Low zinc levels are present in persons with Alzheimer's disease, although it is not certain if this is a cause or result of the disease.

There has been some speculation about a slow-acting virus causing the neurofibrillary tangles in the brain, but no conclusive evidence exists at present to support this theory. Some risks hypothesized to be associated with Alzheimer's disease include hyperlipidemia, hypertension, smoking, head injury, and physical and mental inactivity. At present, no one theory can explain this complex disease.

Symptoms

The symptoms of this progressive, degenerative disease develop gradually and progress at different rates among affected individuals. The Global Deterioration Scale/Functional Assessment Staging offers a means of staging Alzheimer's disease (Fig. 33-1) (Auer & Reisberg, 1997). Although staging of the disease can help predict its general course and anticipate plans for care, it must be appreciated that many factors affect the progression of the disease and that there will be individual variation.

Early in the disease, the patient may be aware of changes in intellectual ability and become depressed or anxious or attempt to compensate by writing down information, structuring routines, and simplifying responsibilities. It may take some time for symptoms to be detected, even by those close to the patient.

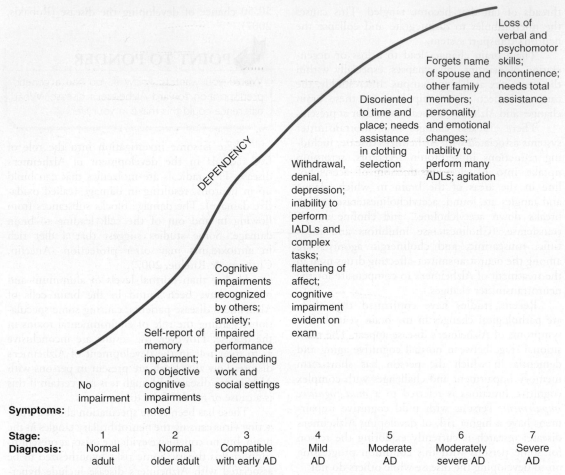

						Loss of verbal and psychomotor skills; incontinence; needs total assistance
					Forgets name of spouse and other family members; personality and emotional changes; inability to perform many ADLs; agitation	
				Disoriented to time and place; needs assistance in clothing selection		
			Withdrawal, denial, depression; inability to perform IADLs and complex tasks; flattening of affect; cognitive impairment evident on exam			
		Cognitive impairments recognized by others; anxiety; impaired performance in demanding work and social settings				
	Self-report of memory impairment; no objective cognitive impairments noted					
Symptoms:	No impairment					
Stage:	1	2	3	4	5	6	7
Diagnosis:	Normal adult	Normal older adult	Compatible with early AD	Mild AD	Moderate AD	Moderately severe AD	Severe AD

FIGURE 33-1 ■ Stages of Alzheimer's disease (AD). IADL, instrumental activities of daily living; ADL, activities of daily living. (Based on Reisberg, B., Ferris, S. H., & de Leon, M. J. (1982). The Global Deterioration Scale for assessment of primary dementia. *American Journal of Psychiatry, 139*, 1136–1139; and Auer, S., & Reisberg, B. (1997). The GDS/FAST staging system. *International Psychogeriatrics, 9*(Suppl. 1), 167–171.)

KEY CONCEPT

The greatest risk of suicide for a person with dementia is in the early stage of the disease when the individual is aware of the changes experienced.

In addition to the history of symptoms from the patient and family members or significant others, diagnosis is aided by brain scans that can reveal changes in the brain's structure that are consistent with the disease, neuropsychological testing that evaluates cognitive functioning, and laboratory tests and neurological examinations.

Treatment

Although currently there is no treatment to prevent or cure Alzheimer's disease, clinical trials are being conducted by the National Institutes of Health and private industry in hopes of finding a means to improve function and slow the progress of the disease. There has been interest in estrogen's role in enhancing cognitive function, with speculation that estrogen has a role in protecting postmenopausal women from developing Alzheimer's disease or other age-related cognitive decline; however, research has produced conflicting results as the women's Health Initiative Memory Study demonstrated an increased risk of dementia in postmenopausal women in women taking estrogen with progestin (Henderson, 2006). Antioxidants, anti-inflammatory agents, supplements (folic acid and vitamins B_6 and B_{12}), gene therapy that adds a nerve growth factor to the aging brain, and the development of a vaccine are among the other areas being investigated in clinical trials (National Institute on Aging, 2006).

Because acetylcholine falls sharply in people with Alzheimer's disease, medications that stop or slow the enzyme (acetylcholinesterase) that breaks down acetylcholine have been developed to help people with Alzheimer's disease; these drugs include donepezil (Aricept), rivastigmine (Exelon), and galantamine (Reminyl).

Other Dementias

In addition to Alzheimer's disease, a variety of other pathologies can cause dementia:

- *Vascular dementia.* results from small cerebral infarctions. Damage to the brain tissue can be diffuse or localized, the onset is more rapid, and the disease progresses more predictably than Alzheimer's disease. It is associated with risk factors such as smoking, hypertension, hyperlipidemia, inactivity, and a history of stroke or cardiovascular disease.

- *Frontotemporal dementia.* is characterized by neuronal atrophy affecting the frontal lobes of the brain rather than by neurofibrillary tangles and plaques as in Alzheimer's disease. A unique characteristic of this dementia is the appearance of behavioral rather than cognitive abnormalities in the early stage. Also, rather than poor memory, early cognitive changes can include impairments in abstract thinking and speech and language skills. Pick's disease is the most common form of frontotemporal dementia.

- *Lewy body dementia.* also known as cortical *Lewy body disease*, is associated with subcortical pathology and the presence of Lewy body substance in the cerebral cortex. People with this dementia have fluctuations in mental status, decompensate rapidly when they experience a medical condition, and often have idiosyncratic reactions to cholinergic-type medications (e.g., sedatives and antipsychotics). About one fourth of the people diagnosed with this dementia have a history of a family member with dementia. Lewy body dementia is often misdiagnosed as other forms of dementia.

- *Creutzfeldt-Jakob disease.* is an extremely rare brain disorder that causes dementia. It has a rapid onset and progression and is characterized by severe neurological impairment that accompanies the dementia. It is believed that this disease can be transmitted through a slow virus; a familial tendency toward the disease is possible. The pathological process displays destruction of neurons in the cerebral cortex, overgrowth of glia, abnormal cellular structure of the cortex, hypertrophy and proliferation of astrocytes, and a spongelike appearance of the cerebral cortex. Symptoms are more varied than with Alzheimer's disease and include psychotic behavior, heightened emotional lability, memory impairment, loss of muscular function, muscle spasms, seizures, and visual disturbances. The disease progresses rapidly, and death typically occurs within 1 year of diagnosis:

- *Wernicke's encephalopathy* and *Parkinson's disease* are responsible for a small percentage of dementias.

- *AIDS.* may lead to the development of dementia in the final phase of the disease.

- *Trauma* and *toxins* are among the other causes of dementia.

These other forms of dementia can present with symptoms similar to those commonly associated with Alzheimer's disease. Without a comprehensive evaluation to identify or exclude other causes of dementia, the label of Alzheimer's disease cannot be accurately given to a dementia.

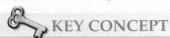
KEY CONCEPT

Other diseases can mimic Alzheimer's disease; therefore, a comprehensive evaluation is essential to rule out other possible causes of dementia before the diagnosis of Alzheimer's disease is made.

Caring for Persons With Dementia

The irreversible nature of dementia and its progressive deteriorating course can have devastating effects on affected individuals and their families. A majority of the care required by persons with dementia falls within the scope of nursing practice.

Ensuring Patient Safety

One of the foremost care considerations is the safety of patients with dementia. Their poor judgment and misperceptions can lead to serious behavioral problems and mishaps. A safe, structured environment is essential. The persons and components of the environment should be consistent (Fig. 33-2). Items to trigger memory are useful to include, such as photographs of the patient or a consistently used symbol (e.g., flower or triangle) on the bedroom door or personal possessions. Noise, activity, and lighting levels can overstimulate the patient and further decrease function; thus, they need to be controlled. This is particularly useful in preventing and managing sundowner syndrome (Box 33-2).

Cleaning solutions, pesticides, medications, and inedible items that could be ingested accidentally must be stored in locked cabinets. Coverings should be applied to unused sockets, electrical

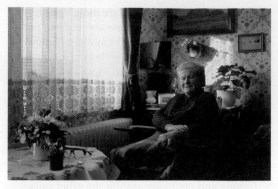

FIGURE 33-2 ■ Familiar objects, a stable environment, and consistency of caregivers can reduce some of the safety risks and behavioral problems associated with dementias.

outlets, fans, motors, and other items into which fingers may be poked. Matches and lighters should not be accessible; if the patient smokes, it must be under close supervision. Windows and doors can be protected with Plexiglas, and non-removable screens can be installed to avoid falls from windows. Wandering is common among patients with dementia; rather than restrain or restrict them, it is more advantageous to provide a safe area in which they can wander. Protective gates can be installed to prevent patients from wandering away; alarms and bells on doors can signal when they are attempting to exit. With the great risk of patients wandering away and not being able to give their names or residence when found, it is beneficial for them to wear identification bracelets at all times and to have a recent photograph available.

The prevention of abuse is another safety consideration. In addition to being taken advantage of due to their poor cognitive function, older persons with dementias may be abused by caregivers who become stressed by the behavior and care needs of the affected individuals. It is important to assess how well caregivers are managing and coping with the persons they care for and to provide support and assistance to prevent them from becoming overwhelmed.

Promoting Therapy and Activity

Various therapies and activities can be offered to the patient with dementia, depending on the patient's level of function. Occupational therapy and expressive therapies can benefit those with early dementia. Various degrees of reality orientation, ranging from daily groups to reminding the patient who he or she is during every interaction, can be used. Even the most regressed patient can maintain contact and derive stimulation through activities, such as listening to music, petting an animal, and touching various objects. Being touched is also a pleasurable and stimulating experience.

Modified communication techniques can facilitate activity. Some useful strategies include:

- Using simple sentences that contain only one idea or instruction
- Speaking in a calm manner using an adult tone (not baby talk)
- Avoiding words or phrases that can be misinterpreted or sarcasm
- Offering opportunities for simple decisions
- Avoiding arguments (distractions can help)
- Recognizing efforts with positive feedback
- Observing nonverbal expressions and behaviors

BOX 33-2 **Sundowner Syndrome**

Individuals with cognitive impairments may experience a nocturnal confusion, named sundowner syndrome due to its presentation "after the sun goes down." Some of the factors that increase the risk of this condition include unfamiliar environment (e.g., recent admission to a facility), disturbed sleep patterns (e.g., from sleep apnea), use of restraints, excess sensory stimulation, sensory deprivation, or change in circadian rhythms.

Nurses can prevent and manage sundowner syndrome by:

- placing familiar objects in the person's room
- providing physical activity in the afternoon to help the person expend energy

- adjusting lighting in the environment to prevent the room from becoming dark in the evening
- keeping a nightlight on throughout the night
- having frequent contact with the person to offer reassurance and orientation
- using touch to provide human contact and calm the person
- ensuring the environmental temperature is within a comfortable range for the person
- controlling noise and traffic flow in the evening
- ensuring the person's basic needs are met (e.g., adequate fluids, toileting, and dry clothing)

Providing Physical Care

The physical care needs of patients with dementia must not be overlooked. These individuals may not complain that they are hungry, so no one may notice that they have consumed less than one quarter of the food served; they may not remember to drink water, so they can become dehydrated; they may fight their bath so strongly that they are left unbathed; and pressure ulcers on their buttocks may go unnoticed. These patients need close observation and careful attention to their physical needs. Consideration must be given to their potential inability to communicate their needs and discomforts; a subtle change in behavior or function, a facial grimace, or repeated touching of a body part may give clues that a problem exists. Consistency in caregivers allows the caregivers to become familiar with a patient's unique behaviors and more quickly recognize a deviation from that individual's norm.

Using Complementary and Alternative Therapies

A variety of alternative medical therapies are being used to treat dementias. Nutritional supplements that have been used include vitamins B_6, B_{12}, C, and E; folic acid; zinc; and selenium. The herb ginkgo biloba has been shown to improve circulation and mental function in several clinical trials (Dos Santos-Neto, de Vilhena Toledo, Medeiros-Souza, & de Souza, 2006; Rassamy, Longpre, & Christen, 2007); caution is needed, however, because ginkgo biloba can increase the risk of intraocular hemorrhage and subdural hematoma when taken for an extended period of time or when an anticoagulant drug is being taken concurrently. Chinese medicine, in addition to herbs and nutrition, uses a form of therapeutic exercise called qigong; it is believed that oxygenation to the brain improves by the breathing exercises and visualization used in qigong exercises.

Respecting the Individual

As patients regress, their dignity, personal worth, freedom, and individuality may be jeopardized. Loved ones may view the demented family member as a stranger living inside the body that once housed the person they knew. Staff may see another dependent or total-care patient and have no sense of that person's unique life history. Viewed less and less as a normal human being or as the same person that has been known, the person with dementia may be treated in a dehumanizing manner. Special attention must be paid to maintaining and promoting the following qualities:

- *Individuality.* The nurse should learn the personal history and uniqueness of the patient and incorporate this into caregiving activities.

- *Independence.* Even if it takes three times longer to guide patients through dressing than it would take to dress them, they should be afforded every opportunity for self care.

- *Freedom.* As major freedoms become limited, minor choices and control become especially important. Nurses must be careful that, in the name of efficiency and safety, such severe restrictions to freedom are not imposed that the quality of life becomes minimal.

- *Dignity.* To become angry or laugh at the behaviors of a demented person is no less cruel than reacting in a similar fashion to a stroke victim who falls during ambulation. These patients should be afforded the respect given to any adult, including attractive clothing, good grooming, adult hairstyles, use of their names, privacy, and confidentiality.

- *Connection.* Persons with dementia continue to be valued human beings who are members of families, communities, and the universe. Interaction and connection with other people and nature show recognition and respect for the spiritual beings that live within the altered bodies and minds.

Supporting the Patient's Family

Assistance and support to the families of patients are integral parts of nursing care for persons with dementia. The physical, emotional, and socioeconomic burden of caring for a cognitively impaired relative can be immense. It should not be assumed that family members understand basic care techniques. The nurse needs to review basic, specific care techniques, including lifting, bathing, and managing inappropriate behaviors. The nurse can also help prepare families for the guilt, frustration, anger, depression, and other feelings that normally accompany this responsibility. Helping families plan respite, network with support groups, and obtain counseling may be beneficial. Most states now have chapters of the Alzheimer's Association to which nurses can refer families (see Resources listing).

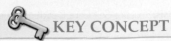

KEY CONCEPT

It cannot be assumed that family members understand feeding, bathing, lifting, and other basic caregiving skills.

Nursing Care Plan 33-1 describes a care plan for a person with Alzheimer's disease.

A home health nurse is making an initial home visit to evaluate 69-year-old Mr. S, who has Alzheimer's disease, and to assist his wife in developing effective caregiving plans. Mr. S was diagnosed approximately 1 year earlier as a result of an evaluation initiated by the university where he taught. University sources stated that Mr. S was behaving inappropriately: entering other professors' classrooms and beginning to lecture, forgetting to be present for classes and meetings, failing to bathe or change his clothes for days, addressing his class in an incoherent manner, and asking coworkers for assistance in operating office equipment that he had used for years without difficulty. After observing Mr. S's condition progressively worsen over time, the dean of the university telephoned Mrs. S to discuss the situation. Mrs. S claims that she noticed that her husband was acting unusually (forgetting names and appointments, bouncing checks, arguing for no reason, making unkind comments to friends, and confusing days off with work days) but thought this could be related to "getting older" and job stress. When the dean spoke with her, Mrs. S realized that a serious problem might exist and accompanied her husband for an evaluation, the result of which was the establishment of a diagnosis of Alzheimer's disease. Mr. S retired immediately from the university and has been with his wife for 24 hours each day since. Mrs. S offered no complaints until this past month, when she repeatedly called the physician to discuss the new problems of incontinence, eating difficulties, and wandering that Mr. S was exhibiting. These new problems have devastated Mrs. S; she looks fatigued and claims to be eating and sleeping poorly. She firmly states that she "will never consider placing her husband in an institution" and that she'll take care of him at home even "if it kills her."

THINK CRITICALLY

- What needs do both Mr. and Mrs. S have at this time?
- What resources could be helpful to Mrs. S to assist her in coping with the demands of caregiving?

THE OLDER ADULT WITH ALZHEIMER'S DISEASE

Nursing Diagnosis: Feeding Self-Care Deficit related to altered cognition

Goals	Nursing Actions
The patient maintains weight within ideal range; is free from signs of malnutrition.	■ Weigh patient to establish baseline weight and advise wife to weigh patient weekly and report weight loss of 5 lb or more.
	■ Review with patient and family patient's food likes and dislikes; assist family in planning meals that incorporate patient's preferences; consult with dietitian as necessary.
	■ Advise family to provide nutritious snacks, finger foods, and soft/pureed foods for patient.
	■ Discourage patient's eating of nuts, hard candy, popcorn, or other foods that could easily be aspirated.
	■ Suggest that patient eat in the same location (preferably a room with minimal distractions) at consistent times daily.
	■ Instruct family to guide patient through meals by placing appropriate utensil in his hand, giving him one-stage instructions, and praising good eating habits.
	■ Discuss with family referral to Meals on Wheels or similar service in community.

Nursing Diagnosis: Toileting Self-Care Deficit and Altered Urinary Elimination: Functional Incontinence related to altered cognition

Goals	Nursing Actions
The patient establishes toileting routine to prevent incontinence (if possible); is free from complications associated with incontinence.	■ Assess urinary elimination pattern and attempt to determine whether incontinence is a result of altered cognition or another problem; refer for evaluation if indicated.

- Assist family in identifying length of time between voiding episodes and develop plan to toilet patient half an hour prior to anticipated voiding time.
- Ensure that bathroom is easily accessible; arrange to obtain commode chair and urinal if necessary.
- Reinforce proper cleansing technique and skin care to prevent irritation.
- Suggest clothing that is easy for patient to remove for toileting; replacement of pants' buttons and zippers with Velcro.
- Supply with information regarding urine containment products and availability in community.

Nursing Diagnosis: Risk for Injury due to wandering, poor judgment secondary to altered cognition

Goal	Nursing Actions
The patient is free from injury.	■ Inspect home with family for potential safety hazards and make appropriate recommendations.
	■ Ensure that home is equipped with smoke alarm and fire extinguisher.
	■ Recommend preventive measures, such as storing chemicals, medications, and other potentially hazardous substances in locked cabinet, setting hot water heater temperature below 120°F, alarming doors to signal patient's wandering from home, keeping environment well lighted and clutter free, capping electrical outlets, locking and securing windows, keeping spare key with neighbor. Assist in locating stores to purchase safety equipment.
	■ Instruct family to administer medications for patient.
	■ Ensure patient wears stable shoes, safe clothing.
	■ Advise family to have current photograph of patient readily available in the event he becomes lost and must be located by persons unfamiliar with him.
	■ Supply with information on obtaining identification bracelet for patient.

Nursing Diagnosis: Disturbed Sleep Pattern related to dementia

Goals	Nursing Actions
The patient sleeps 5 to 7 hours at night; takes one nap during the day; is free from fatigue, insomnia, and other sleep/rest disturbances.	■ Recommend that family maintains a record of patient's sleep and nap times to assess patterns.
	■ Advise family to adhere to simple, consistent bedtime routine; provide soft lighting and music as this facilitates sleep; prevent patient from excess daytime napping; encourage early evening exercise.

Nursing Diagnosis: Impaired Verbal Communication related to Alzheimer's disease

Goals	Nursing Actions
The patient is oriented to person, place, and time (to maximum extent possible); effectively communicates needs.	■ Instruct family in helpful communication techniques, such as:
	• using calm relaxed manner of communication
	• approaching patient from the front and getting his attention
	• before speaking
	• using basic language
	• giving one instruction or comment at a time
	• avoiding overstimulating or overloading patient
	• allowing ample time for patient to respond
	• identifying terms used by patient to describe needs or items
	• using distractions when patient becomes upset
	■ Encourage family to keep patient oriented, place clocks and calendars in rooms used by patient.
	■ Help family to identify and avoid aspects of environment that could promote misperceptions, such as shadows cast by light, radios playing in empty rooms.

(Continues)

NURSING CARE PLAN 33-1 (Continued)

Nursing Diagnosis: Interrupted Family Processes and Caregiver Role Strain related to altered roles and function of patient and demands of caregiving

Goals	Nursing Actions
The family is free from adverse effects from patient's illness; develops effective means of coping with patient's condition.	▪ Assess family's reactions to patient's condition, impact on roles and functions; identify family members' risks and needs. ▪ Discuss realitives of disease and patient's prognosis with family. ▪ Identify other family resources or significant others who can offer support and assistance to family caregiver. ▪ Refer family to local chapter of Alzheimer's Disease and Related Disorders Association, counseling services, and other support services. ▪ Assist in locating respite care; recommend adult day care program for patient. ▪ Discuss potential for nursing home admission; listen to family's concerns; clarify misconceptions and offer facts. ▪ Assist family in identifying their own needs and developing plans for their own lives as patient's condition declines. ▪ Allow and encourage expression of feelings; offer support.

BRINGING RESEARCH TO LIFE

MASSAGE IN THE MANAGEMENT OF AGITATION IN NURSING HOME RESIDENTS WITH COGNITIVE IMPAIRMENT

Holliday-Welsh, D. M., Gessert, C. E., & Renier, C. M. (2009). Geriatric Nursing, 30(2), 109–117.

In this study, a group of nursing home residents were identified as being susceptible to agitation based on their assessment data from the Minimum Data Set report. The subjects were over age 60 with moderate or severe cognitive impairment and with a history of agitation. Baseline data were collected in relation to wandering, verbally and physically abusive behaviors, socially inappropriate or disruptive behavior, and resistance to care. After massage therapy was implemented with the subjects, improvements were seen in all of the behaviors except socially inappropriate or disruptive behaviors, for which there was no effect.

Massage is a well-understood, easy-to-learn, and low-risk intervention that can be provided by nursing staff, family members, and volunteers. It may aid in improving behaviors without the use of medication. Like any intervention, the approach should be individualized and response to the massage monitored and evaluated. Although massage can be a relaxing, pleasant experience for many people, it could trigger agitation in some individuals.

PRACTICE REALITIES

You accept a position at a large nursing home that has a "Special Care Unit" for persons with dementia. There are 25 residents on the unit with moderate to advanced dementia. You notice that the unit looks like any other one and during your orientation ask about the programs and features that make the unit unique. You are told that the Activities Department does a group at 2 P.M. every afternoon and that to prevent wandering off the unit, the doors require punching in a special code to exit.

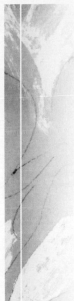

As the days progress you determine that there actually is not anything special about the unit at all. Residents spend most of their day sitting in the hallway or dining room and staff spend most of their time behind the nursing station. You mention to your supervisor that you think there are some interventions that could be used and changes implemented that could provide a higher quality of life and services for the residents and she encourages you to offer ideas.

What are the environmental changes and programming that could support effective care of residents with dementia on this unit? How could you implement them?

CRITICAL THINKING EXERCISES

1. Describe situations that an older patient could experience during a hospitalization for surgery that could cause delirium.

2. Discuss the impact of an older person's diagnosis of Alzheimer's disease on the spouse, adult children, and grandchildren.

3. In what ways could a person show denial of a spouse's signs of dementia? What behaviors by the well spouse could delay the diagnosis of the affected spouse?

4. What risks would an older adult with a mild dementia face if he or she lived alone in the community?

RESOURCES

Alzheimer's Association
http://www.alz.org

National Institute on Aging, Alzheimer's Disease Education and Referral Center
http://www.nia.nih.gov/alzheimers

REFERENCES

Alzheimer's Association. (2007). *Alzheimer's disease: Causes and risk factors.* Retrieved October 10, 2007 from http://www.alz.org/alzheimers_disease_causes_risk_factors.asp

Ancelin, M. L., Christen, Y., & Ritchie, K. (2007). Is antioxidant therapy a viable alternative for mild cognitive impairment? Examination of the evidence. *Dementia and Geriatric Cognitive Disorders, 24*(1), 1–19.

Auer, S., & Reisberg, B. (1997). The GDS/FAST staging system. *International Psychogeriatrics, 9*(Suppl 1), 167–171.

Dos Santos-Neto, L. L., de Vilhena Toledo, M.A., Medeiros-Souza, P., & de Souza, G. A. (2006). The use of herbal medicine in Alzheimer's disease—A systematic review. *Evidence Based Complementary and Alternative Medicine, 3*(4), 441–445.

Dykens, E. M. (2007). Psychiatric and behavioral disorders in persons with Down syndrome. *Mental Retardation and Developmental Disability Research Review, 13*(3), 272–278.

Henderson, V. W. (2006). Estrogen-containing hormone therapy and Alzheimer's disease risk: Understanding discrepant inferences from observational and experimental research. *Neuroscience, 138*(3), 1031–1039.

National Institute on Aging. (2006). *Alzheimer's disease: Unraveling the mystery.* Publication No. 02-3782. Rockville, MD: National Institutes of Health.

Pfeiffer, E. (1975). A short portable mental status questionnaire for the assessment of organic brain deficit in elderly patients. *Journal of the American Geriatric Society, 23*(10), 433.

Rassamy, C., Longpre, F., & Christen, Y. (2007). Ginkgo biloba extract (EGb 761) in Alzheimer's disease: Is there any evidence? *Current Alzheimer Research, 4*(3), 253–262.

Robakis, N. K. (2007). The discovery and mapping to chromosome 21 of the Alzheimer's amyloid gene: History revised. *Journal of Alzheimer's Disease, 10*(4), 453–455.

RECOMMENDED READINGS

Recommended Readings associated with this chapter can be found on the web site that accompanies the book. Visit **http://thepoint.lww.com/Eliopoulos8e** to access the recommended readings and other additional resources associated with this chapter.

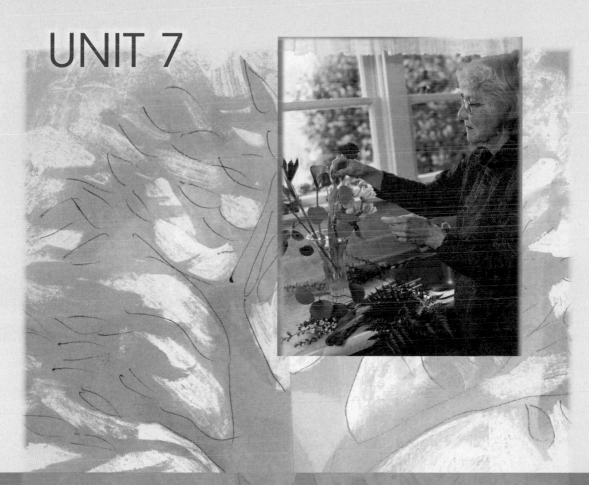

UNIT 7

Gerontological Care Issues

455

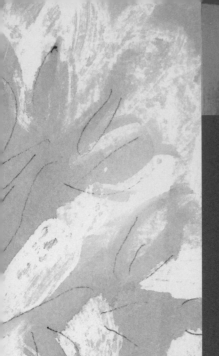

CHAPTER 34

Living in Harmony With Chronic Conditions

CHAPTER OUTLINE

LEARNING OBJECTIVES

After reading this chapter, you should be able to:

1. Discuss the scope of chronic conditions among the older population.

2. Differentiate between healing and curing.

3. List chronic care goals.

4. Outline components of assessment of older adults' chronic care needs.

5. Discuss approaches to maximize the benefits of conventional treatments for older adults with chronic conditions.

6. Identify alternative therapies that could benefit older adults with chronic conditions.

7. Discuss factors affecting the course of chronic care for older adults.

KEY TERMS

Chronic condition: long-term dysfunction or pathology

Defense mechanisms: reactions used to cope with a difficult or stressful situation

Healing: mobilization of body, mind, and spirit to control symptoms, promote sense of well-being, and achieve highest possible quality of life

Illness is not an easy situation to accept. Even a common cold disrupts our lives and makes us uncomfortable, irritable, and unmotivated to work and play. When sick, the basic activities of daily living can become a chore; our appearance may be the least of our worries; and our lives may revolve around the medications, treatments, and doctor's visits that will make us feel better. Fortunately, for most people, illness is an unusual and temporary event; they recover and return to life as usual.

Some illnesses, however, will accompany people for the remainder of their lives—chronic conditions. Potentially every aspect of one's life can be affected by chronic conditions. Because chronic conditions are highly prevalent in the older population, gerontological nurses often are involved in assisting patients with the demands imposed by these conditions. It is important for gerontological nurses to understand the unique challenges and goals for older patients living with chronic conditions. The success with which a chronic condition is managed can make the difference between a satisfying lifestyle in which control of the disease is but one routine component and a life controlled by the demands of the disease.

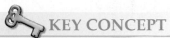

KEY CONCEPT

The manner in which a chronic condition is managed can make the difference between a high-quality, satisfying life and one in which the person is a prisoner to a disease.

CHRONIC CONDITIONS AND OLDER ADULTS

Medical technology has helped many people survive illnesses that once would have killed them; greater numbers of people are reaching old age, in which the incidence of chronic disease is higher. Thus, it should be no surprise that more than 80% of older adults possess at least one chronic disease. There is a profound increase in the rate of most chronic conditions with age (Box 34-1), particularly

BOX 34-1 Major Chronic Conditions of Older Adults

Nearly half of older adults suffer from arthritis.
More than one third of older adults have hypertension.
Nearly one third of older adults have a hearing impairment.
More than one fourth of older adults have a heart condition.
More than one eighth of older adults have a visual impairment.
Nearly another one eighth of older adults have a deformity or orthopedic impairment.
Almost 10% of older adults have diabetes.
Approximately 1 in 12 older adults is affected by hemorrhoids and varicose veins.

considering the impact of these diseases on the individual older person who is affected. The potential nursing diagnoses associated with these chronic conditions (Table 34-1) highlight the disruption to physical, emotional, and social well-being.

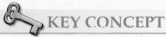

KEY CONCEPT

Most of the chronic conditions that are common in older adults can significantly affect the quality of daily life.

GOALS FOR CHRONIC CARE

Most health professionals were educated in the acute care model, in which care activities focus on diagnosis, treatment, and cure of illness. Within this model, nursing actions are based on interventions that cure patients, and success tends to be judged on how quickly and totally patients are able to recover. Chronic conditions are an entirely different situation. Because chronic diseases cannot be cured, it would be inappropriate to direct care activities down a curative path. Rather, healing is of utmost importance.

Healing implies the mobilization of the body, mind, and spirit to control symptoms, promote a sense of well-being, and enhance the quality of life. The person with a chronic condition can learn to live effectively with the disease and develop a sense of inner peace and harmony through the recognition that he or she is defined by more than the physical body. The nurse serves a healing role in facilitating this process and guiding individuals with chronic conditions to achieve their maximum potential and highest attainable quality of life. Rather than administer care and treatments for or to patients, the nurse stimulates patients' self-healing capabilities by creating a therapeutic human and physical environment; educating; empowering; reinforcing, affirming, and validating; and removing barriers to self-care and self-awareness.

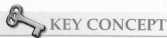

KEY CONCEPT

Healing implies the mobilization of the body, mind, and spirit to control symptoms, promote a sense of well-being, and enhance the quality of life.

Because patients cannot eliminate their disease, care measures focus on helping patients effectively live in harmony with, rather than cure, the condition. Professionals who seek success through the number of patients who recover will be frustrated and disappointed when working with persons who

TABLE 34-1   Potential Nursing Diagnoses Associated With 12 Major Chronic Problems of the Elderly

	Arthritis	Hypertension	Hearing Impairment	Heart Condition	Cataracts	Chronic Sinusitis	Visual Impairment	Deformities, Orthopedic Impairment	Hernia	Diabetes	Varicose Veins	Hemorrhoids
Activity Intolerance	✓	✓		✓	✓			✓	✓	✓	✓	✓
Anxiety	✓	✓	✓	✓	✓	✓	✓	✓	✓	✓	✓	✓
Constipation									✓		✓	
Decreased Cardiac Output												
Impaired Verbal Communication			✓									
Ineffective Coping	✓	✓	✓	✓	✓	✓	✓	✓	✓	✓	✓	✓
Disabled Family Coping	✓	✓	✓			✓	✓	✓	✓	✓	✓	✓
Deficient Diversional Activity	✓	✓	✓	✓	✓	✓	✓	✓	✓	✓	✓	✓
Interrupted Family Processes	✓	✓	✓	✓	✓	✓	✓	✓		✓	✓	✓
Fear	✓	✓	✓	✓	✓	✓	✓	✓		✓	✓	✓
Deficient Fluid Volume								✓				
Excess Fluid Volume					✓							
Grieving												
Ineffective Health Maintenance	✓	✓	✓	✓	✓	✓	✓	✓		✓	✓	✓
Impaired Home Maintenance	✓	✓	✓	✓	✓	✓	✓	✓		✓	✓	✓
Risk of Infection				✓		✓			✓	✓	✓	✓
Risk of Injury	✓	✓	✓	✓	✓	✓	✓			✓		
Knowledge Deficit	✓	✓	✓	✓	✓	✓	✓	✓	✓	✓	✓	✓
Impaired Physical Mobility	✓	✓		✓	✓			✓	✓	✓	✓	
Noncompliance	✓	✓	✓		✓	✓	✓	✓	✓	✓	✓	✓
Imbalanced Nutrition: Less Than Body Requirements	✓				✓	✓	✓	✓	✓	✓		
Imbalanced Nutrition: More Than Body Requirements	✓	✓		✓	✓					✓		
Impaired Oral Mucous Membrane										✓		
Pain	✓	✓		✓		✓		✓	✓		✓	✓
Powerlessness	✓		✓	✓	✓		✓	✓				
Ineffective Breathing Pattern				✓		✓		✓				
Self-Care Deficit	✓	✓	✓	✓	✓		✓	✓		✓	✓	✓
Disturbed Body Image	✓	✓	✓	✓	✓		✓	✓		✓	✓	✓
Disturbed Sensory Perception	✓		✓				✓	✓				
Ineffective Sexuality Patterns	✓	✓		✓				✓		✓		
Impaired Skin Integrity					✓			✓		✓	✓	✓
Disturbed Sleep Pattern	✓	✓		✓		✓		✓	✓	✓	✓	✓
Impaired Social Interaction	✓	✓	✓	✓	✓	✓	✓	✓		✓		
Social Isolation	✓	✓	✓	✓	✓		✓	✓				
Spiritual Distress												
Disturbed Thought Processes		✓	✓	✓			✓			✓		
Ineffective Tissue Perfusion				✓								
Impaired Urinary Elimination				✓						✓		

have chronic conditions; they must reorient themselves to a new set of care goals (Box 34-2). The following goals are appropriate to chronic care:

- *Maintain or improve self-care capacity.* Chronic conditions often place additional demands on people. They may need to eat special diets, modify their activities, administer medications, perform treatments, or learn to use assistive devices or equipment. Nurses may need to assist patients in increasing their abilities to meet these needs. Actions toward achieving this goal include education about the disease and its management, stabilization and improvement of health status, promotion of interest and motivation for self-care, use of assistive devices, and provision of periodic assistance with care.

- *Manage the condition effectively.* Individuals need to be knowledgeable about their conditions and related care. Skills may need to be mastered, such as injecting medications, changing dressings, or applying prostheses. However, motivation is essential to mobilize knowledge and skills in effective self-care, so assessing motivational factors and planning and implementing strategies to enhance motivation are crucial aspects.

- *Boost the body's healing abilities.* The body's tremendous potential to fight disease and heal naturally is often underestimated. Helping patients mobilize natural resources is an important nursing function. Stress management, guided imagery, exercise, immune-boosting nutrients, and biofeedback are among the strategies that can promote self-healing.

- *Prevent complications.* Chronic diseases and conventional treatments used to manage them can increase the risk of infections, injuries, and other complications. Potential risks should be identified and actively prevented, recognizing that risks change over time. Complications must be prevented because they risk weakening

self-care capacity, increasing disability, and hastening decline. Whether a patient with diabetes lives an active life or becomes a blind amputee is largely determined by the extent to which treatment plans are followed and complications are actively prevented.

- *Delay deterioration and decline.* By their nature, chronic conditions often progressively worsen. For example, a person with Alzheimer's disease will demonstrate a progressive decline in status even if highly effective care is provided. However, preventive practices can influence whether that individual is ambulatory or bed bound at the end of a period. A conscious effort must be made to reinforce the importance of preventive care measures and identify problems early.

- *Achieve the highest possible quality of life.* Sitting in bed attached to an oxygen tank may keep the body functioning but offers little stimulation to the mind and spirit. Consideration should be given to helping patients participate in activities that bring pleasure, stimulation, and reward. The nurse should assess the extent to which recreational, social, spiritual, emotional, sexual, and family needs are met and provide assistance to fulfill those needs (e.g., introduction to new hobbies, counseling for alternate positions for intercourse, provision of transportation by specially equipped vehicles, and arrangements for home visits by clergy). A positive self-concept needs to be promoted. It is important for health professionals to periodically evaluate the extent to which treatment of the condition promotes or prohibits a satisfying lifestyle.

- *Die with comfort and dignity.* As health status declines and patients face their final days of life, they will need increasing physical and psychosocial support. Pain relief, preservation of energy, provision of comfort, and assistance in meeting basic needs become crucial. Nurses also must be sensitive to the importance of listening and talking to dying persons, anticipating their needs, assuring spiritual support, and, most importantly, instilling a feeling that the nurse can be depended on for support through this period.

The success and progress of goals of chronic care must be measured differently from acute care. A deterioration of a patient from ambulatory to wheelchair status can be judged a success if, without nursing intervention, that patient may have become bedridden or died. Likewise, a physically and emotionally comfortable death that left positive memories for the patient's family can be a significant accomplishment. These determinants of success are different from those of acute care but are no less important.

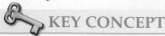

KEY CONCEPT

Successes in chronic care are measured differently from those in acute care.

ASSESSMENT OF CHRONIC CARE NEEDS

Self-care capacities can vary considerably among persons who have chronic conditions. The self-care capacity of the same individual will also vary at different times throughout the course of the illness. Keen assessment and reassessment are thus necessary. The nurse should review the individual's capacity to fulfill each of the health-related requirements, as well as the person's capacity to meet the demands imposed by illness (e.g., medication administration, dressings, and special exercises). From this, the nurse can determine deficits in fulfilling care needs.

A majority of people with chronic conditions manage their conditions in a community setting, most likely with family support or involvement; therefore, assessment must consider not only the capacity of the individual to fulfill the care demands but also the capacity of the family to assist and cope with caregiving. For example, a man with diabetes and severe arthritis in his hands may not be able to manipulate a syringe for his insulin injections, but his wife may be able to give him injections; thus, he does not have a deficit in this area. Likewise, a victim of Alzheimer's disease may not be able to protect herself from safety hazards, but if she lives with a daughter who supervises her activities, this patient may not have a deficit in her ability to protect herself. Within this framework, *the family is the patient*, and the capacities and limitations of the total family unit must be evaluated. Remember that family is not limited to relatives but can include a variety of significant others.

The nurse cannot assume, however, that the presence of family members guarantees compensation for the patient's care deficits. Sometimes the caregivers may not have the physical, mental, or emotional abilities to meet the patient's care needs. For instance, the patient's caregiver daughter may be a frail older adult herself. Likewise, the family may not want to provide care because of the imposition on their lifestyle or their feelings toward the patient. These factors must be considered before care is delegated to family members.

Once identified, care needs should be reviewed with the patient and family members. This not only helps to validate data but also promotes understanding by all parties involved as to what the actual care needs are. Methods of meeting care needs should be identified jointly (e.g., the daughter will assist with bathing, the son will provide transportation to the clinic for monthly visits, the daughter-in-law will call twice daily to remind the patient to take medications). The nurse should inform the family of the services available in their community to supplement their efforts. In fairness to the family, the costs and limitations of community services must be included in this discussion.

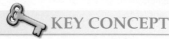

KEY CONCEPT

The patient and family caregivers should validate care plan priorities and goals.

Identified care needs direct goals and plans for care. Setting goals is important in helping patients and their families understand the realistic direction of the condition. For instance, a long-term goal of restoring ambulation sets a different tone from a goal of preventing complications as function deteriorates. Acceptance of long-term goals may require acceptance of the realities of the condition, which is not an easy task for patients and their families. It may take time and considerable nursing support for families to come to the understanding that the patient's physical or mental status will decline over time. This is not to suggest that hope should be destroyed, but rather that it be tempered with a realistic sense of what the future may hold. Short-term goals offer a means of evaluating ongoing efforts and serve as benchmarks in care; these goals can be set on a daily, weekly, or monthly basis, depending on the situation.

Finally, written care plans are beneficial to patients and their families. Having the plans in writing avoids discrepancies between perceptions and reality. It also prevents directions from being forgotten and ensures that anyone who participates in the patient's care will have the same understanding.

POINT TO PONDER

How would your life change if you learned that you had a chronic condition that would progressively worsen? What would you do differently? From where and whom would you draw emotional and spiritual support?

MAXIMIZING THE BENEFITS OF CHRONIC CARE

With similar diagnoses and care requirements, one individual may remain an active participant in society, enjoying a high quality of life, whereas another may become a homebound prisoner to the disease. The difference can depend on how the person approaches and manages care activities.

Selecting an Appropriate Physician

Because chronic conditions demand long-term medical supervision, selection of a physician becomes a significant issue for the patient. The patient should have contact with a specialist who is knowledgeable about state-of-the-art practices related to the condition. The nurse may assist the patient by providing the names of specialists for the patient to consider. In addition to qualifications and expertise in the field, the patient should feel at ease with the physician; a good chemistry between physician and patient will allow the patient to ask questions freely, discuss concerns, and report problems. Some factors that promote a positive physician–patient relationship include accessibility of the physician, sufficient time allocation for office visits and telephone consultations, comfortable and patient-appropriate communication style, respect for patient's involvement and decision-making, consideration of needs of entire family unit, openness to alternative and complementary therapies, and attitude of hope and optimism.

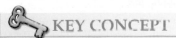

KEY CONCEPT

In addition to expertise in treating the specific condition, the physician should have a style with which the patient is comfortable because the relationship will be long term.

Patients have a responsibility to use their health care provider's time effectively. Patients can be advised to prepare for office visits by writing down questions, symptoms, and concerns and to maintain their own records of laboratory tests, vital signs, and other relevant medical data.

Using a Chronic Care Coach

Anyone who has attempted a weight reduction diet or exercise program appreciates the benefits of having a friend with whom the experience can be shared. Likewise, the person who must face life adjustments every day for the rest of his or her life can benefit from a buddy or coach who can provide support and assistance. The chronic care coach can be a spouse, child, friend, or someone with a similar condition who cares about and has regular contact with the patient (Fig. 34-1). The coach may accompany the patient to diagnostic tests or routine office visits and check on the patient's status routinely. The coach can provide feedback and positive reinforcement, as well as a listening ear when the patient

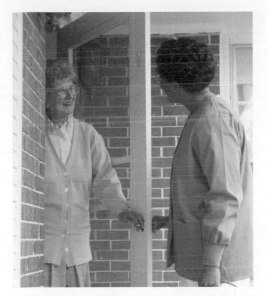

FIGURE 34-1 ■ A chronic care coach, whether a friend, spouse, or someone with a similar condition, has regular contact with the older person and can provide support and assistance.

has "slipped off" the treatment regimen or regressed (Box 34-3). Also, the coach can help the patient stay current about the disease by clipping articles from magazines and sharing information gained through media features. Gerontological nurses can advise and support persons who function as chronic care coaches to older individuals by outlining some of the basic steps of this process (Box 34-4).

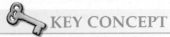

KEY CONCEPT

A chronic care coach provides support, encouragement, reinforcement, assistance, and feedback.

Increasing Knowledge

An informed patient is well equipped to manage the chronic condition successfully and prevent complications. Also, knowledge helps empower the patient. Various organizations for virtually every health condition can provide useful educational materials, often free of charge (see the Resources lists throughout this book). Most newspapers carry regular health columns that provide current information on health conditions and treatments. Local libraries not only possess a wealth of information on their shelves but also can assist people with literature searches. Also, ever-increasing numbers of individuals use the Internet to learn about new information and share knowledge. (If patients do not own a computer, they often can use one

BOX 34-3 Functions of a Chronic Care Coach

- Maintain regular contact with the patient.
- Become informed about the chronic condition and its related care requirements; keep abreast of new information, and share this with the patient; gather information as needed.
- Reinforce the care plan.
- Help patient prioritize and organize care activities.
- Assist patient in developing daily, weekly, and monthly goals.
- Remind the patient of appointments, activities.
- Acknowledge the realities of the condition.
- Listen to concerns and accept reaction without judgment.
- Offer feedback.

- Use humor therapeutically. Engage in fun activities with patient.
- Assist patient in locating and using resources.
- Reframe problems into opportunities; challenge patient to consider changes, new approaches.
- Observe changes or signs that could indicate complications or changes in condition; encourage patient to consult with health care provider promptly.
- Accompany patient to health care providers' office visits as needed.
- Recognize patient's efforts at self-care and compliance and give positive reinforcement.
- Encourage patient to comply with care demands. Provide inspiration and hope.

provided at public libraries.) Nurses should encourage patients to obtain as much information as they can and to maintain a file on their condition.

Locating a Support Group

Support groups can be important for persons with chronic conditions; they provide the opportunity not only for obtaining valuable information but also in gaining perspectives from those living with similar situations. Patients may be more willing to ask questions and express concerns with their peers than with health care professionals. Most support groups can be located through local telephone directories or the information and referral services of the local agency on aging; national headquarters of organizations also can direct patients to local chapters.

Making Smart Lifestyle Choices

Patients with lifelong health conditions need to commit to smart lifestyle choices to maximize their health and quality of life, such as compliance

with the prescribed treatment plan, sound dietary practices, regular exercise, stress management, assertiveness in protecting one's own needs, and development of a healing attitude and mind-set to live positively with the condition.

Using Complementary and Alternative Therapies

Growing numbers of Americans use complementary and alternative therapies for health promotion and illness management, and there is increasing evidence of the effectiveness of these measures. Such therapies use the body's capacity to heal itself and place the patient in charge of the healing process. Box 34-5 lists some of the alternative therapies that can be used to complement conventional therapies. In some cases, complementary and alternative therapies can replace conventional treatments, as when an analgesic is replaced by the use of acupuncture or guided imagery. The fact that complementary and alternative therapies have not been widely used

BOX 34-4 Steps in Chronic Care Coaching

Contact: Schedule regular telephone or face-to-face contact to check on the patient's status.

Observe: Be attentive to comments, mood, body language, energy, general status, presence of symptoms, compliance.

Affirm: Reinforce care plan and actions, recognize patient's efforts and accomplishments.

Clarify: Ask questions, validate observations, correct misconceptions, reinforce information.

Help: Offer assistance when self-care capacity is diminished; locate and negotiate resources.

Inspire: Encourage patient to comply with care plan, build on positive experiences and accomplishments; offer hope.

Nurture: Provide education, information, support.

Guide: Assist in setting realistic goals, developing plans, prioritizing, seeking resources.

Eliopoulos, C. (1997). Chronic care coaches: Helping people to help people. *Home Healthcare Nurse, 15*(3), 188.

BOX 34-5 Complementary and Alternative Therapies for People With Chronic Conditions

Acupressure	Massage therapy
Acupuncture	Meditation
Aromatherapy	Naturopathic medicine
Ayurvedic medicine	Nutritional supplements
Biofeedback	Osteopathy
Chiropathy	Progressive relaxation
Guided imagery	Qigong
Herbal medicine	Sound therapy
Homeopathy	T'ai chi
Hydrotherapy	Therapeutic touch
Hypnotherapy	Yoga
Light therapy	

in this country in the past does not mean that they are ineffective; people in other countries have used some of these measures successfully for centuries. Furthermore, the scarcity of research supporting the use of some of these therapies does not mean that they are useless. (Consider that researchers stand a better chance of obtaining funds for well-understood conventional therapies than for less familiar alternatives; pharmaceutical companies are not going to invest large sums of money testing herbal remedies that cannot be patented for their exclusive use; and most medical researchers have been educated in a system that perpetuates the use of conventional practices.)

This is not to say that there are not charlatans eager to take advantage of people who have chronic conditions. The nurse plays a significant role in helping the patient evaluate the validity of complementary and alternative therapies and use only sound, safe practices. Patients should be encouraged to discuss these therapies with their physicians and other health care providers. (In some circumstances, patients may need to provide literature about complementary and alternative therapies to their providers to educate them about these practices!) Ideally, patients should be able to use the best of both complementary/alternative and conventional health care practices.

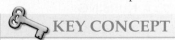

KEY CONCEPT

Many individuals can benefit from using a combination of conventional and complementary and alternative health practices for the care of their conditions.

FACTORS AFFECTING THE COURSE OF CHRONIC CARE

Anyone who has dieted can appreciate the difficulty of sustaining the initial weight loss behaviors (e.g., food restrictions and exercise) on a long-term basis without regular reinforcement and support. The same is true for the new behaviors associated with managing a chronic condition. Persons with chronic conditions cannot be given their instructions for care, discharged, and forgotten. They will need periodic contact and reevaluation of their capacity, resources, and motivation to manage their conditions.

A variety of factors can change patients' abilities to manage their illnesses. The status of the illness may change, placing more or different demands on the patient. The status of the patient may change, reducing self-care ability. The status of the caregiver may change, limiting the degree to which the patient's deficits can be compensated. All the factors affecting the patient's ongoing care must be evaluated regularly.

Defense Mechanisms and Implications

The lifestyle changes, frustrations, and losses commonly experienced by persons who must live with chronic conditions may cause certain reactions to emerge that could disrupt the flow of care. These reactions are defense mechanisms, used when the situation at hand may be too much for the patient to cope with, and include:

- *Denial:* making statements or taking actions that are not consistent with the realities of the illness (e.g., abandoning a special diet, discontinuing medications independently, committing to responsibilities that cannot be fulfilled)

- *Anger:* acting in a hostile manner, having violent outbursts

- *Depression:* making statements regarding the hopelessness of a situation, refusing to engage in self-care activities, withdrawing, questioning the purpose of life

- *Regression:* becoming increasingly dependent unnecessarily, abandoning self-care behaviors

These and other reactions are indications that the patient's ego strength is threatened and that extra support is needed. Rather than reacting to the patient's behavior, caregivers need to understand its origin and help the patient work through it (e.g., by providing an opportunity to vent frustrations and offering respite from the routines of care by doing for the patient until he or she feels psychologically able to resume self-care).

Psychosocial Factors

Chronic conditions can have a profound impact on psychosocial function; in turn, psychosocial function can impact the degree to which the individual lives effectively with the chronic condition. Older adults who are dealing with losses and changes may feel overwhelmed and powerless when faced with chronic conditions. Self-concept can be altered as older persons receive diagnoses that they had associated with old age. They may feel that having chronic conditions causes them to be viewed as different, less competent, or unattractive; they may be stigmatized due to the perception others have of persons with specific diagnoses or due to behaviors that foster stigmatization (e.g., feeling ashamed of their disease or identifying themselves as inadequate due to having a specific diagnosis). They may begin to identify themselves by their diagnosis or limitations (real or perceived); others may impose such identities on them.

Patients need support as they adapt to their condition and encouragement to adapt the chronic condition to their lives, rather than having their lives turned upside down by their chronic condition. Many of the recommendations discussed earlier will equip these individuals to live effectively with their conditions and achieve optimum psychosocial health. Specific psychosocial symptoms and history that could affect adaptation to the chronic condition (e.g., expressions of hopelessness, attention-getting benefits of sick role behaviors, poor coping capacity, and lack of support system) should be considered during the assessment and interventions planned to address them. Support groups can prove beneficial as they offer contact with persons experiencing similar issues who can share successful strategies, answer questions in a peer-to-peer manner, and provide examples of living effectively with the condition.

Impact of Ongoing Care on the Family

In the home management of a chronic illness, the entire family is the patient; therefore, in evaluating care, the impact on the total family must be considered. The patient with Alzheimer's disease may be well groomed, well nourished, and free from complications; looking at the patient in isolation, an evaluation could be made that her home care has been successful. However, the patient's status may have been achieved at great cost to the entire family. For example, her husband may have had to forfeit his job to care for her during the day; her daughter's family life may have been disrupted because she needs to sleep at her parents' home to assist her father in controlling her mother's night wandering; the son's plans to expand his business may have

been postponed because he began subsidizing his parents' income. Some sacrifices and compromises are common when family members assume caregiver roles, but serious disruption to their health or their lives should not result. Families may be so embroiled in the situation that they are unable to see the full impact that the caregiving situation is having on their own lives. Sometimes they feel that they must be a "bad" spouse or child to feel that the patient's care is a burden. Nurses can assist by helping family members realistically evaluate their caregiving responsibilities and identify when other caregiving options should be considered. For instance, the family may sense that it is in the patient's best interest to enter a nursing home, but they need the health care professional to introduce the suggestion and help them through the process of making this difficult decision.

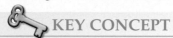

KEY CONCEPT

In chronic care, the entire family is the patient.

The Need for Institutional Care

Although only 5% of the older population is in a nursing home or other institutional setting at any given time, nearly one half of all older women and one third of all older men will spend some time in a long-term care facility during their lives (American Association of Homes and Services for the Aging, 2012). Most families seek assisted living or nursing home care after having attempted caregiving of their elder relative at home, not as a first choice. By the time they seek such assistance, their physical, emotional, and socioeconomic resources can be significantly depleted, and they may require special support and assistance from nurses. (Chapter 37 discusses the care of individuals who are in long-term care facilities.)

POINT TO PONDER

What would you do if a parent, spouse, or child needed considerable care? How much care could you realistically provide, and what resources would you have available?

CHRONIC CARE: A NURSING CHALLENGE

Effective chronic care is not an easy nursing challenge. It requires knowledge and skills related to the management of multiple medical problems, skilled assessment and planning, individualized promotion of self-care capacity, monitoring of family health, and a variety of other demands. The patient's comfort, independence, and quality of life are largely influenced by the type of services rendered; in chronic care, most of those services will fall within the scope of nursing. Perhaps this type of care, more than any other, provides an opportunity for nursing to demonstrate its facets of independent practice and full leadership potential.

BRINGING RESEARCH TO LIFE

DETERMINANTS OF FREQUENCY, DURATION, AND CONTINUITY OF HOME WALKING IN PATIENTS WITH COPD

Donesky, D. A., Lanson, S. L., Nguyen, H. O., Neuhaus, J., Neilands, T. B., & Carrieri-Kohlman, V. (2011). Geriatric Nursing, 32(3), 178–187.

The purpose of this study was to determine factors that influenced the frequency, duration, and continuity of home walking exercise in patients who participated in a dyspnea self-management program. Patients maintained logs and were telephoned biweekly by the intervention nurse. It was found that patients walked more frequently if they had been exercising prior to entering the study, did not have depressive symptoms, and were living with friends or family. The minutes that they exercised (duration) were influenced by receiving supervised exercise training, physical condition, and living with family or friends. The continuation of the exercise over a 1 year period was associated with having more supervised exercise sessions as part of the program and having exercised regularly before entering the program.

From these findings nurses could conclude that prior behaviors influence compliance with behaviors that are recommended to patients to promote management of a chronic condition and that support, either through a formal program or family and friends, influences positive outcomes. As part of the plan to teach strategies for self care and health promotion to people who have chronic conditions, exploring past behaviors can yield valuable insights into potential compliance with plans, as can the availability of support from family and friends. For example, patients who live alone and have a history of poor dietary habits may be less likely to comply with a newly prescribed diet than those who have been conscientious about eating habits and live in a household with people who can support their efforts. Patient education alone may be insufficient to enable people to adapt self-care practices necessary to live effectively with their conditions. Special assistance (e.g., referral to organized programs or support groups and regular phone calls to remind and encourage) may be needed for individuals who lack support or have not had a history of behaviors that may be required of them to address the needs imposed by a chronic condition.

PRACTICE REALITIES

You are joining a new geriatric specialty medical practice with a team of nurses, nurse practitioners, and physicians. The team recognizes that chronic conditions are a major challenge for the population they are targeting and want to offer services addressing this challenge. They want to "think outside the box" in developing innovative approaches and assign you the task of designing an assessment tool that evaluates the holistic needs of the person who has a chronic condition.

Describe the components of the assessment tool you would develop.

CRITICAL THINKING EXERCISES

1. Discuss the way in which your life would be affected if you developed a chronic disease. What additional issues exist for an older adult faced with this same situation?

2. Review the major chronic illnesses affecting the older population and identify the threats to the quality of life that could be associated with each.

3. Describe factors that cause most nurses and physicians to be ill-informed of or resistant to alternative therapies.

4. Identify measures that could help empower an older adult who has a chronic condition.

REFERENCE

American Association of Homes and Services for the Aging. (2012). *Nursing Home Statistics*. Retrieved April 15, 2012 from http://www.aahsa.org/aging_services/default.asp

RECOMMENDED READINGS

Recommended Readings associated with this chapter can be found on the web site that accompanies the book. Visit **http://thepoint.lww.com/Eliopoulos8e** to access the recommended readings and other additional resources associated with this chapter.

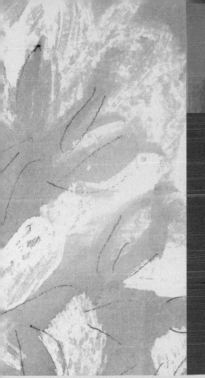

CHAPTER 35

Rehabilitative Care

CHAPTER OUTLINE

LEARNING OBJECTIVES

After reading this chapter, you should be able to:

1. Discuss the challenges for older adults living with a disability.
2. Describe the principles of rehabilitative nursing.
3. List components of the assessment of activities of daily living and instrumental activities of daily living for older adults.
4. Identify positions for proper body alignment.
5. Describe types of range-of-motion exercises.
6. List considerations in older adults' proper use of mobility aids.
7. Describe measures to promote mental function in older adults.
8. Identify resources to assist in older patients' rehabilitation.

TERMS TO KNOW

Activities of daily living (ADLs): toileting, feeding, dressing, grooming, bathing, and ambulating
Assistive technology: technological tools that enable a person to maximize independence
Disability: inability to perform activities normally
Frailty: condition in which a person has poor endurance and weakness
Handicap: limitation to fulfill a role
Impairment: physical or psychological restriction

(Continued)

Instrumental activities of daily living (IADLs): tasks required for community living, such as shopping, meal preparation, laundry, housekeeping, use of telephone, money management, medication management

Sarcopenia: age-related loss of muscle mass

The prevalence of chronic conditions, frailty, and disability among older adults is significant. Many older persons must learn to live with limited mobility, pain, impaired communication, and multiple risks to their safety and well-being. As increasing numbers of people achieve advanced years, surviving once-fatal conditions but with residual disabilities, the prevalence of disability among older adults will rise. The emphasis on saving lives must be balanced with an emphasis on preserving the quality of the lives that have been saved. The advantages of modern technology in diagnosing and treating disease and improving life expectancy may be minimized if older adults must live with disabilities that result in discomfort, dependency, and distress.

POINT TO PONDER

Advances in health care technology have enabled people to be saved from serious illnesses, although in some cases they are left with significantly limited function and discomfort. Would you want every effort made to save your life regardless of the consequences? Why or why not?

THE NEED FOR REHABILITATION

Rehabilitation must be defined broadly in geriatric care. It may be regarded as those efforts that help individuals improve their functional capacity so that they can better cope, be maximally independent, have a sense of well-being, and enjoy a satisfying life. Older adults may be in need of rehabilitative nursing when their functional capacity is compromised due to disabilities or frailty that results from aging, chronic conditions, or accidents.

Many of older adults' disabilities cannot be eliminated or, in many cases, significantly improved. Damaged lungs, amputations, diseased heart muscle, partial blindness, presbycusis, and deformed joints may accompany patients for the remainder of their lives. Often these chronic disabilities receive the least intervention; reimbursement and aggressive attention are given to restore the function of someone who has suffered a stroke or fracture, but those with "no rehabilitation potential"

often are overlooked in their need to maintain function and prevent further decline.

Frailty is a particular challenge to older persons that must be considered in rehabilitative care. Some of the frailty is the result of sarcopenia—age-related changes to the skeletal muscle tissues. Immobility and lack of exercise, increased levels of proinflammatory cytokines, increased production of oxygen free radicals or impaired detoxification, low anabolic hormone output, malnutrition, and reduced neurological drive are thought to be responsible for sarcopenia (Di Iorio et al., 2006). There is a vicious cycle in that conditions that contribute to frailty can foster the development of sarcopenia, and in turn, sarcopenia can lead to the development of conditions that further threaten function and quality of life.

A person is considered frail if he or she has at least three of the following symptoms (Fried et al., 2001):

- unplanned weight loss (10 or more pounds in the past year)
- slow walking speed
- low grip strength
- fatigue, poor endurance
- low levels of activity

Older adults who meet the criteria for frailty are at high risk for falls, disability, hospitalization, nursing home admission, and death. Positive health practices and effective management of health conditions, however, are beneficial in helping older adults to avoid becoming frail. Early recognition and intervention for symptoms of frailty (e.g., correcting weight loss and assisting with muscle-strengthening exercises) can prevent or delay some of the frailty older adults' experience. For this reason, it is especially useful to review symptoms of frailty during nursing assessments of older adults.

Although disability differs from frailty, handicap, and impairment (Table 35-1), the term *disability* will be used throughout this chapter to discuss rehabilitative needs.

LIVING WITH DISABILITY

An accident or a stroke may bring sudden disability to a previously independent, functional adult, or perhaps a chronic condition progressively worsens

TABLE 35-1	Terminology Used to Describe Functional Status	
Term[a]	**Definition**	**Examples**
Disability	Inability to perform an activity in a normal manner	Inability to cut food due to arthritic fingers Abnormal gait related to hemiplegia
Frailty	Three or more of the following symptoms: progressive weight loss, slow walking speed, low grip strength, fatigue, low activity levels	Self-care neglect due to weakness, fatigue Frequent falls due to unsteady gait and weakness
Impairment	Psychological, physiologic, or anatomic loss or abnormality	Loss of limb due to amputation Altered thought processes related to dementia
Handicap	Limitation in ability to fulfill role (possible consequence of disability or impairment)	Loss of job related to amputation Forfeiture of participation in family activities due to altered cognition

[a]Although often used interchangeably, these terms each describe a different status.

and its disabling impact is more acutely realized. Whatever the circumstances, few of us are prepared to deal with disability. It is difficult to accept in ourselves and our loved ones. Relationships, roles, and responsibilities are disrupted; disfigurement and dysfunction alter body image and self-concept. Losses and limitations cause a new vulnerability to emerge and make death seem more real and close. Concern arises over potential physical and emotional pain, and frustration occurs in wanting to eliminate the cause of the problem and knowing we cannot. Disability can be an extremely difficult and devastating mountain to climb.

POINT TO PONDER

What examples have you seen within your own family of differences in the way people respond to health challenges?

Importance of Attitude and Coping Capacity

The severity of the disability can be less important to rehabilitation efforts than the attitude and coping capacity of disabled patients and their families. Someone with a mild cardiac problem may confine himself to his home, become preoccupied with his illness, and demand to be waited on, whereas a patient with hemiplegia could return to independent living in his modified apartment, find a job, and cultivate new friends and interests. Previous attitudes, personality, and lifestyle have a strong influence on reactions to disability. A person who has always felt that life has dealt her a bad hand could view a disability as the last straw and give up all hope. An optimistic person who has approached problems as new challenges to overcome, however, may be determined not to allow

a disability to control her life. Individuals who relish independence and refuse to let illness slow their lifestyles will respond to disability differently from those who use real or exaggerated ills for other gains.

The family's response to the disabled person will also influence that person's reactions. Families that reinforce sick role behaviors and insist on doing everything for the disabled person can cripple him physically and psychologically, whereas families that promote self-care and treat the disabled person as a responsible family member can help him to feel like a normal, useful human being.

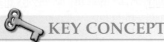

KEY CONCEPT

Previous attitudes, personality, experiences, and lifestyle influence reactions to a disability.

Losses Accompanying Disability

Many losses may accompany disability, such as the loss of function, role, income, status, independence, or perhaps a body part. Disabled persons mourn these losses, often demonstrating the same reactions experienced during the stages of dying. They may deny their disabilities by making unrealistic plans and not complying with their care plans. They may have angry outbursts and become impatient with those who are trying to help them. They may shop for medical advice that will offer them a more optimistic outlook or invest their hopes in any faith healer they can find. On one day they may optimistically state that their disability has given them a new perspective on life, yet the very next day they tearfully question what they have to live for. These reactions can fluctuate; it is the rare individual who accepts a disability without some periods of regret or resentment.

KEY CONCEPT

Disability can be accompanied by many losses, including function, role, income, status, independence, and anatomic structure.

PRINCIPLES OF REHABILITATIVE NURSING

The principles guiding gerontological nursing care are of particular significance in rehabilitation and include the following actions:

- increase self-care capacity
- eliminate or minimize self-care limitations
- act for or do for when the person is unable to take action for himself or herself

KEY CONCEPT

Improving the functional capacity of older adults can promote a sense of well-being and a higher quality of life.

Efforts to increase self-care capacity could include building the patient's arm muscles to enable better transfer to and propelling of a wheelchair or teaching the patient how to inject insulin with the use of only one hand. Relieving pain and having a ramp installed for easier wheelchair mobility are efforts that minimize or eliminate limitations. Obtaining a new prescription from the pharmacy and assisting with range-of-motion exercises are ways in which nurses act for or do for the patient. Whenever nurses act or do for patients, they need to question what could be done to enable patients to perform the action independently. Patients may always be dependent on others for some activities, but for other actions patients can assume responsibility with sufficient education, time allocation, encouragement, and assistive devices.

The following guidelines should be remembered in rehabilitative nursing:

- Know the unique capacities and limitations of the individual. Assess the patient's self-care capacity, mental status, level of motivation, and family support.
- Emphasize function rather than dysfunction and capabilities rather than disabilities.
- Provide time and flexibility. At times, institutional routines (e.g., having all baths completed by 9 A.M., collecting all food trays 45 minutes after delivery) cause caregivers to do tasks for patients so that they may be completed efficiently. Staff desires for efficiency and orderliness should never supersede the patient's need for independence.

- Recognize and praise accomplishments. Seemingly minor acts, such as combing hair or wheeling themselves to the hallway, can be the result of tremendous effort and determination on the part of disabled persons.
- Do not equate physical disability with mental disability. Treat disabled persons as mature, intelligent adults.
- Prevent complications. Recognize potential risks (e.g., skin breakdown, social isolation, and depression) and actively prevent them.
- Demonstrate hope, optimism, and a sense of humor. It is difficult for disabled persons to feel positive about rehabilitation if their caregivers appear discouraged or disinterested.
- Keep in mind that rehabilitation is a highly individualized process, requiring a multidisciplinary team effort for optimal results.

FUNCTIONAL ASSESSMENT

When a person suffers from a disability, functional status, rather than diagnosis, directs rehabilitative care. Among older individuals, functional status varies widely. Some older adults actively hold down jobs and regularly provide volunteer service, others are able to perform activities of daily living (ADLs) if some assistance is provided, and a portion of them are so severely impaired that total care is required. Furthermore, functional status can change within an individual from time to time, depending on the factors such as control of symptoms, progression of the disease, and mood.

Assessment of functional status involves determining an individual's level of independence in performing ADLs and instrumental activities of daily living (IADLs). This information is essential for understanding the rehabilitation needs of the patient. An assessment of ADLs explores the skills the patient possesses to meet basic requirements such as eating, washing, dressing, toileting, and moving. The nurse can use an assessment tool such as the Katz Index of Independence in ADLs. Some assessment tools, such as the Cleveland Scale for Activities of Daily Living, have been developed to assess ADLs in persons with impaired cognition, which may aid in revealing the impact that cognitive deficits have had on function (Mack & Patterson, 2006). Assessment of IADLs examines the skills beyond the basics that enable the individual to function independently in the community, such as the ability to prepare meals, shop, use a telephone, safely use medications, clean, travel in the community, and manage finances. Persons can be totally independent, partially independent, or dependent in their ability to perform these activities (Table 35-2).

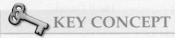

KEY CONCEPT

Assessing a person's functional status involves evaluating his or her ability to perform both ADLs and IADLs.

When a deficit in ADL capacity exists, the underlying cause must be identified so that appropriate interventions can be planned. For example, a person who is partially dependent in bathing because he needs to have a basin of water brought to him will have different nursing requirements than one who forgets what he is doing as he bathes and needs to be reminded of the next action to take.

INTERVENTIONS TO FACILITATE AND IMPROVE FUNCTIONING

When functional assessment reveals disabilities and impairments, nurses should identify areas of functioning that could be improved through

TABLE 35-2	Assessing Capacity to Perform Activities of Daily Living	
Total Independence	**Partial Independence**	**Dependence**
Eating		
Uses all utensils	Needs tray to be set up	Needs to be fed
Cuts meats	Cannot cut foods or butter bread	
Butters bread	Needs encouragement,	
Drinks from cup or glass	reminders to eat	
Hygiene		
Transfers in or out of tub	Reaches some body parts to cleanse	Needs complete bathing
or shower	Unable to brush teeth or dentures	assistance
Reaches and bathes all	Unable to turn faucets or flush toilet	
body parts	Needs assistance transferring in or	
Brushes teeth or dentures	out of tub or shower	
Brushes or combs hair	Needs assistance to comb or brush hair	
Cleanses self after toileting	Must have basin brought	
Turns faucets, flushes toilet	Needs reminders, encouragement to bathe	
Dressing		
Selects appropriate garments	Needs assistance with some garments,	Needs to be fully dressed
Puts on all clothing	zippers, buttons, snaps	
Slips on shoes, socks, stockings	Unable to select appropriate garments	
Ties shoelaces	Needs encouragement, reminders	
Able to manage zippers,	to dress	
buttons, snaps		
Continence		
Continent of bladder and bowels	Incontinent less than once daily	Totally incontinent
Toileting		
Uses bedpan or toilet without	Needs to be taken to toilet or	Needs assistance getting on or
assistance	have bedpan brought or taken	off bedpan or commode
Able to reach or transfer to	Needs encouragement or reminders	Unable to use bedpan or
and from bedpan or toilet	to toilet	commode
Manages ostomy or catheter	Needs assistance with ostomy or	Unable to perform ostomy or
independently	catheter care	catheter care
Mobility		
Ambulates with no assistance	Ambulates with assistance	Bedbound
Turns corners	Climbs stairs with assistance	Needs to be pushed in
Climb stairs	Transfers with assistance	wheelchair
Sits or lifts from chair and bed	Propels wheelchair but needs	Unable to transfer
Uses wheelchair, cane, walker	to be assisted in and out	Unable to climb stairs
with no assistance	Wanders in limited area	Wanders away if not supervised

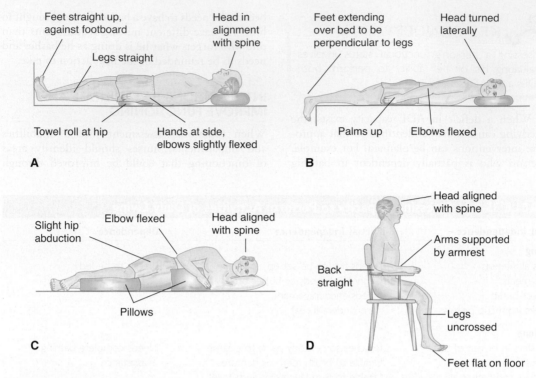

FIGURE 35-1 ■ **A.** Supine position. **B.** Prone position. **C.** Lateral position. **D.** Chair position.

interventions. Some examples of these interventions include positioning, range-of-motion exercises, use of mobility aids, bowel and bladder training, and activities to promote mental function.

Facilitating Proper Positioning

Correct body alignment facilitates optimal respiration, circulation, and comfort and prevents complications such as contractures and pressure ulcers. When patients are unable to position their bodies independently, nurses must be attentive to keeping their bodies properly aligned. Figure 35-1 demonstrates proper alignment in various positions.

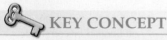 **KEY CONCEPT**

Correct body alignment facilitates the optimal function of major systems, promotes comfort, and prevents complications.

Assisting With Range-of-Motion Exercises

Exercise is an essential component of the health maintenance and promotion plan of every adult and is particularly significant for older adults. Range-of-motion exercises have many benefits, including the promotion of joint motion and muscle strength,

stimulation of circulation, maintenance of functional capacity, and prevention of contractures and other complications. Teaching the older adult how to perform range-of-motion exercises or assisting them with these exercises is an important component of rehabilitative nursing.

Exercises can be done in the following degrees:

■ active—independently by patients

■ active assistive—with assistance to the patient

■ passive—with no active involvement of the patient

During the assessment, all joints should be put through a full range of motion to determine the degree of movement possible actively, with active assistance, and passively. The most significant concern is the degree to which range of motion is sufficient to participate in ADLs. Box 35-1 lists some of the terms used in describing joint motion.

Patients should be encouraged to put all joints through a full range of motion at least once daily. Figure 35-2 demonstrates the basic range-of-motion exercises that should be incorporated into the older adult's daily activities. When nurses need to assist patients with these exercises, they should remember the following points:

■ First, offer support below and above the joint being exercised.

BOX 35-1   Terms Used to Describe Joint Motion

Flexion: bending
Extension: straightening
Hyperextension: extending beyond normal range
Abduction: moving away from body
Adduction: moving toward body
Pronation: rotating down, toward back of body

Supination: rotating up, toward front of body
Internal rotation: turning limb inward, toward center
External rotation: turning limb outward, from center
Inversion: turning joint inward
Eversion: turning joint outward
Circumduction: moving in a circular manner

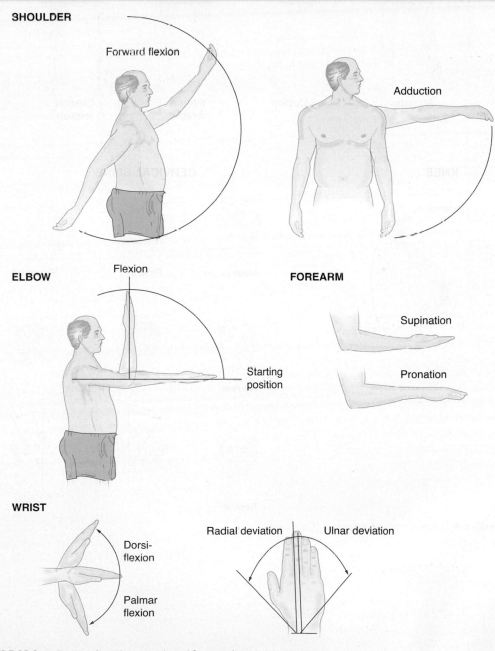

SHOULDER
Forward flexion
Adduction

ELBOW   Flexion
Starting position

FOREARM
Supination
Pronation

WRIST
Dorsi-flexion
Palmar flexion
Radial deviation   Ulnar deviation

FIGURE 35-2 ■ Range-of-motion exercises. (*Continues*)

HIP

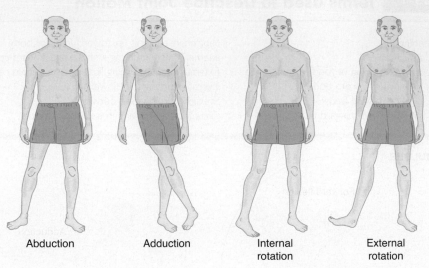

Abduction   Adduction   Internal   External
                                       rotation   rotation

KNEE

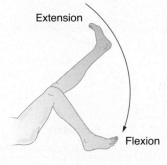

Extension

Flexion

CERVICAL SPINE

  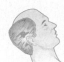

Neutral   Flexion   Extension

  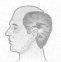

Neutral   Rotation

 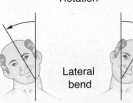

Neutral   Lateral
                                   bend

FIGURE 35-2 ■ Range-of-motion exercises. (*Continues*)

THUMB

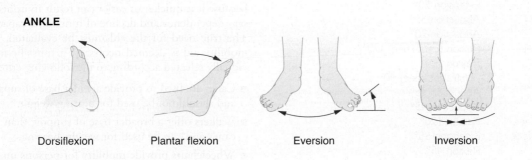

Adduction

Abduction

Opposition

FINGERS

Adduction

Abduction

Extension

Neutral

ANKLE

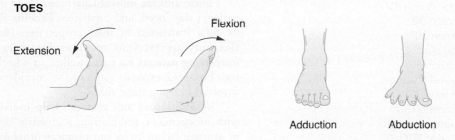

Dorsiflexion

Plantar flexion

Eversion

Inversion

TOES

Flexion

Extension

Adduction

Abduction

FIGURE 35-2 ■ *(Continued)*

- Next, move the joint slowly and smoothly, exercising it at least three times.
- Third, do not force the joint past the point of resistance or pain.
- Finally, document joint mobility.

Table 35-3 offers a tool that can be used to document the patient's range of motion.

With any exercise program, caution must be taken to ensure that the physical activity does not overexert the older patient. Some of the signs that would warrant stopping an exercise include the development of:

- a resting heart rate greater than or equal to 100 beats/minute
- an exercise heart rate greater than or equal to 35% above the resting heart rate
- increase or decrease in systolic blood pressure by 20 mm Hg

- angina
- dyspnea, pallor, cyanosis
- dizziness, poor coordination
- diaphoresis
- acute confusion, restlessness

TABLE 35-3 **Tool for Assessing and Documenting Range of Motion**

Joint	Normal Range	Patient's Range
Shoulder	Flexion 160°	
	Extension 50°	
Elbow	Flexion 160°	
	Extension from 160° to 0°	
Wrist	Flexion 90°	
	Extension 70°	
	Abduction 55°	
	Adduction 20°	
Hip	Flexion (bent knee) 120°	
	Flexion (straight knee) 90°	
	Abduction 45°	
	Adduction 45°	
Knee	Flexion 120°	
Neck	Extension 55°	
	Flexion 45°	
	Lateral bending 40°	
	Rotation 70°	
Ankle	Dorsiflexion 20°	
	Plantar flexion 45°	
	Inversion 30°	
	Eversion 20°	
Great toe	Distal phalange: Flexion 50°	
	Proximal phalange: Flexion 35°	
	Extension 80°	
Finger	Proximal phalange: Flexion 90°	
	Extension 30°	
	Middle phalange: Flexion 120°	
	Distal phalange: Flexion 80°	
Thumb	Proximal phalange: Flexion 70°	
	Distal phalange: Flexion 90°	

From Eliopoulos, C. (1991). Range of motion exercises. *Long-Term Care Educator, 2*(9), 3.

Assisting With Mobility Aids and Assistive Technology

Wheelchairs, canes, and walkers can make the difference between older persons living full lives or being confined to their immediate environments. Mobility aids can enable patients to independently fulfill their universal needs and enhance functional capacity. If misused, however, these aids can present significant safety risks; thus, nurses must ensure that these pieces of equipment are used properly.

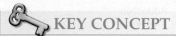
KEY CONCEPT

Inappropriately used canes, walkers, and wheelchairs can subject the older adult to falls and other injuries.

The first principle in using mobility aids is to use them only when necessary. Using a wheelchair because it is quicker or easier can result in unnecessary dependency and decline of functional capacity. The true need for the aid must be evaluated. If a mobility aid is deemed necessary, it must be individually selected according to the following criteria:

- Canes are used to provide a wider base of support and should not be used for bearing weight.
- Walkers offer a broader base of support than canes and can be used for weight-bearing.
- Wheelchairs provide mobility for persons unable to ambulate because of various disabilities, such as paralysis or severe cardiac disease.

These aids are individually fitted based on the patient's size, need, and capacities. Patients should be fully instructed in their proper use. Physical therapists are excellent resources for sizing and instructing patients for cane, walker, or wheelchair use. Box 35-2 explains some of the considerations involved in using these aids.

In addition to aids that can help individuals with independent ambulation, a growing amount of assistive technologies can promote other aspects of independent function. These can include splints, utensil grips, Velcro attachments, computers, voice synthesizers, Braille readers, remote control devices, and robotic arms. Research and testing is being conducted on the expanded use of artificial intelligence, robots, and other technologies to compensate for physical and mental limitations. These devices not only will enable older adults to care for themselves and function within the community but also afford them the opportunity to remain in the workforce despite having a disability. Nurses need to keep abreast of technological advances to be

BOX 35-2   Proper Use of Mobility Aids

CANES

Depending on the disability, various canes may be recommended. Canes should be individually fitted, usually based on the distance from the greater trochanter to a distance 6 inches from the side of the person's foot.

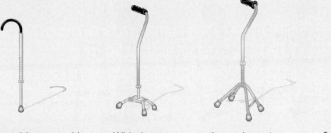

| Adjustable cane with standard handgrip | Wide-base quad cane | Large-based quad cane | Small-based quad cane |

The cane is used on the *unaffected* side of the body and is advanced when the affected limb advances. For example, if the right leg is affected, the person holds the cane in his or her left hand and advances it with the advance of the right leg.

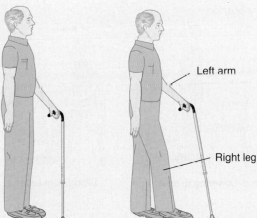

Left arm

Right leg

WALKERS

A variety of walkers can provide support and stability during ambulation. Walkers are sized by the measurement from the patient's trochanter to the floor.

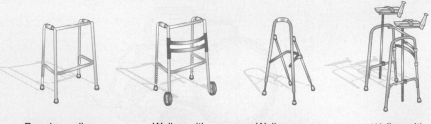

| Regular walker | Walker with wheels | Walker-cane | Walker with forearm attachments |

(Continues)

BOX 35-2 **Proper Use of Mobility Aids** (continued)

The person should place his or her hands on the sides of the walker, with the elbows slightly flexed. During ambulation, the person advances the walker and then steps forward.

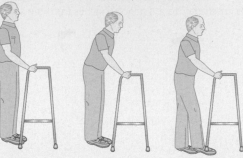

Person standing
with walker

Walker
advanced

Person advancing
to walker

Appropriate use should be followed during transfer activities also. When lowering to a seat, the person should back the walker to the seat. When lifting from a seat, the person's hands should be on the arm of the chair. The person pushes on the arms of the chair to a standing position; the person should not use the walker to pull himself or herself to a standing position.

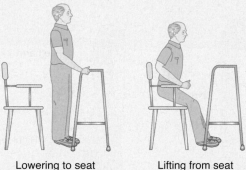

Lowering to seat

Lifting from seat

WHEELCHAIRS

A wheelchair should be individually fitted. The seat should be slightly larger than the person's width to prevent pressure and friction. The person's arm should be able to reach the wheels easily, and footrests should be adjusted to support the patient's foot in a flat position. Removable or fold-down armrests facilitate transfer.

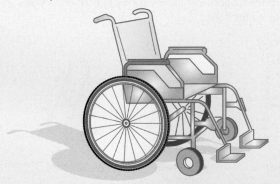

Wheelchairs should be checked routinely for ease of wheeling; function of brakes; and freedom from jagged edges, tears in upholstery, and broken or missing hardware.

able to understand and utilize them in enhancing independent function.

Teaching About Bowel and Bladder Training

Bowel and bladder elimination are important ADLs. Incontinence can have a profound impact on a person's general health and well-being. Skin breakdown can result from the moisture and irritation to which the skin is subjected. Urine or feces on the floor can cause falls. Soiled, odorous clothing can lead to embarrassment and social isolation. Infections, fractures, depression, altered self-concept, anorexia, and other problems can stem from poor bladder and bowel control.

Educating older adults with incontinence about bowel and bladder training can help them improve continence. However, the nurse must evaluate the physical and mental capacity of the patient to achieve continence before a training program is begun. Some patients may not have the functional capacity to control their elimination despite good intentions; to initiate a training program with them would be unrealistic and frustrating. If the patient has the capacity to be continent, training should begin as early as possible. Nursing Care Plans 21-2 and 22-1 provide information about bowel and bladder training programs. Consistency is a crucial factor in training programs; the gains of the day shift in keeping the patient continent are lost if the evening and night shifts do not toilet the patient at the appropriate intervals. Success should be recognized and praised; patients should not be chastised for accidents, but the reasons for the incontinent episodes should be discussed with them. Encouraging patients to wear street clothes promotes a positive self-image and normality and often discourages regression. Accurate documentation can assist in determining the effectiveness of the plan.

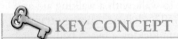

KEY CONCEPT

Consistency and adherence to the toileting schedule by all caregivers on all shifts is essential to bladder and bowel retraining programs.

Maintaining and Promoting Mental Function

Promoting physical functioning is only one aspect of rehabilitation. Equally important are efforts to restore, maintain, and promote mental function. In institutional settings where the contact patients have with staff mainly revolves around illness-related issues, or in their own homes where they may be socially

isolated, healthy mental stimulation may be sorely lacking. Like any other function, mental function can deteriorate if not exercised; thus, all rehabilitative efforts include the promotion of mental activity.

Mental stimulation is a highly individualized process, based on the unique intellectual and educational level of the patient. Some people enjoy reading the classics; others are barely interested in reading the local newspaper. Some people thrive on large social events, whereas others could spend days alone solving a crossword puzzle. Some people maintain a large network of contacts through social media, though others are challenged using the phone. Some people want to make things happen; others derive pleasure from watching them happen. This diversity, present in all age groups, reinforces the need to gear mental activities to the unique capacities and interests of the individual. Patients can take part in a wide range of intellectual, recreational, and social activities.

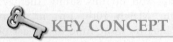

KEY CONCEPT

Like younger adults, older individuals show variation in activities that bring them intellectual stimulation and enjoyment.

Reminiscence

Reminiscence is one mentally stimulating activity that has a therapeutic aim. Since Butler and Lewis first described reminiscence, or life review (Butler & Lewis, 1982), studies have supported the value of this process as a means of validating existence, resolving past conflicts, and finding meaning in remaining life (Hsieh & Wang, 2003).

Nurses can guide patients in reminiscing through individual or group means (see also discussion of life review in Chapter 4). Often, patients can supply meaningful themes for reminiscence. For example, a patient may comment, "Kids today have it a lot easier than I did when I was young," which could lead the nurse to explore the patient's youth and feelings associated with that period of his or her life. Knowing something of the patient's personal history can help nurses find relevant topics for reminiscence, such as the patient's immigration to America, development of a business, or efforts to assist the country during war time. Themes can be selected for group reminiscing, including playing old records and asking participants what their lives were like when those records were popular, showing old photographs and asking participants what memories arise, and asking them to describe the important pieces of history they have witnessed. Perhaps the most important skill for nurses to use in reminiscing activities is listening.

As the patient discusses the topic, questions can be asked and comments made to encourage greater exploration. If the patient begins to ramble aimlessly, he or she can be redirected to the topic by comments such as, "Yes, you've mentioned that before ... I can tell it was important to you. Now tell me what happened after that."

Reality Orientation

Patients with moderate-to-severe memory loss, confusion, or disorientation require therapeutic efforts to keep them mentally integrated with the world around them. For these patients, reality orientation is an effective tool. More than just a simple review of day, date, weather, next meal, and next holiday, reality orientation is a total approach to keeping the patient oriented. Every nurse–patient contact can enhance orientation. For example, when passing medications, the nurse can state, "Hello, Mr. Richards. I'm Nurse Jones with your medicine. How are you on this sunny Tuesday? It's very warm for March 10th, isn't it?" This simple exchange adds no more time to the act of administering the medications but provides helpful orientation. Misinformation and misperceptions of

the patient should be clarified simply, for instance: "No, your son will not be visiting today. He comes on Sunday and today is Wednesday." Chastising or becoming frustrated with the patient for not remembering serves no therapeutic value. Clocks, calendars, holiday theme decorations, and reality boards enhance, but do not substitute for, staff interactions. Consistency is crucial to promoting orientation; it makes little sense for the day shift to reinforce to the patient that she is in a nursing home if the evening shift agrees with the patient's claim that she is on her grandfather's farm.

Using Community Resources

Every community has its unique resources for persons with rehabilitative needs; such resources provide education, support, and various forms of assistance to the disabled and their caregivers. Social workers, physical therapists, occupational therapists, speech and hearing therapists, and rehabilitation and vocational counselors are among the professionals who can offer guidance in locating appropriate resources. Local libraries, health departments, and information and referral services for older people can also provide valuable assistance.

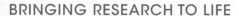

BRINGING RESEARCH TO LIFE

ENHANCING FUNCTIONAL BALANCE AND MOBILITY AMONG PEOPLE LIVING IN LONG-TERM CARE FACILITIES

Nitz, J. C., & Josephson, D. L. (2011). Journal of Gerontological Nursing, 32(2), 106–113.

Evidence exists that exercise programs and balance training can impact functional mobility. Postural stability and balance rely on intact sensory and motor systems and the function of these systems can impact the ability of older adults to participate in and benefit from balance-strategy training programs. Balance-strategy training programs have proven to reduce falls in community-dwelling older adults, but studies showing the effectiveness of these programs for long-term care residents did not exist. In this prospective study, residents from long-term care settings were invited by physiotherapists to participate in a balance-strategy training program. Residents had to be able to walk with a walking aid and understand simple directions to participate in the program. The balance-strategy training program activities consisted of a variety of exercises, including kicking a beach ball, tossing bean bags, sitting and standing, arm movements, and deep breathing. The program was conducted for 12 weeks, during which time resident performance was evaluated; evaluation continued for a 12-week period thereafter. The program proved successful in improving functional mobility and balance, which can reduce the risk of falls.

Knowing the risk of falls is extremely high in the older population, gerontological nurses need to be proactive in fall prevention strategies. Basic exercises that can be done in any setting can prove valuable for improving mobility and balance and should be considered for every older individual. This study demonstrates that nursing home and assisted living residents can also benefit from basic rehabilitation programs that can reduce the risk of falls and enhance physical function. Even for residents not receiving rehabilitation services, function can be sustained and improved by implementing balance-strategy training programs and similar activities.

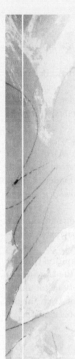

PRACTICE REALITIES

Sixty-nine-year-old Mr. Barr had a below-the-knee amputation several weeks ago and this week began receiving instruction in the use of his prosthesis. He has been making progress but still has difficulty with transfers. Mr. Barr gives the impression of a tough guy who has it all under control, but you have observed him at times looking frightened and depressed when he is unable to navigate smoothly with his new prosthesis.

At the team meeting that Friday, the social worker reports that Mr. Barr's insurance will no longer reimburse for inpatient rehabilitation after Monday. On Saturday afternoon the physician visits Mr. Barr and asks him if he wants to go home. Mr. Barr responds that he would and the doctor writes the order for discharge that day.

You know that Mr. Barr lives alone in a two-story townhouse. Arrangements have been made for a physical therapist from a home health agency to visit him on Monday. You have concerns about Mr. Barr managing over the weekend.

What could you do to assist Mr. Barr until the home health agency visits?

CRITICAL THINKING EXERCISES

1. Discuss the way in which a disability can impact a person's body, mind, and spirit.

2. Consider the way in which your average routine would be altered if you possessed a disability. What resources could you use?

3. Describe the way in which prejudices and misinformed attitudes regarding disabilities can affect disabled persons.

4. Identify resources to assist persons in your community who have aphasia, blindness, bilateral amputation, and alcoholism.

RESOURCES

Amputations

National Amputation Foundation
http://www.nationalamputation.org

Arthritis

Arthritis Foundation
http://www.arthritis.org

General Disability and Rehabilitation

Disabled American Veterans
http://www.dav.org

Federal Government Disability Information
http://www.DisabilityInfo.gov

National Rehabilitation Information Center
http://www.naric.com

Paralyzed Veterans of America
http://www.pva.org

Sister Kenny Rehabilitation Institute
http://www.allina.com/ahs/ski.nsf

Head Injuries

National Head Injury Foundation
http://www-nmcp.med.navy.mil/Neurology/dzchi.asp

The Brain Injury Association Inc.
http://www.biausa.org

Hearing Impairments

Dogs for the Deaf
http://www.dogsforthedeaf.org

Independent Living Aids
http://www.independentliving.com

National Institute of Neurological and Communicative Disorders
http://www.nidcd.nih.gov

National Association for the Deaf
http://www.nad.org

Self-Help for Hard of Hearing People
http://www.shhh.org

Neurologic Diseases

American Parkinson's Disease Association
http://www.apdaparkinson.org

Epilepsy Foundation of America
http://www.epilepsyfoundation.org

Myasthenia Gravis Foundation
http://www.mysathenia.org

National Huntington's Disease Association
http://www.hdsa.org

National Multiple Sclerosis Society
http://www.nmss.org

National Stroke Association
http://www.stroke.org

Ostomies

United Ostomy Association
http://www.uoa.org

Spinal Cord Disorders

National Spinal Cord Injury Foundation

http://www.spinalcord.org

Paralyzed Veterans of America
http://www.pva.org

Visual Impairments

American Foundation for the Blind
http://www.afb.org

Blinded Veterans Association
http://www.bva.org

Guide Dogs for the Blind
http://www.guidedogs.com

Guiding Eyes for the Blind
http://www.guiding-eyes.org

Leader Dogs for the Blind
http://www.leaderdog.org

National Association for the Visually Handicapped
http://www.navh.org

National Braille Association
http://www.members.aol.com/nbaoffice

National Eye Institute
http://www.nei.nih.gov

National Library Service for the Blind and Physically
   Handicapped
http://www.loc.gov/nls

Recordings for the Blind
http://www.rfbd.org

REFERENCES

Butler, R. N., & Lewis, M. I. (1982). *Aging and mental health* (p. 58). St. Louis: Mosby.

Di Iorio, A., Abate, M., DiRenzo, D., Russolillo, A., Battaglini, C., Ripari, P., Abate, G., et al. (2006). Sarcopenia: Age-related skeletal muscle changes from determinants to physical disability. *International Journal of Immunopathology and Pharmacology, 19*(4), 703–719. Review.

Fried, L. P., Tangen, C. M., Walston, J., Newman, A. B., Hirsch, C., Gottdiener, J., McBurnie MA, et al.; Cardiovascular Health Study Collaborative Research Group. (2001). Frailty of older adults: Evidence for a phenotype. *Journals of Gerontology: Biological Sciences and Medical Sciences, 56A*(3), M146–M156.

Hsieh, H. F., & Wang, J. J. (2003). Effect of reminiscence therapy on depression in older adults: A systematic review. *International Journal of Nursing Studies, 40*(4), 335–345.

Mack, J. L., & Patterson, M. B. (2006). An empirical basis for domains in the analysis of dependency in the activities of daily living (ADL): results of a confirmatory factor analysis of the Cleveland Scale for Activities of Daily Living (CSALD). *Clinical Neuropsychologist, 20*, 662–667.

RECOMMENDED READINGS

Recommended Readings associated with this chapter can be found on the web site that accompanies the book. Visit **http://thepoint.lww.com/Eliopoulos8e** to access the recommended readings and other additional resources associated with this chapter.

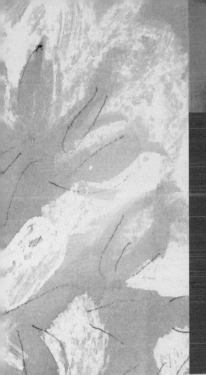

CHAPTER 36

Acute Care

CHAPTER OUTLINE

LEARNING OBJECTIVES

After reading this chapter, you should be able to:

1. List measures to minimize risks faced by acutely ill older adults.

2. Describe risks and precautions for older patients undergoing surgery.

3. Discuss common geriatric emergencies and related nursing actions.

4. Identify measures to reduce the risk of infection in older adults.

5. Discuss the importance of early discharge planning for hospitalized older adults.

6. Describe factors that influence postdischarge outcomes for older adults.

TERMS TO KNOW

Iatrogenic complications: complications inadvertently caused by practitioners or by medical treatments or procedures

Nosocomial infections: hospital-acquired infections

Today's acute care hospitals play a significant role in geriatric care. Older adults have a higher rate of hospitalization and longer length of hospital stay as compared with other age groups (Centers for Disease Control and Prevention, 2012). Furthermore, older people are significant consumers of outpatient hospital services. Many age-related changes increase the risk of injuries and infections and can cause complications with the chronic conditions that are common in older adults. Further, technology has opened the door for new diagnostic procedures, enabled malfunctioning older organs to be repaired and replaced, and made new treatment options available. Acute care settings are definitely in the geriatric care business, and nurses in these settings must be familiar with the unique care needs of older adults.

RISKS ASSOCIATED WITH HOSPITALIZATION OF OLDER ADULTS

Many older adults who have lived independently in their homes prior to a hospital admission are not discharged with the same level of function; in some circumstances, nursing home transfer is needed. The decline in status can sometimes be attributed to the effects of aging on the older adult's ability to withstand the stress of an acute condition; however, during hospitalization older individuals are at high risk for nosocomial infections (hospital-acquired infections) and iatrogenic complications (complications inadvertently caused by practitioners or by medical treatments or procedures). Examples of complications include delirium, falls, pressure ulcers, dehydration, incontinence, constipation, and loss of functional dependence (Table 36-1).

TABLE 36-1 **Potential Risks of Older Adults During Hospitalization**

Risk	Contributing/Causative Factors
Delirium	New environment
	Sensory deprivation
	Inaccessible eyeglasses, hearing aid
	Altered cognition or level of consciousness
	Excess stimuli
	Adverse drug reactions
	Physiologic disturbance
Falls	Dizziness
	Orthostatic hypotension
	Weakness, fatigue
	Unfamiliar environment
	Altered cognition or level of consciousness
	Presence of equipment, supplies
	Chemical or physical restraints
	Failure to use bed rails
	Effects of medications
	Lack of assistance
Pressure ulcers	Age-related changes to skin
	Immobilization
	Shearing forces
	Sedation
	Pain
	Weakness
	Debilitating condition
	Lack of assistance
Dehydration	Age-related decrease in thirst sensation
	Sedation
	Nausea, vomiting
	Altered cognition or level of consciousness
	Inaccessible fluids
	Lack of assistance
Incontinence	Diuresis
	Sedation
	Weakness
	Inaccessible commode, bedpan
	Indwelling catheterization
	Lack of assistance
Constipation	Age-related changes to gastrointestinal system
	Effects of medications
	Effects of surgery
	Dietary modifications
	Reduced activity
	Poor positioning during defecation
	Inaccessible commode, bedpan
	Lack of toileting assistance
Loss of functional independence	Stereotypical expectations by staff
	Unnecessary restrictions
	Insufficient time for self-care
	Knowledge deficit
	Immobility
	Development of complications
	Failure to ambulate, mobilize early

Nurses should anticipate and minimize the common risks faced by acutely ill older persons in an effort to promote optimal functional independence. Some useful measures include:

- careful assessment to identify problems and risks
- early discharge planning
- encouragement of independence
- close monitoring of medications and assurance that age-adjusted dosages are used
- reminders and assistance to patient with frequent repositioning, coughing, deep breathing, toileting

- early identification and correction of complications, recognizing that atypical signs and symptoms may be present
- avoidance of urinary catheterization if possible
- strict adherence to aseptic techniques and infection control practices
- close monitoring of intake and output, vital signs, mental status, and skin status
- environmental modifications to accommodate older patients' needs (e.g., room temperature of 75°F, noise control, use of nightlights, and avoidance of glare)
- assistance, as necessary, with activities of daily living
- patient and family education
- reality orientation as necessary
- referral to resources to promote self-care ability and independence

POINT TO PONDER

What do you perceive to be the rewards and challenges of caring for older adults during an acute hospitalization?

SURGICAL CARE

Because of improved surgical procedures and the increasing number of persons living to old age, nurses today are caring for many more surgical patients of advanced age. Also, people are no longer denied the benefit of surgery based on their age alone. Surgical intervention has provided many older people not only with more years to their lives but also with more functional years. Successful surgical management of an older person's health problems depends on the nurse's understanding of the age-related factors that alter normal surgical procedures.

KEY CONCEPT

Surgical intervention not only can add years to an older adult's life but also can improve the quality and functional independence of those added years.

Special Risks for Older Adults

In general, older adults have a smaller margin of physiologic reserve and are less able to compensate for and adapt to physiologic changes. Infection, hemorrhage, anemia, blood pressure changes, and fluid and electrolyte imbalances are more problematic in older people. Unfortunately, inelasticity of blood vessels,

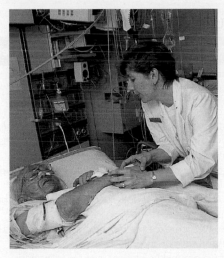

FIGURE 36-1 ■ The hospitalized older adult requires nursing interventions to prevent complications and to promote a return to wellness.

malnourishment, increased susceptibility to infection, and reduced cardiac, respiratory, and renal reserves cause complications to occur more frequently in older persons, especially during emergency or complicated surgical procedures. By strengthening older adults' capacities preoperatively, maintaining these capacities postoperatively, and being alert to early signs of complications, the nurse can help reduce the risk of surgical complications (Fig. 36-1). Nursing Diagnosis Table 36-2 lists diagnoses that may be identified in older adults who have undergone surgery.

Preoperative Care Considerations

The gerontological nurse must be sensitive to the fears that many older patients have concerning surgery. Throughout their lifetimes, today's older adults may have witnessed severe disability or death in older persons having surgery, and they may worry about similar outcomes from their operation. Patients need to understand the increased success of surgical procedures through the following advances:

- better diagnostic tools facilitating earlier diagnosis and treatment
- improved therapeutic measures, including surgical techniques and antibiotics
- increased knowledge concerning the unique characteristics of older adults

In addition to offering reassurance, the nurse teaches patients and their families what to expect before, during, and after the operative procedure, including the following information:

- preoperative preparation—scrubs, medications, nothing to eat by mouth (NPO)

NURSING DIAGNOSIS

| TABLE 36-2 | Nursing Diagnoses Related to Surgery |

Causes or Contributing Factors	Nursing Diagnosis
Altered oxygen transport, pain	Activity Intolerance
Fear of death or disability, pain, lack of knowledge	Anxiety
Anesthesia, immobility, actual or perceived pain, analgesics	Constipation
Shock, fluid and electrolyte imbalances, sepsis, anesthesia	Decreased Cardiac Output
Diagnostic tests, positioning, tissue trauma, immobility	Acute Pain
Decreased cerebral blood flow, endotracheal intubation, pain, anesthesia, central nervous system depressants	Impaired Verbal Communication
Concern about loss of body function or part, death, outcome of surgery	Fear
Shock, infection, excessive wound drainage, NPO status, electrolyte imbalance, blood loss	Deficient Fluid Volume
Excessive or rapid IV infusion, venous pooling/stasis	Excess Fluid Volume
IV therapy, intubation, break in aseptic technique, catheterization	Risk for Infection
Altered cerebral function, pain	Risk for Injury
Lack of knowledge of surgical procedure, expected outcome, risks, postoperative care	Deficient Knowledge
Pain, weakness, altered cognition, restrictions	Impaired Physical Mobility
Anorexia, nausea, vomiting, pain, inability to feed self	Imbalanced Nutrition: Less Than Body Requirements
Trauma from endotracheal tube, NPO status, mouth breathing, inadequate oral hygiene	Impaired Oral Mucous Membrane
Inability to help self, lack of knowledge	Powerlessness
Anesthesia, narcotics, immobility, pain, secretions	Impaired Gas Exchange
Immobility, weakness, restrictions from IV apparatus	Self-Care Deficit (Bathing, Dressing, Feeding, Toileting)
Change in body function or part, pain, dependency	Disturbed Body Image
Immobility, pressure from operating table, edema, dehydration	Impaired Skin Integrity
Immobility, anxiety, pain, new environment, drugs	Disturbed Sleep Pattern
Anesthesia, drugs, confusion, dehydration, indwelling catheter	Impaired Urinary Elimination

IV, intravenous; NPO, nothing by mouth.

- types of reactions to anesthesia
- length of the surgery and a brief description of it
- routine recovery room procedures
- expected pain and its management
- turning, coughing, and deep-breathing exercises
- rationale for and frequency of dressing changes, suctioning, oxygen, catheters, and other anticipated procedures

The nurse documents any patient education in the patient's record so that this information is available to other health care providers. During assessment and preoperative preparation, the nurse identifies concerns, questions, and fears and makes the physician aware of these findings.

The nurse also reviews with the physician the medications the patient is receiving to determine those that must be continued throughout the hospitalization. The patient's routine medications may

need to be administered despite NPO restrictions. For instance, sudden interruption of steroid therapy can cause cardiovascular collapse. The nurse may learn that the patient has been taking antihypertensive, tranquilizing, or other medications before hospitalization. Occasionally, patients forget or are reluctant to tell the physician about these drugs. Because cardiac and pulmonary functions can be altered by certain drugs, it is important to make sure this information is communicated to the physician. Likewise, the physician needs to know about herbal medications that the patient may be using because some (such as ginseng and gingko biloba) can affect clotting.

Nurses should ensure that basic preoperative screening has been completed, including the following:

- analysis of blood samples: creatinine clearance, glucose, electrolytes, complete blood counts, total plasma proteins, arterial blood gases, cardiac enzymes, lymphocyte count, serum albumin, hemoglobin, hematocrit, total iron-binding capacity, transferrin

- chest x-ray
- electrocardiogram (ECG)
- pulmonary function testing: for obese individuals and those with a history of smoking or pulmonary disease
- nutritional assessment: height, weight, midarm circumference, triceps skin-fold, diet history
- mental status

Because of the direct nature of the care they provide, nurses may be the only health care professionals to recognize certain problems. For example, they may discover loose teeth, which can become dislodged and aspirated during the surgical procedure, causing unnecessary complications. Such a problem should be brought to the physician's attention to ensure preoperative dental correction.

If prolonged surgery is anticipated, another precaution during surgery preparation is to pad the bony prominences of older patients. Because they will be lying on a hard operating room table, padding will help prevent pressure ulcers or muscle and bone discomfort following surgery.

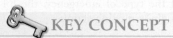

KEY CONCEPT

Careful positioning of the patient and padding of bony prominences can reduce some of the postoperative muscle and bone soreness that older adults may experience with prolonged surgery.

Infection control must be at the forefront of the nurse's mind during the entire hospitalization and begins early during the preoperative preparation. Promoting a good nutritional state and correcting existing infections are important preoperative considerations. To further reduce the risk of infection, three preoperative bathings—in the morning and at bedtime on the day before surgery and on the morning of surgery, using an antiseptic—are recommended, as is performing preoperative shaving as close to the time of surgery as possible.

Finally, although it is the physician's legal responsibility, nurses can ensure that the patient's informed consent has been obtained preoperatively (see Chapter 8 for discussion of informed consent).

Operative and Postoperative Care Considerations

Anesthesia use must be considered carefully in older adults. Because anesthesia produces depression of the already compromised functions of the cardiovascular and respiratory systems of the older patient, it must be carefully selected. Close monitoring by the anesthesiologist during surgery can detect and prevent difficulties in the patient's vital functions. Prolonged surgery for the older patient is discouraged. Rough, frequent handling of the tissue during surgery is usually avoided because this stimulates reflex activity, increasing the demand for anesthesia. If inhaled agents are used for anesthesia, the nurse should be aware that the patient may remain anesthetized for a longer time because of the older body's slower elimination of these agents; turning and deep breathing will facilitate faster elimination of inhaled agents.

Hypothermia is one of the major complications older adults face intraoperatively and postoperatively. Factors that contribute to this problem include the lower normal body temperatures of many older persons, the cool temperature of operating rooms, and the use of medications that slow metabolism. The cool environment and shivering that may result can increase cardiac output and ventilation and deprive the heart and brain of necessary oxygen; however, shivering occurs less frequently in older individuals. Furthermore, the slowing of metabolism that occurs with hypothermia delays awakening and the return of reflexes. Close monitoring of body temperature is essential. Some hypothermia may be preventable with proper warming measures; research has demonstrated that warming during the intraoperative and early postoperative periods resulted in higher core temperatures and a lower incidence of hypothermia (Grossman, Bautista, & Sullivan, 2002; Horn et al., 2012; Yang et al., 2012).

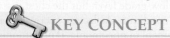

KEY CONCEPT

Hypothermia is a major intraoperative and postoperative risk to older patients.

Frequent, close postoperative observation and monitoring are extremely important. The decreased ability of older people to manage stress reinforces the need to detect and treat symptoms of shock and hemorrhage promptly. Although not fully conscious after surgery, the older person may demonstrate restlessness as the primary symptom of hypoxia. It is important that this restlessness not be mistaken for pain; administration of a narcotic could deplete the body's oxygen supply even more. Prophylactic administration of oxygen may be a beneficial component of the postoperative therapy. Blood loss should be accurately measured and, if excessive, promptly corrected. Frequent checking of urinary output can help reveal the onset of serious complications. Finally, fluid and electrolyte imbalances can be avoided and detected through strict recording of intake and output. Output should include drainage, bleeding, vomitus, and all other sources of fluid loss.

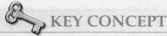

> **KEY CONCEPT**
>
> Postoperative restlessness could indicate hypoxia, not pain; inappropriate administration of a narcotic analgesic could further deplete the body's oxygen supply.

Because the older patient has a greater risk of developing infections, strict attention must be paid to caring for wounds and changing dressings. A good nutritional status is beneficial to tissue healing and should be encouraged. To conserve the patient's energy and provide comfort, relief of pain is essential. Maintaining regular bowel and bladder elimination, keeping joints mobile, and helping the patient achieve a comfortable position can aid in pain control. If medications are used for pain relief, nurses should pay attention to the reduced activity that may result and to the prevention of the ill effects of such immobilization. The nurse should also be aware that positioning on the hard operating room table and pulling and moving of the unconscious patient may cause muscle and bone soreness for several days postoperatively. Finally, it is vital to observe the patient for respiratory depression if narcotic analgesics are administered.

Older patients are particularly subject to several postoperative complications. Respiratory complications include pneumonia, pulmonary emboli, and atelectasis. With atelectasis there may be decreased lung sounds and a low-grade fever, but the chest x-ray may not show the condition. Atelectasis increases the risk for the development of pneumonia. If pneumonia develops in an older individual, it is more problematic than it would be for a younger adult and requires a longer recovery period. Cardiovascular complications include embolus, thrombus, myocardial infarction, and arrhythmias. Cerebrovascular accident and coronary occlusion occur, but they are less common than other complications. Reduced activity and lowered resistance can cause pressure ulcers to develop easily. Drug-induced renal failure is common; drugs that commonly cause this complication include cimetidine, digoxin, aminoglycosides, cephalosporins, ampicillin, and neuromuscular-blocking agents. Older postoperative patients, particularly those with hip repair, tend to have a higher incidence of delirium than the general adult population. Paralytic ileus, accompanied by fever, dehydration, abdominal tenderness, and distention, is an additional postoperative complication that the aged may experience. Table 36-3 lists other complications.

The nurse is in a key position to help the older patient achieve the maximal benefit from surgery. The most sophisticated surgical procedure in the world performed by the most skillful surgeon is of little value if poor rehabilitative care causes disability or death from avoidable complications. To combine the principles and practices of surgical nursing with the unique characteristic of the older patient is an immense challenge to the gerontological nurse. However, to see the increased capacity and more meaningful life many older adults derive from the benefits of surgery is an immense satisfaction.

EMERGENCY CARE

Emergencies in older persons are particularly problematic. First, they occur frequently because of the age-related changes that lower resistance and make the body more susceptible to injury and illness. Second, they often present an atypical picture that complicates diagnosis. Third, they can be more difficult to treat or stabilize because of older persons' altered response to treatment. Finally, they carry a greater risk of causing serious complications and death. By recognizing emergency situations and intervening promptly, nurses can spare considerable discomfort and disability to older patients and, in many situations, save their lives.

Regardless of the type of emergency, the following basic goals guide nursing actions:

- maintain life functions
- prevent and treat shock
- control bleeding
- prevent complications
- keep the patient physically and psychologically comfortable
- observe and record signs, treatments, and responses
- assess for causative factors

Whenever there is a question regarding whether a true emergency exists, nurses should err on the side of safety. It is far better to obtain an x-ray or ECG that results in a negative finding than to believe it would be an unnecessary bother or expense and have the patient suffer from a delayed diagnosis.

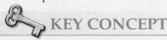

> **KEY CONCEPT**
>
> When an emergency condition is suspected, it is better to err on the safe side and obtain diagnostic tests rather than risk delaying the diagnosis.

Box 36-1 highlights some of the emergency conditions that may be encountered with older adults and related nursing measures.

TABLE 36-3 Common Complicating Conditions in Older Surgical Patients

Complicating Condition	Medical-Surgical Factors	Aging Processes	Nursing Interventions
Fluid and electrolyte imbalance	Blood, fluid losses during surgery; cool operating room, fluids evaporate from tissues, surgery and anesthesia stimulate ADH and aldosterone, overhydration with IV infusion	Decreased renal function—nephron loss, GFR, decreased renal blood flow and creatinine clearance; decreased cardiopulmonary function	Careful monitoring of intake and output, assessment of skin turgor—over sternum or forehead, assess for signs of hypervolemia and hypovolemia, determine urinary status, note nonmeasured fluid losses such as diaphoresis, assess for sacral edema, correct imbalances with isotonic IV infusions and electrolytes
Malnutrition	NPO for test preparations, decreased intake postoperatively, psychosocial influences, operative site, stress of surgery increases nutritional needs	Decreased secretion, motility, and absorption; decreased basal metabolic rate; taste bud atrophy; loss of appetite; reduced absorption of iron, B_{12}, calcium; sensory losses	Preoperative nutritional assessment, monitor weight, fluid balance, food intake and laboratory values, preoperative nutritional preparation, calorie and protein increases postoperatively, hyperalimentation if indicated, use of nutritional support team, maintain positive nitrogen balance postoperatively; vitamin/mineral supplements
Pneumonia, atelectasis	Heavy smokers with cough, obesity, bronchitis, chronic pulmonary disease, thoracic or upper abdominal surgery, anesthesia and pain medication reduce functional residual capacity, lung expansion and gas exchange	Reduced bronchopulmonary movement, decreased pulmonary function—tidal volume, loss of protective airway reflexes	*Preoperatively*—cease smoking for 1 week, weight reduction, pulmonary function testing; if bronchitis present, give antibiotics, expectorants, and bronchodilators, teach pulmonary maneuvers: cough (tongue extended to loosen secretions), deep breathing, incentive spirometer *Postoperatively*—position change hourly, monitor blood gases, off ventilator as soon as possible, continue pulmonary maneuver; O_2 to ensure adequate oxygenation, early ambulation, chest physiotherapy
Pressure ulcers	Malnutrition; chronic disease (e.g. diabetes, CHF, PVD); length of time on OR table	Moisture loss, thinning epidermis, capillary loss in dermis, loss of sensory receptors, loss of subcutaneous fat	Frequent turning, correct positioning, pressure-relieving devices, avoidance of shearing forces, early movement and ambulation, good skin hygiene, lotions gentle massage nutritional supplements, increase fluid intake, high-protein, high-calorie diet
Wound dehiscence, wound evisceration	Malnutrition; large, sudden weight loss	Delayed immune response, delayed wound healing—slowing of inflammatory response, mitosis, cell proliferation, abnormal collagen formation causing poor tensile strength in wound, decreased muscle strength	1–3 weeks preoperative nutritional preparation, hyperalimentation, vitamin supplements; strict aseptic wound care, encourage rest—slow-wave sleep aids wound healing, inspiratory breathing exercises, coughing only if secretions present, prevent/reduce vomiting; discharge teaching, proper wound care and observation for complications, diet instructions

(continues)

TABLE 36-3	Common Complicating Conditions in Older Surgical Patients (Continued)		
Complicating Condition	**Medical-Surgical Factors**	**Aging Processes**	**Nursing Interventions**
Incidental hypothermia	Cold operating rooms, room temperature infusions, exposure of skin for draping and preparation, exposure of peritoneum/pleura during surgery, peripheral vasodilation	Impaired thermoregulatory mechanisms, decreased cardiopulmonary reserves, impaired ability to increase basal metabolic rate	Temperature monitoring in OR, careful cardiac monitoring, hyperthermia blanket, warm top blankets after incision closure, warm IV fluids, transfer from OR quickly, thermal top blankets in RR, transfer blankets with patient to surgical unit
Joint stiffness, contractures	Presence of degenerative joint disease, osteoporosis, reduced mobility during preoperative preparation, immobility during surgery, pain-limiting motion in postoperative period	Decreased muscle strength and wasting, decreased bone mass, ossification of cartilage in joints, flexion of joints, stooped posture, slowed movement, gait changes	Assess prior functioning level, leg exercises preoperatively; early ambulation, proper positioning and movement in bed, active/passive range of motion, encourage active movement by patient
Acute confusional states, delirium	Type of anesthesia, penetration of blood–brain barrier by certain drugs, presence of preexisting depression or dementia, environmental factors, number of medications taken, hypoxemia, psychosocial factors	Loss of neurons, brain atrophy, decreased cerebral blood flow and oxygen consumption, decreased renal function, slowed clearance of drugs from system, sensory losses, decreased cardiopulmonary reserves	*Preoperatively*—baseline assessment of mental status and emotional state, psychological support, allow time for questions and verbalization of fears, provide pastoral care if desired, correct electrolyte imbalances, anemia *Postoperatively*—monitor level of consciousness, avoid restraints, provide calm environment, avoid use of indwelling catheters, orient to environment, progressive mobility, small doses of haloperidol (Haldol) if organic causes, reassurance from all staff, need special attention if have hearing loss, monitor electrolytes and fluid balance, ensure adequate oxygenation
Cardiac failure	Existing cardiac disease, hypertension, anesthesia effects on blood pressure, stress of surgery increases metabolic needs and increases workload on heart	Decreased cardiac output, altered O_2 transport, fatty accumulations in heart valves, atherosclerosis of vessels, widening pulse pressure	*Preoperatively*—risk assessment, correct, treat existing conditions; low dosage heparinization; improved nutritional status will improve cardiac function *Postoperatively*—continuous CVP monitoring; assess JVD and breath sounds hourly; continuous ECG monitoring; close observation of vital signs, level of consciousness and urinary output, maintain infusion rates; check intake and output; observe peripheral circulation, color; maintain cardiovascular functions; careful, early mobilization, rest periods

ADH, antidiuretic hormone; CHF, congestive heart failure; CVP, central venous pressure; ECG, electrocardiogram; GFR, glomerular filtration rate; IV, intravenous; JVD, jugular vein distention; NPO, nothing by mouth; OR, operating room; PVD, pulmonary vascular disease; RR, recovery room.

From Palmer, M.A. (1990). Care of the older surgical patient. In Eliopoulos, C. (Ed.), *Caring for the elderly in diverse care settings* (pp. 350–372). Philadelphia, PA: J.B. Lippincott.

BOX 36-1   Selected Emergencies for Older Adults

ACUTE CONFUSION/DELIRIUM

Clinical manifestations: rapid decline in cognitive function, disturbed intellectual function, disorientation to time and place, diminished attention span, poorer memory, labile mood, meaningless chatter, poor judgment, altered level of consciousness, restlessness, insomnia, personality changes, and suspiciousness.

Goal: identify and correct causative factor.
Nursing Actions:

- Assess for changes in physical health, stresses, lifestyle changes, medications taken, dietary intake, or other problems.
- Obtain blood samples for evaluation.
- Monitor vital signs, intake and output, and behaviors.
- Support treatment plan, for example, electrolyte replacement, medication change, and fever control.

Goal: protect from injury and complications.
Nursing Actions:

- Supervise activities closely.
- Remove hazardous substances, medications, and machinery from patient's immediate environment.
- Ensure adequate nutritional intake, toileting, and hygiene.

Goal: reduce confusion.
Nursing Actions:

- Limit number of staff who provide care. Offer consistency of approach.
- Maintain stable, calm environment. Avoid bright lights, excessive noise, and extreme room temperatures.
- Offer orienting statements, such as "Mr. Jones, you are in the hospital. It is Tuesday evening. Your wife is at your side."
- Clarify misconceptions.

Note: A thorough evaluation is crucial when confusion exists. This problem can result from a wide range of disturbances such as hypoglycemia, hypercalcemia, malnutrition, infection, trauma, and drug reactions.

DEHYDRATION

Clinical manifestations: concentrated urine, decreased or excessive urine output, weight loss, output exceeds intake, increased pulse rate, increased temperature, decreased skin turgor, dry-coated tongue, dry skin and mucous membrane, weakness, lethargy, confusion, nausea, and anorexia; thirst may or may not be present.

Goal: restore lost fluids.
Nursing Actions:

- Obtain blood sample for the analysis of electrolytes.
- Force fluids unless contraindicated. Administer intravenous solutions as ordered.
- Monitor and record intake and output, weight, and vital signs.

Goal: minimize or eliminate causative factors.
Nursing Actions:

- Assess for possible causes (e.g., insufficient intake, fever, vomiting, diarrhea, and wound drainage).
- Correct underlying cause.
- Monitor and encourage good fluid intake.

Note: The reduction in intracellular fluid that occurs with age contributes to less total body fluids; thus, any fluid loss is more significant in older adults. Unless there is a medical need for restriction, fluid intake should range between 2,000 and 3,000 mL daily. Assess for special factors that can lead to dehydration, such as diminished thirst sensations, disabilities that restrict independent fluid intake, altered mental status, and desires to minimize urinary frequency and nocturia.

FALLS

Clinical manifestations: patient found on floor or reports falling.
Goal: evaluate and treat injury sustained from fall.
Nursing Actions:

- Do not move patient until status is evaluated.
- Request x-ray if fracture is suspected.
- Control bleeding.
- Relieve patient's anxiety.
- Assess vital signs, mental status, and functional capacity. Note signs and symptoms (e.g., incontinence, tremors, and weakness).
- Review events preceding fall (e.g., position change, medication administration, pain, and dizziness).
- Observe and monitor patient's status for the next 24 hours.

Goal: prevent future falls.
Nursing Actions:

- Assess and correct factors contributing to falls (e.g., gait disturbances, poor vision, confusion, improper use of assistive device, medications, and environmental hazards).
- Teach patient how to fall safely (e.g., protect head and face and do not move until checked).

(continues)

BOX 36-1   Selected Emergencies for Older Adults (Continued)

- Teach patient how to reduce the risk of falls.
- Teach patient to wear safe shoes; avoid long robes.
- Teach patient to sit on the edge of bed for a few minutes before rising.
- Teach patient to use rails, particularly in tubs and stairways.
- Teach patient to walk only in well-lighted areas.
- Eliminate clutter and loose rugs from environment.

Note: An older person who falls once is at greater risk of falling again; thus, active prevention is necessary. Falls are the second leading cause of accidental death; the morbidity and mortality associated with falls increase with age.

MYOCARDIAL INFARCTION

Clinical manifestations: acute confusion/delirium, dyspnea, reduced blood pressure, pale skin, and weakness; chest pain may or may not be present.
Goal: aid in prompt diagnosis.
Nursing Actions:

- Identify signs early. Signs may be missed or attributed to other problems.
- Even with the slightest suspicion that a myocardial infarction exists, proceed with a diagnostic evaluation.
- Obtain an ECG and blood specimen— sedimentation rate will be elevated.

- Monitor vital signs.

Goal: reduce cardiovascular stress.
Nursing Actions:

- Support prescribed treatment. Administer antiarrhythmics as ordered.
- Provide oxygen. Monitor blood gases. Observe for signs of carbon dioxide retention.
- Support limbs.
- Control stress.
- Relieve pain and anxiety.

Goal: prevent and promptly identify complications.
Nursing Actions:

- Perform range-of-motion exercises. Ensure frequent change of position.
- Monitor intake and output. Anuria can develop; straining due to constipation can produce strain on heart.
- Evaluate response to medications. Note adverse reactions (e.g., bleeding, bradycardia, and hypokalemia).
- Observe for signs of congestive heart failure (e.g., dyspnea, cough, rhonchi, and rales).
- Observe for signs of shock (e.g., drop in blood pressure, increased pulse, cool moist skin, decreased urine output, and restlessness).

INFECTIONS

Infections are common acute conditions that demand prompt attention. A variety of factors can be responsible for the high risk of infection in older adults (Box 36-2).

As discussed in Chapter 30, not only do infections develop more easily in older people but they also are more difficult to identify early because of altered symptomatology. That is, the atypical presentation of symptoms can complicate early identification and correction. For example, lower body temperature can cause fever to appear atypically; reduced cough efficiency can prohibit the productive cough that can give a clue to a respiratory infection; and anorexia, fatigue, and altered cognition can be ascribed to other health problems or "old age."

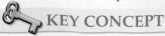 **KEY CONCEPT**

Gerontological nurses should suspect an infection when there is any abrupt, unexplained change in physical or mental function in the older adult.

The most common infection in the older population is urinary tract infection (UTI). In older adults, signs of UTI could include confusion, incontinence, vague abdominal pain, anorexia, nausea, and vomiting. Patients with diabetes may experience a loss of glycemic control. Diagnosis can be confirmed by laboratory tests.

Bacterial pneumonia is the leading cause of infection-related death in older adults. As with other infectious processes, symptoms can be atypical and include confusion, lethargy, and anorexia, in addition to the typical signs associated with pneumonia in any age group. Serum and blood testing are done to confirm the diagnosis.

Careful attention must be paid to infection prevention in older adults. Measures that assist in this effort include:

- promoting good hydration and nutritional status
- monitoring vital signs, mental status, and general health status
- maintaining intact skin and mucous membrane

Factors Contributing to the High Risk of Infection in Older Adults

- Age-related changes
  - altered antigen–antibody response
  - decreased respiratory activity
  - reduced ability to expel secretions from lungs
  - weaker bladder muscles facilitating urinary retention
  - prostatic hypertrophy
  - increased alkalinity of vaginal secretions
  - increased fragility of skin and mucous membrane
- High prevalence of chronic disease
- Immobility
- Greater likelihood of malnutrition, urinary catheter use, invasive procedures, hospitalization, and institutionalization

- avoiding immobility
- ensuring pneumococcal and influenza vaccines have been administered (unless contraindicated)
- maintaining a clean environment
- restricting contact with persons who have infections or suspected infections
- storing foods properly
- preventing injuries
- adhering to infection-control practices

A variety of vitamins and herbs have been promoted for the prevention and management of infections. Vitamin C and vitamin A supplements are recommended, as is the elimination of refined sugar from the diet. The herbs *Echinacea*, goldenseal, and garlic can prevent and treat infections; in small doses, they are believed to boost resistance to infection, and in larger doses, they may fight pathogens. Siberian ginseng can protect the body from the hazardous effects of stress and boost resistance to infection. Patients should be advised to consult with their health care providers before using an alternative therapy.

Chapter 30 provides a more complete discussion of infections.

DISCHARGE PLANNING FOR OLDER ADULTS

Hospitalized older adults require early and competent discharge planning to prevent complications, reduce the risk of re-hospitalization, and minimize stress to themselves and their caregivers. Effective discharge planning is particularly significant in this era of abbreviated hospital stays that cause patients to leave the hospital in sicker, more debilitated states.

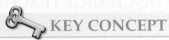 **KEY CONCEPT**

In this era of patients being discharged sooner and sicker, early discharge planning is essential.

Many factors can influence postdischarge outcomes of hospitalized older people, such as:

- patients' perceptions of health status and prognosis
- number and complexity of medical conditions
- prior history of self-care practices
- family or social supports and resources

The nurse should assess and anticipate the patient's postdischarge needs as early as possible in order to have time before discharge to ade-

Eighty-two-year-old Mrs. H is brought to the emergency department by her daughter, with whom she lives. Mrs. H had been ambulatory and able to perform all self-care activities until 6 days ago, when she became increasingly confused and weak; she has also lost weight and begun to experience urinary incontinence. She is diagnosed with bacterial pneumonia and is admitted to the hospital.

THINK CRITICALLY

- What risks does Mrs. H face during her hospitalization?
- What can be done to minimize these risks?
- What plans would you make to assist her daughter in caregiving activities after Mrs. H's discharge?

quately educate the patient and caregivers, make referrals, and suggest home preparation. Some acute care settings use an interdisciplinary geriatric team that consults with staff and develops discharge plans. A gerontological nurse specialist in the acute care setting may also perform this activity.

Discharge plans must take into account the needs of the family or significant others who provide support and caregiving assistance (Fig. 36-2). The plan must be one that works for all parties involved, not just the patient, to be fully successful. (A more complete discussion of family caregiving is provided in Chapter 38.)

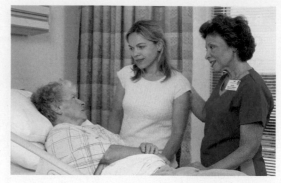

FIGURE 36-2 ■ In discharge planning for the older adult, the nurse must also consider the needs of family members who may provide care at home.

BRINGING RESEARCH TO LIFE

AGE-RELATED DIFFERENCES IN PERCEPTION OF QUALITY OF DISCHARGE TEACHING AND READINESS FOR HOSPITAL DISCHARGE

Bobay, K. L., Jerofke, T. A., Weiss, M. E., & Yakusheva, O. (2010). Geriatric Nursing, 31(3), 178–187.

This study investigated differences in the perceptions of the quality of discharge teaching and readiness for hospital discharge and their relationship to the use of the emergency department after discharge and hospital readmission. Nearly 2,000 older adults discharged from 16 medical-surgical units in 4 midwestern hospitals participated in the study. Questionnaires were administered that assessed patients' perception of their discharge teaching and their perception of readiness to go home. Emergency department visits and hospital readmissions within 30 days post discharge were recorded.

There was found to be an association between discharge teaching and discharge readiness in patients younger than 85 years. Older patients reported receiving less discharge information; reasons for this were not explored, although possibly thought to be related to these patients having prior hospitalizations for similar problems and requiring additional time for the teaching.

Older adults account for one third of all hospital admissions, and nearly one fifth are readmitted within 30 days. Inadequate discharge preparation plays a role in patient and family readiness to manage care postdischarge and the risk of readmission. Gerontological nurses need to not only provide discharge teaching but also assess readiness and recognize that there can be age-related differences in readiness and required teaching styles.

PRACTICE REALITIES

Mrs. Davis, a relatively active 84-year-old, had a total hip replacement. Her recovery was complicated by a reaction to an analgesic that caused her dizziness, severe sedation, and vomiting. Her symptoms caused her to be less active and to stay in bed, sleeping most of the time. Except for her daily visits to physical therapy, she spent most of her time resting in bed.

Mrs. Davis was discharged to a nursing home for continued rehabilitation. Within 48 hours she was readmitted with pneumonia and stage 3 pressure ulcers that the nursing home claimed were present upon admission, although this was not documented in the hospital record. Her condition is now more serious than it was at any time during her initial hospital stay.

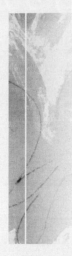

What could have been done to prevent Mrs. Davis' complications and readmission? What can a nursing home do to facilitate a patient's transition to this setting so that hospital readmissions can be avoided?

CRITICAL THINKING EXERCISES

1. A new gerontological nurse specialist on an inpatient surgical unit has been given the task of implementing nursing interventions to help reduce the older person's risk of complications during hospitalization. What protocols, staff development activities, and other actions could this nursing specialist consider?

2. Develop an outline of concepts you would review in teaching community-based older adults measures to prevent infection.

3. What prejudices or misinformed views could jeopardize the health and well-being of acutely ill older people?

REFERENCES

Centers for Disease Control and Prevention (2012). Hospital utilization. Retrieved June 19, 2012 from http://www.cdc.gov/nchs/fastats/hospital.htm

Grossman, S., Bautista, C., & Sullivan, L. (2002). Using evidence-based practice to develop a protocol for postoperative surgical intensive care unit patients. *Dimensions of Critical Care Nursing, 21*(5), 206–214.

Horn, E. P., Dein, B., Bohm, R., Steinfath, M., Sahili, N., & Hocker, J. (2012). The effect of short time periods of pre-operative warming in the prevention of peri-operative hypothermia. *Anaesthesia, 67*(6), 612–617.

Yang, H. L., Lee, H. F., Chu, T. L., Su, Y. Y., Ho, L. L., & Fan, J. Y. (2012). The comparison of two recovery room warming methods for hypothermia patients who had undergone spinal surgery. *Journal of Nursing Scholarship, 44*(1), 2–10.

RECOMMENDED READINGS

Recommended Readings associated with this chapter can be found on the web site that accompanies the book. Visit **http://thepoint.lww.com/Eliopoulos8e** to access the recommended readings and other additional resources associated with this chapter.

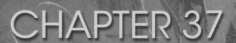

Long-Term Care

LEARNING OBJECTIVES

After reading this chapter, you should be able to:

1. Describe the development of long-term institutional care.

2. Discuss the problems resulting from the lack of a unique model for long-term care.

3. Identify major categories of standards described in nursing home regulations.

4. List various roles of nurses in long-term care facilities.

5. Describe the hygiene, holism, and healing needs of long-term care facility residents.

TERMS TO KNOW

Almshouse: institution for poor persons

Regulations: minimum standards developed by government agencies that must be met to comply with the law and qualify for licensure and reimbursement

Subacute care: level of care in which continued management of acute condition along with assistance with basic care is needed and provided in a long-term care setting

The long-term care facility is becoming a complex and dynamic clinical setting for nursing practice. Increasingly, such facilities are caring for a more medically complex population than ever before; many nursing homes are establishing subacute care units that provide ventilator care, hyperalimentation, and other services that were once confined to hospital settings. Consumers are more informed of the standards of good care and quality living environments, giving them higher expectations of providers than previously. Also, for many nurses who have become frustrated with the caregiving limitations of abbreviated hospital stays and fragmented care, such facilities offer an opportunity to establish long-term relationships and practice nursing's healing arts.

Although the number of facilities providing long-term care has declined since the implementation of tougher standards, the number of residents who are served in long-term care facilities has grown along with the growth of the older population. Among the current generation of people entering their senior years, a majority will need some type of facility-based or community long-term care, and about half of all older women and one third of all older men will spend some time in a long-term care facility during their lives (Centers for Disease Control and Prevention, 2012).

DEVELOPMENT OF LONG-TERM INSTITUTIONAL CARE

The many positive aspects of geriatric nursing in nursing homes are often overshadowed by an uncomplimentary image of this care setting, influenced by a history laden with scandals and the media's readiness to highlight the abuses and substandard conditions demonstrated by a small minority. This negative image is compounded by reimbursement policies that significantly limit the ability to provide high-quality care. Reviewing the manner in which nursing home care developed helps to clarify some of the reasons for the current challenges nurses face in working in this setting and to avoid similar problems in the future.

Before the 20th Century

Institutions to care for persons who were mentally ill, developmentally disabled, aged, orphaned, poor, or suffering from a contagious disease were common in most European countries by the end of the 17th century. Typically, all of these individuals were housed together, often with criminals. With limited funds and low public interest in these populations, care was custodial at best.

In the United States, any type of inpatient care, acute or long term, was scarce until the 19th century because it was expected that respectable people would be cared for at home by private help or family. Even when the number of hospitals increased after 1800, these facilities discouraged long-term stays by poor persons with chronic conditions. Communities responded by developing almshouses, which became the primary source of institutional care. With limited resources, care was basic at best.

Residents who were able were expected to work in the institution. Many recovered residents with no better option in the community remained in the institution and received room, board, and a very small salary in exchange for caring for residents, cooking, and cleaning.

The primary concern of the managers was running an efficient operation; this was done through the establishment of rules and routines that offered residents minimal autonomy and individuality of care. During this era, sociologist Erving Goffman offered a profile of these facilities, which he labeled "total institutions," when he characterized them as follows (Goffman, 1961):

- all activities conducted in the same manner, in the same place
- all individuals treated in the same manner and required to comply with the same activities and schedules
- strict, inflexible schedule of activities
- numerous and heavily enforced rules
- activities that furthered the aims of the institution more than serving the needs of its residents

This approach to care cast residents as inmates rather than as unique individuals in need of assistance and, in combination with the isolation of residents from mainstream society, led to an erosion of their identities and development of apathy, inactivity, and maladaptive and stereotypical behaviors.

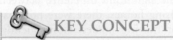

KEY CONCEPT

The many rules and routines that were implemented to keep the poorly funded early institutions operating efficiently resulted in residents developing abnormal behaviors.

During the 20th Century

By the early 1900s, public and charitable institutions began to replace almshouses. Residents lived in institutions dedicated to their specific population. Funding remained scarce, so care improved little.

It is significant to note that there was no careful assessment of the special needs of persons requiring long-term institutional care. There was no strategic planning and no thought given to the differences between facilities housing frail, dependent individuals for an extended period and other types of institutions. There was neither a model of long-term care nor a set of standards describing the unique care expectations for this special population. Instead, facilities providing long-term care modeled themselves after hospitals, prisons, and other institutions of the period. Patterning themselves after institutions that served very different populations for very different purposes was like trying to fit a square peg into a round hole; the absence of a clear model of long-term institutional care laid a weak foundation that affected the growth of this clinical setting.

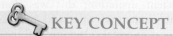

KEY CONCEPT

Long-term care facilities were fashioned after prisons, hospitals, and other institutions rather than on a model based on the unique needs of the population served.

In 1935, the enactment of Social Security provided a means for many older people to seek alternatives to the public and charitable institutions. In response, small facilities began to develop, offering room, board, and some personal care. Some of these facilities were operated by nurses or persons who called themselves nurses; thus the term "nursing home" became popularized. In 1946, the government contributed to nursing home growth by granting funds to help construct these facilities through the Hill-Burton Hospital Survey and Construction Act. As the name implies, the grant's original intent was to assist in the construction of hospitals; therefore, the physical plant standards attached to the funding reflected characteristics desirable in an acute hospital setting. Indeed, despite the significant difference between hospitals and nursing homes, there were no separate standards for nursing homes. Consequently, nursing homes constructed during this time, and for many years thereafter, were replicas of hospitals. Nursing homes modeled hospitals not only in their architectural features but also in their style of operation. Starched white linens and uniforms, rigid schedules, passive residents, strict visitation policies, and restriction of pets were among the similarities.

In the 1960s, the growing older population began to exercise its political power by requesting increased and improved health care services. The enactment of Medicaid and Medicare not only helped ease the hospitals' frustration with the growing numbers of older patients filling their beds for extended periods but also reimbursed nursing homes for providing this care. As a result, between 1960 and 1970 the number of nursing homes more than doubled and the number of residents served in this setting more than tripled. Unfortunately, most nursing home owners and operators were business-oriented individuals with minimal experience and understanding of nursing care. Federal standards

(regulations) were minimal, and monitoring and enforcement systems were lax.

Because of deplorable nursing home conditions and resulting public outrage, the Department of Health and Human Services commissioned the Institute of Medicine (IOM) to study long-term care facilities and recommend changes. The IOM study reported widespread problems with the quality of care and recommended strengthening nursing home regulations (Institute of Medicine, Committee on Implications of For-Profit Enterprise in Health Care, 1986). In response, highly stringent nursing home regulations were developed under legislation known as the Omnibus Budget Reconciliation Act of 1987 (OBRA '87). OBRA required the use of a standardized assessment tool, called the Minimum Data Set (MDS); timely development of a written care plan; reduction in the use of restraints and psychotropic drugs; increase in staffing; protection of residents' rights; and training for nursing assistants.

POINT TO PONDER

What perceptions of nursing homes have you heard family, friends, and other health care professionals express? How has this affected your thoughts about employment in this setting?

Lessons to Be Learned From History

As this history demonstrates, the lack of a vision and a clear model for long-term care contributed to disorganization and confusion regarding the purpose, function, and standards for nursing homes. When nursing fails to exercise leadership, non-nurses will determine nursing practice. The essence of long-term care is nursing care; therefore, who better than nurses to define nursing facility care? Unfortunately, nurses took a reactive, passive role and allowed persons with minimal understanding of caregiving to dictate nursing practice.

When nurses do not attempt to correct problems in the health care system, others will, and public perception will be that nurses are part of the problem. When conditions in long-term care facilities reached scandalous proportions, it was not the nursing community that was outraged and demanded change, but the public. Nurses who worked in nursing homes witnessed and complained of substandard conditions but took no organized public action to effect change. Nurses who did not work in nursing homes often were critical of the conditions that caused them to stay away from this practice setting, yet they did nothing to improve the situation. When they are not part of the solution, nurses create the perception that they are part of the problem.

Entrepreneurial thinking can benefit nursing and patients. In the era of rapid nursing home growth, many entrepreneurs saw the opportunity to reap considerable financial gains by owning and operating long-term care facilities; many did become millionaires as a result. These businesspeople were not necessarily brighter, richer, or harder working than nurses, but they were more apt to see opportunities and take risks. By not being entrepreneurs and owning and operating nursing homes themselves, nurses not only missed the opportunity to benefit financially but also—and more importantly—were not in positions of power from which they could influence the quality of care, staffing levels, salaries, and other critical aspects of nursing home care.

These lessons should have meaning for nurses and students today, as they observe financial professionals making decisions that determine clinical practice, work in settings in which staffing and services are below acceptable standards, and see new services and agencies develop in response to income potential rather than need.

POINT TO PONDER

What would you do if you worked in a setting in which care was substandard?

FACILITY-BASED LONG-TERM CARE TODAY

Conditions in nursing homes, now commonly referred to as long-term care facilities, have improved, largely due to federal regulations and increased professional interest in this care setting. Licensed staff must be on duty around the clock, nursing assistants must complete a certification process, the use of chemical and physical restraints has declined, and documentation has improved. However, problems do remain. Issues such as insufficient and inconsistent staffing and high staff turnover and conditions such as pressure ulcers, dehydration, and malnutrition continue to plague this care setting.

Nursing Home Standards

Most nursing homes are concerned with complying with regulations. Regulations describe minimal standards that a nursing home must meet in order to comply with the law and qualify for reimbursement (Box 37-1). It must be emphasized that these

BOX 37-1 Regulations Related to Nursing Homes

- Resident rights
- Admission, transfer, and discharge rights
- Resident behavior and facility practices
- Quality of life
- Nursing services
- Dietary services
- Physician services
- Specialized rehabilitation services
- Dental services
- Pharmacy services
- Infection control
- Physical environment
- Administration

standards are the minimum ones that must be fulfilled for facilities to comply with the law and be licensed and certified.

States can add to the basic federal regulations and create higher standards that facilities are obliged to meet. Also, the Joint Commission publishes higher standards that facilities can voluntarily choose to follow (standards are published in accreditation manuals that are available for purchase). It is crucial for nurses working in this setting to be familiar with the regulations pertaining to nursing homes in their specific states.

Nursing Home Residents

People who seek nursing home care are those who are functionally dependent on a long-term basis as a result of physical or mental impairment. It is the level of function, therefore, not the medical diagnosis, that influences the need for long-term care. Typically, residents of nursing homes have dependencies in their ability to fulfill activities of daily living; many are incontinent and cognitively impaired. Most nursing home residents are older adults, with the average age being 85 years (National Center for Health Statistics, 2007). Fifty-five percent of nursing home residents are over age 65 years, 42% are adults under age 65 years, and 3% are children. At any given time, only 5% of the older adult population resides in a nursing home, although as mentioned, a higher percentage will need this form of care at some point in their lives (National Center for Health Statistics, 2007).

For most of these residents, admission to a nursing home was not the first or most desirable choice. In many situations, family members tried to assist in caregiving but found that caregiving needs exceeded the family's capacities. By the time the decision to seek nursing home care is made, many families are physically, emotionally, and financially drained, adding to whatever guilt, depression, and frustration they feel about the situation. Often, a crisis triggers the need for placement in a nursing home, placing families in the position of having to seek and decide on a facility under less than ideal circumstances. An important function of the gerontological nurse is to help residents and their families as they face the challenges of selecting and adjusting to a nursing home (Boxes 37-2 and 37-3).

Nursing Roles and Responsibilities

As mentioned earlier, regulatory changes since OBRA '87 placed new demands on nursing homes for competent resident assessment, care planning, quality assurance, and protection of residents' rights. The increased demands and complexities of nursing homes necessitate that highly competent nurses be employed in this setting.

Unlicensed nursing personnel currently deliver most care in the nursing home setting. This imposes greater demands on licensed staff; not only must nurses oversee the status of residents, but

---

BOX 37-2   Factors to Consider When Selecting a Nursing Home

COST
- daily rate
- type of health insurance accepted
- out-of-pocket costs necessary to supplement health insurance
- services covered and excluded in daily rate
- charge for services not covered in daily rate
- policy regarding care of resident when reimbursement limits are reached

PHILOSOPHY OF CARE
- custodial vs. restorative/rehabilitative
- promotion of independence and individuality
- encouragement of residents and families to be active participants in care

ADMINISTRATION
- organizational structure
- ownership
- accessibility and availability of administrator, director of nursing, medical director, department heads
- existence of regularly scheduled meetings between administration and residents and families

SPECIAL SERVICES
- availability of podiatry, speech therapy, occupational therapy, physical therapy, transportation, beauty/barber shop
- cost for special services
- conditions and arrangements for transfer to hospital

STAFF
- number of caregivers available on typical shift
- ratio of RNs, LPNs, nursing assistants to residents
- number of supervisory staff on duty on typical shift
- frequency and type of in-service education offered to staff
- appearance, image portrayed by staff
- quality of staff–resident interactions
- courtesy, helpfulness of staff

RESIDENTS
- cleanliness, grooming, general appearance
- type of clothing worn (pajamas, street clothes, clean, wrinkled)
- activity level
- ease of interaction with staff and other residents

PHYSICAL FACILITY
- cleanliness, attractiveness, fresh-smelling
- ease of use for disabled and frail
- lighting
- noise control
- safe areas for walking
- general fire and safety precautions
- proximity of bathrooms, dining rooms, activity rooms, nursing stations, and exits to residents' rooms
- visibility of residents to staff
- outdoor areas for residents' use

MEALS
- meal schedule
- type of food served
- attractiveness, temperature of food served
- availability of staff to assist residents at mealtime
- location where residents dine (e.g., bedroom, communal dining hall)
- availability of dietitian or nutritionist for consultation
- range of special diets
- ability to have meal substitutions, ethnic preferences
- availability of snacks between meals

ACTIVITIES

- posted activity schedule
- range and frequency of activities
- ability of families and visitors to participate in activities with residents
- existence of resident council
- mechanisms for residents to have input into planning and evaluation of activities
- opportunity for residents to engage in activities off facility grounds
- range of bedside activities

CARE

- basic daily care provided
- frequency of contact with licensed staff
- management of special problems; incontinence, confusion, wandering, immobility
- efforts to increase mobility and function
- dignity, privacy, individuality afforded residents

- frequency at which complications develop (e.g., pressure ulcers, dehydration, infections)
- management of unusual incidents, emergencies
- evaluations by regulatory agencies

FAMILY INVOLVEMENT

- preadmission preparation offered to families
- orientation and ongoing support to families
- frequency of family conferences
- mechanisms for communicating with families, involving families in care
- visitation policies

SPIRITUAL NEEDS

- religious affiliation of facility, if any
- availability of chapel, synagogue, meditation room
- visitations from clergy
- measures to assist residents in meeting spiritual needs

BOX 37-3 **Measures to Help Families With Nursing Home Admission of a Relative**

PRIOR TO ADMISSION

- Encourage the family to visit the facility and allocate a block of uninterrupted time to spend with them. Review basic information about the facility and its routines without overloading. Introduce the family to the director of nursing, medical director, administrator, and other key personnel.
- Ask for information about the resident that will enable staff to understand the resident's unique history, needs, and preferences. Demonstrate an interest in the resident as an individual.
- Accompany the family to a private area and offer them an opportunity to express their concerns and feelings. Communicate to them that it is normal for families to feel guilty, angry, and depressed at having a loved one enter a long-term care facility; assure them that these feelings will improve in time. Advise them that it is not unusual for the resident initially to be angry at them, beg to go home, or reject them; assure them that as the resident adjusts to the facility, these reactions usually diminish.

- Describe the rights and responsibilities of families within the facility.
- Provide written description of facts communicated verbally.

AT ADMISSION

- Attempt to have a staff member who has met the family prior to admission meet the family and accompany them through the admission process.
- Inform family members of the location of cafeteria, vending machines, and rest rooms. If possible, order a snack or lunch tray for family members so that they may share the resident's first meal time in the facility.
- Arrange for staff who will be caring for the resident to introduce themselves to the family. It is beneficial for staff to write their names on a paper that the family can consult for future reference.
- Introduce the family to another resident's family member and encourage them to develop a "buddy system." Often families can provide significant support to each other and make visitations more pleasurable.

(continues)

BOX 37-3 Measures to Help Families With Nursing Home Admission of a Relative (continued)

- Advise the family of the anticipated sequence of events for the resident (e.g., the resident will be examined by the physician this afternoon, attend a group activity this evening, visit physical therapy tomorrow morning). Inform the family of the dates and times for care planning conferences and other events in which they are invited to participate.
- Encourage the family to go home at a reasonable time. Reinforce to them that the admission process is tiring to both them and the resident and that both could benefit from some rest. Express understanding that they and the resident may have many uncomfortable feelings at this time, but that these feelings normally improve with time.

DURING VISITATIONS

- Encourage the family to be actively involved in care planning and care activities. Instruct family members on care activities that they can perform, such as feeding, back rubs, range-of-motion exercises, and grooming.

- Suggest activities that the family can share with the resident during visits (e.g., card games, bringing in a pet, compiling a photo album, reading, puzzles, decorating a bulletin board). If possible, take the resident to an activity room or outdoors for the visit and encourage the family to take the resident off the premises for short periods.
- Encourage touch between the family and the resident.
- Offer and respect privacy during visits.

IN GENERAL

- Be courteous and patient. Remember that having a relative in a health care facility is difficult and can cause various reactions that can be displaced to staff.
- Call the family when there is a change in status or an incident involving the resident.
- Listen to and investigate complaints. Encourage families to discuss problems and concerns with unit-level staff.
- Invite the family's participation in care planning and delivery to the fullest extent possible.

Eliopoulos, C. (1990). Understanding and supporting families. *Long-Term Care Educator, 1*(5), 6.

they also must monitor the competency and performance of unlicensed caregivers (Fig. 37-1). Staff education, role modeling, good supervision, coaching, performance evaluation, and correction of performance problems are responsibilities of most

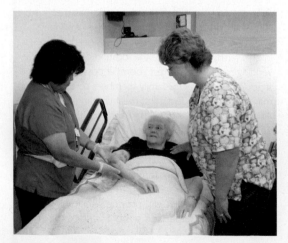

FIGURE 37-1 ■ Nurses work with other members of the health care team to ensure quality of care for residents in long-term care facilities.

long-term care nurses in addition to their major clinical and administrative duties.

Gerontological nurses have increasing opportunities for role variety in the nursing facility. They can fill administrative and management roles as director of nursing, supervisor, unit nurse coordinator, or charge nurse. They can fill specialized roles, such as staff development director, quality assurance coordinator, infection control coordinator, geropsychiatric nurse specialist, or rehabilitative nurse. Of course, nurses can also be direct care providers to residents. Each of these roles requires competencies beyond basic nursing, thereby challenging nurses to obtain additional education and experience to assure competent fulfillment of these specialized roles. The American Association for Long Term Care Nursing has developed position descriptions and core competencies for the major roles in long-term care; to learn more visit http://www.ltcnursing.org.

Nurses influence the quality of care provided to residents in a variety of ways. Admission assessments and the completion of the MDS assessment tool are coordinated by a registered nurse, and most of the entries on the MDS rely on nursing assessment. Problems identified through the MDS

BOX 37-4 Major Responsibilities of Gerontological Nurses in Long-Term Care Facilities

- Assist residents and their families in the selection of and adjustment to the facility.
- Assess and develop an individualized care plan based on assessment data.
- Monitor residents' health status.
- Recommend and use rehabilitative and restorative care techniques when possible.
- Evaluate the effectiveness and appropriateness of care.
- Identify changes in residents' conditions and take appropriate action.
- Communicate and coordinate care with the interdisciplinary team.
- Protect and advocate for residents' rights.
- Promote a high quality of life for residents.
- Assure residents' preferences and choices are honored.
- Ensure and promote the competency of nursing staff.

assessment tool direct care planning activity. The written care plan guides nursing actions; staffs are held accountable by regulatory agencies for ensuring that care plans are accurate and followed. Nurses ensure that nursing assistants provide care appropriately and monitor residents to evaluate the effectiveness of care and to recognize changes in status. Box 37-4 lists some of the major responsibilities of nurses in this setting.

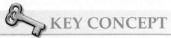

KEY CONCEPT

The Minimum Data Set is a standardized assessment tool that must be completed on admission, whenever there is a change in the resident's status, and annually.

Unlike many other clinical settings, the average nursing home does not have physicians and other professionals on-site at all times. Although this places a greater burden on nurses for assessment and management of problems, it does offer the opportunity for nurses to function independently and use a wide range of knowledge and skills. Independent nursing practice and the ability to develop long-term relationships with residents and their families are among the exciting features of nursing in this setting.

Assisted Living Communities

In recent years, there has been a growth in assisted living communities as an option for individuals who need some assistance with activities of daily living, but whose needs are not complex enough to warrant 24/7 nursing attention. Assisted living facilities do not have the stringent regulations that nursing homes are required to meet and have fewer licensed nurses available. While the number of nursing home beds has been declining, the number of assisted living beds has increased, supporting a trend toward this type of care. At the present time, most assisted living care is paid for privately. Gerontological nurses are challenged to ensure that appropriate standards of care are developed and practiced in this setting to avoid the scandalous conditions that plagued the early development of nursing homes and to advocate for payment options for assisted living for those individuals who lack private funds to afford this care.

LOOKING FORWARD: A NEW MODEL OF LONG-TERM CARE

As this chapter's discussion about the development of long-term care reflected, facility-based long-term care emerged without a clearly defined model. Rather than a tapestry of a wide range of therapeutic interventions that enable persons relying on others for long-term assistance to achieve optimum physical, psychosocial, and spiritual health and well-being, long-term care facilities are more like a patchwork quilt of poorly fitted fragments of traditional medical care loosely held together by weak threads of regulations and institutional rules.

Because most resident needs and care activities in long-term care settings fall within the realm of nursing, nurses are the logical choice of professionals to define the model of long-term care. Recognizing the limitations of the medical model in nursing homes, the themes of the new model could be holism and healing. Figure 37-2 offers a hierarchy of residents' needs that can help nurses and nurses-to-be envision this new model and challenge them to consider a design for long-term care services that exceeds the minimum requirements. The levels of needs shown include hygiene, holism, and healing.

Hygiene encompasses the most basic needs including physiologic needs, assurance of safety of the human and physical environment, treatment of medical conditions, and restoration and/or stabilization of physical and mental health. Basic survival depends on the fulfillment of these needs; however, having these needs met does not ensure a satisfying, fulfilling life.

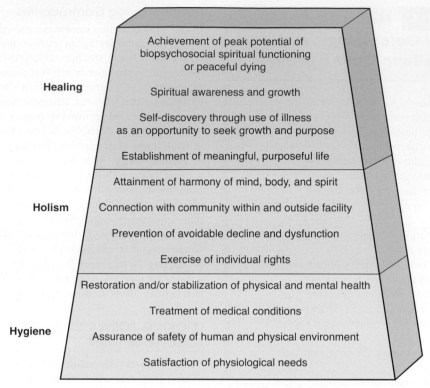

FIGURE 37-2 ■ Hierarchy of nursing home residents' needs. (From Eliopoulos, C. (2007). *Transforming nursing homes into healing centers: A holistic model for long-term care.* Glen Arm, MD: Health Education Network.)

At the *holism* level, psychological, social, and spiritual aspects are considered. To attain harmony and balance among mind, body, and spirit, individuals need to exercise individual rights, assume responsibility for self-care to the fullest extent possible, prevent avoidable declines and dysfunction, and experience a dynamic relationship with the community inside and outside the facility.

The fulfillment of hygiene and holism needs provides the foundation for *healing* to occur. Healing does not imply cure but, rather, the establishment of a meaningful and purposeful life, using illness as an opportunity for self-discovery, deepening spiritual awareness and growth, and transcending the physical being.

Woven within this model of holism and healing are the following assumptions (Eliopoulos, 2007):

■ Psychological, social, and spiritual well-being are of equal and sometimes greater importance than physical well-being.

■ Medical supervision and treatment are only one component of the overall needs of residents.

■ Many of the needs resulting from chronic conditions can be effectively and safely met with the use of alternative and complementary therapies.

■ Caregivers' presence and interactions affect health, healing, and the quality of nursing facility life.

■ The physical environment can be used as a therapeutic tool.

■ The nursing home is an integral and active member of the community at large.

The *culture change* movement has been a positive step in the direction of supporting this new model of long-term care. Key elements of culture change typically include creating a physical environment that is more home-like than institutional, providing consistent assignments of staff, individualizing care to meet the specific needs and desires of residents, nurturing positive relationships, offering educational opportunities for staff, and empowering residents and their caregivers. The Eden Alternative was one of the early culture change programs that cast a vision for a different quality of life for nursing home residents. Its founder, Dr. Bill Thomas, planted the seed that nursing homes needed to offer residents a life worth living. Many nursing homes have adapted Eden principles to provide an environment that is more home-like, encourage and respect resident decision making, and foster higher quality relationships between residents and their caregivers. Several years after the Eden Alternative's appearance, the Wellspring Program was launched. With an emphasis on quality improvement measures, Wellspring attempted to advocate for greater resident and direct care worker empowerment and an improved quality of life for residents. In 2012, the Wellspring Program joined the Eden Alternative family to offer the culture change movement expanded programming, emerging from the synergy of these two dynamic programs.

Continuing his impact in redefining nursing home care, Dr. Bill Thomas in 2003 conceptualized The Green House Project with the intent of designing the ideal nursing home from scratch. The model consists of small, self-contained homes, in which each home with eight to ten residents receives individualized care and enjoys a more home-like setting. Direct care staff are cross-trained in roles so that the same direct care worker may fix breakfast in the home, run a load of laundry through the washer and dryer, and offer personal care to residents.

In addition to enhancing the quality of life, research has shown that these homes reduce complications and avoidable hospitalizations.

There is openness to redesigning long-term care. The challenge will be to offer a high quality of life for older adults who need increasingly complex long-term care services in environments that are more home-like than institutional. Nursing services are a crucial, essential component of any long-term care model; thus, nurses should exercise leadership in the redevelopment of this form of care. Gerontological nurses must reclaim nursing's healing role and cast a new vision for long-term care that can enable residents of nursing facilities to experience the highest possible quality of life and care for the remaining time in their lives.

POINT TO PONDER

If you could design a long-term care facility that promoted holism and healing, what would it look like?

BRINGING RESEARCH TO LIFE

CHANGES IN DEPRESSIVE SYMPTOMS, SOCIAL SUPPORT, AND LONELINESS OVER 1 YEAR AFTER A MINIMUM 3-MONTH VIDEOCONFERENCE PROGRAM FOR OLDER NURSING HOME RESIDENTS

Tsai, H. H., & Tsai, Y. F. (2011). Journal of Medical Internet Research, 13(4), 93–95.

This study evaluated the long-term effects of videoconference intervention in improving nursing home residents' social support, loneliness, and depressive symptoms over 1 year. Using laptops and with the help of a research assistant, residents were asked to use the Internet at least 5 minutes each week for videoconferencing with a family member or significant other.

Whereas in a previous study videoconferencing was not shown to make a difference in depression and loneliness, in this study videoconferencing was shown to alleviate loneliness and improve depression when evaluated at 3-, 6-, and 12-month intervals. A factor responsible for this difference was believed to be that residents not only were shown how to use the Internet but also had appointments scheduled to communicate with family members and significant others. The use of videoconference visits decreased over time, attributed to the novelty wearing off, a lack of staff to help residents use the computers, and the lack of reminders to family to use videoconferencing.

As increasing numbers of people enter nursing homes and assisted living communities with experience using the Internet, videoconferencing as a means to stay connected with family and friends will become an important activity for residents. It is important for nurses not only to advocate that this technology be available for residents but also to assist residents with computer use and scheduling of videoconferencing as their independent capacity to do so diminishes. The quality of life for residents can be enhanced by maintaining a connection with contacts in the community.

PRACTICE REALITIES

Nurse Rogers had worked at a nonprofit nursing home that had implemented culture change programming. Residents were able to go to the dining room whenever they desired and select from a large menu. Generous staffing patterns allowed for not only high-quality care but also individualized activities. Residents were assisted in decorating their bedrooms in a manner that reflected individual preferences, down to the selection of a color theme.

Due to family relocation, Nurse Rogers had to find new employment. She accepted a position as a director of nursing at a nursing home in town. The nursing home was for profit, constructed in the 1960s with little modification since. Due to very basic staffing levels, care was task-oriented and residents had to comply with a rigid meal and bathing schedule. Concerned, Ms. Rogers met with the administrator and reviewed the benefits of culture change. She proposed staffing and operational changes that could support this transformation. The administrator was sympathetic but told Ms. Rogers that there were no funds for these changes. "How come the last nursing home I worked at could offer these things for residents?" Ms. Rogers asked.

The administrator responded, "They were a nonprofit facility with additional funding from a religious organization. We admit only Medicaid and Medicare residents and have to rely on those funds. The reimbursement we receive barely covers the basic services we offer."

Ms. Rogers is concerned about this inequality and feels all residents should have access to the best care possible.

What would you do if you were Ms. Rogers?

CRITICAL THINKING EXERCISES

1. Consider the expectations baby boomers will have when they use long-term care facilities in the future and outline the environmental features, services, and operations that will accommodate them.

2. Imagine that you are a director of nursing in a long-term care facility and describe:
   - activities that could be planned to encourage the local community to become involved in facility activities
   - services the facility could offer persons living in the neighboring community
   - programs and services that could be provided for families of residents

3. Describe actions nurses can take to improve long-term care facilities.

RESOURCES

American Assisted Living Nurses Association
http://www.aalna.org

American Association for Long-Term Care Nursing
http://www.ltcnursing.org

American Health Care Association
http://www.ahca.org

American Nurses Association, Inc., Council on Nursing Home Nurses
http://www.nursingworld.org

Eden Alternative
http://www.edenalt.org

Geriatric Advanced Practice Nurses Association
http://www.gapna.org

Green House Project
http://thegreenhouseproject.org

Leading Age (formerly American Association of Homes and Services for the Aging)
http://www.leadingage.org

National Association of Directors of Nursing Administration in Long-Term Care (NADONA)
http://www.nadona.org

National Consumer Voice for Quality Long Term Care
http://www.theconsumervoice.org

National Gerontological Nursing Association
http://www.ngna.org

Pioneer Network
http://www.pioneernetwork.net

REFERENCES

Centers for Disease Control and Prevention. (2012). *Fast facts, nursing home care.* Retrieved June 19, 2012 from http://www.cdc.gov/nchs/fastats/nursingh.htm

Eliopoulos, C. (2007). *Transforming nursing homes into healing centers: A holistic model for long-term care* (Rev. ed.). Glen Arm, MD: Health Education Network.

Goffman, E. (1961). *Asylums.* Garden City, NY: Anchor Books.

Institute of Medicine, Committee on Implications of For-Profit Enterprise in Health Care. (1986). Profits and health care: An introduction to the issues. In B. H. Gray (Ed.), *For-profit enterprise in health care* (pp. 3–18). Washington, DC: National Academy Press.

National Center for Health Statistics. (2007). *Nursing home residents age 65 and older by age, sex, and race.* Retrieved April 20, 2007 from http://www.cdc.gov/nchs/data/hus/hus06.pdf#102

RECOMMENDED READINGS

Recommended Readings associated with this chapter can be found on the web site that accompanies the book. Visit **http://thepoint.lww.com/Eliopoulos8e** to access the recommended readings and other additional resources associated with this chapter.

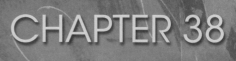

Family Caregiving

LEARNING OBJECTIVES

After reading this chapter, you should be able to:

1. List the various structures and functions of families.

2. Discuss various roles that family members can assume.

3. Describe classic family relationships.

4. Identify risks to caregivers and ways to reduce them.

5. Identify signs of elder abuse.

6. Discuss interventions to reduce family dysfunction.

TERMS TO KNOW

Caregiver burden: stresses, challenges, and negative consequences associated with providing assistance to a person in need

Elder abuse: the infliction of physical or emotional harm, neglect, financial exploitation, sexual mistreatment, or abandonment of an older adult

Sandwich generation: middle-aged persons who are caring for their own children and their parents

Skipped-generation household: household in which grandparent is raising minor grandchild with no parent present

Aging is a family affair. Whether it is the retiree's concern about living and supporting his family on a pension, a middle-aged daughter's decision to accept her mother into her household, or a sister's attempt to care for her dying brother at home, the impact of one individual's aging process has a ripple effect on the entire family unit. This impact is also felt when older members of the family require assistance with daily needs and care. Families are absorbing more complex responsibilities for caregiving for longer periods of time than ever before. With growing numbers of people reaching the old-old years and the trend toward maintaining very ill older individuals in the community, the burdens faced by family caregivers will likely continue to grow. The increase of women in the workforce, mobility of families, and complexity of family structures resulting from divorce and remarriage complicate family relationships and caregiving. Nurses need to understand the various family structures, roles, and relationships in order to work most effectively with older adults and their caregivers.

KEY CONCEPT

Greater numbers of families are providing more complex care for their older members for longer periods of time than ever before.

THE OLDER ADULT'S FAMILY

Almost every individual is part of a family unit, although that family may not reflect the stereotypical nuclear family. In fact, one may find among older adults a diversity of family structures, including:

- couples (married, unmarried, heterosexual, and homosexual)
- couples with children (heterosexual, homosexual, married, and unmarried)
- parent and child or children
- siblings
- groups of unrelated individuals
- multigenerations

When interviewing older adults, it is important to explore all persons who are "significant others" to an individual and fulfill a family role, regardless of whether they are unrelated or reside in different households. For example, a widow can have a friend with whom she shares a close emotional tie or a cousin in a neighboring community who provides assistance and support.

KEY CONCEPT

Persons beyond traditional family members can serve significant caregiver roles.

Identification of Family Members

One can identify family members by looking for those individuals who fulfill family functions. In aging families, family functions are somewhat modified to address the special needs of older persons and focus on the following:

- ensuring fulfillment of physical needs
- providing emotional support and comfort
- maintaining connections with family and community
- handling financial affairs
- instilling a sense of meaning to life
- managing crises

Asking older adults the following questions can also facilitate the identification of significant persons who perform family functions for them:

- Who checks on them regularly?
- Who shops with or for them?
- Who escorts them to the clinic or physician?
- Who assists with or manages their problems?
- Who takes care of them when they are ill?
- Who helps them make decisions?
- Who assists them with banking, paying bills, and managing financial matters?
- Who do they seek for emotional support?

All persons fulfilling significant family functions should be included in the development and evaluation of the care plans of older adults.

Family Member Roles

Frequently, family members assume certain roles as a result of their socialization process and family needs and expectations. Possible roles include the following:

- *Decision-maker:* the person who is granted or assumes responsibility for making important decisions or is called on in times of crisis; may not be geographically close or involved in daily activities but is consulted for problem solving
- *Caregiver:* the person who provides direct services, looks after, or assists with personal care and home management of another family member
- *Deviant:* the "problem child" who has strayed from family norms; may be the family scapegoat or may provide a sense of purpose for family members who "rescue" or compensate for this individual
- *Dependent:* an individual who depends on the other members of the family for economic or caregiving assistance
- *Victim:* a person who forfeits his or her legitimate rights and may be physically, emotionally, socially, or economically abused by the family.

POINT TO PONDER

What are the dynamics within your own extended family? What different roles and functions do various members fulfill?

The impact of these roles should be explored when assessing the family unit. Nurses must be sensitive to the fact that certain "negative" roles may not have the adverse effects on the family unit that would be anticipated; likewise, "positive" roles may not be welcomed by the family. For example, the middle-aged son who drifts from town to town, regularly contacting his older parents for funds to pay off his latest indulgences, may not function as a responsible, mature adult, but he may bring excitement and a sense of being needed to his parents' lives, thereby bringing them some rewards. However, his financially secure, responsible brother who takes care of his parents' affairs may be less popular within the family because of his dullness and practicality.

KEY CONCEPT

Even seemingly negative roles can be fostered by and meet certain needs of the family.

Family Dynamics and Relationships

The dynamics among family members can have positive or negative effects on older individuals. In assessing the family unit it is useful to explore the following issues:

- *How family members feel about each other*. Do they love but not like, admire, respect, or enjoy each other? How do they express affection?
- *The manner of communication*. Do they share daily events or have contact only on holidays? Is their style of interaction parent–child or adult–adult?
- *Attitudes, values, and beliefs*. Do they feel that the young should take care of the old or that children owe their parents nothing? What are their expectations of family members, friends, and society? Does their faith imply certain responsibilities?
- *Links with organizations and the community*. How involved are they with persons outside the family unit? Is the family similar to others in the community?

As discussed in Chapter 1, the majority of older people are not abandoned by their children; most

do enjoy regular contact with them. Nevertheless, lifestyles, housing, and societal expectations in Western culture are not conducive to parents and their adult children living together. Most older people want to live in their own residences, if possible, and the majority do. The arrangement of generations living under separate roofs but within a 30-minute trip of each other is often the most satisfactory. It is understood that parents and children will provide assistance and share a household if an unusual circumstance arises.

KEY CONCEPT

Most older people and their families prefer to live near but not with each other.

More than 9 of 10 older people are grandparents. Grandparenting can be a positive experience for older adults because they obtain enjoyment, affection, and a sense of purpose from caring for their grandchildren without the 24-hour stress of child-rearing responsibilities. In some cases grandparents do assume parenting responsibilities; in fact, there has been an increase in what is referred to as skipped-generation households in which grandparents are raising grandchildren with no parent present. Grandchildren can provide new interests and meaning to life. In turn, grandchildren usually receive the benefit of unconditional love and attention (Fig. 38-1). As grandchildren grow into adulthood, their involvement with grandparents often lessens, but a strong bond continues to exist.

The relationship between siblings is a strong one. The typical pattern is for siblings to drift apart during young and middle adulthood but then reestablish strong ties in later life. Siblings can provide socialization, emotional support, and financial and household assistance. Usually, earlier conflicts and differences become insignificant as siblings develop mutually supportive relationships in later life.

Older couples have a low rate of divorce, although it is increasing. Rocky marriages often stabilize in later life as the couple faces a new interdependency. Older spouses look to each other for security, support, and safety in an imperfect world. After years of experiencing and reinforcing one another's behaviors, the couple can understand, anticipate, and complement one another's actions. Spouses look after the care and welfare of their mates and derive security in having someone available to care about them.

Relationships in old age are affected by the forms of relationships experienced throughout life. Parents who ignored or abused their children early in life may produce children who want nothing

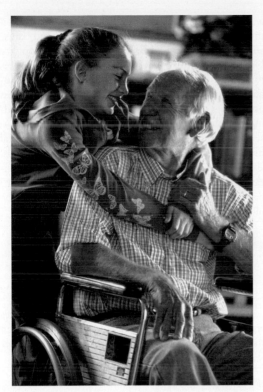

FIGURE 38-1 ■ Caring family relationships are beneficial for both grandparents and grandchildren.

to do with them in adulthood. Siblings who have unresolved anger over favoritism displayed by their parents may refuse to assist when the favored child is in need. Couples who never shared intimacy and friendship may exist in separate worlds under the same roof. Nurturing relationships during every stage of life is an investment in having meaningful, supportive relationships in later life.

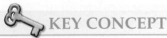 **KEY CONCEPT**

Children who feel their parents were insensitive to their needs throughout their lives may be reluctant caregivers to these parents in old age.

SCOPE OF FAMILY CAREGIVING

Most of the home care of older persons is provided by family members, not formal agencies. It is estimated that more than 10 million people are involved in parent care, approximately half of whom provide care on a regular basis. More than 45% of caregivers are 65 years of age or older themselves. Nearly half of the caregivers for older adults are wives; the next largest group of caregivers is daughters and daughters-in-law. Indeed, today

the average woman will spend more time providing care for her parents than for her children; often, these women are responsible for care of their parents and children concurrently, causing them to be named the "sandwich generation." Growing numbers of people employed full-time also carry family caregiving responsibilities.

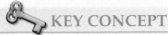 **KEY CONCEPT**

Most of the home care of older adults is provided by family members, not formal agencies.

Families provide many types of assistance to their older members (Box 38-1). Often, the provision of assistance is a subtle, gradual process. For example, a daughter may begin by telephoning her mother after the mother has returned from a physician's visit and inquiring about medication changes. As time progresses, the daughter may accompany her mother to the physician's office, discuss the medications directly with the physician, and telephone her mother to monitor the response to the drugs. Eventually, the daughter may need to lift her mother in and out of the car, push her into

BOX 38-1 **Types of Assistance Families Provide to Their Older Members**

Maintaining and cleaning the home
Managing finances
Shopping
Transporting
Providing opportunities for socialization
Advising
Explaining
Troubleshooting
Reassuring
Accompanying to physician's office and hospital
Negotiating services
Cooking and providing meals
Reminding to take medications, keep appointments, and take actions
Monitoring and administering medications
Performing treatments
Supervising
Protecting
Bathing and dressing
Feeding
Toileting
Assisting with decision making

the physician's office in a wheelchair, undress her for the examination, and administer the medications to her on a regular basis.

POINT TO PONDER

If you suddenly faced the situation of having to provide care to a parent or older relative, how would your life change and how would you manage the added responsibilities?

PROTECTING THE HEALTH OF THE OLDER ADULT AND CAREGIVER

A family is a strong chain of human experience that bonds its members through life's challenges and joys; however, that chain is only as strong as its weakest link. Effective gerontological nursing recognizes that the health of all family members must be maintained and promoted.

Maintaining older persons' independence facilitates normality in family relationships. Having to live with or be cared for by family members can threaten the status and roles of older persons and cause anger, resentment, and other feelings to develop (see Nursing Diagnosis Highlight). Sound health practices to prevent disease and disability are crucial to maintaining self-care ability and independence. If illness occurs, aggressive attention should be paid to avoiding complications and restoring the affected person to a healthy state. Interventions such as environmental modifications, financial aid, home-delivered meals, assistance with chores, transportation for the physically disabled, telephone reassurance, or a home companion can supplement deficits and strengthen the older person's reserves for independent living.

KEY CONCEPT

Caregivers of older persons frequently are senior citizens themselves.

If the caregiver is a spouse or sibling, chances are that he or she is of advanced age as well. Even the children of the older person can be older

---

NURSING DIAGNOSIS HIGHLIGHT

INTERRUPTED FAMILY PROCESSES

Overview
An interruption in family processes exists when the family's normal functions are altered due to a transition, crisis, or uncertainly of outcome. When this problem is present, the family may be unable to meet the physical, emotional, socioeconomic, or spiritual needs of its members, may deal with stress ineffectively, may communicate ineffectively or inappropriately, and may refuse to seek or accept help from others. They may be fearful, guarded, or suspicious when visited or interviewed.

Causative or Contributing Factors
Illness or injury of family member; change in dependency level of member; change in role or function of family member; addition or loss of family member; relocation, reduced income, added expenses, social or sexual deviance by family member; break in religious or cultural practices by family members.

Goal
The family will demonstrate support and assistance to members in their fulfillment of physical, emotional, and socioeconomic needs; the family will seek and accept assistance from external sources as appropriate.

Interventions
- Collect a comprehensive family history that includes profile of family (include significant others who fill family functions as family members); age, health, and residence of members;

roles and responsibilities of each member; typical patterns of communication, problem solving, and crisis management; recent changes in composition of the family and members' roles, responsibilities, and health statuses; new burdens; and the family's assessment of problem.
- Identify factors related to family dysfunction and plan appropriate interventions such as family therapy, financial aid, family conference, visiting nurse, or clergy visit.
- Facilitate open, honest communication among family members; assist in planning family conferences, promoting discussion by all members, developing realistic goals and plans, and allocating responsibility; provide privacy for family.
- When a member is receiving health services, explain care activities and expected outcomes, prepare for changes, and involve the family in care to the maximum extent possible.
- Provide caregiver education and support; help caregivers identify community resources; and emphasize the importance of respite for caregivers.
- Make the family aware of support and self-help groups that can assist them, such as Alzheimer's Disease and Related Disorders Association, American Cancer Society, Alcoholics Anonymous, and American Diabetes Association.

adults themselves. The physical, emotional, and social health of the caregivers must be evaluated periodically to ensure that they are competent to provide the required services and are not jeopardizing themselves in the process. Provisions must be made for what gerontological nurses refer to as caregivers' TLC:

T—training in care techniques, safe medication use, recognition of abnormalities, and available resources

L—leaving the care situation periodically to obtain respite and relaxation and maintain their normal living needs

C—caring for themselves via adequate sleep, rest, exercise, nutrition, socialization, solitude, support, financial aid, stress reduction, and health management.

Gerontological nurses should review the TLC needs of caregivers during every contact to ensure their continued effectiveness.

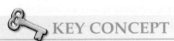

KEY CONCEPT

Caregivers need TLC: training, leave, and care for self.

A particularly vulnerable group of caregivers is middle-aged daughters who are a likely caregiver group. After years of sacrificing and struggling with child-rearing, they are beginning to taste some freedom as their children gain independence and begin to leave home. They are concerned for their children's success and well-being and experience ambivalence over the less intense parental role. Ever-increasing numbers of them are in the workforce, perhaps resuming delayed careers. Some may be coping with spouses who are experiencing midlife crises, having mixed feelings about their marriage, or reacting to undesirable changes in their physical appearance. They are clouded with the "superwoman" myth and desperately try to be the supportive parent, understanding wife, exciting lover, interesting friend, and aspiring employee. In short, they are overwhelmed. At this point in life, the final straw may be dependent parents and their demands. These daughters feel that they certainly cannot deprive their parents, trust their care to strangers, or institutionalize them. However, what will this mean to their careers, income, marital relationships, friendships, leisure pursuits, and energy? As a growing number of middle-aged women confront this dilemma, special nursing intervention is warranted. Box 38-2 describes some ways in which nurses can aid family caregivers.

BOX 38-2   Nursing Strategies to Assist Family Caregivers

- *Guide the family to view the situation realistically.* Perhaps a leave of absence rather than resignation from a job is warranted to assist a parent or spouse through convalescence. Perhaps the needs are such that a lay caregiver (e.g., family member) will not be able to care for them adequately. Often an objective outsider can guide the family in viewing the real situation and understanding the extent of care needs.

- *Provide information that can assist in anticipating needs.* Caregivers need to be guided in exploring the various scenarios that can arise and developing plans before a crisis occurs. Encourage the expression of feelings. Raised with an abundance of "shoulds" and "oughts" regarding the treatment of older persons, families need to know that the guilt, anger, resentment, and depression they feel are neither uncommon nor bad.

- *Assess and monitor the impact of the caregiving on the total family unit.* Although caregivers may feel they alone are assuming responsibility for care, they need to examine the effects on the total family unit.

How will their children's tuition be paid if they quit their jobs to care for a parent? Will someone have to forfeit a bedroom if the relative moves in? What is the relationship of the spouse with the in-laws? Who will help lift grandma into the tub? Will the family be able to take vacations and entertain at home? Is someone available to relieve them if they want to go out for a special occasion?

- *Introduce and promote a review of care options.* Often family members believe that care must be one of two extremes: institutionalization or total care provided solely by the caregiver. Although these are options, other possibilities exist within these extremes, including home health aides, live-in companions, geriatric day care, or shared family care in which the elder lives at specific times with various relatives, or relatives spend designated days at the elder's home. Caregivers also should be aided in identifying their limitations and the need for institutional care when necessary. See Chapter 35 for more information about services for the elderly and their caregivers.

FAMILY DYSFUNCTION AND ABUSE

Many factors can threaten the healthy functioning of the family unit; the gerontological nurse must be skilled in identifying such problems and providing interventions for them (see the Nursing Diagnosis Highlight). Family dysfunction occurs in many forms, ranging from an older parent's domination and manipulation of an adult child, to incestuous relationships. A lifelong history of dysfunction may exist, or the dysfunction may be a recent problem, associated with a wide range of factors (e.g., divorce, loss of income, increased dependency of older family member, and illness of caregiver). Families experiencing dysfunction may be:

- less able to fulfill the physical, emotional, socio-economic, and spiritual needs of their members
- rigid in roles, responsibilities, and opinions
- unable or unwilling to obtain and use help from others
- composed of members with psychopathology or behavioral disorders
- inexperienced or ineffective at managing crises
- ineffective or inappropriate with their communication and behavior (including learned violence patterns)

One form of dysfunction that has gained increased visibility in recent years is elder abuse. It is estimated that more than 2 million older adults suffer some form of abuse annually in the United States, primarily by a close family member (Acierno et al., 2010). The profile of the older adult at greatest risk for abuse is a disabled woman, older than 75 years of age, who lives with a relative and is physically, socially, or financially dependent on others. It is important to remember that abuse occurs in all sorts of families, regardless of social, financial, or ethnic background, and can present in many forms, including:

- infliction of pain or injury
- withholding of food, money, medications, or care
- confinement, physical or chemical (drug) restraint
- theft or intentional mismanagement of assets
- sexual abuse
- verbal or emotional abuse
- neglect

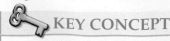

KEY CONCEPT

Both the actual commission of a harmful act and the threat of committing it are considered abuse.

The older adult may be reluctant to report or admit to mistreatment. Subtle clues of abuse include malnutrition, failure to thrive, injuries, oversedation, and depression. Nurses can assess for abuse using a tool such as the Elder Assessment Instrument developed by Fulmer, Street, and Carr (1984) and currently recommended by the Hartford Institute for Geriatric Nursing (see Resource listings). Nurses must manage potentially abusive situations tactfully. Once abuse is detected, the nurse needs to assess the degree of immediate danger and take appropriate actions. Abused persons must be assured that their plight will not be worsened by making the abuse public; they may prefer being verbally threatened or having their money taken to the alternative of living in an institution or foster home. (See Chapter 8 for legal considerations regarding elder abuse.)

The family needs empathy, not judgment, from the nurse. Although some individuals are consciously malicious and abusive for their own gain, most abusers are distressed persons who find themselves in stressful caregiving situations and are coping ineffectively. Abuse can also be associated with a family pattern of violence, emotional or cognitive dysfunction of the abused or the abuser, a history of dependency of the abuser on the victim, or retaliation for a history of earlier abuse. A good family history can be helpful in gaining insight into the family dynamics that could contribute to abuse.

Abuse may be stopped and family health salvaged by helping the family find effective ways to manage its situation, such as counseling or respite care. The nurse must consider that caregiving burdens often increase over time; therefore, ongoing interventions are necessary to prevent future abuse after the immediate episode has been resolved.

REWARDS OF FAMILY CAREGIVING

A caring, interested family is one of the most valuable resources an individual can possess in old age. In turn, the love and richness of experience offered by older persons adds a unique depth and meaning to the family. Caregiving experiences provide opportunities for relatives to learn more about each other as individuals and to obtain gratification in the young giving something back to the aged who may have sacrificed for them. Gerontological nurses must view older adults in the context of their family units and structure care to enhance the functional capacity of all family members.

CONSIDER THIS CASE

Mary K is a 45 year old single parent who is the sole wage earner for herself and her three teenage children. Several years ago, when Ms. K's father was diagnosed with dementia, she arranged to have him move into an apartment in the same apartment complex where she lives. His condition has since deteriorated, and he is now incontinent and unable to eat or dress without assistance; he has also started fires in his apartment and has been found wandering around the complex grounds at all hours of the night. Ms. K has decided to take her father into her own three-bedroom apartment. Ms. K's two daughters share one bedroom, her son has his own room, and she has one bedroom for herself; therefore, she has moved her father into her son's room, much to her son's resentment. In fact, her son states that he cannot stand the urine odor and noise made by his grandfather, so he has begun sleeping on the living room sofa and staying at friends' homes whenever possible. Ms. K's father's pension is not sufficient to pay the additional cost for a larger apartment because of the expense of his medication and incontinence care supplies.

Between the stress and her father's nighttime activity, Ms. K is unable to obtain adequate rest and has been late for work and "nodding off" at work as a result. Her employer knows of her situation but states that Ms. K's job could be in jeopardy if she is unable to perform her duties and be dependable. Although Ms. K's children understand that their grandfather has no one else to care for him, they are angry at how this situation has disrupted their lives: They no longer feel comfortable bringing friends home, they forfeit social activities to help with their grandfather's care, and they have less money to spend. Together, the children confront Ms. K and suggest that their grandfather be placed in a nursing home. Ms. K becomes upset and responds, "How can you even suggest putting your own flesh and blood in a place like that? If it kills me, I'll never put your grandfather in a nursing home."

THINK CRITICALLY

- Describe the actual and potential problems associated with caring for Ms. K's father.
- Discuss the impact of this situation on each family member.
- Describe approaches that could be used to introduce Ms. K to other caregiving options, including nursing home care of her father.
- Develop a care plan to assist this family.

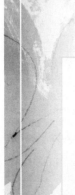

BRINGING RESEARCH TO LIFE

CHAOS AND UNCERTAINTY: THE POST-CAREGIVING TRANSITION

Ume, E. P., & Evans, B. C. (2011). Geriatric Nursing, 32(4), 288–293.

The caregiving trajectory has some predictable stages that include the *pre-caregiving phase*, in which minimal support is needed; the *active caregiving phase*, which includes active caregiving commitment; and the *post-caregiving phase*, which is the period following the termination of caregiving, resulting from the person's death or placement in a nursing home. The post-caregiving phase has not been well studied; in this article the authors have summarized studies that address this period.

Some studies show that the emotional impact of caregiving lasts beyond the termination of formal caregiving roles. Caregivers have been found to experience a post-caregiving void, a period of closing down, in which there is a termination of the financial and legal matters and a construction of life post-caring that involves a re-establishment of roles and development of a new identity. Research varies as to the physical consequences to post-caregivers, with some studies showing increases in blood pressure, weight loss, and other stress-related effects whereas other studies show a marked improvement in caregiver health. Although the studies have had a majority of Caucasian samples, African Americans have been found to report less caregiving stress and seldom attend post-caregiving support groups.

Post-caregiving transition is poorly understood and in some cases, results have been conflicting. Additional research in this area is needed. Nurses need to appreciate that responses of caregivers in the post-caregiving period can vary, warranting assessment to identify individual needs so that interventions to support caregiver health can be properly planned.

PRACTICE REALITIES

Seventy-year-old Mr. Warren has recently been discharged from the hospital with a new colostomy. At the first home visit the nurse finds Mr. Warren living alone in an extremely dirty house; roaches and mouse droppings are evident. The house is cluttered and in desperate need of repair.

Concerned, the nurse asks Mr. Warren if he has any family or friends who can assist him. "No," he responds, "I don't associate with any of my neighbors and I've been divorced for over 30 years. I've got two kids but they are too wrapped up in their own lives to help me."

When Mr. Warren mentions the names of his son and daughter the nurse recognizes them as affluent leaders of the community. She asks Mr. Warren if she can contact them and he agrees, adding, "It won't do any good, though. They are selfish snobs."

When the nurse phones Mr. Warren's children she is surprised by their reaction. The son says he has no interest in talking with her. The daughter does speak with the nurse. "My father is not a nice man," the daughter contributes. "He was abusive to my mother and did nothing to help us. There were times we had no food and were evicted because he gambled and drank his money away. It is hard to describe how cruel he was to us. My mother left him as soon as we were out of the house. Had she stayed with him, he probably would've killed her. My father never wanted to have anything to do with us once we were grown. I'm sorry to hear of his situation, but my brother and I wrote him out of our lives years ago."

What would you do if you were this nurse?

CRITICAL THINKING EXERCISES

1. Describe the potential changes the average family would face if they suddenly had to provide care for an older relative.
2. Discuss satisfactions and benefits family members can derive from caring for older relatives.
3. Identify resources in your community to assist families with caregiving.

RESOURCES

Clearinghouse on Abuse and Neglect of the Elderly
http://www.elderabusecenter.org

ElderWeb
http://www.elderweb.com

Hartford Institute for Geriatric Nursing
Try This: Best Practices in Nursing Care to Older Adults
Elder Mistreatment and Abuse: Detection of Elder Mistreatment
http://consultgerirn.org/topics/elder_mistreatment_and_
    abuse/want_to_know_more

National Association of Professional Geriatric Care Managers
http://www.caremanager.org

National Center on Elder Abuse
http://www.ncea.aoa.gov

National Council on Family Relations
http://www.ncfr.com

National Eldercare Locator
http://www.eldercare.gov

National Family Caregivers Association
http://www.nfcacares.org

REFERENCES

Acierno, R., Hernadez, M. A., Amstadter, A. B., Resnick, H. S., Steve, K., Muzzy, W., & Kilpatrick, D. G. (2010). Prevalence and correlates of emotional, physical, sexual, and financial abuse and potential neglect in the United States: The National Elder Mistreatment Study. *American Journal of Public Health, 100*(2), 292–297.

Fulmer, T., Street, S., & Carr, K. (1984). Abuse of the elderly: Screening and detection. *Journal of Emergency Nursing, 10*(3), 131–140.

RECOMMENDED READINGS

Recommended Readings associated with this chapter can be found on the web site that accompanies the book. Visit **http://thepoint.lww.com/Eliopoulos8e** to access the recommended readings and other additional resources associated with this chapter.

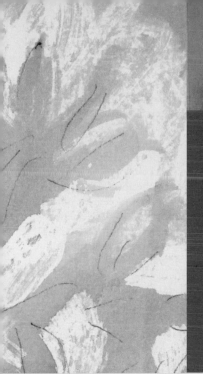

CHAPTER 39

End-of-Life Care

LEARNING OBJECTIVES

After reading this chapter, you should be able to:

1. Discuss the difficulty people may experience in facing death.

2. Describe the stages people commonly go through when facing death and describe related nursing interventions.

3. List physical care needs of dying individuals and related nursing interventions.

4. Discuss ways in which nurses can support family and friends of dying individuals.

5. Discuss ways in which nurses can support other nursing staff dealing with dying patients.

TERMS TO KNOW

Do not resuscitate (DNR): medical order advising providers not to initiate cardio-pulmonary resuscitation in the event of cardiac or respiratory arrest

End of life: period when recovery from illness in not expected, death is anticipated, and focus is on comfort

Hospice care: program that delivers palliative care to dying individual and support to dying person and that person's family and caregivers

Palliative care: care that relieves suffering and provides comfort when cure is not possible

(Continued)

Death is an inevitable, unequivocal, and universal experience, common to all. Despite the reality that it touches every person's life at one time or another, death is difficult for many individuals to face. Although a certainty, the cessation of life is often dealt with in terms of fury and fear. Humans can be very reluctant to accept their mortality.

Gerontological nurses commonly face the reality of death because more than 80% of deaths occur in old age.

In addition to facing this reality, gerontological nurses must learn to deal with the entire dying process—the complexity of experiences that dying individuals, their family, their friends, and all others involved with them go through. Working with those who undergo this complicated process requires a blend of sensitivity, insight, and knowledge about the complex topic of death in order to diagnose nursing problems and effectively intervene.

DEFINITIONS OF DEATH

The final termination of life, the cessation of all vital functions, the act or fact of dying—these are definitions the dictionary offers concerning death—attempts at succinct explanations of this complex experience. But we are often reluctant to accept such simple descriptions. For example, the world of literature contains many eloquent words on the topic of death:

> Do not go gentle into that good night,
> Old age should burn and rave at close of day
> Rage, rage against the dying of the light.
> *Dylan Thomas*

> Each person is born to one possession which
> outvalues all the others—his last breath.
> *Mark Twain*

> Death is fortunate for the child,
> bitter to the youth,
> too late to the old.
> *Publilius Syrus*

> A man can die but once:
> We owe God a death.
> *Shakespeare, Henry IV*

Current scientific literature does not provide much more in the way of specific definitions of death. The United Nations Vital Statistics Division defines death as the cessation of vital functions without capability of resuscitation. However, terms such as brain death (the death of brain cells determined by a flat electroencephalogram [EEG]); somatic death (determined by the absence of cardiac and pulmonary functions); and molecular death (determined by the cessation of cellular function) confuse the issue. The controversy lies in deciding at which level of death a person is considered dead. In some situations, an individual with a flat EEG still has cardiac and respiratory functions; could this individual be considered dead? In other situations, individuals with flat EEGs and no cardiopulmonary functions still have living cells that permit their organs to be transplanted; are individuals really dead if they possess living cells? The answers to these questions are not simple. Much current thought and investigation are focused on the need for a single criterion in the determination of death.

FAMILY EXPERIENCE WITH THE DYING PROCESS

In today's Western culture, many people have very limited experiences with death or the dying process, but this was not always the case. This change is due in part to decreases in the mortality rate over the years (Fig. 39-1). In the past, a higher mortality rate made experiences with the dying process more common. In addition, there were fewer hospitals and other institutions in which people could die. Today, health and medical care are easily available and accessible, and new medications, therapeutic interventions, and lifesaving technologies have lowered the number of deaths.

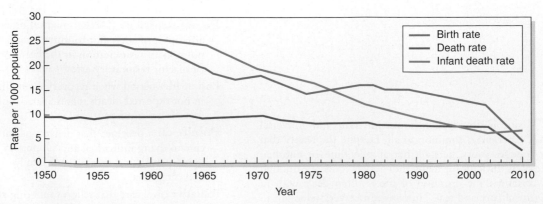

FIGURE 39-1 ■ Changes in birth and death rates from 1950 to 2010. (Data from the U.S. Bureau of the Census (2012). *Births, Deaths, Marriages, & Divorces.* 2012 Statistical Abstract of the United States. Available at: http://www.census.gov/compendia/statab/cats/births_deaths_marriages_divorces.html)

Perhaps even more significant for limiting exposure to the dying process are changes in the site and circumstances of death. Previously viewed as natural processes, most births and deaths were managed by familiar faces in familiar surroundings. Perhaps the family felt a certain comfort and closeness by being with and doing for the person whose life was about to begin or end.

Today, nuclear families are mobile and frequently composed of young members; older parents and grandparents live in different households, often in different parts of the country. Furthermore, more deaths occur in an institutional or hospital setting. Rarely do family and friends remain with the individual or witness the dying process.

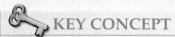

KEY CONCEPT

With fewer people dying at earlier ages than in the past and most deaths occurring in hospitals or nursing homes, most people have minimal direct involvement with dying individuals.

The separation of individuals from their loved ones and familiar surroundings during the dying process seems discomforting, stressful, and unjust. How inhumane to remove dying persons from intimate involvement with their support systems at the time of their greatest need for support. As direct experiences with dying and death are lessened, death becomes a more impersonal and unusual event. Its reality is difficult to internalize.

Perhaps this explains why many persons have difficulty accepting their own mortality. Avoiding discussions about death and not making a will or other plans related to one's own death are clues to the lack of internalization of one's mortality.

POINT TO PONDER

Do you have a will that outlines your desires for the care of your children, the distribution of your assets, and your funeral arrangements? If not, why not?

Nurses who understand their own mortality are more comfortable helping individuals through the dying process. In denying their own mortality or feeling angry about it, nurses may tend to avoid dying persons, discourage their efforts to deal realistically with their death, or instill false hope in them and their families. The difficult process of confronting and realizing one's own mortality need not be viewed as depressing by the nurse; it can provide a fuller appreciation of life and the impetus for making the most of every living day.

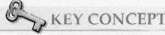

KEY CONCEPT

Understanding one's own mortality can be therapeutic to the nurse personally, as well as helpful in the care of dying patients.

SUPPORTING THE DYING INDIVIDUAL

For a long time, nurses were more prepared to deal with the care of a dead body than with the dynamics involved with the dying process. Not only was open discussion of an individual's impending death rare, but also it was typical for the dying person to be moved to a separate and often isolated location during the last few hours of life. If the family was present, they were frequently left alone with the dying person, without benefit of a professional's support. Rather than planning for additional staff support for the dying person and the family, nurses were concerned with whether a patient would live until their next shift and require postmortem care. When death did occur, the body was removed from the unit in secrecy so that other patients would be unaware of the event. Nurses were discouraged from showing emotion when a patient died. A detached objectivity was promoted as part of nursing the dying patient.

Nursing now offers a more humanistic approach to end-of-life care. Emphasis on meeting the total needs of the patient in a holistic manner has stimulated greater concern for the psychosocial and spiritual care of the dying. In addition, there is now recognition that family members and significant others play a vital role in the dying process and must be considered by the nurse. Knowledge has increased in the field of thanatology (i.e., the study of death and dying), and more nurses are exposed to this body of knowledge. Hospice care has developed into a specialty (Box 39-1). The nursing profession has come to realize that professionalism does not preclude human emotions in the nurse–patient relationship. These factors have contributed to increased nursing involvement with the dying individual.

Because the dying process is unique for every human being, individualized nursing intervention is required. Patients' previous experiences with death, religious and spiritual beliefs, philosophy of life, age, and health status are among the multitude of complex factors affecting the dying process. Nursing Diagnosis Table 39-1 lists a variety of nursing diagnoses related to death and dying along

---

BOX 39-1   **Hospice**

Hospice is a way of caring for terminally ill individuals and their families. Although most hospice care is provided in the home, these services are required to be provided in nursing home settings also. The first hospice program was St. Christopher's Hospice in London. In the United States, the first hospice began at Hospice, Inc., in New Haven, Connecticut, in 1974. The National Hospice Organization has developed standards for hospice care to guide local hospice programs; however, individuality and autonomy of each program are encouraged.

Hospice care aids in adding quality and meaning into the remaining period of life. The care involves interdisciplinary efforts to address physical, emotional, and spiritual needs, including:

- pain relief
- symptom control
- coordinated home care and institutional care
- bereavement follow-up and counseling

For more information, contact the National Hospice & Palliative Care Organization (NHPCO), 1700 Diagonal Road, Suite 625, Alexandria, VA 22314, 703-837-1500, HelpLine: 800-658-8898, http://www.nhpco.org.

---

with contributing factors. The nurse must carefully assess the particular experiences, attitudes, beliefs, and values that each individual brings to his or her dying process. Only through this assessment can the most therapeutic and individualized support be given to the dying person.

KEY CONCEPT

Patients' reactions to dying are influenced by previous experiences with death, age, health status, philosophy of life, and religious, spiritual, and cultural beliefs.

Stages of the Dying Process and Related Nursing Interventions   WATCH & LEARN

Although the dying process is a unique journey for each individual, common reactions that have been observed to occur provide a basis for understanding the process. After several years of experiences with dying patients, Elisabeth Kübler-Ross developed a conceptual framework outlining the coping mechanisms of dying in terms of five stages that has now become classic (Kübler-Ross, 1969). It behooves the nurse to be familiar with these stages and to understand the most therapeutic nursing

interventions during each stage. Not all dying persons will progress through these stages in an orderly sequence. Neither will every dying person experience all of these stages. However, an awareness of Kübler-Ross' conceptual framework can help the nurse support dying individuals as they demonstrate complex reactions to death. A brief description of these stages, along with pertinent nursing considerations, follows.

Denial

On becoming aware of their impending death, most individuals initially react by denying the reality of the situation. "It isn't true" and "There must be some mistake" are among the comments reflective of this denial. Patients sometimes "shop" for a physician who will suggest a different diagnosis or invest in healers and fads that promise a more favorable outcome. Denial serves several useful purposes for the dying person. It is a shock absorber after learning the difficult news that one has a terminal condition, it provides an opportunity for people to test the certainty of this information, and it allows people time to internalize the information and mobilize their defenses.

Although the need is strongest early on, dying persons may use denial at various times throughout their illness. They may fluctuate between wanting to discuss their impending death and denying its reality. Although such a contradiction may be confusing, the nurse must be sensitive to the person's need for defenses while also being ready to participate in discussions on death when the person needs to do so. The nurse should try to accept the dying person's use of defenses rather than focus on the conflicting messages. An individual's life philosophy, unique coping mechanisms, and knowledge of the condition determine when denial will be replaced by less radical defense mechanisms. Perhaps the most important nursing action during this stage is to accept the dying individual's reactions and to provide an open door for honest dialogue.

Anger

The stage of denial and the "No, not me" reaction is gradually replaced by one of "Why me?" This second stage, anger, is often extremely difficult for individuals surrounding the dying person because they are frequently the victims of displaced anger. In this stage, the dying person expresses the feeling that nothing is right. For example, nurses do not answer the call light soon enough; the food tastes awful; the doctors do not know what they are doing; and visitors either stay too long or not long enough. Seen through the eyes of the dying person,

NURSING DIAGNOSIS

TABLE 39-1 Nursing Diagnoses Related to Death and Dying

Causes or Contributing Factors	Nursing Diagnosis
Depression, fatigue, pain, treatments, immobility	Activity Intolerance
Separation from loved one, loss of body function or part, realization of impending death, concern about treatment prior to and at death	Anxiety
Narcotics, immobility, diet, stress	Constipation
Stress, antibiotics, tube feedings, cancer, fecal impaction	Diarrhea
Congestive heart failure, cardiogenic shock, anemia, fluid and electrolyte imbalances, drugs, stress	Decreased Cardiac Output
Cancer, diagnostic tests, poor positioning, overactivity	Pain (Acute, Chronic)
Pain, drugs, fatigue	Impaired Verbal Communication
Changes in body integrity, separation from loved one, ineffective family coping, helplessness, powerlessness	Ineffective Coping
Impending death of loved one, lack of knowledge or support	Disabled Family Coping
Hospitalization, treatment demands, depression	Deficient Diversional Activity
Loss of family member, changes in roles, care costs	Interrupted Family Processes
Treatments, pain, death	Fear
Shock, fever, infection, anorexia, inability to drink independently, depression	Deficient Fluid Volume
Loss of body function or part, pain, separation from family	Chronic Sorrow
Cancer, renal failure, treatments, immobility, lowered resistance, drugs (e.g., antibiotics, steroids), malnutrition	Risk of Infection
Altered ability to protect self, pain, drugs, fatigue	Risk of Injury
Diagnostic tests, treatments, drugs, pain management	Deficient Knowledge
Weakness, pain, bed rest	Impaired Physical Mobility
Denial, lack of knowledge, impaired functional capacity	Noncompliance
Anorexia, depression, pain, treatments, nausea, vomiting	Imbalanced Nutrition: Less Than Body Requirements
Cancer, infection, drugs, malnutrition, dehydration, mouth breathing, poor hygiene	Impaired Oral Mucous Membrane
Dependency, disability, institutional constraints, inability to reverse condition	Powerlessness
Thick secretions, pain, anxiety, drugs, immobility, decreased lung elasticity and activity, mouth breathing	Ineffective Breathing Pattern
Pain, weakness, disability	Self Care Deficit (Bathing, Dressing, Feeding, Toileting)
Loss of body function or part, institutionalization, pain	Disturbed Body Image
Separation from partner, pain, fatigue, depression, drugs, treatments, hospitalization	Sexual Dysfunction
Immobility, infections, edema, dehydration, emaciation	Impaired Skin Integrity
Immobility, pain, anxiety, depression, drugs, new environment	Disturbed Sleep Pattern
Loss of body function or part, depression, anxiety	Impaired Social Interaction
Hospitalization, disability, deformity, discomfort of others	Social Isolation
Loss of body function or part, barriers imposed by treatments or hospitalization, feelings toward dying process	Spiritual Distress
Depression, anxiety, fear, isolation	Disturbed Thought Processes

such anger is understandable. Why wouldn't people resent not having what they want when they want it when they don't have much time? Why wouldn't they be envious of those who will enjoy a future they will never see? Their unfulfilled desires and the unfinished business of their life may cause outrage. Perhaps their complaints and demands are used to remind those around them that they are still living beings.

During this time, the family may feel guilt, embarrassment, grief, or anger in response to the dying person's anger. They may not understand why their intentions are misunderstood or their actions unappreciated. It is not unusual for them to question whether they are doing things correctly. The nurse should help the family gain insight into the individual's behavior, which can relieve their discomfort and, thus, create a more beneficial environment for the dying person. If the family can come to realize that the person is reacting to impending death and not to them personally, it may facilitate a more supportive relationship.

The nurse should also guard against responding to the dying person's anger as a personal affront. The best nursing efforts may receive criticism for not being good enough; cheerful overtures may be received with scorn; the call light goes on the minute the nurse leaves the room. It is important that the nurse assess such behavior and understand that it may reflect the anger of the second stage of the dying process. Instead of responding to the anger, the nurse should be accepting, implying to the dying person that it is fine to vent these feelings. Anticipating needs, remembering favorite things, and maintaining a pleasant attitude can counterbalance the anticipated losses that are becoming more apparent to the dying individual. It may be useful for nurses to discuss their feelings about the patient's anger with an objective colleague who can serve as a sounding board so that the nurse–patient relationship continues to be therapeutic.

Bargaining

After recognizing that neither denial nor anger changes the reality of impending death, dying persons may attempt to negotiate a postponement of the inevitable. They may agree to be a better Christian if God lets them live through one more Christmas; they may promise to take better care of themselves if the physician initiates aggressive therapy to prolong life; they may promise anything in return for an extension of life. Most bargains are made with God and usually kept a secret. Sometimes such agreements are shared with members of the clergy. The nurse should be aware that dying persons may feel disappointed at not having their bargain honored or guilty over the fact that, having gained time, they want an additional extension of life even though they agreed that the request would be their last. It is important that these often covert feelings be explored with the dying person.

Depression

When a patient is hospitalized with increasing frequency and experiences declining functional capacity and more symptoms, the reality of the dying process is emphasized. The older patient may already have had many losses and experienced depression. Not only may lifetime savings, pleasurable pastimes, and a normal lifestyle be gone, but also bodily functions and even body parts may be lost. Understandably, all this may lead to depression. Unlike other forms of depression, however, the depression of the dying person may not benefit from encouragement and reassurances. Urging dying persons to cheer up and look at the sunny side of things implies that they should not contemplate their impending death. It is unrealistic to believe that dying people should not be deeply saddened by the most significant loss of all—their life.

The depression of the dying person is usually a silent one. It is important for the nurse to understand that cheerful words may be far less meaningful to dying individuals than holding their hand or silently sitting with them (Fig. 39-2). Being with the dying person who openly or silently contemplates the future is a significant nursing action during this stage. An interest in prayer and a desire for visits from clergy are commonly seen during this stage. The nurse should be particularly sensitive to the dying person's religious needs and facilitate the clergy–patient relationship in every way possible.

The nurse may need to help the family understand this depression, explaining that their efforts to cheer the dying person can hinder rather than enhance the patient's emotional preparation. The family may require reassurance for the helplessness they feel at this time. The nurse may emphasize that this type of depression is necessary for the individual to be able to approach death in a stage of acceptance and peace.

Acceptance

For many dying persons, a time comes when the struggling ends and relief ensues. It is as though a final rest is being taken to gain the strength for a long journey. This acceptance should not be mistaken for a happy state; it implies that the individual has come to terms with death and has

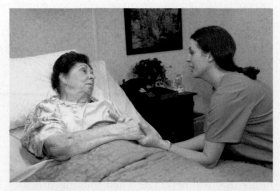

FIGURE 39-2 ■ Touching, comforting, and being near the dying individual are significant nursing actions.

found a sense of peace. During this stage, patients may benefit more from nonverbal than verbal communication. It is important that their silence and withdrawal not result in isolation from human contact. Touching, comforting, and being near the person are valuable nursing actions. An effort to simplify the environment may be required as the dying person's circle of interests gradually shrinks. It is not unusual for the family to need a great deal of assistance in learning to understand and support their loved one during this stage.

Significantly, hope commonly permeates all stages of the dying process. Hope can be used as a temporary but necessary form of denial, as a rationalization for enduring unpleasant therapies, and as a source of motivation. It may provide a sense of having a special mission to comfort an individual through the last days. A realistic confrontation of impending death does not negate the presence of hope.

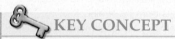 **KEY CONCEPT**

The five stages of the dying process include denial, anger, bargaining, depression, and acceptance.

Physical Care Challenges

Pain

Concern regarding the degree of pain that will be experienced and its management may be a considerable source of distress for dying individuals; nurses can reduce distress for patients by supplying them with realistic information regarding pain. Patients with cancer are more likely to experience severe pain than persons dying from other causes, and even among terminally ill cancer patients, pain can be managed effectively.

Gerontological nurses must be aware that patients will perceive and express pain differently based on their medical diagnosis, emotional state, cognitive function, cultural background, and other factors. Complaints of pain or discomfort, nausea, irritability, restlessness, and anxiety are common indicators of pain; however, the absence of such expressions of pain does not mean it does not exist. Some patients may not overtly express their pain; in these individuals, signs such as sleep disturbances, reduced activity, diaphoresis, pallor, poor appetite, grimacing, and withdrawal may provide clues to the presence of pain. In some circumstances, confusion can be associated with pain.

Nurses must regularly assess pain because it can increase or decrease over time. Patients should be encouraged to report their pain in a timely manner and openly discuss their concerns about pain.

It can be useful for patients to rate their pain on a scale of 0 to 10 (0 being no pain and 10 the most severe pain); nursing staff can record patients' self-appraisal of pain along with other factors on a flow sheet.

For the dying patient, the goal of pain management is to *prevent* pain from occurring rather than to respond to it after it occurs. Pain prevention not only helps patients avoid discomfort but also ultimately reduces the amount of analgesics they use. After the pattern of pain has been assessed, a schedule for the administration of analgesics can be developed. The type of analgesic used will depend on the intensity of the pain, ranging from aspirin or acetaminophen for mild pain to codeine or oxycodone for moderate pain to morphine or hydromorphone for severe pain. Meperidine and pentazocine are contraindicated for pain control in older adults because of their high incidence of adverse effects, particularly psychosis, at relatively low dosages. Nurses should note and instruct patients to report ineffectiveness of analgesics or their schedule of administration, overdosage, and adverse reactions (Box 39-2).

 KEY CONCEPT

For the dying patient, the goal of pain management is to prevent pain from developing rather than treat it once it occurs.

Alternatives to medications should be included in the pain control program of dying patients. Such measures include guided imagery, hypnosis, relaxation exercises, massage, acupressure, acupuncture, therapeutic touch, diversion, and the application of heat or cold. Even if these measures cannot substitute for medications, they could reduce the amount of drugs used or potentiate the drugs' effects.

Respiratory Distress

Respiratory distress is a common problem in dying patients. In addition to the physical discomfort resulting from dyspnea, patients can experience tremendous psychological distress associated with the fear, anxiety, and helplessness that results from the thought of suffocating. The causes of respiratory distress can range from pleural effusion to deteriorating blood gas levels. Interventions such as elevating the head of the bed, pacing activities, teaching the patient relaxation exercises, and administering oxygen can prove beneficial. Atropine or furosemide may be administered to reduce bronchial secretions; narcotics may be used for their ability to control respiratory symptoms by blunting the medullary response.

BOX 39-2 Pain Management for the Dying Patient

Mr. Lugio is a terminally ill nursing facility resident who is suffering from pain secondary to metastasis of his lung cancer to his spine. His pain has been managed with a nonsteroid anti-inflammatory drug that he receives PRN, but nursing staff feel that the drug may be ineffective because Mr. Lugio is seen grimacing with pain periodically throughout the day. A review of his medication administration record reveals that he sometimes asks for his pain medication at 6- to 8-hour intervals, although he is able to have the drug every 4 hours. The nurses observe that he complains of pain more frequently during the week than on weekends when his family visits.

Nursing staff could consider the following in helping to achieve improved pain control for Mr. Lugio:

- Assess the pattern and severity of pain. Provide Mr. Lugio with a chart to record his pain. Instruct him to rate his pain on a scale of 0 to 10, in which 0 indicates no pain and 10 indicates severe pain. Analyze the pattern.
- Recommend that Mr. Lugio take his analgesic on a regular basis rather than sporadically. Rather than change the type or dosage of analgesic at this time, determine if a regular schedule of administration

could improve pain control. Often, regularly scheduled doses can maintain an analgesic level that prevents pain and provides greater relief. If regularly scheduled doses prove ineffective, a change in dosage or the type of analgesic can be considered.
- Assess Mr. Lugio's understanding of analgesic use. He should understand that addiction or "overuse" of the analgesic is not a primary concern and be encouraged to inform nursing staff of the need for pain relief when necessary.
- Consider the impact of psychological factors on his physical pain. The worsening of his pain when his family is not present could be related to anxiety, boredom, or other psychosocial factors. Psychosocial discomfort can intensify or exacerbate physical discomfort. Mr. Lugio may benefit from a listening ear, counseling, diversional activities, or more frequent visits from his family.
- Use nonpharmacologic pain relief measures. Back rubs, therapeutic touch, guided imagery, relaxation exercises, and counseling could prove effective in managing pain. Trained practitioners could provide acupressure, acupuncture, and hypnosis. These measures should be reviewed with the physician.

Constipation

Reduced food and fluid intake, inactivity, and the effects of medications cause constipation to be a problem for most dying patients—a problem that can add to the discomfort these patients already are experiencing. Knowing that the risk of this problem is high, nursing staff should take measures to promote regular bowel elimination in terminally ill patients. Increasing activity and the intake of fluids and fibers are beneficial. Laxatives usually are administered on a regular schedule, and bowel elimination patterns should be recorded and assessed. It must be remembered that what may appear to be diarrhea may actually be seepage of liquid wastes around a fecal impaction.

Poor Nutritional Intake

Many dying patients experience anorexia, nausea, and vomiting that can prevent the ingestion of even the most basic nutrients. Additionally, fatigue and weakness can make the act of eating a monumental task. Serving small-portioned meals that have alluring appearances and aromas can stimulate the appetite, as can providing foods that are patients' favorites. An alcoholic drink before meals can boost

the appetite of some persons. Nausea and vomiting can be controlled with the use of antiemetics and antihistamines; ginger has been used successfully by many individuals as a natural antiemetic. Also useful are basic nursing measures, such as assisting with oral hygiene, offering a clean and pleasant environment for dining, providing pleasant company during mealtime, and assisting with feeding as necessary.

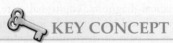

KEY CONCEPT

The herb ginger has been effective in controlling nausea for some individuals without the side effects of antiemetic drugs.

Spiritual Care Needs

Americans hold a diversity of religious beliefs. Each religion has its own practices related to death, and nursing staff must respect these practices to promote the fulfillment of patients' spiritual needs. Nursing Diagnosis Table 39-2 lists some basic differences among religions in beliefs and practices related to death. Nursing staff must be sensitive to

NURSING DIAGNOSIS

| TABLE 39-2 | Religious Beliefs and Practices Related to Death |

Religious Affiliation	Beliefs and Practices Related to Death
Baptist	Prayer, communion
Buddhist	Last rites by Buddhist priest
Catholic	Prayer, last rites by priest
Christian Scientist	Visit from Christian Science reader
Episcopal	Prayer, communion, confession, last rites
Friends (Quakers)	Individual communicates with God directly, no belief in afterlife
Greek Orthodox	Prayer, communion, last rites by priest
Hindu	Visit by priest to perform ritual of tying thread around neck or wrist, water put in mouth, family cleanses body after death, cremation accepted
Jewish	After death, body washed by religious person
Lutheran	Prayer, last rites
Mormon	Baptism and preaching to deceased
Muslim	Confession, family prepares body after death, deceased must face Mecca
Pentecostal	Prayer, communion
Presbyterian	Prayer, last rites
Russian Orthodox	Prayer, communion, last rites by priest
Scientologist	Confession, visit with pastoral counselor
Seventh Day Adventist	Baptism, communion
Unitarian	Prayer, cremation accepted

differences and ensure that they do not inadvertently disrespect the religious beliefs of patients and their families.

Because it is likely that the importance of religion in patients' lives as they are dying will be a reflection of the role of religion throughout their lives, assessment should explore not only their religious affiliation but also their individual religious practices. Furthermore, nurses must recognize that religion and spirituality are not synonymous (see Chapter 13). Religion is but one aspect of spirituality; patients can be highly spiritual without religious affiliation. To determine the significance of spirituality and the spiritual needs of patients, nurses can ask questions such as the following:

- What gives you the strength to face life's challenges?
- Do you feel a connection with a higher being or spirit?
- What gives your life meaning?

Clergy and congregation members of the faith group to which the patient belongs should be invited to be actively involved with the patient and family, according to their wishes. If nursing staff feel comfortable with the practice, they can offer to pray with patients or read to them from religious texts; of course, nursing staff should

ensure that prayers offered are consistent with a patient's belief system.

Signs of Imminent Death

When death is near, bodily functions will slow and certain signs and symptoms will occur, including:

- decline in blood pressure
- rapid, weak pulse
- dyspnea and periods of apnea
- slower or no pupil response to light
- profuse perspiration
- cold extremities
- bladder and bowel incontinence
- pallor and mottling of skin
- loss of hearing and vision

Identifying the approach of death enables nursing staff to assure family is notified and given the opportunity to share the last minutes of the patient's life. If the family is unavailable, a staff member should remain with the patient. Depending on the wishes of the patient and family, clergy may be called to visit the patient at this time. It is important that the patient not be alone during this period; even if it appears that the patient is unresponsive, he or she should be spoken to and touched.

Advance Directives

A patient can express desires regarding terminal care and life-sustaining measures through the legal document of an advance directive. All health care facilities and agencies that receive Medicare and Medicaid funding must provide information to patients about the Patient Self-Determination Act, which gives individuals the right to express their choice regarding medical and surgical care and to have those preferences honored at a later time if they are unable to communicate it. Nurses should review this issue with patients as they are admitted to a hospital or nursing home setting and discuss the importance of the patient expressing his or her desires in a legally sound manner. For many older adults and their families, discussing issues pertaining to dying is uncomfortable; by introducing and guiding the discussion with sensitivity, nurses can assist older adults in confronting these important issues and assuring their wishes are known. If an advance directive exists, the nurse should review it with the patient to assure it continues to reflect the patient's preference and place a copy in the medical record to inform all members of the interdisciplinary team. (Chapter 8 provides more discussion on legal issues pertaining to death and dying.)

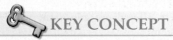

KEY CONCEPT

An advance directive protects the patient's right to make decisions about terminal care and eases some of the burden of family members during this difficult time.

SUPPORTING FAMILY AND FRIENDS

Thomas Mann's comment that "a man's dying is more the survivors' affair than his own" is a reminder that the family and friends need to be considered in the nursing care of the dying person. They too may have needs requiring therapeutic intervention during the dying process of their loved one. Offering appropriate support throughout this process may prevent unnecessary stress and provide immense comfort to those involved with the dying person.

Supporting Through the Stages of the Dying Process

Just as dying persons experience different reactions as they cope with the reality of their impending death, so may family and friends pass through the stages of denial, anger, bargaining, and depression before they are ready to accept the fact that a special person in their lives is going to die.

In the denial stage, family and friends may discourage patients from talking or thinking about death; visit patients less frequently; state that patients will be better as soon as they return home, start eating, have their intravenous tube removed, and so forth. They may shop around for a doctor or hospital to find a special cure for the terminal illness.

Reactions during the anger stage may include criticizing staff for the care they are giving, reproaching a family member for not paying attention to the patient's problem earlier, and questioning why someone who has led such a good life should have this happen.

Family and friends may try to bargain to avoid or delay their loved one's death. They may tell the staff that if they could take the patient home they know they could improve his or her condition. Through prayers or open expression they may agree to take better care of the patient if given another chance. They may consent to some particular action (e.g., going to church regularly, volunteering for good causes, or giving up drinking) if only the patient could live to a particular time.

When entering the depression stage, family and friends may become more dependent on the staff. They may begin crying and limiting contact with the patient.

In the acceptance stage, people may react by wanting to spend a great deal of time with the dying person and telling the staff of the good experiences they have had with the patient and how they are going to miss the person. They may request the staff to do special things for the patient (e.g., arrange for favorite foods, eliminate certain procedures, and provide additional comfort measures). They may frequently remind the staff to be sure to contact them "when the time comes." They may begin making specific arrangements for their own lives without the patient (e.g., change of housing, plans for property, and strengthening other relationships for support).

Obviously, the type of nursing support will vary depending on the stage at which a family member or friend is assessed to be. Although the nursing actions described for the dying individual during each stage may be applicable for family and friends, the stages experienced by those involved with the dying person may not coincide with the patient's own timetable for these stages. For instance, patients may already have worked through the different stages, come to accept the reality of death, and be ready to openly discuss the impact of their death and make plans for their survivors. However, family members and friends may be at different stages and not be able to deal with the patient's acceptance. The nurse must be aware of these discrepancies in states and provide individualized therapeutic interventions. While providing appropriate support to family and friends as they pass through the stages, the nurse can offer opportunities for dying people to discuss their death openly with a receptive party.

Helping Family and Friends After a Death

When patients die, it is useful for the nurse to be available to provide any needed support to family and friends. Some people wish to have several minutes in private with deceased patients to view and touch them. Others want the nurse to accompany them as they visit the deceased. Still others may not want to enter the room at all. Nurses must respect the personal desires of the family and friends and be careful not to make value judgments of the family's reaction based on their own attitudes and beliefs. It is beneficial to encourage the family and friends to express their grief openly. Crying and shouting may help people cope with and work through their feelings about the death more than suppressing their feelings to achieve a calm composure.

Funeral and burial arrangements may require guidance by a professional. The survivors of the deceased may be experiencing grief, guilt, or other reactions that place them in a vulnerable position. At this time, they are especially susceptible to sales pitches equating their love for the deceased to the cost of the funeral. The family may need to have the extravagant plans presented by a funeral director counterbalanced by realistic questions concerning the financial impact of such a funeral. Whether it is the nurse, a member of the clergy, or a neighbor, it is valuable to identify some person who can be an advocate for the family at this difficult time and prevent them from being taken advantage of. People should be encouraged to learn about the funeral industry and plan in advance for funeral arrangements. In addition to books on the topic, a number of memorial societies can assist individuals in their planning.

After the agitation of the funeral has diminished and fewer visitors are calling to pay their respects, the full impact of the death may first be realized. At the time when the most intense grief occurs, fewer resources may be available to provide support. The gerontological nurse can arrange for a visiting nurse, a church member, a social worker, or someone else to check on the family members several weeks after the death to make sure they are not experiencing any crisis. Widow-to-widow and similar groups can support individuals through the grieving process. It may also be beneficial to provide the telephone number of a person whom the family can contact if assistance is required.

Decades ago Edwin Schneidman, who did considerable "postventive" work with survivors, offered the following concise guidance in working with the family and friends of the deceased. His guidance remains relevant today (Schneidman, 1994):

- Total care of a dying person needs to include contact and rapport with the survivors-to-be.
- In working with survivor-victims of dire deaths, it is best to begin as soon as possible after the tragedy, within the first 72 hours if possible.
- Remarkably little resistance is met from survivor-victims; most are willing to talk to a professional person, especially one who has no ax to grind and no pitch to make.
- The role of negative emotions toward the deceased—irritation, anger, envy, guilt—needs to be explored, but not at the beginning.
- The professional plays the important role of reality tester—not so much the echo of conscience as the quiet voice of reason.
- Medical evaluation of the survivors is crucial. One should be alert for possible decline in physical health and in overall mental well-being.

SUPPORTING NURSING STAFF

The staff members working with the dying individual have their own set of feelings regarding this significant experience. It may be extremely difficult for staff not only to accept a particular patient's death but also to come to terms with the whole issue of death. Some nursing staff share the difficulty that many persons have in realizing their own mortality. Their experiences with death may be limited, as may their exposure to the subject through formal education. In a health profession in which the emphasis is primarily on "curing," death may be viewed as a dissatisfying failure. Nursing staff may feel powerless as they realize that their best efforts can do little to overcome the reality of impending death. It is not unusual for a nursing caregiver who is involved with a dying patient to also experience the stages of the dying process described by Elisabeth Kübler-Ross. Staff members are commonly observed to avoid contact with dying patients, tell a patient to "cheer up" and not think about death, continue to practice "heroic" measures although a patient is nearing death, and grieve at the death of a patient. Nursing staff may be limited in their ability to support patients and their families if they are at a different stage from them.

The staff working with a dying patient requires a great deal of support. Colleagues should help coworkers explore their own reactions to dying patients and recognize when those reactions interfere with a therapeutic nurse–patient relationship. The attitude of colleagues and the environment should be such that nursing staff can retreat from a situation that is not therapeutic either for them or for the patient. To encourage the nurse to cry or show emotions in other forms may be extremely beneficial. The use of thanatologists, hospice staff, and other resource people may also be valuable in providing support to nurses as they assist an individual through the dying process.

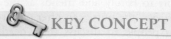

KEY CONCEPT

Nursing staff should be encouraged to express their own feelings about patients' deaths.

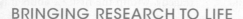

BRINGING RESEARCH TO LIFE

DETECTING AND MANAGING DEPRESSED PATIENTS: PALLIATIVE CARE, NURSES' SELF-EFFICACY, AND PERCEIVED BARRIERS TO CARE

McCabe, M. P., Mellor, D., Davison, T. E., Hallford, D. J., & Goldhammer, D. L. (2012). Journal of Palliative Medicine, 15(4), 463–467.

Although highly prevalent, depression is underrecognized and undertreated in individuals receiving palliative care. Nurses, due to their direct work with patients, are in an ideal position to identify depression and assist patients in obtaining treatment, but research indicates that their confidence and competencies in doing so are low. This study investigated factors influencing why this may be the case. Findings indicated that nurses had difficulty differentiating depression from grief, were not able to detect signs and symptoms of depression in many patients, and lacked skill in discussing depression with patients and families.

This study supports the need for nurses to be better educated in the assessment and care of depression in persons receiving palliative care. Addressing depression can provide comfort that can alleviate suffering and add quality to the final days of life.

PRACTICE REALITIES

Seventy-eight-year-old Mr. Harod has been a long-term resident of a retirement community. Although mentally sharp, his physical condition has declined in the past several months and he has been diagnosed with pancreatic cancer. He has declined treatment, stating that he understands his poor prognosis and would rather spend whatever life he has left unbothered by the stress and side effects of treatment.

Last month Mr. Harod was transferred to the nursing home section of the retirement community. You have noticed several individuals regularly visiting him and learn from another resident that these people are part of a group who support assisted suicide.

A few days later, when entering Mr. Harod's room for morning rounds, you find him deceased. By his bed are several papers that describe who to contact and what plans to make. You are aware that the people who had been visiting had been there the evening before and spent considerable time in a private meeting with Mr. Harod.

One of the residents comments that Mr. Harod "went out on his own terms." It appears several of the residents support his choice; it was, in fact, suicide.

What should you do in this situation?

CRITICAL THINKING EXERCISES

1. Discuss factors that cause Americans to have difficulty discussing and planning for death.

2. In addressing a group of older adults at a senior citizen center, what examples could you offer to support the benefits of developing an advance directive?

3. State some examples of behaviors that could demonstrate reactions of nursing staff to the death of a long-term patient.

RESOURCES

Advance Directives (by State)
http://www.caringinfo.org

American Hospice Foundation
http://www.americanhospice.org

End of Life/Palliative Education Resource Center
www.eperc.mcw.edu/elnec/curriculum.htm

Family Hospice & Palliative Care
http://www.familyhospice.com

Hospice
http://www.hospicenet.org

Hospice Foundation of America
http://www.hospicefoundation.org

International Association for Hospice & Palliative Care
http://www.hospicecare.com

National Hospice and Palliative Care Organization
http://www.nhpco.org

REFERENCES

Kübler-Ross, E. (1969). *On death and dying*. New York, NY: Macmillan.

Schneidman, E. S. (1994). Postvention and the survivor-victim. In E. S. Schneidman (Ed.), *Death: Current perspectives* (4th ed.). New York, NY: Aronson Jason.

RECOMMENDED READINGS

Recommended Readings associated with this chapter can be found on the web site that accompanies the book. Visit **http://thepoint.lww.com/Eliopoulos8e** to access the recommended readings and other additional resources associated with this chapter.

Index